CLINICAL PATHOPHYSIOLOGY

A FUNCTIONAL PERSPECTIVE

A systems approach to understanding and reversing disease processes

Joseph E. Pizzorno Jr., ND
Joseph Katzinger, ND

Clinical Pathophysiology—A Functional Perspective

A systems approach to understanding and reversing disease processes

Mind Publishing
Our focus is education

For information contact:

Mind Publishing Inc.
PO Box 57559,
1031 Brunette Avenue
Coquitlam, BC Canada V3K 1E0
Tel: 604-777-4330 Toll free: 1-877-477-4904
Fax: 1-866-367-5508
Email: info@mindpublishing.com
www.mindpublishing.com

ISBN: 978-1-927017-04-3

Printed in Canada

Design: FWH Creative

Editor: Sheila Quinn

Knowledge and best practice in this field are constantly changing. As new research and experience broaden our knowledge, changes in practice, treatment, and drug therapy may become necessary or appropriate. Readers are advised to check the most current information provided (i) on procedures featured or (ii) by the manufacturer of each product to be administered, to verify the recommended dose or formula, the method and duration of administration, and contraindications. It is the responsibility of the practitioner, relying on their own experience and knowledge of the patient, to make diagnoses, to determine dosages and the best treatment for each individual patient, and to take all appropriate safety precautions. To the fullest extent of the law, neither the Publisher nor the Editors assume any liability for any injury and/or damage to persons or property arising out or related to any use of the material contained in this book.

Library and Archives Canada Cataloguing in Publication

Pizzorno, Joseph E.

Clinical pathophysiology : a functional perspective : a systems approach to understanding and reversing disease processes / Joseph E. Pizzorno Jr., Joseph Katzinger.

Includes bibliographical references and index.
ISBN 978-1-927017-04-3

1. Physiology, Pathological. I. Katzinger, Joseph, 1975- II. Title.

RB113.P59 2012 616.07 C2012-905150-0

Table of Contents

DEDICATION

We dedicate this textbook to the scientists and clinicians whose courage and vision have made this evolution in medicine possible. Roger Williams, PhD, whose understanding of "biochemical individuality" and the connections between individual physiological variation and health paved the way for personalized medicine. Royal Lee, DDS, for his leadership in the field of nutrition, recognition of the significance of whole foods, and early conceptualization of systems healing. John Bastyr, DC, ND, who always taught us to treat the person, not the disease, using the wisdom of nature to support the body's own healing systems. Bruce Ames, PhD, whose insights and research have been critical, especially his discovery of nutritional triage. Jeffrey Bland, PhD, the tireless and brilliant educator whose 30 years of functional medicine updates and articulation of systems biology have greatly contributed to the evolution of the functional medicine model. Sidney Baker, MD, whose remarkable ability to distill the complexities of human physiology into concepts meaningful to clinicians, and to convey the limitations of "disease-naming-based medicine", has so substantively advanced the understanding of this new medicine. David Jones, MD, whose leadership and commitment to incorporating a functional approach into the standard of medicine is unparalleled. Lastly, we would like to express our deep appreciation to Michael Murray, ND, for his seminal and relentless work bringing science to naturopathic medicine.

All of these pioneers have shaped the evolution of medicine—for both health care professionals and their suffering patients. They have helped establish and make understandable the scientific basis which underlies the core principles of curative medicine, and bring about a real change in the way we think about health and disease.

Joseph Pizzorno would like to also thank all the dedicated students who have taken my Healing Systems class since 1980 when I first started teaching this way of thinking about patients. Their patience and feedback helped me refine and expand my ideas over the decades.

Joseph Katzinger would like to thank Paula Davey, MD, for showing me what excellent medicine looks like, and giving me the gift of lifelong inspiration.

Joseph E. Pizzorno Jr., ND

Joseph Katzinger, ND

FOREWORD

One of the key aspects of practicing good medicine is addressing the underlying cause of the pathophysiology. For some health conditions this goal is easily achieved, but in many situations the disturbance of normal physiology or structure is the result of complex interrelationships, many of which are influenced by a combination of genetic and nutritional aspects. This book provides the guidance that we as physicians need in order to address underlying pathophysiology via diet, lifestyle, and natural products, rather than simply trying to suppress symptoms with the use of drug therapy. It provides a clear understanding of the gap between normal physiology and overt pathology, and explains how to restore physiology back to the normal state. Unfortunately, this subject is rarely discussed in conventional medical textbooks. Instead the focus is on the use of drugs that artificially arrest the pathophysiology instead of effectively reversing it.

There is no question that most chronic health conditions reflect some basic alterations in physiology. This alteration in function most often occurs first at the cellular level. Not surprisingly, restoring health and homeostasis via natural medicine often focuses on the cellular level as well. In a systems approach to health there is a deep recognition that the external and internal environment of a cell and its membrane composition, communication and signaling pathways, enzymatic activity, and cellular energy production all impact the function of each individual cell and, in turn, the tissues, organs, and entire human body.

While this milieu is complex, what Drs. Pizzorno and Katzinger provide is an amazingly clear path for improving the health of the systems discussed in the book. This goal is achieved by impacting the underlying function of the individual cells composing that system. I have known Dr. Pizzorno for over 30 years and have always appreciated his ability to see the connections between the individual components of systems. This talent allowed him to play an enormous role in the growth and success of not only Bastyr University, but the naturopathic "system" as a whole. In collaboration with Joseph Katzinger, he has applied this skill in *Clinical Pathophysiology—A Functional Perspective* to help us better understand how we can take advantage of the ability to influence systems in the body by enhancing the function of the components within that system. It is truly a masterful approach for practicing clinical medicine that will undoubtedly lead to more effective interventions by followers of this important work.

Michael T. Murray, ND

September 2012

INTRODUCTION

Contents

Many Diseases—Few Causes

Reviewing our many years of experience researching, teaching, treating patients, and writing books, we realized that, although thousands of diseases have been named, the overwhelming majority of these diseases owe their origin to a relatively few underlying causes. The actual symptoms or diseases a person manifests are determined by the constellation of genetic, psychological, dietary, lifestyle, and environmental factors. The role of the advanced physician is to identify these underlying causes rather than focus only on symptom alleviation or disease treatment.

Every organism on the planet, from the simplest single-celled amoeba to the complex human being, relies on the internal mechanism of homeostasis to sustain life. If the homeostatic mechanism cannot overcome disruptive forces, the result is disease—a disturbance in the ability of a body system or part to carry out its normal function. By focusing on reestablishing proper homeostasis, patients can reverse disease and enjoy the benefits of health.

Henry David Thoreau said, *"Nature is doing her best each moment to make us well. She exists for no other end. Do not resist."* What Thoreau was undoubtedly referring to is the innate healing presence within each of us that seeks to reestablish proper homeostasis. Unfortunately, there are often obstacles that must first be removed before a person can experience full restoration of balance and health.

Our goal for *Clinical Pathophysiology—A Functional Perspective* is to focus on key methods of assessment to identify underlying core factors that are responsible for disease, along with effective interventions using natural medicines and patient monitoring to provide a truly individualized approach. To reach this goal, we have reviewed thousands of research articles and extracted the most current, relevant information for practicing clinicians, and organized it by physiological systems.

We have created this clinical guide to provide health care providers with a practical tool to better understand their patients' unique physiology and identify the causes of underlying dysfunction. Although this guide should also be used to enhance the treatment of previously diagnosed illness, we have used our solid background in functional and natural medicine to focus on physiology and function to better address the causes of disease, rather than its myriad manifestations. We believe these underlying dysfunctions are the antecedents to frank disease and its associated signs and symptoms.

For example, inflammation is now considered to be a feature of many acute and chronic diseases, and it is often treated by targeting the enzymes that produce inflammatory mediators. In our chapter devoted to inflammation, we discuss how factors such as organelle dysfunction and gastrointestinal permeability trigger the pathological inflammation found in many chronic diseases, as well as treatments which brings about a natural resolution to inflammation, rather than its suppression.

We've reviewed the latest research for the most effective diet and lifestyle interventions and clinically proven natural products that help to restore normal function. For instance, in our chapter reviewing the spectrum of insulin resistance, we discuss the powerful impact that dietary changes and physical activity have on restoring insulin sensitivity and glycemic control. We also review the clinical research for the unique combination product of viscous fibers, PGX®, shown to reduce appetite, restore insulin sensitivity, and perhaps most importantly, reduce postprandial hyperglycemia. Given recent evidence that postprandial hyperglycemia is a greater risk factor than fasting glucose for the development of cardiovascular disease, and both morbidity and mortality in patients with type 2 diabetes, this is of tremendous importance to restoring optimal health.

We are committed to providing exceptional and sophisticated educational tools, like this guide, to health care providers. By utilizing our in-depth reviews of the physiological etiology of disease and dysfunction, and providing a guide to assessment and restoration of healthy function, practitioners can benefit from our many hours of research and years of experience in providing personalized, exceptional natural medicine.

Vision Statement

We have developed *Clinical Pathophysiology—A Functional Perspective* from a strong philosophical foundation:

1. Physiological normalization rather than disease treatment
2. Research driven
3. Clinically proven interventions
4. Curative vs. symptom palliation
5. Measure–treat–measure

We believe this provides a very distinct clinical approach: we have the clear intent of physiological normalization; the interventions are based on strong peer-reviewed medical research; and we recommend objective tests to accurately determine the physiological problem and then measure the efficacy of the interventions. Our goal is the restoration of optimal function, and is not limited to the simpler paradigm of disease treatment.

Organization

With a strong foundation in functional medicine, we have mapped out the causes of and contributors to disease, organized by system rather than by diagnosis. The guide is organized into ten chapters. Each of the chapters covers a primary area of physiological function. The basic structure of each chapter includes:

Introduction/Overview

Review of normal function

Description of most common dysfunctions

Typical associated diseases

Assessment/Diagnosis

Treatment

As you read and utilize the guide, you will notice that the content is fully referenced. While we are "true believers" in natural medicine philosophy and therapies, we know that the only way to apply these approaches effectively and responsibly is to use good science.

The following diagram depicts how the foundation of our clinical recommendations is normalization of the core physiological functions.

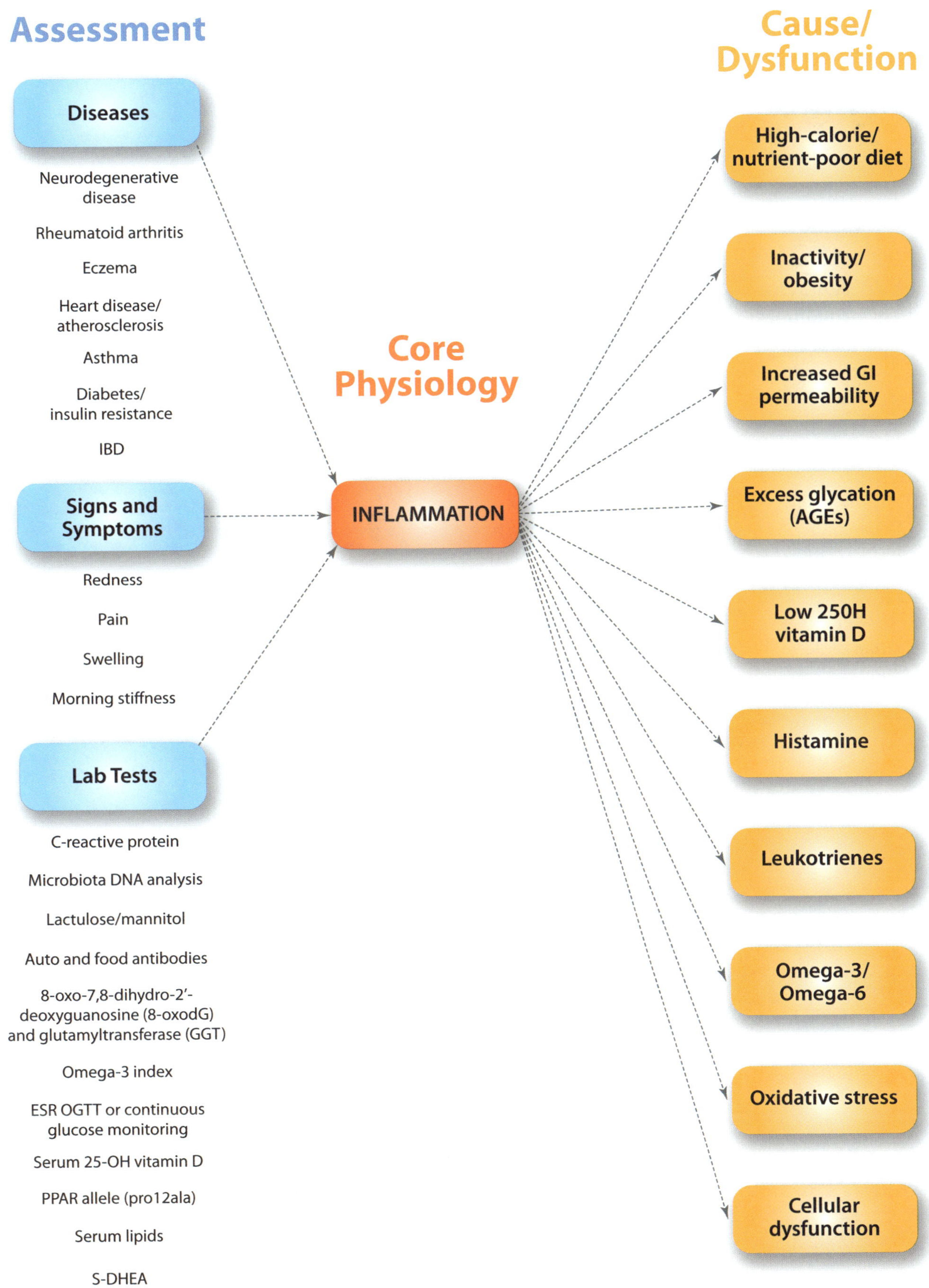
Assessment
Diseases
Neurodegenerative disease
Rheumatoid arthritis
Eczema
Heart disease/ atherosclerosis
Asthma
Diabetes/ insulin resistance
IBD
Signs and Symptoms
Redness
Pain
Swelling
Morning stiffness
Lab Tests
C-reactive protein
Microbiota DNA analysis
Lactulose/mannitol
Auto and food antibodies
8-oxo-7,8-dihydro-2′-deoxyguanosine (8-oxodG) and glutamyltransferase (GGT)
Omega-3 index
ESR OGTT or continuous glucose monitoring
Serum 25-OH vitamin D
PPAR allele (pro12ala)
Serum lipids
S-DHEA
Core Physiology
INFLAMMATION
Cause/ Dysfunction
High-calorie/ nutrient-poor diet
Inactivity/ obesity
Increased GI permeability
Excess glycation (AGEs)
Low 250H vitamin D
Histamine
Leukotrienes
Omega-3/ Omega-6
Oxidative stress
Cellular dysfunction

Tables

To help clinicians determine which physiological dysfunctions are most likely involved in a specific patient's conditions, we have created two tables, one for Diseases and the other for Symptoms. The basic format is to indicate for a particular disease or symptom the systemic dysfunction most likely to be implicated, and refer practitioners to the appropriate chapter. Below is an abbreviated example of each table, which can be found in the appendices at the end of the book.

System Implicated	Cellular	Digestion	Insulin Resistance	Inflammation	Immune	Cardiovascular
Disease						
Irritable bowel syndrome		•				
Peripheral arterial disease				•		•
Symptom						
Dyslipidemia			•	•		•
Food hypersensitivity		•			•	

Chapter Contents

Clinical Focus 7—Immune Function

- Overview
- Innate Immunity
- Adaptive Immunity
- Causes of Immune Dysfunction
- Assessment
- Interventions

Clinical Focus 8—Endocrine Balance

- Overview
- Thyroid
- Adrenal
- Reproductive Endocrinology
- Assessment
- Highlights/Interventions

Clinical Focus 9—Cardiovascular Disease

- Overview
- Epidemiology
- Pathophysiology of CVD
- Assessment
- Interventions

Clinical Focus 10—Regeneration/Healthy Aging

- Overview
- Causes of Excessive Degeneration
- Telomeres
- Mitochondrial DNA
- Neurological Degeneration
- Assessment
- Therapies and Prevention

A Cellular Approach to Health

Overview

The etiology of many diseases, especially chronic degenerative diseases, owes its origin to basic cellular dysfunction.[1] A cellular approach to health reflects a recognition that the external and internal environment of a cell, membrane composition, communication and signaling pathways, enzymatic activity, and mitochondrial energy production all impact the function of an individual cell and, in turn, the tissues, organs, and body systems which they comprise. Identifying suboptimal cellular function and improving it with targeted interventions helps to address underlying cellular pathology, thus forming a stronger basis for optimal health.

External and Internal Environment

One of the key basic functions of a cell is to create a homeostatic internal environment. In fact, every organism on the planet, from the simplest single-celled amoeba to the human being, relies on achieving cellular homeostasis to sustain life. One of the key mechanisms of achieving cellular homeostasis is the sodium-potassium pump (Na+/K+-ATPase). This active transport system pumps three sodium ions out of the cell for every two potassium ions pumped in. In doing so, it helps maintain resting potential and regulate cellular volume. It also functions as signal transducer/integrator to regulate MAPK pathway (a chain of proteins in the cell that communicates a signal from a receptor on the surface of the cell to the DNA in the nucleus of the cell), antioxidant protection, as well as intracellular calcium. This simple pump utilizes about 33% of most cells' energy expenditure. For neurons, it is even more critical and is responsible for nearly 70% of the nerve cell's energy expenditure. Obviously, damage to the Na+/K+-ATPase or impaired activity is severely detrimental to the health of the cell.

The external environment of the cell plays a major role in cellular function as it is the source of nutrients and oxygen required for the cell to function properly. It is also the source of hormones, physiological mediators, and other compounds that influence the functional performance of the cell. The external as well as the internal environment of the cell are capable of damaging cellular function, thereby leaving the cell in a compromised position to experience structural damage. For example, hyperglycemia is known to induce the production of inflammatory proteins, increase oxidative damage, lead to glycosylation of membrane-bound receptor proteins, and severely alter extracellular and intracellular signals that lead to programmed cell death (apoptosis). Oxygen plays a central role both in the health of a cell and cellular damage. Oxygen is required for normal cellular function. When oxygen is lacking, tissue hypoxia causes what has been termed the "oxidative stress paradox." During periods of hypoxia or anoxia, there is actually an increase in oxidative damage best characterized by the severe damage of a stroke or myocardial infarction. Much of the damage in anoxia or hypoxia is due to an increase in reactive nitrogen species (and a smaller increase in reactive oxygen species). When oxygen is in limited supply to mitochondria they produce nitric oxide, from which peroxynitrite forms. Peroxynitrite both damages cellular enzymes and DNA as well as upregulates "hypoxia genes," changing the cell's function.[2]

Basic support of cellular health involves first supplying essential critical nutrients required for cellular function, and secondly supplying key protective antioxidants to protect the cellular structures from damage as well as mitigating cellular damage due to hyperglycemia, toxins, and inflammation. For example, glutathione plays a crucial role in shielding cellular macromolecules from endogenous and exogenous reactive oxygen/nitrogen species. Interventions including flavonoids (e.g., catechin, ECGC, and quercetin) and antioxidants (CoQ10, acetyl-L-carnitine, and N-acetylcysteine) have been shown to reduce the damage caused by such external influences.[3,4,5,6,7]

Cell Membranes and Messaging

Cell membranes are comprised of lipid bilayers, highly controlled barriers that separate the cytoplasm of the cell from the external world and internally compartmentalize organelles. They direct the flow of molecules into and out of the cytoplasm, as well as the flow of intracellular traffic and energy production in cellular organelles, making them key components of sensory and signaling pathways. Without a healthy membrane, cells lose their ability to hold water, vital nutrients, and electrolytes. They also lose their ability to communicate with other cells and be controlled by regulating hormones. They simply do not function properly. An alteration in cell membrane function is the central factor in the development of cell injury and death that contributes to a number of chronic diseases. Cell membranes are composed chiefly of phospholipids derived from the diet. As a result, the composition of cell membranes and their resulting structure, function, and integrity can be influenced by dietary changes. A diet composed mostly of saturated fat, animal fatty acids, cholesterol, and trans-fatty acids produces cell membranes that are much less fluid in nature than the membranes of people who eat optimum levels of mono-unsaturated fat and essential fatty acids, especially the omega-3 fatty acids.

Since cell membranes also act as a phospholipid pool from which fatty acids are transformed into eicosanoids (Figure 1.1), regulating a wide variety of cellular processes, (including inflammation, platelet aggregation, and vasoconstriction/dilation, as well as cardiovascular, digestive, and renal function), changing the type or ratio of dietary fat can produce significant changes in physiology. For example, a higher ratio of omega-3 to omega-6 fatty acid content in cell membranes leads to a greater production of anti-inflammatory, anti-arrhythmic, neuroprotective, and platelet-inhibiting compounds, such as PGE3, PGI3, LTB5, as well as the recently discovered classes of compounds known as resolvins and protectins.[8]

In addition to providing the precursors for eicosanoid synthesis, the fatty acid content of cellular membranes also strongly influences their fluidity, which affects protein function and trafficking, vesicle budding and fusion, and

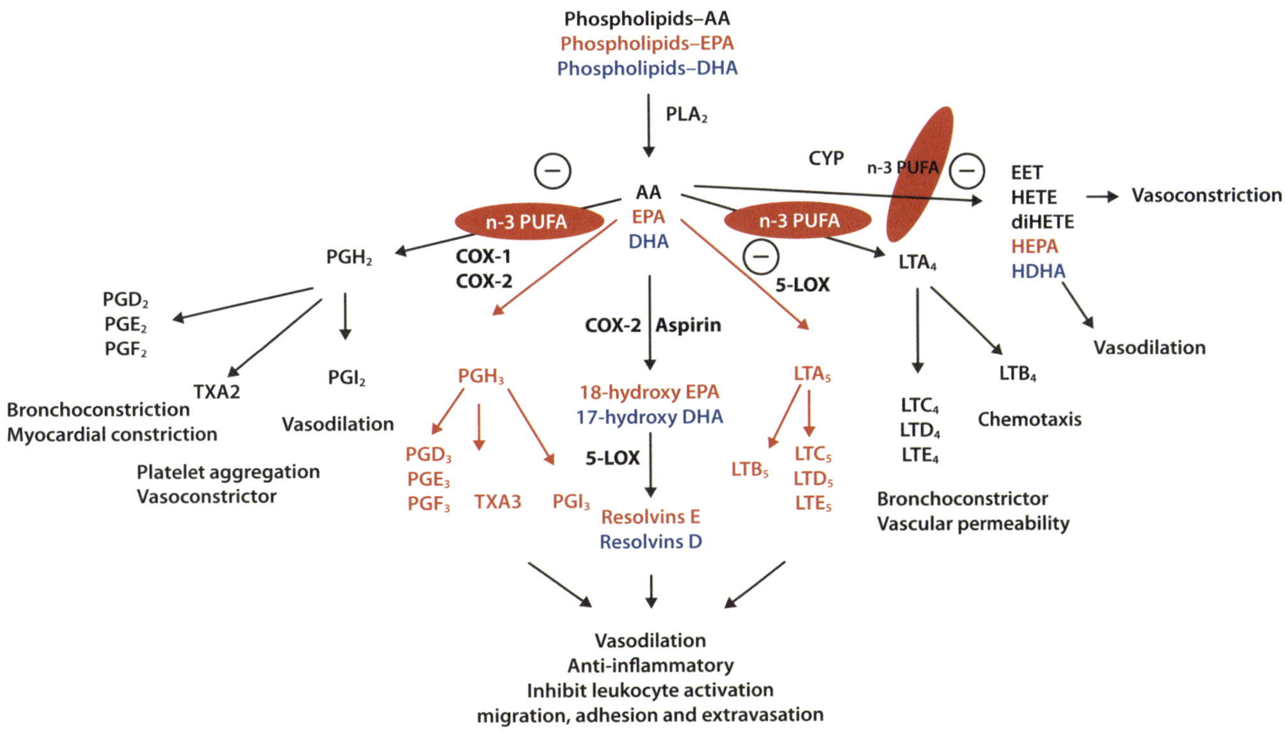

Figure 1.1 Generation of omega 3 & 6 derived eicosanoids and their cardiovascular effects. From: Siddiqui RA, Harvey KA, Zaloga GP. Modulation of enzymatic activities by n-3 polyunsaturated fatty acids to support cardiovascular health. *J Nutr Biochem.* 2008 Jul;19(7):417-37. Reproduced with permission from Elsevier.

signaling pathways with other cells and intracellular organelles. Regulating hormones such as insulin are also affected. Fatty acid membrane content influences gene expression by inducing or inhibiting transcription factors such as NF-KappaB, peroxisome proliferator activated receptors (PPARs), and retinoid X receptors. Fortunately, it is well-established that an increase in omega-3 fatty acid consumption leads to an increase in the cellular membrane content of these beneficial fatty acids.[9]

In addition to lipids, specialized proteins embedded in the membranes span the full width of the bilayer. Indeed, membrane proteins constitute more than a quarter of all known proteins, and range from a single transmembrane-spanning domain in receptor tyrosine kinases, to the multi-subunit ATP synthase.[10,11] These proteins carry out many tasks, including signal transduction, transport of small molecules, and catalysis of enzymatic reactions; they respond to a variety of stimuli, including nutrients, hormones, light, voltage, and membrane tension.[12]

Our knowledge of the structure and function of biological membranes has grown tremendously since the “fluid mosaic model” was initially proposed in 1972. Originally, it was assumed that the proteins in a membrane are dispersed at very low concentrations in an unperturbed sea of lipids, with only peripherally exposed hydrophobic side chains. We now know that most of these assumptions were incorrect, that instead, membranes are very crowded structures with varying bilayer thickness, and its proteins are arranged in functional complexes, or patches, some which have large structures outside the lipidic region, such as ATP synthase (Figure 1.2).[13]

Not only do we now believe membranes to be “patchy” structures, with segregated regions of structure and function and lipid regions varying in thickness and composition, but the discovery of the communication and connections between membranes and intracellular organelles has been quite astounding. For example, the endoplasmic reticulum, an intracellular organelle, extends from the nucleus across the entire intracellular space to the plasma membrane. Thus, it is spatially intertwined with virtually all cellular organelles, including the mitochondria, peroxisomes, and the Golgi, and may be a bridge of communication between them.[14] One of the ways these organelles communicate with each other is through second messengers, often with Ca^{2+} as the mediator. As will be discussed below, Ca^{2+} signaling is a dynamic interaction which occurs between the plasma membrane, mitochondria, and endoplasmic reticulum, and is a key regulator of both cellular metabolism and cell death.

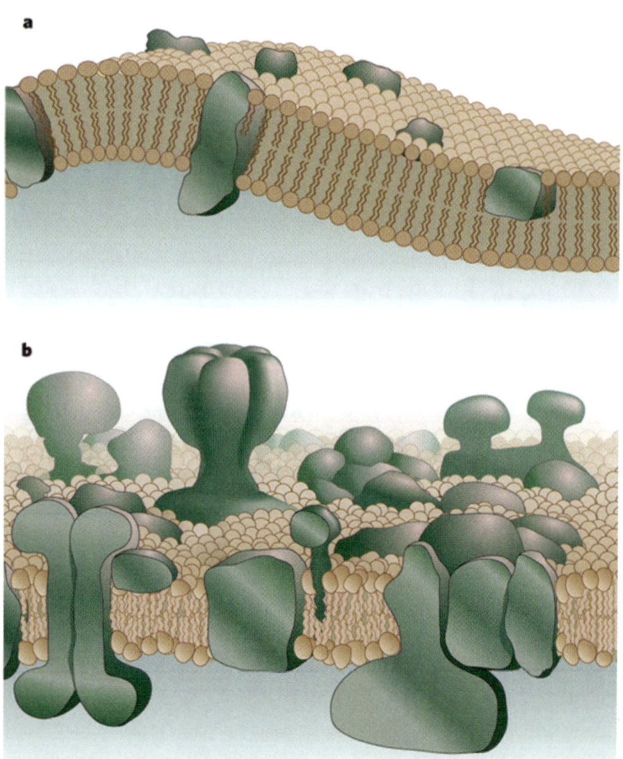

Figure 1.2 Models for membrane structure (original fluid mosaic and an updated model). From: Engelman DM. Membranes are more mosaic than fluid. *Nature.* 2005 Dec 1;438(7068):578-80. Reprinted with permission from Macmillan Publishers Ltd.

Research has documented that the lipid composition of cell membranes has direct clinical consequences. For example, in a case-control study of over 300 patients, those with a higher (mean of the third quartile) omega-3 fatty acid content in their red blood cell (RBC) membranes had a 70% reduction in risk of cardiac arrest compared to those with lower (mean of the lowest quartile) omega-3 content.[15] In a 2008 case-control study of over 700 individuals, a similar reduction in risk for acute coronary syndrome was reported for those with the highest amount of EPA and DHA content of RBC membranes.[16] The total trans fat content of cell membranes has also been found to affect risk of cardiovascular disease, with a 3-fold increase in the risk of primary cardiac arrest found in those with higher levels of the trans isomers of linoleic acid.[17]

A recent hypothesis has been suggested that the incorporation of trans and partially oxidized polyunsaturated fatty acids, as well as a high ratio of omega-6 to omega-3 fatty acids, leads to chronic hypoxia, which may be a major contributor to cancer initiation.[18] While this has not been confirmed, it has been established that membranes with higher contents of DHA have structural properties that influence cellular membrane function, as well as activity of intra-membrane proteins.[19] Given the strikingly different effects that omega-3 fatty acids and both omega-6 and trans fatty acids have on membrane function, it should be no surprise that trans fat consumption has clearly been shown to increase insulin resistance, leading to an increased risk for both diabetes and cardiovascular disease.[20] Indeed, one study estimated that substituting polyunsaturated vegetable oils for margarine containing hydrogenated vegetable oil would reduce the likelihood of developing type 2 diabetes by 40%![21]

A number of studies have also shown that an increase in omega-3 fatty acid intake combined with a decrease in overall calorie intake improves insulin sensitivity, and is a significant predictor of fasting insulin and insulin resistance.[22,23,24] Fish oil supplementation has also been shown to improve endothelial function in those without diabetes who have an increased risk for its development.[25] In animal models, fish oil has been shown to reduce body weight and improve the efficiency of glucose uptake by cells,[26] and recently fish oil has been shown to reverse atherosclerotic plaque formation in mice genetically predisposed to diabetes.[27] This was a particularly interesting study, because not only was atherosclerosis induced by the effects of insulin resistance on foam cell formation (i.e., macrophage apoptosis), but this effect could be prevented by supplemental fish oil. A transgenic mouse, which endogenously produces omega-3 fatty acids, was shown to have enhanced insulin secretion and also greater protection against cytokine-induced beta-cell destruction.[28]

Insulin Resistance, Hyperglycemia, and Impaired Nutrient Transport

One of the most important hormonal cellular regulators is insulin. Insulin facilitates the proper utilization of glucose, but it also plays a role in other aspects of cellular function and nutrition. For example, vitamin C (or its reversibly oxidized metabolite dehydroascorbic acid (DHAA)) has been shown to cross the plasma membrane primarily through facilitated diffusion and active transport, in large part through facilitative glucose transporters, such as GLUT1 that require insulin for activation.[29] Hence, the cellular uptake of DHAA is promoted by insulin and inhibited by hyperglycemia, because DHAA competes with glucose for uptake via GLUT transporters. This resultant cellular deficiency, sometimes known as tissue scurvy, has been associated with a number of clinical consequences. Decreased uptake of DHAA in osteoblasts lowers the production of collagen, and is thought to contribute to the increased incidence of osteopenia seen in diabetes.[30] It has also been associated with an increased risk of hypertension and cardiovascular disease,[31] and the reduced uptake in the brain and retina may contribute to diabetic retinopathy.[32] Indeed, cells that rely more heavily on GLUT transport of DHAA may be most prone to injury, suggesting a common etiology in the nephropathy, retinopathy, and neuropathy characteristic of diabetes.[33]

Vitamin C is not the only nutrient whose transport across cell membranes is affected by insulin resistance and/or hyperglycemia. Insulin has also been shown to affect protein metabolism, as well as the transport of a number of amino acids, neurotransmitters (GABA), and other macromolecules across the cell membrane.[34,35,36,37] Additionally, insulin influences the activity of transporters other than the GLUT proteins, including the Na(+),K(+)-ATPase and the Na+/K+/Cl- cotransporters, affecting renal electrolyte and water reabsorption, as well as blood pressure regulation.[38,39] Insulin's action and release from pancreatic beta cells are thought to be closely tied to mitochondrial function and mitochondrial calcium signaling (more below).[40] Thus, improving insulin sensitivity and plasma glucose levels has the potential to benefit a wide range of cellular nutrient levels and processes.

As mentioned earlier, hyperglycemia is also known to affect cellular function, at least partly by altering cell membranes and membrane-bound proteins. A recent animal-based study found that N-acetylcysteine significantly improved lipid composition and restored membrane fluidity and the activity of intra-membrane enzymes.[41] It has also had similar effects on membrane lipid and enzymatic activity in cells exposed to other toxins, suggesting it may be a potent protector of lipid membranes.[42]

Calcium as an intracellular messenger

Many studies in the past decade have focused on calcium as an intracellular messenger for a wide variety of processes, including energy production and apoptosis. Perhaps most important is the influence calcium has on mitochondrial activity. The overall effect of elevated mitochondrial calcium is the coordinated upregulation of the entire oxidative phosphorylation (OXPHOS) process, resulting in faster respiratory chain activity and higher ATP output. A physiological example of this upregulation is demonstrated by the beta-adrenergic stimulation in cardiomyocytes signaling the demand for increased contractility. The concomitant upregulation of OXPHOS via mitochondrial calcium elevation provides the ATP needed for increased contractile force.[43]

However, an elevation in calcium in the presence of oxidative stress may also open the mitochondrial permeability transition pore, an event linked to programmed cell death.[44] This dual potential of a calcium influx (i.e., increased energy production or cell death) has even been called the yin/yang of mitochondrial calcium.[45] The difference between these two outcomes appears to depend on some other variable—the presence or absence of a second pathological factor, such as an increase in reactive oxygen species. This model is sometimes referred to as the "two-hit hypothesis"[54] (Figure 1.3).

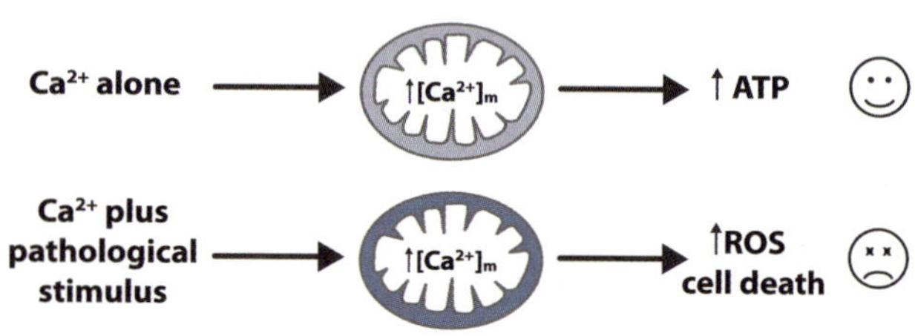

Figure 1.3 Dual potential of mitochondrial calcium elevation in oxidative phosphorylation. From: Brookes PS, Yoon Y, Robotham JL, et al. Calcium, ATP, and ROS: a mitochondrial love-hate triangle. *Am J Physiol Cell Physiol.* 2004 Oct;287(4):C817-33. Reproduced with permission from the American Physiological Society.

The induction of apoptosis also appears to be closely tied to the influence of the endoplasmic reticulum on mitochondrial function. For example, initiation of the "unfolded protein response" (an event which occurs when the endoplasmic reticulum detects cellular dysfunction) increases mitochondrial calcium, and is likely to drive the induction of apoptosis.[46]

This effect on mitochondrial activity has significant clinical relevance. A recent review indicates that the endoplasmic reticulum and the unfolded protein response are implicated in the pathophysiology of various cardiovascular diseases, including heart failure, ischemic heart disease, the development of atherosclerosis, and plaque rupture.[47] The effects are not limited to cardiovascular disease, but may also be seen in neurodegenerative disorders, diabetes, obesity, intestinal inflammation, and cancer (Figure 1.5).[48,49]

EPA/DHA to improve membrane/signaling

The association between a reduction in cardiovascular disease and an increase in cell membrane omega-3 content indicates value in prescribing supplemental DHA/EPA, which increases membrane n-3 content (Figure 1.4), is likely to improve membrane fluidity and lower risk, and influences a number of cellular processes.[50]

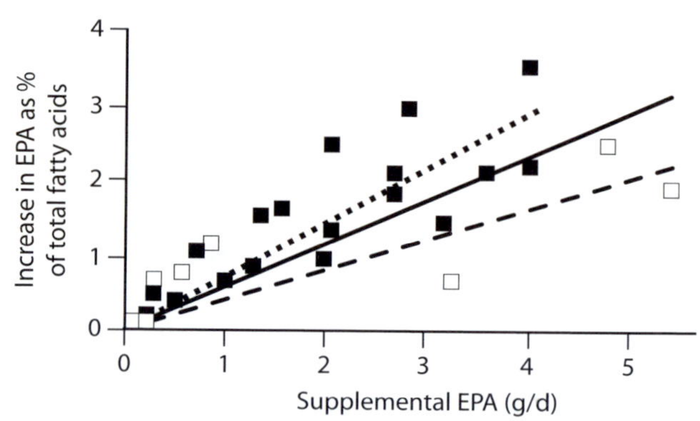

Figure 1.4 Dose-dependent incorporation of EPA into human immune cells. From: Calder PC. The relationship between the fatty acid composition of immune cells and their function. *Prostaglandins Leukot Essent Fatty Acids.* 2008 Sep-Nov;79(3-5):101-8. Reproduced with permission from Elsevier.

A recent study found that the erythrocyte content of DHA and EPA was similarly improved by either twice weekly consumption of fatty fish or a daily supplement of fish oil.[51] If fish is being consumed rather than fish oil, a greater potential for mercury and PCB exposure exists. A 2008 survey by the EPA found that 100% of fish tested had detectable mercury and PCBs, and 81% had dioxins and furans. Over half of the lakes tested had fish with levels of mercury higher than considered safe by the EPA, and 16.8% had PCBs above the EPA threshold value (Figure 1.6).

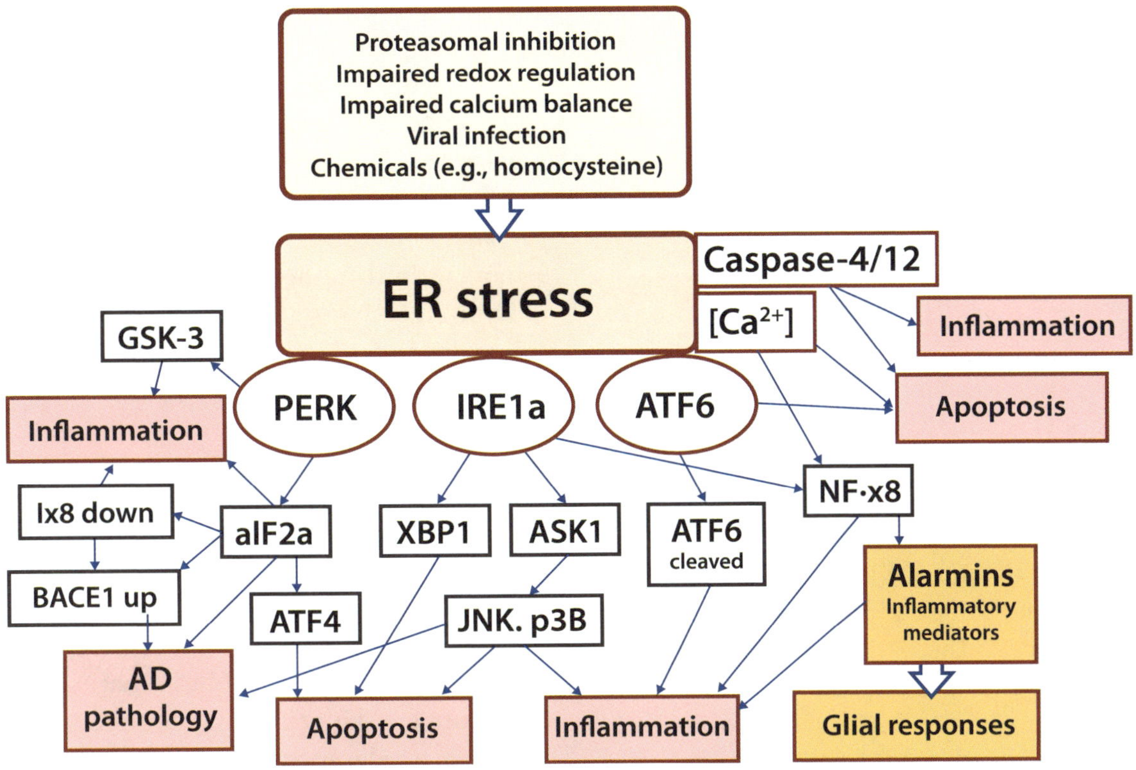

Figure 1.5 The unfolded protein response in Alzheimer's disease pathology. From: Salminen A, et al. ER stress in Alzheimer's disease: a novel neuronal trigger for inflammation and Alzheimer's pathology. *J Neuroinflammation*. 2009 Dec 26;6:41. Reproduced from Open Access article under Creative Commons Attribution License.

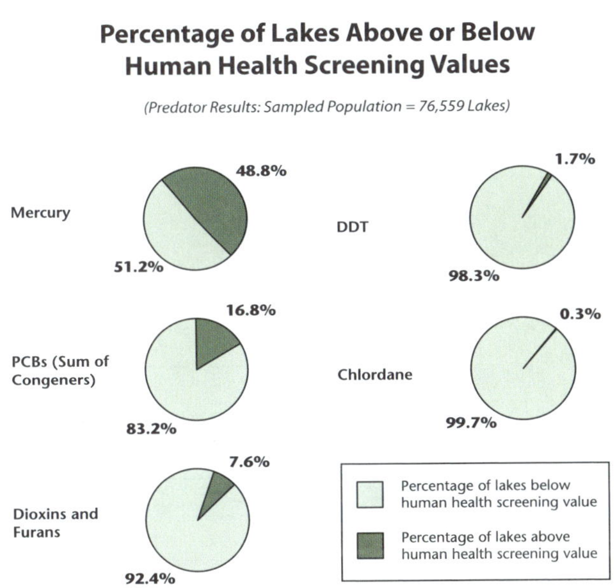

Figure 1.6 Percentage of lakes above or below human health screening values for a variety of toxins. Reproduced from: U.S. Environmental Protection Agency (USEPA). The National Study of Chemical Residues in Lake Fish Tissue. 2009. EPA-823-R-09-006. U.S. Environmental Protection Agency, Office of Water, Washington, DC.

Vitamin D

Vitamin D deficiency or insufficiency is relatively common and clinically important.[52] Vitamin D's involvement in calcium signaling and intracellular messaging may also explain its benefit in treating obesity and cancer. In cancer cells, vitamin D induces a sustained increase in intracellular calcium, an effect which leads to apoptosis of these cells. Fortunately, this is a selective death of cancer cells, because normal cells only have a transient increase in calcium, which does not induce apoptosis.[53] This effect of vitamin D has also been seen in adipocytes, indicating the potential of vitamin D in the treatment of obesity.[54] Selectively inducing apoptosis in adipocytes is one mechanism for reducing adipose tissue mass, and thus obesity.

Antioxidants

Quercetin has recently been shown to avert the consequences of stress to the endoplasmic reticulum and calcium influx in an *in vitro* study of intestinal cells.[55] Quercetin has also been found to be taken up by mitochondria; it protects against reactive oxygen and nitrogen species.[56] Other antioxidants, including curcumin, NAC, and acetyl-L-carnitine, have all been found to protect against oxidative damage, and mitigate the effects of the cellular stress response.[57]

Intracellular pH

Diet-induced "acidosis" has long been a controversial subject, and one which research is only beginning to clarify. It is fairly well accepted that food contributes either a net base or a net acid effect to the intracellular pH, determined by constituents such as protein, potassium, and sodium chloride.[58] The 3rd U.S. National Health and Nutrition Examination Survey (NHANES III) found the average American diet to be acid producing, with an NEAP (net endogenous acid production) of positive 48 mEq/d.[59] In comparison, 87% of 159 pre agricultural diets were estimated to be base-producing, with a mean NEAP of negative 88 mEq/d. This chronic low-grade acidosis appears to impact cellular function and over time could lead to disease, the most well documented of these being osteoporosis and kidney stone formation.[89,90,91]

Acidification has been shown to increase cellular calcium levels and induce pathways that lead to cell growth in tumor cells.[60] Immune cells are also affected; many conditions with frank acidemia are accompanied by immunodeficiency, and some evidence has emerged that an acidic pH impairs lymphocyte cytotoxicity and proliferation.[61] But even without a frank acidemia, i.e., a pH less than 7.35 in the extracellular fluid, effects on cellular function that have significant clinical consequences can be observed.

Metabolic response to acidosis

Several physiological mechanisms provide a buffer for chronic dietary acidosis; the most prominent is the release of alkaline salts of calcium from the skeleton. This loss of bone mass has long been thought to be a passive process, but recent research has determined that it is actually an active one, involving the activation of osteoclastic resorption of bone. *In vitro* experiments show that while osteoclasts are almost inactive at a pH above 7.4, very small reductions in pH (e.g., ≤0.1) are sufficient to cause a doubling of resorption pit formation, removing both mineral and organic components of bone and having an inhibitory action on matrix mineralization.[62,63,64,65] The same mechanism may be involved in calcium nephrolithiasis.[66,67,68]

Assessment of acid/base status

While many laboratory tests such as plasma pH, bicarbonate, standard base excess, and arterial pCO_2 are appropriate for critical care and frank acidemia, they are not sensitive enough to detect the chronic metabolic acidosis that is analogous to the impaired glucose tolerance preceding frank blood sugar elevation. While there is no widely accepted gold standard for estimating diet-induced acidosis load, several research methods are available with a relatively high degree of accuracy. The analyzed RNAE (renal net acid excretion) is one of the more accurate tests, but one of several calculations based on dietary components is often used clinically.[69] A 24-hour urine also appears to be a reasonable tool for assessment, and compares well with the calculated values (Figure 1.7).[70]

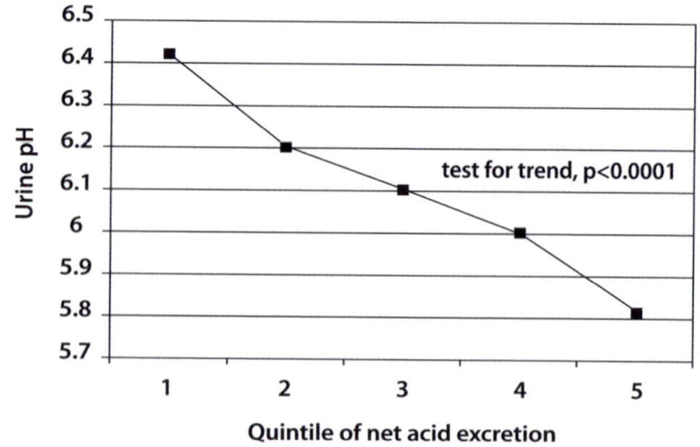

Figure 1.7 Estimates of renal net acid excretion and mean urine pH values. From: Michaud DS, Troiano RP, Subar AF, et al. Comparison of estimated renal net acid excretion from dietary intake and body size with urine pH. *J Am Diet Assoc.* 2003 Aug;103(8):1001-7. Reproduced with permission from Elsevier.

Clinical effects of acidosis

A considerable body of research has now documented that diet-induced acidosis increases bone loss, osteoporosis and fractures, as well as renal stone formation.[71] In one of the largest trials, a lower dietary intake of acid-producing foods was correlated with greater spine and hip bone mineral density among more than 1000 women ages 45–54, even after adjusting for age, weight, height, and menstrual status.[72] Perhaps as a result of the same mechanism, the acid load of the diet had the strongest association to stone risk (among a variety of variables) in a trial of 200 renal stone formers.[73] With less conclusive results, there may also be a connection between insulin resistance and acid-base equilibrium. In a study of 148 adults with no kidney stones, highly acidic urine appears to be a feature of the metabolic syndrome and is associated with the degree of insulin resistance.[74,75]

Treatment and prevention

A number of trials have shown that increasing dietary alkali through diet and/or supplementation normalizes diet-induced acidosis, documented by an increase in bone mineralization. For example, a randomized, prospective, double-blind trial of 161 postmenopausal women with osteopenia detected a bone mass increase over a 12-month period of increasing their daily alkali intake through supplementation with potassium citrate.[76] Consumption of other minerals bound to citrate would produce the same benefit. Potassium bicarbonate supplementation reduced daily urinary calcium excretion in a trial of 170 postmenopausal women, with the greatest benefit seen among those who had the largest urinary calcium loss prior to supplementation.[77] Increased fruit and vegetable consumption and potassium and magnesium intake has also been consistently associated with a greater bone mineral density.[78] A healthy vegetarian diet has a considerably lower NEAP than both a high and moderate omnivorous protein intake,[79] and reducing protein consumption down to the U.S. dietary recommended intake in a trial of 39 healthy premenopausal women was found to reduce calcium excretion and raise urinary pH, as well as reduce markers of bone resorption.[80] However, a protein-deficient diet is not recommended. Renal NH_4 formation is dependent upon adequate protein intake, so a protein-deficient diet may also increase acidosis.[81] Dietary sodium chloride appears to be independently associated with bone loss and should be minimized.[82] Several research studies have shown that supplementation with potassium and magnesium salts improves acid/base balance and prevents the bone resorption found in acidosis.[83,84]

Recommendations to prevent and treat diet-induced acidosis

In summary, the most effective means for preventing diet-induced acidosis is to choose foods that have an alkaline-inducing effect. Essentially, this means increasing dietary fruits and vegetables while decreasing animal protein and sodium chloride. Additionally, for those at increased risk or with associated pathology, supplementation with potassium, magnesium, and other minerals preferably as citrates, is indicated.

Mitochondrial Function/ Energy Production

Overview of mitochondrial function

Mitochondria are among the most important organelles within a cell. They are essential for numerous cellular processes, most prominent among them being energy production, but they also have active roles in programmed cell death (apoptosis), cell signaling, and metabolic pathways. Found in almost all cells (erythrocytes lack mitochondria), on average there are 300–400 mitochondria per cell. More active cells such as brain, muscle, and liver cells have hundreds of thousands of mitochondria per cell and comprise 40% of the cells' cytoplasm.[85]

Mitochondria also have their own DNA (mtDNA), which is quite unique, considering it is inherited

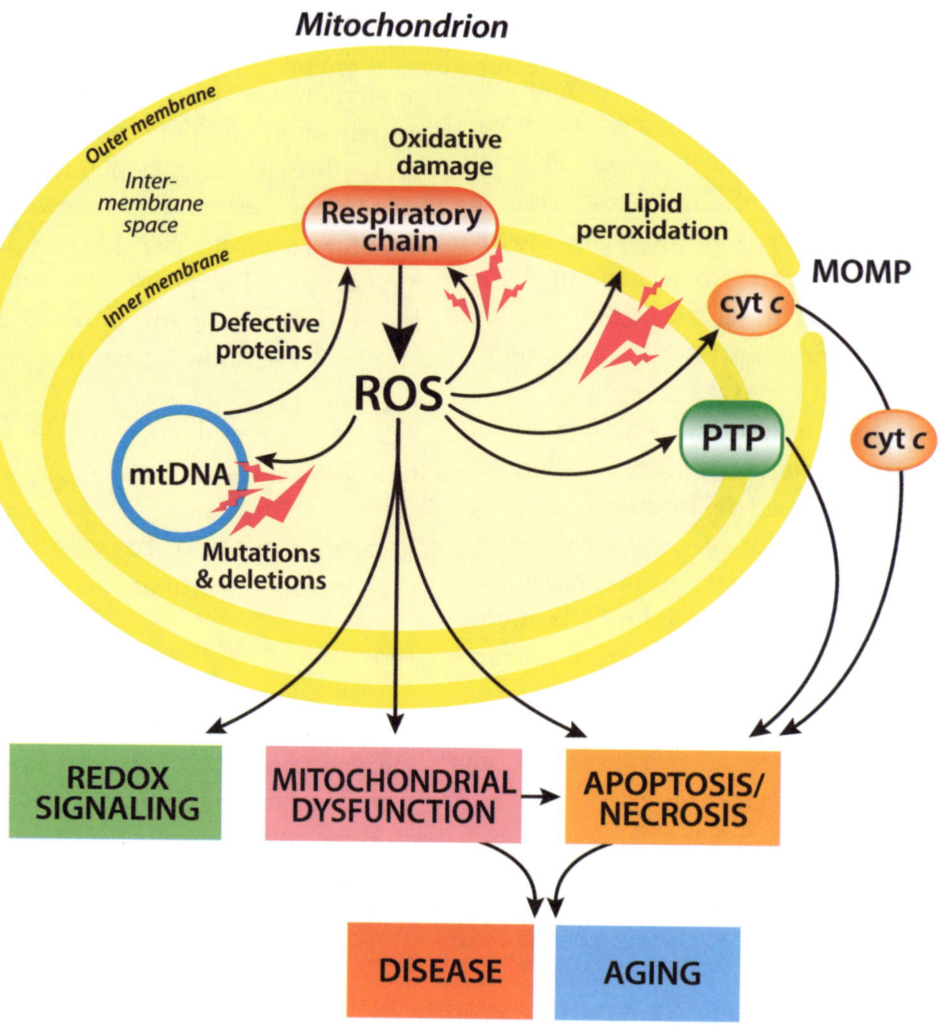

Figure 1.8 Overview of mitochondrial reactive oxygen species production. From: Murphy MP. How mitochondria produce reactive oxygen species. *Biochem J.* 2009 Jan 1;417(1):1-13. Reproduced from Open Access article under terms of Creative Commons Attribution License.

maternally, has its own genetic code, and (in contrast to nuclear DNA) it displays non-Mendelian inheritance patterns. OXPHOS, the metabolic process that provides most of the energy usable by cells, is an astonishing coordination between the nuclear and the mitochondrial genomes.[86]

The vast majority of cellular energy produced through aerobic metabolism occurs through OXPHOS—the conversion of energy from nutrient-derived substrates into the energy stored in ATP, the cellular energy currency. OXPHOS reflects the orchestrated action of five respiratory enzyme complexes packaged in a special structure of the inner mitochondrial membrane. Two main reactions operate in an integrated fashion: (1) the transfer of electron equivalents from the reduced electron carriers NADH and $FADH_2$ to molecular oxygen, and (2) ATP synthesis, driven by energy primarily stored as an electrochemical proton gradient.[87] For example, in the heart, 97% of ATP is generated by OXPHOS within the mitochondria, with the remaining 3% produced by glycolysis.[88] The tremendous gain in efficiency of energy production due to cellular incorporation of mitochondria has been proposed as a possible driver of new species formation,[89] though this increase in efficiency may also play a role in obesity, the metabolic syndrome, and cardiovascular disease in populations that are now less physically active and eating high-calorie

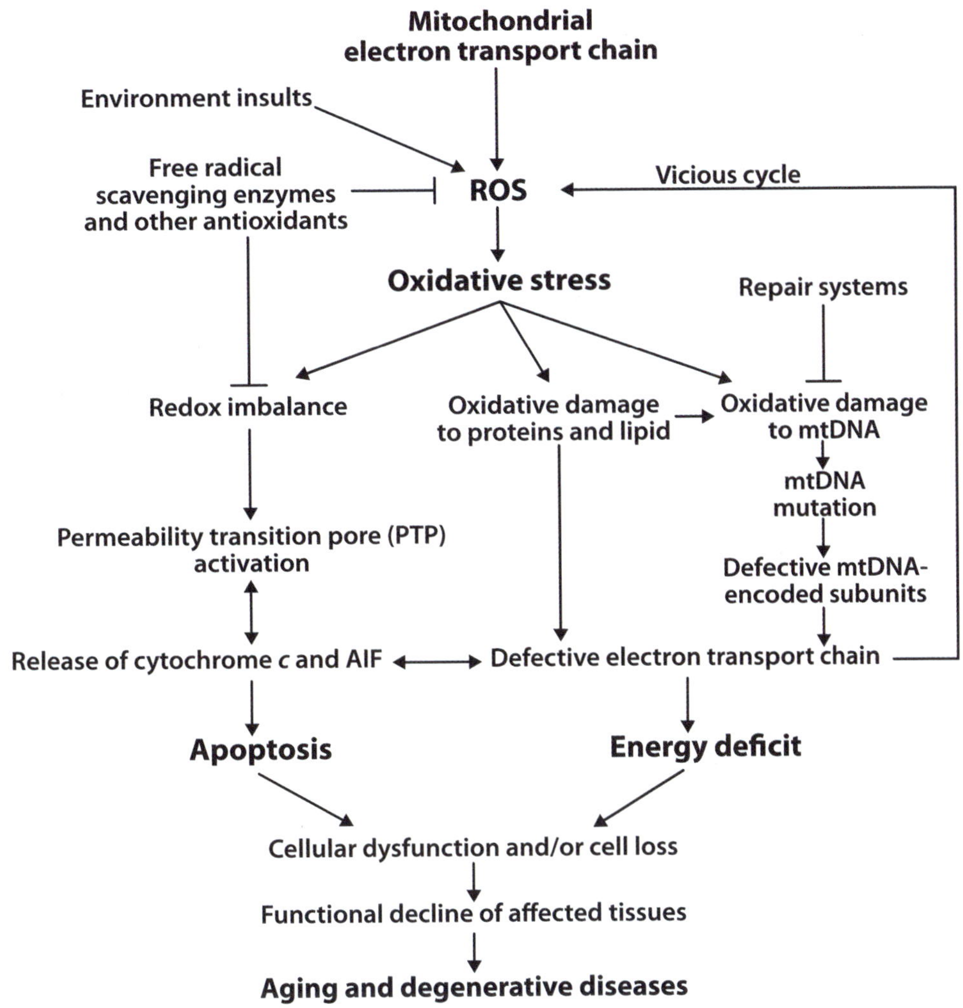

Figure 1.9 Mitochondrial role in human aging and age-related degenerative diseases. From: Wei YH, Lee HC. Oxidative stress, mitochondrial DNA mutation, and impairment of antioxidant enzymes in aging. *Exp Biol Med (Maywood).* 2002 Oct;227(9):671-82. Reproduced with permission from the Society for Experimental Biology and Medicine.

diets, an unfavorable combination for a genotype well-suited to scarcity.[103]

mtDNA oxidative damage

As discussed above, one consequence of OXPHOS is the production of reactive oxygen species, including the superoxide anion and the hydroxyl radical (Figure 1.8).

Perhaps because of the proximity to these reactive oxygen species, mtDNA is thought to be damaged at a frequency nearly 20 times greater than that for nuclear DNA.[90] This increased damage, combined with a lack of histones (protective molecules surrounding nuclear DNA) and mammal DNA repair activity, leads to a 17-fold higher mutation rate in mtDNA than in nuclear DNA. The progressive accumulation of mutations over a lifetime is thought to lead to a decline in mitochondrial energy production, and has been proposed as a theory behind the aging process (Figure 1.9).[91]

Mitochondria and aging

When the accumulation of damage to mitochondrial tissue and mtDNA leads to loss of mitochondrial energy production (and the aging of humans and animals), the stage is set for a vicious cycle. As oxidative damage causes mutations in mtDNA and alterations in cell signaling

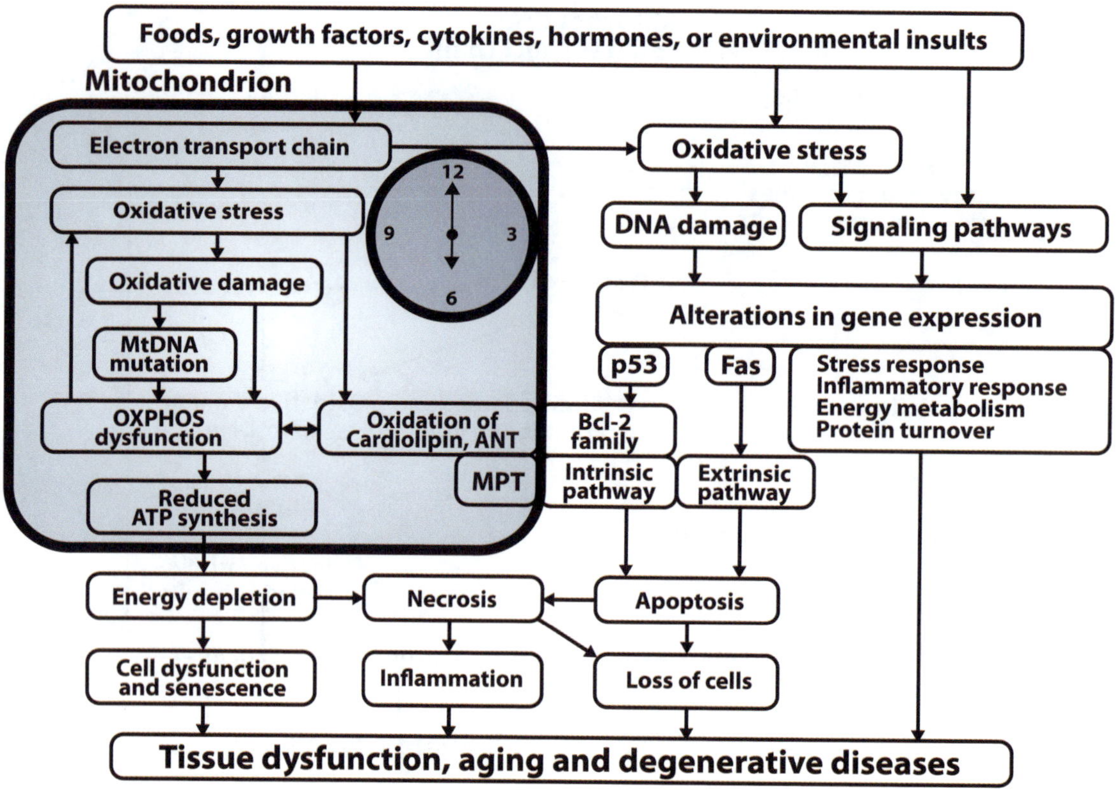

Figure 1.10 Mechanisms for mitochondria as etiology for human aging. From: Lee HC, Wei YH. Oxidative stress, mitochondrial DNA mutation, and apoptosis in aging. *Exp Biol Med (Maywood)*. 2007 May;232(5):592-606. Reproduced with permission from the Society for Experimental Biology and Medicine.

pathways, OXPHOS efficiency is reduced and ATP production decreases. As a result, energy depletion, with consequent cellular dysfunction, apoptosis, and inflammation, leads to tissue dysfunction, aging, and degenerative disease (Figure 1.10), as well as an increase in reactive oxygen species and depletion in cellular antioxidants such as glutathione. Clinically, many diseases (including several neurodegenerative diseases) have been associated with mitochondrial damage: Alzheimer's disease, Parkinson's disease, dementia,[92] autism,[93] chronic fatigue syndrome,[94] cardiovascular disease, diabetes, and migraine headache.[95,96]

Assessment of Cellular Function

While much of the assessment of cellular function is based on clinical data, i.e., the syndromes and conditions known to have cellular dysfunction, many laboratory tests that give a more targeted analysis, particularly in regard to mitochondrial function, are now becoming available. These range from minimally invasive tests to invasive diagnostic procedures and genetic testing. Our review of the available research has determined that some factors have higher predictability than others in determining mitochondrial health (see Table 1.1).

Minimally invasive tests of mitochondrial function include blood levels of lactate and pyruvate, which reflect the NADH/NAD+ cytoplasmic redox state. These tests, however, are not very sensitive or specific, and are technically challenging because the blood must be transferred and analyzed quickly. While more invasive, stress tests such as carbohydrate loading prior to lactate, pyruvate, and alanine analysis or exercise may also reveal mitochondrial dysfunction. Urinary organic acid analysis has also been used to evaluate mitochondrial disorders, and may detect impaired fatty acid metabolism (i.e., beta-oxidation).[97]

Table 1.1 Predictability of factors associated with mitochondrial health

HIGH PREDICTABILITY	
AIDS/HIV	Hepatitis B
Alzheimer's disease	Parkinson's disease
CoQ10 deficiency	
MEDIUM PREDICTABILITY	
Atherosclerosis	Doxorubicin (Adriamycin)
Cadmium exposure	Glutathione depletion
Copper deficiency	Mercury exposure
Diabetes type 2	Vitamin B2 deficiency
LOW PREDICTABILITY	
Arsenic exposure	Dieldrin exposure
Chloroform, chronic exposure	Iron deficiency
DDT, chronic exposure	Macular degeneration

A recently developed "ATP profile" test is a combination profile which claims to determine the availability of ATP in neutrophils, the fraction complexed with magnesium, the efficiency of oxidative phosphorylation, and the transfer efficiencies of ADP into the mitochondria and ATP into the cytosol. When used among patients with chronic fatigue syndrome, it appeared to have a remarkable correlation with severity of illness, with only 1 of 71 patients testing in the "normal" range.[98]

More invasive testing involves biopsy; it is much more revealing and can be used to assess CoQ10 levels, fibroblasts, and other morphological and biochemical signs of mitochondrial dysfunction in the tissues from which they are taken. However, selection of the appropriate tissue is critical; for example, deficits in cardiac tissue may not be present in skeletal muscle.[115] DNA testing from both mitochondrial and nuclear DNA is also starting to emerge, though it currently has a number of drawbacks.[115]

Assessment of oxidative damage is also important for determining cellular and mitochondrial health. Markers of lipid and DNA oxidation may indicate the level of oxidative stress and the need for protective substances. For example, 8-oxo-7,8-dihydro-2'-deoxyguanosine has been used as a marker of endogenous oxidative damage to DNA, as well as a risk factor for many diseases including cancer.[99] Similarly, the thiobarbituric acid (TBA) assay measures the lipid peroxidation end-product, malondialdehyde (MDA).

Mitochondrial optimization strategies

To optimize mitochondrial function and maintain OXPHOS production of ATP over the lifespan, a three-part strategy is recommended: reducing exposure to damaging factors, providing nutrients needed for optimal mitochondrial function, and providing protection from oxidative damage. Unfortunately the list of factors damaging to mitochondria is quite extensive: cyanide, carbon monoxide, ozone, heavy metals such as cadmium and mercury,[100] synthetic substances such as triazine herbicides (atrazine),[101] persistent organic pollutants, and organochlorine pesticides.[102] Cadmium and mercury have been shown to increase reactive oxygen species via a mechanism that may directly promote neurodegeneration.[103] Additionally, many drugs are known to poison mitochondria, including rotenone, amytal, malonate, antimycin, minocycline, myxothiazol, oligomycin, aurovertin, sumatriptan, propranolol, L-dopa, and statins.[104,105]

Statin drugs are particularly controversial because of their widespread usage. They are well known to inhibit the production of CoQ10, with some but not all trials showing a benefit of supplemental CoQ10 for those patients that develop myalgia.[106] Evidence is also mounting for additional statin-associated adverse effects related to mitochondrial dysfunction, including cognitive loss, neuropathy, pancreatic and hepatic dysfunction, cancer, and sexual dysfunction.[107] Given these potential adverse effects it seems prudent to correct the deficiency of this important cellular antioxidant.

Aging, cigarette smoke, hyperglycemia, excessive arachidonic acid, and excessive exercise are all thought to contribute to mitochondrial damage.[108,109,110] Interestingly, the amino acid methionine may specifically increase mitochondrial reactive oxygen species production as well as mtDNA oxidative damage, while carnitine has the opposite relationship, at least in animal studies.[111] A summary of mitochondrial injuries from drugs and toxins can be found in Table 1.2.

Table 1.2 Mitochondrial injuries from drugs and toxins

DRUG OR TOXIN	MECHANISM OF ACTIVITY
Acetaminophen	Poisons mitochondria
Arachidonic acid	Inhibits Complex I
Aspirin	Uncouples electron transport
AZT	Inhibits mitochondrial replication
Cocaine, ethanol	Uncouples OXPHOS, ↑radical production
Griseofulvin	Interferes with mitochondrial replication
Methamphetamine	Uncouples electron transport chain
L-dopa	Inhibits Complex I
NSAIDs	Uncouples electron transport chain
Rotenone and other pesticides	Inactivates Complex I NADH dehydrogenase
Statins	Interferes with synthesis of CoQ10
Tobacco	Uncouples OXPHOS, ↑free radical production
Valproic, adipic, and benzoic acids	Increases mitochondrial permeability

Nutrients Needed for Mitochondrial Energy Production and the Protection of Mitochondria Against Oxidative Damage

The largest contributor to intracellular reactive oxygen species is the mitochondrial respiratory chain under both normal physiologic and pathologic conditions, with approximately 1–5% of the oxygen consumed by mitochondria converted to ROS. Nutrients that protect against oxidative damage reduce the damage done to both intracellular proteins and mtDNA, allowing for continued and efficient energy production.

Ribose

Ribose is a naturally occurring 5-carbon sugar produced in the body from glucose. In addition to serving as the carbohydrate backbone for ribonucleic acid (RNA) and deoxyribonucleic acid (DNA), ribose is also an essential ingredient in the manufacture of ATP. In fact, the availability of ribose in the muscle mitochondria is a limiting factor for the rate of re-synthesis of ATP. Mitochondria utilize two methods for building or conserving cyclic nucleotides like ATP, ADP, and AMP. The first process is via synthesis from ribose. The second, faster pathway, is the salvage pathway, in which the mitochondria "pick up the pieces" of ATP metabolites to form new ATP. In this manner ribose enables the cells to quickly and efficiently recycle the end products formed by the breakdown of ATP to form new ATP molecules.

Oral or intravenous ribose can rapidly restore ribose levels and dramatically improve recovery of falling ATP levels during and following acute or chronic anoxia or ischemia or exercise. Research has shown that taking ribose has a positive effect on ATP production in all muscle fiber types, especially the heart. Ribose supplementation increases the de novo production of ATP through oxidative phosphorylation by 340–430%. Ribose also activates the salvage pathway, causing nucleotides to be revitalized into the manufacture of ATP by over 700%.[112]

In one human double-blind crossover trial, the effect of oral ribose supplementation on the resynthesis of adenine nucleotides and performance after 1 week of intense intermittent exercise was examined. The subjects performed cycle training consisting of 15 x 10 seconds of all-out sprinting twice per day for 7 days. After training the subjects received either ribose (200 mg/kg body weight) or placebo three times per day for 3 days. An exercise test was performed at 72 hours after the last training session. Immediately after the last training session, muscle ATP was lowered by 25% in the placebo and Ribose groups, respectively. After 72 hours, muscle ATP was similar to pre-training in the ribose group, but still lower in the placebo group. The results indicate that the availability of ribose in the muscle is a limiting factor for the rate of re-synthesis of ATP.[113]

Several studies have shown ribose supplementation to improve cardiac energy production in congestive heart failure.[114] Typically at a dosage of 5 g of ribose, three times daily. Improvements were noted in many parameters, including walking distance, stroke volume index, ejection fraction, and left ventricular systolic volume. Ribose has also been shown in other studies to improve the efficiency of energy production, as evidenced by reduction of oxidative stress during vigorous exercise.[115]

Lastly, ribose supplementation improved symptoms in fibromyalgia and/or chronic fatigue syndrome patients. Forty-one patients with a diagnosis of FMS and/or CFS were given D-ribose, at a dose of 5 g three times per day. D-ribose was well-tolerated, resulted in a significant improvement in all five visual analog scale (VAS) categories: energy; sleep; mental clarity; pain intensity; and well-being, as well as an improvement in patients' global assessment. Approximately 66% of patients experienced significant improvement while on D-ribose, with an average increase in energy on the VAS of 45% and an average improvement in overall well-being of 30%.[116]

Magnesium

Magnesium is stored within the mitochondria, and acts as an important cofactor for mitochondrial enzymes, playing a pivotal role in ATP synthase.[117,118] Magnesium supplementation can be beneficial for a number of clinical conditions with suspected mitochondrial dysfunction. For example, a growing body of evidence points to mitochondrial dysfunction as part of the pathophysiology of diabetes, which is characterized by intracellular magnesium depletion. Most clinical trials have demonstrated a therapeutic benefit in using magnesium for both the prevention and treatment of type 2 diabetes.[119,120]

B vitamins

Several B vitamins (B1, B2, B3, B6) and NADH are essential to mitochondrial function. Riboflavin, for example, is the major cofactor for the flavoproteins FAD and FMN, which shuttle energy from the citric acid cycle and beta-oxidation to complex II of the electron transport chain.[121] This also means riboflavin has the potential to bypass complex I in those patients with complex I dysfunction. It has been used with benefit for several clinical conditions in which mitochondrial function is impaired; both pediatric and adult migraines, for example, have shown a reduction in frequency in response to riboflavin.[122,123] One trial in children did not show benefit, but an unusually high placebo response complicated that finding.[124]

Vitamin A

Fascinating research has emerged regarding the role of vitamin A in mitochondrial energy production. A recent animal-based study found that retinol is essential for the metabolic fitness of mitochondrial energy production.[125] Not only is it a cofactor for protein kinase C, but it may also act as nutrient sensor, regulating the amount of pyruvate that is funneled through the Krebs cycle. The authors suggest this previously unknown role of vitamin A as an explanation for the pathologies that are uncorrected by retinoic acid and require vitamin A for optimal function, such as immune deficiencies and male infertility.[143]

Creatine

Creatine is also necessary for mitochondrial ATP production. The formation of phosphocreatine from creatine is catalyzed by creatine kinase, and participates in efficient recycling of ATP from ADP by supplying a reserve of phosphate groups. Supplemental creatine is beneficial for a number of clinical conditions, and has recently been proposed as part of a treatment for several neurodegenerative disorders, particularly Huntington's disease and Parkinson's disease, known to have defective cellular energy production as part of their pathogenesis.[126,127]

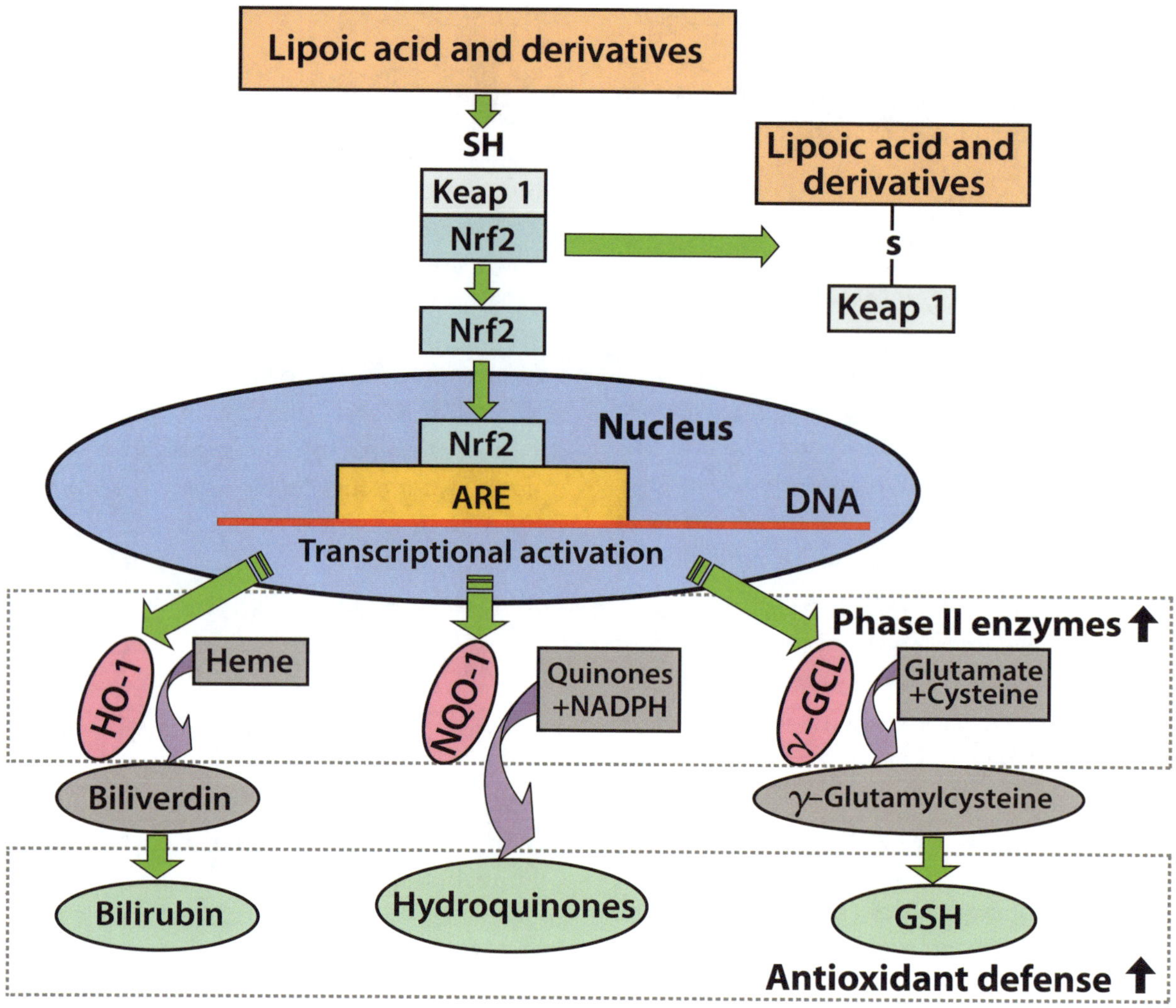

Figure 1.11 Possible mechanism of neuroprotective effects of lipoic acid. From: Liu J. The effects and mechanisms of mitochondrial nutrient alpha-lipoic acid on improving age-associated mitochondrial and cognitive dysfunction: an overview. *Neurochem Res.* 2008 Jan;33(1):194-203. Reproduced with permission from Springer Science+Business Media and Dr. Stuart Lipton.

L-carnitine and acetyl-L-carnitine

Acetyl-L-carnitine and L-carnitine are both involved in mitochondrial function. Carnitine transports short, medium, and long-chain fatty acids toward or across the inner mitochondrial membrane, thereby facilitating beta-oxidation. It also promotes gluconeogenesis, and modulates the activity of several mitochondrial enzymes, particularly pyruvate dehydrogenase.[128] Acetyl-L-carnitine facilitates the uptake of acetyl-CoA into the mitochondria during fatty acid oxidation, and appears to be of clinical benefit for a number of conditions, including Alzheimer's dementia, chronic fatigue syndrome, depression, diabetic neuropathies, ischemia, and reperfusion.[146] In a recent trial of acetyl-L-carnitine in elderly patients with fatigue, significant improvements were seen in physical and mental fatigue, as well as in muscle pain, cognitive function, and sleep disorders.[129]

CoQ10

CoQ10 may be one of the most well-researched nutrients needed for mitochondrial function; the level of CoQ10 in cardiac mitochondria has been directly correlated with the maximum lifespan across species.[130] Its ability to protect mitochondria from toxins and drugs has been well-established, including a recent animal-based study in which CoQ10 prevented damage from a dopaminergic mitochondrial toxin.[131] It has also been shown to protect against exercise-induced muscle injury in a placebo-controlled trial of athletes taking 300 mg CoQ10 per day.[132] A second trial found it to augment fat oxidation during exercise.[133] Compared to placebo, 300 mg per day of CoQ10 preoperatively also improved mitochondrial efficiency and mitigated the oxidative damage from reoxygenation following cardiac surgery.[134]

Lipoic acid

Lipoic acid has a powerful role as a mitochondrial nutrient; it has been shown to protect and improve mitochondrial function (Figure 1.11).[135] In addition to its role as an antioxidant, it upregulates phase II enzymes that provide additional support against oxidative damage, including those involved in glutathione production.[136] A recent animal-based study reported that it may protect against diabetic cardiomyopathy by its upregulation of protective factors, including glutathione and superoxide dismutase.[137] It also shows promise for the prevention of migraine headaches.[138]

Acetyl-L-carnitine and alpha-lipoic acid

Some nutrients also appear to have a synergistic effect when taken together. For example, lipoic acid and acetyl-L-carnitine increase mitochondrial function and reduce oxidative stress to a greater degree than with either nutrient used alone (Figure 1.12); the combination has also been shown to increase glutathione in old mice comparable to those levels found in young ones (Figure 1.13).[139,140] These two nutrients, when taken together, have also demonstrated improved cognitive function in an animal model of Alzheimer's disease.[141]

Ginkgo biloba

A standardized extract of *Ginkgo biloba* has been shown to protect against oxidative damage and stabilize mitochondrial function, with a recent study demonstrating its ability to protect complexes I, IV, and V of OXPHOS against a number of mitochondrial poisons.[142] A second cell-based study found that it may also protect against intracellular glutathione deprivation.[143]

Resveratrol

Resveratrol has demonstrated a number of mitochondrial benefits, including protection from oxidative damage caused by iron and arachidonic

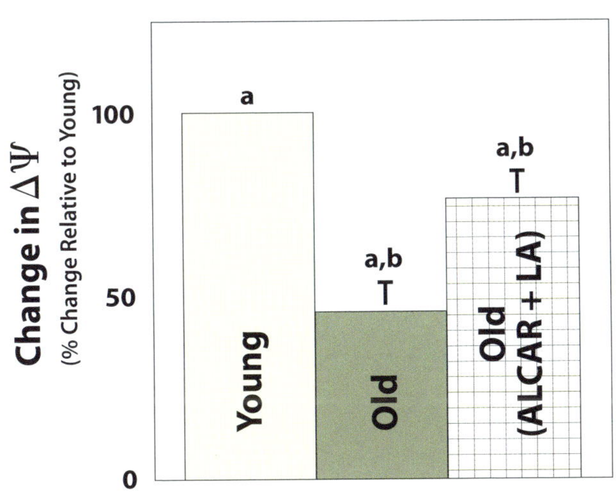

Figure 1.12 Partial reversal of age-related decline (as mitochondrial membrane charge) in rats with dietary supplementation of acetyl-L-carnitine and lipoic acid. From: Hagen TM, et al. Feeding acetyl-L-carnitine and lipoic acid to old rats significantly improves metabolic function while decreasing oxidative stress. *Proc Natl Acad Sci* 2002; 99: 1870–5. Reproduced by kind permission of Dr. Ames.

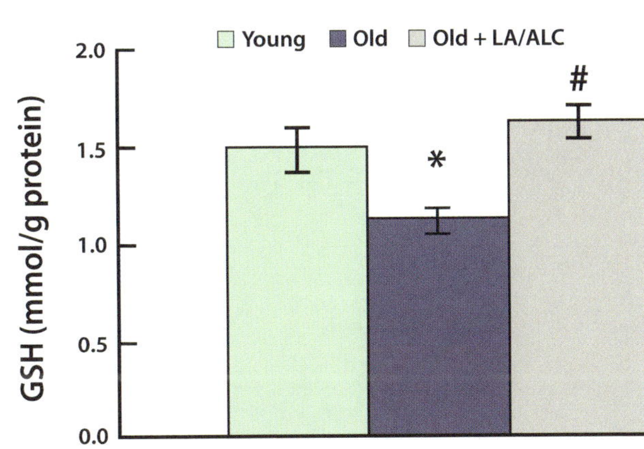

Figure 1.13 GSH level in the mitochondria of rat brain, with restoration by LA/ALC. From: Long J, Gao F, Tong L, Mitochondrial decay in the brains of old rats: ameliorating effect of alpha-lipoic acid and acetyl-L-carnitine. *Neurochem Res.* 2009 Apr;34(4):755-63. Reproduced with permission from Springer Science+Business Media.

acid[144] and the upregulation of antioxidant defense mechanisms.[145] It has even induced the biogenesis of mitochondria in endothelial cells of diabetic mice.[146] This increased biogenesis has been associated with increased running time and oxygen consumption in muscle fibers of mice.[147] Its potential for use in Alzheimer's disease was also highlighted by an animal-based study which found it helped to clear beta-amyloid from Alzheimer's disease cells (Figure 1.14).[148]

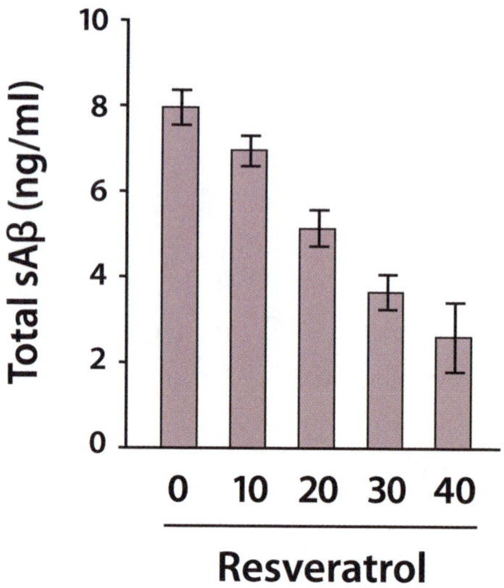

Figure 1.14 Effect of resveratrol on Aβ levels in APP695-HEK293 cells. From: Marambaud P, et al. Resveratrol promotes clearance of Alzheimer's disease amyloid-beta peptides. *J Biol Chem.* 2005;280:37377-82. Reproduced with permission from the American Society for Biochemistry & Molecular Biology.

Melatonin

Melatonin has a long history as an antioxidant, and appears to be a potent one for mitochondria. A recent study found that it reduced reactive oxygen species in the mitochondria, while maintaining OXPHOS activity and ATP production.[149] It has also been shown to prevent heart ischemia reperfusion injury by inhibiting the mitochondrial permeability transition pore opening, an event associated with calcium release and programmed cell death.[150] This prevention of apoptosis lends support to its use in a number of neurodegenerative disorders, including Parkinson's disease and Alzheimer's disease.[151]

Summary

Optimal cellular function is an essential component of restoring and maintaining optimal health and vitality. Additionally, the root causes of many of today's illnesses begin by impairing basic cellular functions, such as mitochondrial energy production and intercellular signaling, or by inducing structural changes to cell membranes, such as those caused by a diet low in omega-3 fatty acids. Not only do Western diets and lack of physical activity damage these cellular functions, but many modern environmental toxins and medications do as well. In the first chapter of this guidebook, we've outlined the physiology of the involved cellular mechanisms, how they influence many chronic diseases, as well as fully referenced strategies to assess cellular dysfunction and more effectively treat it. Healthy cellular function provides the foundation for healthier lives.

References

1. Di Donato S. Multisystem manifestations of mitochondrial disorders. *J Neurol.* 2009 May;256(5):693-710.
2. Poyton RO, Castello PR, Ball KA, et al. Mitochondria and hypoxic signaling: a new view. *Ann N Y Acad Sci.* 2009 Oct;1177:48-56.
3. Wu CH, Wu CF, Huang HW, et al. Naturally occurring flavonoids attenuate high glucose-induced expression of proinflammatory cytokines in human monocytic THP-1 cells. *Mol Nutr Food Res.* 2009 Aug;53(8):984-95.
4. Allen CL, Bayraktutan U. Antioxidants attenuate hyperglycaemia-mediated brain endothelial cell dysfunction and blood-brain barrier hyperpermeability. *Diabetes Obes Metab.* 2009 May;11(5):480-90. Epub 2008 Feb 18.
5. Kumar S, Sitasawad SL. N-acetylcysteine prevents glucose /glucose oxidase-induced oxidative stress, mitochondrial damage and apoptosis in H9c2 cells. *Life Sci.* 2009 Mar 13;84(11-12):328-36.
6. Jantzie LL, Cheung PY, Johnson ST, et al. Cerebral Amino Acid Profiles after Hypoxia-Reoxygenation and N-Acetylcysteine Treatment in the Newborn Piglet. *Neonatology.* 2009 Oct 28;97(3):195-203.
7. Barhwal K, Hota SK, Prasad D, et al. Hypoxia-induced deactivation of NGF-mediated ERK1/2 signaling in hippocampal cells: neuroprotection by acetyl-L-carnitine. *J Neurosci Res.* 2008 Sep;86(12):2705-21.
8. Schmitz G, Ecker J. The opposing effects of n-3 and n-6 fatty acids. *Prog Lipid Res.* 2008 Mar;47(2):147-55.
9. Calder PC. The relationship between the fatty acid composition of immune cells and their function. *Prostaglandins Leukot Essent Fatty Acids.* 2008 Sep-Nov;79(3-5):101-8.
10. Anson L. Membrane protein biophysics. *Nature.* 2009 May 21;459(7245):343.
11. Engelman DM. Membranes are more mosaic than fluid. *Nature.* 2005 Dec 1;438(7068):578-80.
12. Phillips R, Ursell T, Wiggins P, et al. Emerging roles for lipids in shaping membrane-protein function. *Nature.* 2009 May 21;459(7245):379-85.
13. Engelman DM. Membranes are more mosaic than fluid. *Nature.* 2005 Dec 1;438(7068):578-80.
14. Lebiedzinska M, Szabadkai G, Jones AW, et al. Interactions between the endoplasmic reticulum, mitochondria, plasma membrane and other subcellular organelles. *Int J Biochem Cell Biol.* 2009 Oct;41(10):1805-16.
15. Siscovick DS, Raghunathan TE, King I, et al. Dietary intake and cell membrane levels of long-chain n-3 polyunsaturated fatty acids and the risk of primary cardiac arrest. *JAMA.* 1995 Nov 1;274(17):1363-7.
16. Block RC, Harris WS, Reid KJ, et al. EPA and DHA in blood cell membranes from acute coronary syndrome patients and controls. *Atherosclerosis.* 2008 Apr;197(2):821-8. Epub 2007 Sep 17.
17. Lemaitre RN, King IB, Raghunathan TE, et al. Cell membrane trans-fatty acids and the risk of primary cardiac arrest. *Circulation.* 2002 Feb 12;105(6):697-701.
18. Peskin BS, Carter MJ. Chronic cellular hypoxia as the prime cause of cancer: what is the de-oxygenating role of adulterated and improper ratios of polyunsaturated fatty acids when incorporated into cell membranes? *Med Hypotheses.* 2008;70(2):298-304. Epub 2007 Jul 25.
19. Gawrisch K, Soubias O, Mihailescu M. Insights from biophysical studies on the role of polyunsaturated fatty acids for function of G-protein coupled membrane receptors. *Prostaglandins Leukot Essent Fatty Acids.* 2008 Sep-Nov;79(3-5):131-4.
20. Mozaffarian D, Aro A, Willett WC. Health effects of trans-fatty acids: experimental and observational evidence. *Eur J Clin Nutr.* 2009 May;63 Suppl 2:S5-21.
21. Salmeron J, Hu FB, Manson JE, et al. Dietary fat intake and risk of type 2 diabetes in women. *Am J Clin Nutr* 2001;73:1019-26.
22. Rivellese AA, De Natale C, Lilli S. Type of dietary fat and insulin resistance. *Ann N Y Acad Sci.* 2002;967:329-35.
23. Ramel A, Martinéz A, Kiely M, et al. Beneficial effects of long-chain n-3 fatty acids included in an energy-restricted diet on insulin resistance in overweight and obese European young adults. *Diabetologia.* 2008 Jul;51(7):1261-8.
24. Abete I, Parra D, Crujeiras AB, et al. Specific insulin sensitivity and leptin responses to a nutritional treatment of obesity via a combination of energy restriction and fatty fish intake. *J Hum Nutr Diet.* 2008 Dec;21(6):591-600. Epub 2008 Aug 27.
25. Rizza S, Tesauro M, Cardillo C, et al. Fish oil supplementation improves endothelial function in normoglycemic offspring of patients with type 2 diabetes. *Atherosclerosis.* 2009 Oct;206(2):569-74.
26. Steerenberg PA, Beekhof PK, Feskens EJ, et al. Long-term effect of fish oil diet on basal and stimulated plasma glucose and insulin levels in ob/ob mice. *Diabetes Nutr Metab.* 2002 Aug;15(4):205-14.
27. Li S, Sun Y, Liang CP, et al. Defective phagocytosis of apoptotic cells by macrophages in atherosclerotic lesions of ob/ob mice and reversal by a fish oil diet. *Circ Res.* 2009 Nov 20;105(11):1072-82.
28. Wei D, Li J, Shen M, et al. Cellular Production of {omega}-3 PUFAs and Reduction of {omega}-6/{omega}-3 ratios in the Pancreatic {beta}-cells and Islets Enhance Insulin Secretion and Confer Protection against Cytokine-induced Cell Death. *Diabetes.* 2009 Nov 23. Epub ahead of print.
29. Wilson JX. Regulation of vitamin C transport. *Annu Rev Nutr.* 2005;25:105-25.
30. Qutob S, Dixon SJ, Wilson JX. Insulin stimulates vitamin C recycling and ascorbate accumulation in osteoblastic cells. *Endocrinology.* 1998 Jan;139(1):51-6.

31. Ng LL, Ngkeekwong FC, Quinn PA, et al. Uptake mechanisms for ascorbate and dehydroascorbate in lymphoblasts from diabetic nephropathy and hypertensive patients. *Diabetologia.* 1998 Apr;41(4):435-42.

32. Minamizono A, Tomi M, Hosoya K. Inhibition of dehydroascorbic acid transport across the rat blood-retinal and -brain barriers in experimental diabetes. *Biol Pharm Bull.* 2006 Oct;29(10):2148-50.

33. Root-Bernstein R, Busik JV, Henry DN. Are diabetic neuropathy, retinopathy and nephropathy caused by hyperglycemic exclusion of dehydroascorbate uptake by glucose transporters? *J Theor Biol.* 2002 Jun 7;216(3):345-59.

34. Biolo G, Williams BD, Fleming RY, et al. Insulin action on muscle protein kinetics and amino acid transport during recovery after resistance exercise. *Diabetes.* 1999 May;48(5):949-57.

35. Christensen NJ, Hilsted J. Insulin facilitates transport of macromolecules and nutrients to muscles. *Int J Obes Relat Metab Disord.* 1993 Dec;17 Suppl 3:S83-5.

36. Bonadonna RC, Saccomani MP, Cobelli C, et al. Effect of insulin on system A amino acid transport in human skeletal muscle. *J Clin Invest.* 1993 Feb;91(2):514-21.

37. Duarte AI, Santos MS, Seiça R, et al. Insulin affects synaptosomal GABA and glutamate transport under oxidative stress conditions. *Brain Res.* 2003 Jul 4; 977(1):23-30.

38. Longo N. Insulin stimulates the Na+,K(+)-ATPase and the Na+/K+/Cl- cotransporter of human fibroblasts. *Biochim Biophys Acta.* 1996 May 22;1281(1):38-44.

39. Tiwari S, Riazi S, Ecelbarger CA. Insulin's impact on renal sodium transport and blood pressure in health, obesity, and diabetes. *Am J Physiol Renal Physiol.* 2007 Oct;293(4):F974-84.

40. Wiederkehr A, Wollheim CB. Minireview: implication of mitochondria in insulin secretion and action. *Endocrinology.* 2006 Jun;147(6):2643-9. Epub 2006 Mar 23.

41. Kamboj SS, Chopra K, Sandhir R. Hyperglycemia-induced alterations in synaptosomal membrane fluidity and activity of membrane bound enzymes: beneficial effect of N-acetylcysteine supplementation. *Neuroscience.* 2009 Aug 18;162(2):349-58. Epub 2009 May 6.

42. Kamboj A, Kiran R, Sandhir R. N-acetylcysteine ameliorates carbofuran-induced alterations in lipid composition and activity of membrane bound enzymes. *Mol Cell Biochem.* 2006 Jun;286(1-2):107-14.

43. Brookes PS, Yoon Y, Robotham JL, et al. Calcium, ATP, and ROS: a mitochondrial love-hate triangle. *Am J Physiol Cell Physiol.* 2004 Oct;287(4):C817-33.

44. Baumgartner HK, Gerasimenko JV, Thorne C, et al. Calcium elevation in mitochondria is the main Ca2+ requirement for mitochondrial permeability transition pore (mPTP) opening. *J Biol Chem.* 2009 Jul 31; 284(31):20796-803.

45. Rizzuto R, Marchi S, Bonora M, et al. Ca(2+) transfer from the ER to mitochondria: when, how and why. *Biochim Biophys Acta.* 2009 Nov;1787(11):1342-51.

46. Rasheva VI, Domingos PM. Cellular responses to endoplasmic reticulum stress and apoptosis. *Apoptosis.* 2009 Aug;14(8):996-1007.

47. Minamino T, Kitakaze M. ER stress in cardiovascular disease. *J Mol Cell Cardiol.* 2009 Nov 12.

48. Austin RC. The Unfolded Protein Response in Health and Disease. *Antioxid Redox Signal.* 2009 Sep;11(9):2279-2287.

49. Kaser A, Blumberg RS. Endoplasmic reticulum stress in the intestinal epithelium and inflammatory bowel disease. *Semin Immunol.* 2009 Jun;21(3):156-63.

50. Gorjão R, Azevedo-Martins AK, Rodrigues HG, et al. Comparative effects of DHA and EPA on cell function. *Pharmacol Ther.* 2009 Apr;122(1):56-64.

51. Harris WS, Pottala JV, Sands SA, et al. Comparison of the effects of fish and fish-oil capsules on the n 3 fatty acid content of blood cells and plasma phospholipids. *Am J Clin Nutr.* 2007 Dec;86(6):1621-5.

52. Holick MF. Vitamin D deficiency. *N Engl J Med.* 2007 Jul 19;357(3):266-81

53. Sergeev IN. Calcium signaling in cancer and vitamin D. *J Steroid Biochem Mol Biol.* 2005 Oct;97(1-2):145-51.

54. Sergeev IN. 1,25-Dihydroxyvitamin D3 induces Ca2+-mediated apoptosis in adipocytes via activation of calpain and caspase-12. *Biochem Biophys Res Commun.* 2009 Jun 19;384(1):18-21.

55. Natsume Y, Ito S, Satsu H, et al. Protective effect of quercetin on ER stress caused by calcium dynamics dysregulation in intestinal epithelial cells. *Toxicology.* 2009 Apr 28;258(2-3):164-75.

56. Fiorani M, Guidarelli A, Blasa M, et al. Mitochondria accumulate large amounts of quercetin: prevention of mitochondrial damage and release upon oxidation of the extramitochondrial fraction of the flavonoid. *J Nutr Biochem.* 2009 Mar 17.

57. Calabrese V, Cornelius C, Mancuso C, et al. Cellular stress response: a novel target for chemoprevention and nutritional neuroprotection in aging, neurodegenerative disorders and longevity. *Neurochem Res.* 2008 Dec;33(12):2444-71.

58. Frassetto LA, Morris RC Jr, Sebastian A. Dietary sodium chloride intake independently predicts the degree of hyperchloremic metabolic acidosis in healthy humans consuming a net acid-producing diet. *Am J Physiol Renal Physiol.* 2007 Aug;293(2):F521-5.

59. Sebastian A, Frassetto LA, Sellmeyer DE, et al. Estimation of the net acid load of the diet of ancestral preagricultural *Homo sapiens* and their hominid ancestors. *Am J Clin Nutr.* 2002 Dec;76(6):1308-16.

60. Huang WC, Swietach P, Vaughan-Jones RD, et al. Extracellular acidification elicits spatially and temporally distinct Ca2+ signals. *Curr Biol.* 2008 May 20;18(10):781-5.

61. Lardner A. The effects of extracellular pH on immune function. *J Leukoc Biol.* 2001 Apr;69(4):522-30.

62. Brandao-Burch A, Utting JC, Orriss IR, et al. Acidosis inhibits bone formation by osteoblasts *in vitro* by preventing mineralization. *Calcif Tissue Int.* 2005 Sep;77(3):167-74.

63. Bushinsky DA. Metabolic alkalosis decreases bone calcium efflux by suppressing osteoclasts and stimulating osteoblasts. *Am J Physiol.* 1996 Jul;271(1 Pt 2):F216-22.

64. Bushinsky DA. Stimulated osteoclastic and suppressed osteoblastic activity in metabolic but not respiratory acidosis. *Am J Physiol.* 1995 Jan;268(1 Pt 1):C80-8.

65. Arnett TR. Extracellular pH regulates bone cell function. *J Nutr.* 2008 Feb;138(2):415S-418S.

66. Osther PJ. Effect of acute acid loading on acid-base and calcium metabolism. *Scand J Urol Nephrol.* 2006;40(1):35-44.

67. Caudarella R, Vescini F, Buffa A, et al. Bone mass loss in calcium stone disease: focus on hypercalciuria and metabolic factors. *J Nephrol.* 2003 Mar-Apr;16(2):260-6.

68. Osther PJ, Bollerslev J, Hansen AB, et al. Pathophysiology of incomplete renal tubular acidosis in recurrent renal stone formers: evidence of disturbed calcium, bone and citrate metabolism. *Urol Res.* 1993 May;21(3):169-73.

69. Frassetto LA, Todd KM, Morris RC Jr, et al. Estimation of net endogenous noncarbonic acid production in humans from diet potassium and protein contents. *Am J Clin Nutr.* 1998 Sep;68(3):576-83.

70. Michaud DS, Troiano RP, Subar AF, et al. Comparison of estimated renal net acid excretion from dietary intake and body size with urine pH. *J Am Diet Assoc.* 2003 Aug;103(8):1001-7.

71. Sellmeyer DE, Stone KL, Sebastian A, et al. A high ratio of dietary animal to vegetable protein increases the rate of bone loss and the risk of fracture in postmenopausal women. Study of Osteoporotic Fractures Research Group. *Am J Clin Nutr.* 2001 Jan;73(1):118-22.

72. New SA, MacDonald HM, Campbell MK, et al. Lower estimates of net endogenous non-carbonic acid production are positively associated with indexes of bone health in premenopausal and perimenopausal women. *Am J Clin Nutr.* 2004 Jan;79(1):131-8.

73. Trinchieri A, Lizzano R, Marchesotti F, et al. Effect of potential renal acid load of foods on urinary citrate excretion in calcium renal stone formers. *Urol Res.* 2006 Feb;34(1):1-7.

74. Maalouf NM, Cameron MA, Moe OW, et al. Low urine pH: a novel feature of the metabolic syndrome. *Clin J Am Soc Nephrol.* 2007 Sep;2(5):883-8.

75. Abate N, Chandalia M, Cabo-Chan AV Jr, et al. The metabolic syndrome and uric acid nephrolithiasis: novel features of renal manifestation of insulin resistance. *Kidney Int.* 2004 Feb;65(2):386-92.

76. Jehle S, Zanetti A, Muser J, et al. Partial neutralization of the acidogenic Western diet with potassium citrate increases bone mass in postmenopausal women with osteopenia. *J Am Soc Nephrol.* 2006 Nov;17(11):3213-22.

77. Frassetto L, Morris RC Jr, Sebastian A. Long-term persistence of the urine calcium-lowering effect of potassium bicarbonate in postmenopausal women. *J Clin Endocrinol Metab.* 2005 Feb;90(2):831-4.

78. Tucker KL, Hannan MT, Chen H, et al. Potassium, magnesium, and fruit and vegetable intakes are associated with greater bone mineral density in elderly men and women. *Am J Clin Nutr.* 1999 Apr;69(4):727-36.

79. Ball D, Maughan RJ. Blood and urine acid-base status of premenopausal omnivorous and vegetarian women. *Br J Nutr.* 1997 Nov;78(5):683-93.

80. Ince BA, Anderson EJ, Neer RM. Lowering dietary protein to U.S. Recommended dietary allowance levels reduces urinary calcium excretion and bone resorption in young women. *J Clin Endocrinol Metab.* 2004 Aug;89(8):3801-7.

81. Remer T. Influence of nutrition on acid-base balance—metabolic aspects. *Eur J Nutr.* 2001 Oct;40(5):214-20.

82. Teucher B, Dainty JR, Spinks CA, et al. Sodium and Bone Health: The Impact of Moderately High and Low Salt Intakes on Calcium Metabolism in Postmenopausal Women. *J Bone Miner Res.* 2008 Apr 14.

83. Kato Y, Yamaguchi S, Yachiku S, et al. Changes in urinary parameters after oral administration of potassium-sodium citrate and magnesium oxide to prevent urolithiasis. *Urology.* 2004 Jan;63(1):7-11.

84. Ettinger B, Pak CY, Citron JT, et al. Potassium-magnesium citrate is an effective prophylaxis against recurrent calcium oxalate nephrolithiasis. *J Urol.* 1997 Dec;158(6):2069-73.

85. Bhopal RS, Rafnsson SB. Could mitochondrial efficiency explain the susceptibility to adiposity, metabolic syndrome, diabetes and cardiovascular diseases in South Asian populations? *Int J Epidemiol.* 2009 Aug;38(4):1072-81. Epub 2009 May 7.

86. Fernández-Vizarra E, Tiranti V, Zeviani M. Assembly of the oxidative phosphorylation system in humans: what we have learned by studying its defects. *Biochim Biophys Acta.* 2009 Jan;1793(1):200-11.

87. Di Donato S. Multisystem manifestations of mitochondrial disorders. *J Neurol.* 2009 May;256(5):693-710.

88. Stanley WC. Myocardial energy metabolism during ischemia and the mechanisms of metabolic therapies. *J Cardiovasc Pharmacol Ther.* 2004 Sep;9 Suppl 1:S31-45.

89. Gershoni M, Templeton AR, Mishmar D. Mitochondrial bioenergetics as a major motive force of speciation. *Bioessays.* 2009 Jun;31(6):642-50.

90. Richter C, Park JW, Ames BN. Normal oxidative damage to mitochondrial and nuclear DNA is extensive. *Proc Natl Acad Sci U S A.* 1988 Sep;85(17):6465-7.

91. Lee HC, Wei YH. Oxidative stress, mitochondrial DNA mutation, and apoptosis in aging. *Exp Biol Med (Maywood).* 2007 May;232(5):592-606.

92. Aliev G, Palacios HH, Walrafen B, et al. Brain mitochondria as a primary target in the development of treatment strategies for Alzheimer disease. *Int J Biochem Cell Biol.* 2009 Oct;41(10):1989-2004.

93. Palmieri L, Papaleo V, Porcelli V, et al. Altered calcium homeostasis in autism-spectrum disorders: evidence from biochemical and genetic studies of the mitochondrial aspartate/glutamate carrier AGC1. *Mol Psychiatry.* 2008 Jul 8.

94. Myhill S, Booth NE, McLaren-Howard J. Chronic fatigue syndrome and mitochondrial dysfunction. *Int J Clin Exp Med.* 2009;2(1):1-16.

95. Di Donato S. Multisystem manifestations of mitochondrial disorders. *J Neurol.* 2009 May;256(5):693-710.

96. Finsterer J. Central nervous system manifestations of mitochondrial disorders. *Acta Neurol Scand.* 2006 Oct; 114(4):217-38.

97. Haas RH, Parikh S, Falk MJ, et al. Mitochondrial Medicine Society's Committee on Diagnosis. The in-depth evaluation of suspected mitochondrial disease. *Mol Genet Metab.* 2008 May;94(1):16-37.

98. Myhill S, Booth NE, McLaren-Howard J. Chronic fatigue syndrome and mitochondrial dysfunction. *Int J Clin Exp Med.* 2009;2(1):1-16.

99. Valavanidis A, Vlachogianni T, Fiotakis C. 8-hydroxy-2' -deoxyguanosine (8-OHdG): A critical biomarker of oxidative stress and carcinogenesis. *J Environ Sci Health C Environ Carcinog Ecotoxicol Rev.* 2009 Apr;27(2): 120-39.

100. Monroe RK, Halvorsen SW. Environmental toxicants inhibit neuronal Jak tyrosine kinase by mitochondrial disruption. *Neurotoxicology.* 2009 Jul;30(4):589-98.

101. Lim S, Ahn SY, Song IC, et al. Chronic exposure to the herbicide, atrazine, causes mitochondrial dysfunction and insulin resistance. *PLoS One.* 2009;4(4):e5186.

102. Lee HK, Cho YM, Kwak SH, et al. Mitochondrial dysfunction and metabolic syndrome-looking for environmental factors. *Biochim Biophys Acta.* 2009 Nov 13.

103. Monroe RK, Halvorsen SW. Environmental toxicants inhibit neuronal Jak tyrosine kinase by mitochondrial disruption. *Neurotoxicology.* 2009 Jul;30(4):589-98.

104. Przedborski S, Jackson-Lewis V, Muthane U, et al. Chronic levodopa administration alters cerebral mitochondrial respiratory chain activity *Ann Neurol.* 1993;34:715-23.

105. Kupsch K, Hertel S, Kreutzmann P, et al. Impairment of mitochondrial function by minocycline. *FEBS J.* 2009 Mar;276(6):1729-38.

106. Caso G, Kelly P, McNurlan MA, et al. Effect of Coenzyme Q10 on myopathic symptoms in patients treated with statins. *Am J Cardiol.* 2007 May 15;99(10):1409-12.

107. Golomb BA, Evans MA. Statin adverse effects : a review of the literature and evidence for a mitochondrial mechanism. *Am J Cardiovasc Drugs.* 2008;8(6):373-418.

108. Cocco T, Di Paola M, Papa S, et al. Arachidonic acid interaction with the mitochondrial electron transport chain promotes reactive oxygen species generation. *Free Rad Biol Med.* 1999;27: 51-9.

109. Collins M, Renault V, Grobler LA, et al. Athletes with exercise-associated fatigue have abnormally short muscle DNA telomeres. *Med Sci Sports Exerc.* 2003;35:1524-8.

110. Rabøl R, Højberg PM, Almdal T, et al. Effect of hyperglycemia on mitochondrial respiration in type 2 diabetes. *J Clin Endocrinol Metab.* 2009 Apr;94(4):1372-8.

111. Gomez J, Caro P, Sanchez I, et al. Effect of methionine dietary supplementation on mitochondrial oxygen radical generation and oxidative DNA damage in rat liver and heart. *J Bioenerg Biomembr.* 2009 Jun;41(3):309-21.

112. Zimmer HG. Significance of the 5-phosphoribosyl-1-pyrophosphate pool for cardiac purine and pyrimidine nucleotide synthesis: studies with ribose, adenine, inosine, and orotic acid in rats. *Cardiovasc Drugs Ther.* 1998 Sep; 12 Suppl 2:179-87.

113. Hellsten Y, Skadhauge L, Bangsbo J. Effect of ribose supplementation on resynthesis of adenine nucleotides after intense intermittent training in humans. *Am J Physiol Regul Integr Comp Physiol.* 2004 Jan;286(1):R182-8.

114. Omran H, Illien S, MacCarter D, et al. D-Ribose improves diastolic function and quality of life in congestive heart failure patients: a prospective feasibility study. *Eur J Heart Fail.* 2003 Oct;5(5):615-9.

115. Seifert JG, Subudhi AW, Fu MX, et al.The role of ribose on oxidative stress during hypoxic exercise: a pilot study. *J Med Food.* 2009 Jun;12(3):690-3.

116. Teitelbaum JE, Johnson C, St Cyr J. The use of D-ribose in chronic fatigue syndrome and fibromyalgia: a pilot study. *J Altern Complement Med.* 2006 Nov;12(9):857-62.

117. Kubota T, Shindo Y, Tokuno K, et al. Mitochondria are intracellular magnesium stores: investigation by simultaneous fluorescent imagings in PC12 cells. *Biochim Biophys Acta.* 2005 May 15;1744(1):19-28.

118. Ko YH, Hong S, Pedersen PL. Chemical mechanism of ATP synthase. Magnesium plays a pivotal role in formation of the transition state where ATP is synthesized from ADP and inorganic phosphate. *J Biol Chem.* 1999 Oct 8; 274(41):28853-6.

119. Barbagallo M, Dominguez LJ. Magnesium metabolism in type 2 diabetes mellitus, metabolic syndrome and insulin resistance. *Arch Biochem Biophys.* 2007 Feb 1;458(1):40-7.

120. Zorzano A, Liesa M, Palacín M. Role of mitochondrial dynamics proteins in the pathophysiology of obesity and type 2 diabetes. *Int J Biochem Cell Biol.* 2009 Oct;41(10):1846-54.

121. Tarnopolsky MA. The mitochondrial cocktail: rationale for combined nutraceutical therapy in mitochondrial cytopathies. *Adv Drug Deliv Rev.* 2008 Oct-Nov;60(13-14):1561-7.

122. Condò M, Posar A, Arbizzani A, et al. Riboflavin prophylaxis in pediatric and adolescent migraine. *J Headache Pain.* 2009 Oct;10(5):361-5.

123. Schoenen J, Jacquy J, Lenaerts M. Effectiveness of high-dose riboflavin in migraine prophylaxis. A randomized controlled trial. *Neurology.* 1998 Feb;50(2):466-70.

124. MacLennan SC, Wade FM, Forrest KM, et al. High-dose riboflavin for migraine prophylaxis in children: a double-blind, randomized, placebo-controlled trial. *J Child Neurol.* 2008 Nov;23(11):1300-4.

125. Acin-Perez R, Hoyos B, Zhao F, et al. Control of oxidative phosphorylation by vitamin A illuminates a fundamental role in mitochondrial energy homoeostasis. *FASEB J.* 2009 Oct 7.

126. Ryu H, Rosas HD, Hersch SM, et al. The therapeutic role of creatine in Huntington's disease. *Pharmacol Ther.* 2005 Nov;108(2):193-207.

127. Adhihetty PJ, Beal MF. Creatine and its potential therapeutic value for targeting cellular energy impairment in neurodegenerative diseases. *Neuromolecular Med.* 2008;10(4):275-90.

128. Calabrese V, Giuffrida Stella AM, Calvani M, et al. Acetylcarnitine and cellular stress response: roles in nutritional redox homeostasis and regulation of longevity genes. *J Nutr Biochem.* 2006 Feb;17(2):73-88.

129. Malaguarnera M, Gargante MP, Cristaldi E, et al. Acetyl L-carnitine (ALC) treatment in elderly patients with fatigue. *Arch Gerontol Geriatr.* 2008 Mar-Apr; 46(2):181-90.

130. Sohal RS, Forster MJ. Coenzyme Q, oxidative stress and aging. *Mitochondrion.* 2007 Jun;7 Suppl:S103-11.

131. Mitsumoto Y, Kobayashi S, Matsushima H, et al. Oral administration of coenzyme Q(10) prevents cytochrome C release from mitochondria induced by 1-methyl-4-phenylpyridinium ion in mouse brain synaptosomes. *Neurosci Lett.* 2009 Sep 29;463(1):22-5.

132. Kon M, Tanabe K, Akimoto T, et al. Reducing exercise-induced muscular injury in kendo athletes with supplementation of coenzyme Q10. *Br J Nutr.* 2008 Oct;100(4):903-9.

133. Zheng A, Moritani T. Influence of CoQ10 on autonomic nervous activity and energy metabolism during exercise in healthy subjects. *J Nutr Sci Vitaminol* (Tokyo). 2008 Aug;54(4):286-90.

134. Rosenfeldt F, Marasco S, Lyon W, et al. Coenzyme Q10 therapy before cardiac surgery improves mitochondrial function and *in vitro* contractility of myocardial tissue. *J Thorac Cardiovasc Surg.* 2005 Jan;129(1):25-32.

135. Liu J. The effects and mechanisms of mitochondrial nutrient alpha-lipoic acid on improving age-associated mitochondrial and cognitive dysfunction: an overview. *Neurochem Res.* 2008 Jan;33(1):194-203.

136. Hagen TM, Ingersoll RT, Lykkesfeldt J, et al. (R)-alpha -lipoic acid-supplemented old rats have improved mitochondrial function, decreased oxidative damage, and increased metabolic rate. *FASEB J.* 1999 Feb;13(2):411-8.

137. Li CJ, Zhang QM, Li MZ. Attenuation of myocardial apoptosis by alpha-lipoic acid through suppression of mitochondrial oxidative stress to reduce diabetic cardiomyopathy. *Chin Med J* (Engl). 2009 Nov 5;122(21):2580-6.

138. Magis D, Ambrosini A, Sándor P, et al. A randomized double-blind placebo-controlled trial of thioctic acid in migraine prophylaxis. *Headache.* 2007 Jan;47(1):52-7.

139. Hagen TM, Liu J, Lykkesfeldt J, et al. Feeding acetyl-L-carnitine and lipoic acid to old rats significantly improves metabolic function while decreasing oxidative stress. *Proc Natl Acad Sci.* 2002; 99: 1870-5.

140. Long J, Gao F, Tong L. Mitochondrial decay in the brains of old rats: ameliorating effect of alpha-lipoic acid and acetyl-L-carnitine. *Neurochem Res.* 2009 Apr;34(4):755-63.

141. Shenk JC, Liu J, Fischbach K, et al. The effect of acetyl-L-carnitine and R-alpha-lipoic acid treatment in ApoE4 mouse as a model of human Alzheimer's disease. *J Neurol Sci.* 2009 Aug 15;283(1-2):199-206.

142. Abdel-Kader R, Hauptmann S, Keil U, et al. Stabilization of mitochondrial function by *Ginkgo biloba* extract (EGb 761). *Pharmacol Res.* 2007;56:493-502.

143. Shi C, Yao Z, Xu J, et al. Dosage effects of EGb761 on hydrogen peroxide-induced cell death in SH-SY5Y cells. *Chem Biol Interact.* 2009 Aug 14;180(3):389-97.

144. Shin SM, Cho IJ, Kim SG. Resveratrol protects mitochondria against oxidative stress through AMP-activated protein kinase-mediated glycogen synthase kinase-3 beta inhibition downstream of poly (ADP-ribose) polymerase-LKB1 pathway. *Mol Pharmacol.* 2009 Oct;76(4):884-95.

145. Ungvari Z, Labinskyy N, Mukhopadhyay P, et al. Resveratrol attenuates mitochondrial oxidative stress in coronary arterial endothelial cells. *Am J Physiol Heart Circ Physiol.* 2009 Nov;297(5):H1876-81.

146. Csiszar A, Labinskyy N, Pinto JT, et al. Resveratrol induces mitochondrial biogenesis in endothelial cells. *Am J Physiol Heart Circ Physiol.* 2009 Jul;297(1):H13-20.

147. Lagouge M, Argmann C, Gerhart-Hines Z, et al. Resveratrol improves mitochondrial function and protects against metabolic disease by activating SIRT1 and PGC-1α. Cell 27:1109-22.

148. Marambaud P, Zhao H, Davies P, et al. Resveratrol promotes clearance of Alzheimer's disease amyloid-beta peptides. *J Biol Chem.* 2005;280:37377-82.

149. López A, García JA, Escames G, et al. Melatonin protects the mitochondria from oxidative damage reducing oxygen consumption, membrane potential, and superoxide anion production. *J Pineal Res.* 2009 Mar;46(2):188-98.

150. Petrosillo G, Colantuono G, Moro N. Melatonin protects against heart ischemia-reperfusion injury by inhibiting mitochondrial permeability transition pore opening. *Am J Physiol Heart Circ Physiol.* 2009 Oct;297(4):H1487-93.

151. Wang X. The antiapoptotic activity of melatonin in neurodegenerative diseases. *CNS Neurosci Ther.* 2009 Winter; 15(4):345-57.

Digestive Health

Overview

"The gastrointestinal (GI) system is the primary gateway by which the external environment interacts with the body."[1] The largest mucosal surface in the body, the GI tract is responsible for the digestion and absorption of nutrients from food, but its impact extends well beyond the gut. For example, the GI tract contains an extraordinary number of immune cells that must defend against pathogens and toxins (to which we are exposed on a continuous basis), while allowing for tolerance to food and commensal bacteria—a balancing act that has systemic consequences.

In adults, the GI tract is approximately 7 m long with a surface area of approximately 300 m^2, making it the largest exposed mucosal surface of the body. To defend against the daily exposure to pathogens, it has a number of protective mechanisms, including a low pH in the stomach, coverage of the complete GI tract with a mucus layer, an enormous array of immune cells that lie beneath this mucus layer, and the presence of commensal microbes that abundantly colonize the GI tract.[63] The role of digestion is to first separate food into its components by mechanical homogenization and chemical breakdown, followed by absorption of the smaller carbohydrates, lipids, proteins, vitamins, minerals, and other nutrients through a variety of passive and active processes.

While the basic physiology of digestion and absorption is fairly well understood, a significant portion of the population experiences digestive disturbances that remain unresolved. A component of many digestive disturbances is a disruption in one (or more) of the following mechanisms: loss of gastric acidity or digestive enzyme function; altered immune homeostasis due to infection and/or to treatment for infections; loss of commensal microbiota; an increase in intestinal permeability (IP). Increased IP impairs the selective absorption function that is so critical to overall health, causing inflammation which further fuels the pathology. This chapter is designed to review basic digestive physiology, highlight the types of dysfunctions frequently encountered, discuss their assessment, and present clinically valid interventions designed to restore optimal GI health.

Epidemiology

The spectrum of digestive disturbances is quite broad, with many individuals experiencing functional impairment for varying periods of time prior to frank disease. For example, inflammatory bowel disease (IBD), a widely recognized cause of severe intestinal barrier impairment, has an estimated prevalence of nearly 1 million people in the United States (with considerable geographic variation).[2] However, the largest survey of GI symptoms to date found an overall prevalence of ≥1 upper GI symptom in 45% of those surveyed (based on the preceding 3-month period); symptoms included heartburn, early satiety, loss of appetite, and postprandial fullness.[3] A smaller survey of Canadian adults found a prevalence of lower GI symptoms of 5.2% (abdominal pain/bloating, constipation, diarrhea). More recent studies in the U.S. suggest bloating may afflict 19–21% of U.S. adults.[4,5]

Unfortunately, in as many as half of the symptomatic patients seen by gastroenterologists, a cause is not found, and patients are often given a diagnosis of unclear etiology, such as functional dyspepsia or irritable bowel syndrome (IBS).[6] This suggests that the underlying physiology of many gastrointestinal disturbances is not well-understood, or that early stages of dysfunction are overlooked. For example, in recent years the prevalence of celiac disease has been found to be many-fold greater than previously assumed, affecting up to 1% of the U.S. population, or roughly 3 million people. However, a recent report from the UK estimated that only 1 out of every 9 cases of celiac disease has actually been diagnosed (i.e., 8 out of 9 remain undiagnosed)[7]; the time of delayed diagnosis ranges from 4.5–9 years.[8] An earlier study suggested that, in some patients with IBS, celiac disease may be the underlying cause, with an odds ratio (OR) of 7.0 for those with IBS.[9] Indeed, a screening of over 13,000 individuals found that those with digestive complaints such as constipation, diarrhea, and/or abdominal pain had a 1:56 chance of having celiac disease, a risk increase of more than 2-fold that of the general population.[10] Thus, a careful assessment may be particularly important for signs and symptoms of digestive dysfunction.

Underlying Digestive Physiology

The digestive process varies for macronutrients. For example, glucose requires no digestion, while lipid absorption depends on gastric and pancreatic lipases for digestion and bile salts for emulsification and transport of the hydrophobic components. Absorption of these nutrients varies not only by type, i.e., monosaccharide vs. amino acid, but also by the environment. For example, glucose is normally absorbed by active transport, but this may be overridden during a sugar-rich meal.

Carbohydrates

Monosaccharides

No digestion is required for single sugar carbohydrates, such as glucose. It is absorbed in the small intestine primarily by active transport (the sodium-dependent glucose transporter, SGLT1). However, during sugar-rich meals this transport becomes saturated, and a diffusive process provides a major pathway for absorption. This diffusive absorption is facilitated by glucose transporter type 2 (GLUT2), a receptor normally found in the

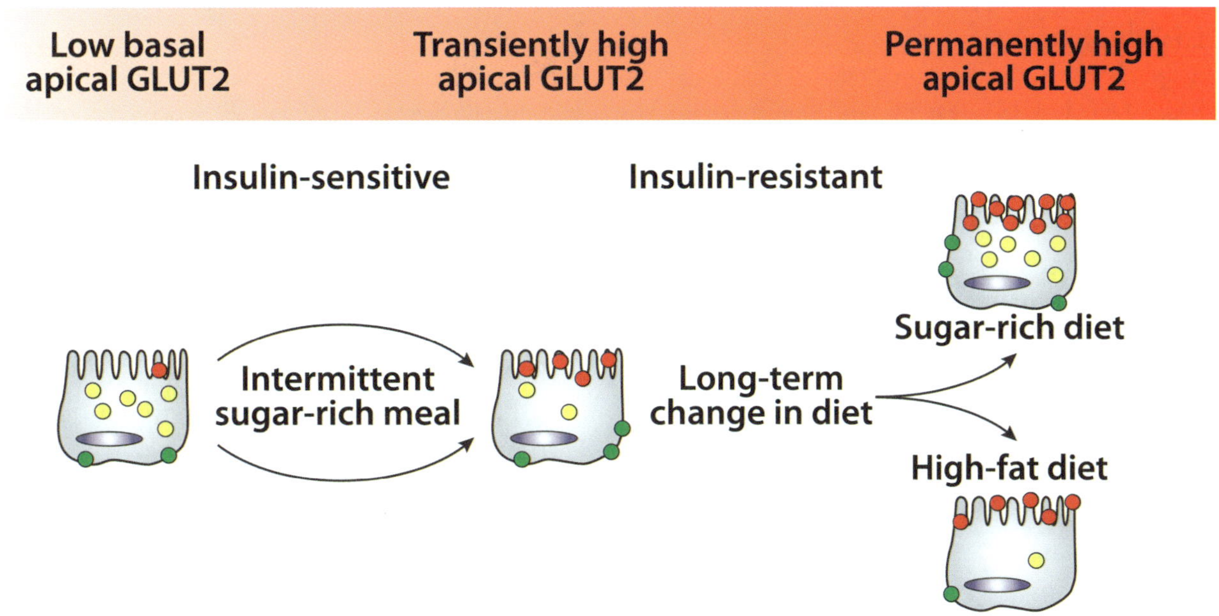

Figure 2.1 Permanent apical GLUT2 elevation due to insulin resistance in response to poor diet. From: Kellett GL, Brot-Laroche E, Mace OJ, et al. Sugar absorption in the intestine: the role of GLUT2. *Annu Rev Nutr.* 2008;28:35-54. Reproduced with permission of Annual Reviews Inc.

basolateral membrane, but one which inserts into the apical membrane within minutes in response to a high-sugar meal.[11]

As a result of a Western diet high in sugar, there is a constant elevation of GLUT2 in the apical membrane, further increasing the absorption of glucose. Artificial sweeteners likely have this same effect, and may also lead to increased absorption of any natural sugars present in the diet (Figure 2.1). GLUT2 may also act as a glucose sensor in the brain, a hypothesis suggested by data showing an increased intake among those with a GLUT2 genetic variant in both diabetic and healthy populations.[12] Flavonoids, particularly quercetin, may have some role in reducing the absorption of glucose by inhibiting GLUT2.[13]

Disaccharides

Disaccharides, such as sucrose and lactose, require small intestinal surface enzymes for hydrolysis to monosaccharides. Digestive enzymes, such as lactase-phlorizin hydrolase and sucrase isomaltase, are anchored to the mucosal surface of the small intestine where the soluble sugars in the lumen are hydrolyzed to free glucose, galactose, and fructose, which are absorbed rapidly from the lumen.[14]

Damage to the intestinal brush border (such as that due to chronic NSAID use, inflammation, trauma, disease, or parasite infection) impairs absorption of disaccharides as a consequence of the loss in enzymatic activity. For example, celiac disease is an important cause of mucosal damage. In patients with lactose intolerance, 24% were found to have celiac disease, compared to 2% of controls, leading the authors to suggest that all individuals with a positive hydrogen lactose breath test be screened for celiac disease.[15]

Carbohydrate malabsorption may also lead to bacterial overgrowth, gas, bloating, and irritable bowel syndrome, as seen in patients with fructose intolerance. Thirty-eight percent of patients with IBS were found to have a positive fructose breath test, and symptoms such as pain, belching, bloating, fullness, indigestion, and diarrhea improved after implementing a fructose-restricted diet.[16] A previous study involving 183 men and women with unexplained abdominal symptoms found that 73% had a positive fructose breath test.[17]

One of the most prevalent cases of disaccharide malabsorption is lactose intolerance, with a wide range of both GI and systemic symptoms (see Table 2.1). Up to 70% of the world population has lactase nonpersistence, with intolerance rates ranging from 5% in a British population to 100% in some Asian countries.[18]

Table 2.1 Symptoms of lactose intolerance

	Number of people with symptom (% of total)
(A) Gut related	
Abdominal pain	100
Gut distension	100
Borborygmi	100
Flatulence	100
Diarrhea	70
Constipation	30
Nausea	78
Vomiting	78
(B) Systemic	
Headache and lightheadedness	86
Loss of concentration and poor short-term memory	82
Long-term severe tiredness	63
Muscle pain	71
Joint pain, and/or swelling and stiffness	71
Allergy	40
Eczema	
Pruritis	
Rhinitis	
Sinusitis	
Asthma	
Heart arrhythmia	24
Mouth ulcers	30
Increased frequency of micturition	<20
Sore throat	<20

Systemic lactose intolerance: a new perspective on an old problem. From: Matthews SB, Waud JP, Roberts AG, et al. *Postgrad Med J.* 2005 Mar;81(953):167-73. Reproduced with permission of BMJ Publishing Group Ltd.

One potential cause of lactose intolerance, in addition to lactase nonpersistence, is small bowel bacterial overgrowth (SBBO), which may explain why lactose malabsorption is known to be more prevalent in the elderly. A recent trial found 50% of elderly subjects to be lactose intolerant compared to 5% of controls, with 90% of those with lactose intolerance having SBBO (determined by biopsy).[19] When the SBBO was treated, the lactose intolerance resolved. This study found that the lactulose breath test, often used to diagnose SBBO, was not reliable (it identified only 18% of those with SBBO).

Bloating is frequently due to poor disaccharide digestion. In a small trial of 36 patients with "functional abdominal bloating," 72% had positive breath tests for carbohydrate malabsorption, and 81% of those patients experienced relief within 1 month after implementing a malabsorbed sugar-free diet.[20]

Lipid digestion

The major form of dietary lipids consumed is long chain triglycerides (TAGs), and a lesser amount of the phospholipid lecithin. The process of digestion converts water-insoluble lipids into an absorbable form that can traverse the aqueous lumen of the GI tract. The first step in the digestion of TAGs, preceding absorption, begins in the stomach with the initiation of emulsification, creating a stable lipid droplet with a large surface area.[21] The droplets consist of a hydrophobic core containing the majority of the triacylglycerol molecules, esterified cholesterol, and fat-soluble vitamins, surrounded by an amphipathic surface monolayer of phospholipids, free cholesterol, and a few triacylglycerol molecules.[22] What follows is a partial hydrolysis of TAGs into diacylglycerol (DAG) and free fatty acids (FFAs), performed by gastric lipase, an enzyme with a surprisingly broad pH range for activity. While optimal pH is about 4–5.5, it retains activity at any acidic pH.[21] Gastric lipase is responsible for 10–30% of lipid hydrolysis.[23]

Upon entering the small intestine, TAG degradation products cause gall bladder emptying of bile acids, pancreatic lipase and co-lipase secretion, and cholecystokinin release.[23] The majority of TAG digestion is due to pancreatic lipase. In patients with congenital absence of pancreatic lipase, 50–60% of dietary fats are not absorbed.[24] Co-lipase mediates the binding of lipase, with the lipase/co-lipase enzyme complex attaching to the triglyceride emulsion. Digestion is also enhanced by the action of phospholipase A_2, which digests the phospholipids on the surface of the emulsion and exposes the TAG core.

Bile acids also play a large role in lipid digestion. Bile acids act as biological detergents, forming aggregates (micelles) that penetrate the water layer, thus playing an essential role as enzyme cofactor and vehicle for effective solubilization of hydrophobic sterols and alcohols. Bile acids are synthesized from cholesterol in the liver, secreted from hepatocytes into the bile canaliculi, and subsequently stored in the gall bladder and released in response to a meal. Bile salts are efficiently absorbed by passive diffusion and active transport in the terminal ileum, and they are transported back to the liver via the portal vein (enterohepatic circulation). Each bile salt may complete 4–12 cycles between liver and intestine per day.[25]

In addition to their classic role in lipid absorption, bile acids have only recently been recognized as versatile signaling molecules that have *systemic endocrine function*. Specifically, bile acids are ligands for a number of receptors, and may regulate triglyceride, cholesterol, energy and glucose homeostasis, and act as an integral "hormonal" component of the response to food ingestions, informing the body of food availability.[26] It is also plausible that they are a bridge between metabolism and food intake, as bile acid levels have been shown to activate the thyroid hormone activating enzyme, type 2 iodothyronine deiodinase, in animal studies.[27,28]

Poor lipid digestion is associated with a number of clinical consequences. For example, pancreatic insufficiency and/or liver dysfunction result in decreased fatty acid and fat-soluble nutrient absorption, which may manifest in a number of ways. A low level of fecal elastase-1, suggestive of pancreatic insufficiency, is more commonly found in patients with osteoporotic fractures.[29] Patients with both type 1 and 2 diabetes mellitus have a high prevalence of exocrine pancreatic insufficiency, which is often associated with steatorrhea.[30] A recent observational study suggests that exocrine insufficiency may precede the beta cell failure seen in diabetes, at least in some patients.[31] And finally, celiac patients with chronic diarrhea are likely to have low fecal elastase, suggesting pancreatic insufficiency, even when following a gluten-free diet.[32]

Protein digestion

Protein digestion proceeds in phases, with an initial gastric phase followed by an intestinal phase. Digestion begins in the stomach with the action of proteases (pepsins) produced by the gastric cells. Pepsins are secreted as inactive precursors, known as pepsinogens (pepsinogen A and C), and are autocatalytically cleaved to pepsin under acidic conditions.[21] Enzyme secretion and HCl production are both triggered primarily by gastrin secretion, which is induced by distention of the stomach.[33]

About 1.5–2.5 liters of gastric juice containing HCl are produced daily by the parietal cells,[34] creating a pH of less than 2. This acidic pH increases the catalytic efficiency of pepsins, creates an acidic pH for activation of pepsinogen, and directly denatures proteins. Because pepsins are not active at a pH above 4, their activity is restricted to the stomach.

Inadequate digestion of protein due to low HCl secretion is thought to *increase the risk of food allergy*. In a recent observational study of 152 patients given anti-ulcer medication for dyspepsia, 25% developed a boost or de-novo IgE formation towards regular constituents of the daily diet, and remained sensitized 5 months after discontinuation of the therapy.[35] This may be especially concerning given that nearly 25% of U.S. adults (NHANES) report taking calcium containing antacids, a number which does not include other types of acid suppressive medication.[36] A recent review describes the increased risk for food allergy with impairment of GI digestion, as well as a decreased threshold dose of allergens needed to elicit symptoms in sensitized individuals.[33] Figure 2.2 depicts this general process.

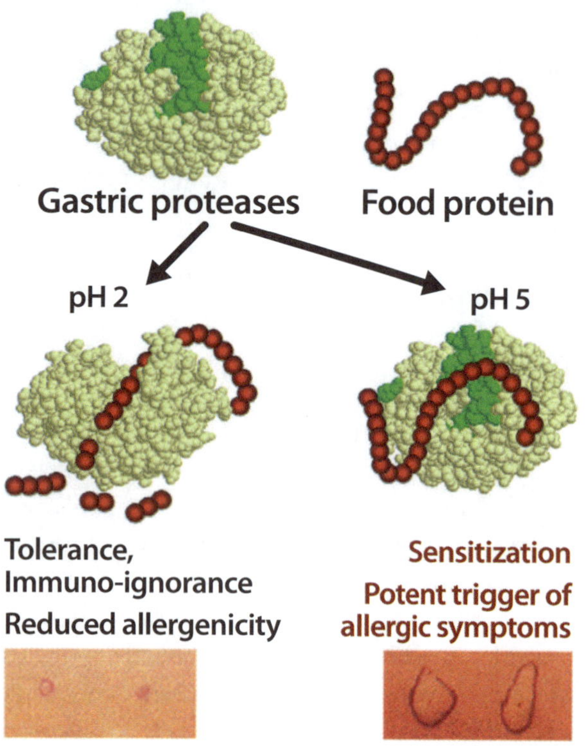

Figure 2.2 Development of allergic symptoms and sensitization from impaired gastric digestion. From: Untersmayr E, Jensen-Jarolim E. The role of protein digestibility and antacids on food allergy outcomes. *J Allergy Clin Immunol.* 2008 Jun;121(6):1301-8. Reproduced with permission of Elsevier.

Following the gastric phase, the intestinal phase of protein digestion consists of a luminal phase, brush border phase, and intracellular phase. In the luminal phase, pancreatic proteases and peptidases (secreted as inactive precursors, or zymogens) are secreted from the pancreas; these include trypsinogen, chymotrypsin, proelastase, and procarboxypeptidases A and B.[21] During the brush border phase, the enzyme enteropeptidase (aka enterokinase) generates trypsin, which in turn activates the remaining zymogens. The brush border is also rich in aminopeptidase activity, and during this next phase of digestion oligopeptides undergo further hydrolysis.

During the intracellular phase, single amino acids or small peptides of up to 3 amino acids in length are actively taken up by enterocytes through a number of distinct transport systems, and further hydrolyzed to free amino acids. While typically thought to be necessary only for lipid absorption, *bile acids* may also accelerate hydrolysis by pancreatic proteins.[37]

Damage to the intestinal brush border may occur from a number of factors (chronic NSAIDs, inflammation, trauma, disease, infection, celiac disease), and lead to incomplete protein digestion and malabsorption.[38] *Incomplete protein digestion* may also be a trigger for antibody formation (see above, food allergies). *Curcumin* and *glutamine* have both shown some potential to reduce the damage, at least by NSAIDs.[39,40] NSAIDs may act by upregulating Toll-like receptor 4 (TLR4), which glutamine has been shown to downregulate in animal studies.[41,42] In addition to food allergies, in susceptible individuals the resistance of dietary gluten to complete digestion leads to large oligopeptides crossing into the enterocyte, triggering an autoimmune response, e.g., celiac disease.[43]

Minerals

Minerals are typically bound to proteins, ligands, phosphates and other organic acids; many (i.e., calcium, iron) require gastric HCl to become more absorbable. For example, calcium must be in a soluble form, ionized (Ca^{++}), at least in the upper small intestine, or bound to a soluble organic molecule before it can cross the wall of the intestine; low gastric pH ionizes calcium.[21,44] While the decrease in calcium absorption that occurs with age has often been attributed to hypochlorhydria, a decrease in the vitamin D receptor concentration, as well as of the calcium channel/transporter TRPV6 may also explain the reduction.[45] Iron absorption varies widely by type, heme vs. non-heme. Heme iron is absorbed more efficiently and is relatively unaffected by dietary factors. Food components have a much greater effect on non-heme iron: black tea has been shown to inhibit iron absorption by 49–59% in both healthy individuals and those with iron deficiency anemia. *Ascorbic acid* increased the absorption by 270–350% in the same populations.[46] Celiac disease may initially present as iron deficiency, indicating the importance of intestinal integrity for iron absorption.[47,48]

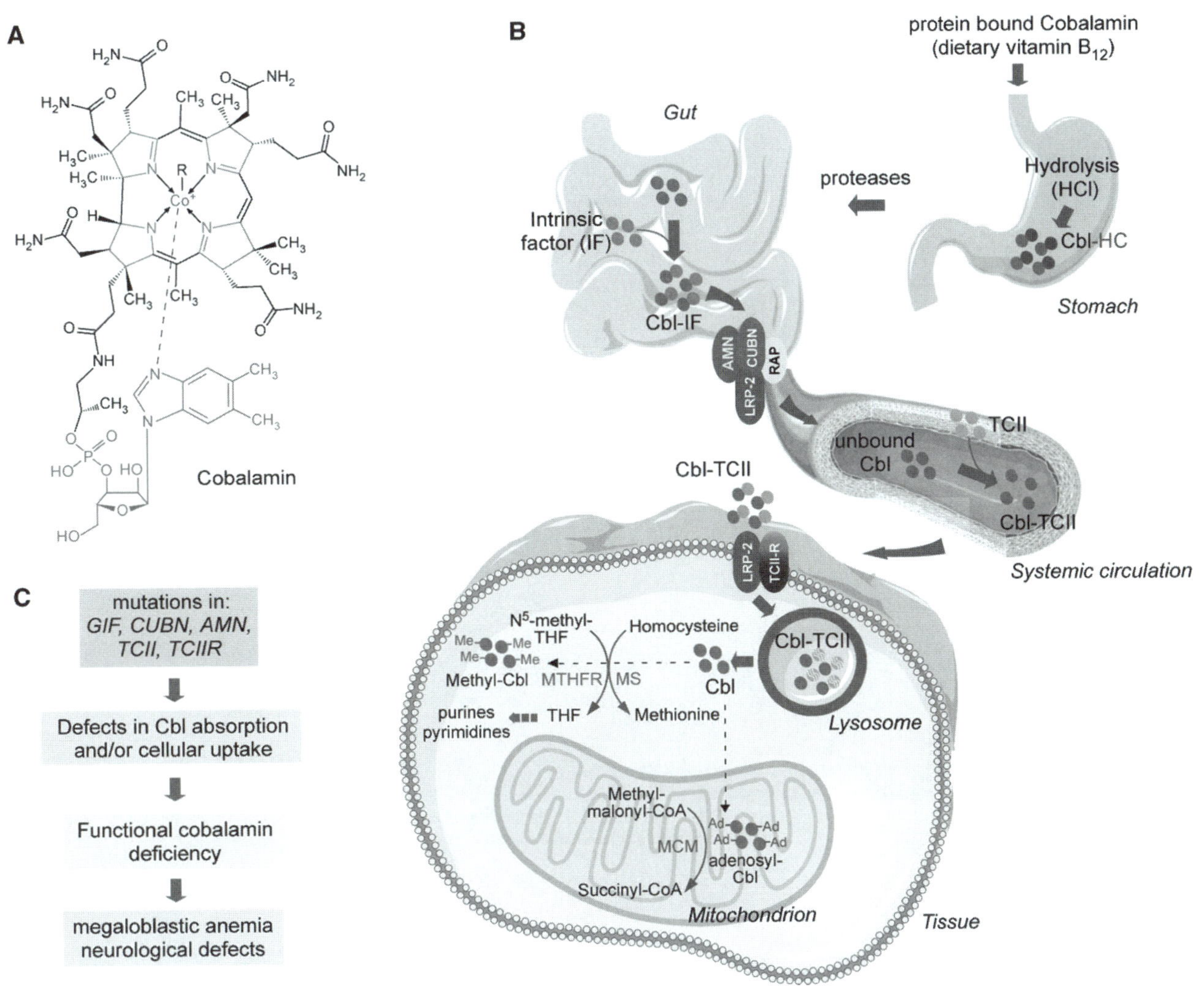

Figure 2.3 Cobalamin absorption and metabolic pathway. From: a. Reproduced with permission of Oxford University Press.

Additionally, several dietary components may also affect mineral absorption. Dietary phytate, for example, inhibits the absorption of most minerals. Zinc absorption is more efficient in low-zinc diets, but this effect is minimal if the diet is also rich in phytate.[49] In phytate-rich diets, the availability of other minerals such as copper and iron is significantly depressed.[50] Iron absorption was found to increase 2–12-fold when a commercial preparation of phytase was used to degrade the phytic acid.[51]

Vitamins

Water-soluble vitamins

Most vitamins are present in foods as part of coenzyme systems, and require protein digestion to separate, with both active and passive (water-soluble) absorption processes. In some cases, high dosages of vitamins can bypass digestive dysfunction. For example, vitamin B12 is bound to dietary animal protein, and its absorption involves gastric, upper intestinal, and ileal stages, as well as an enterohepatic circulation.[21] In the presence of gastric acid and pepsin, cobalamin is released from its protein bond and then transferred to R-binding protein (haptocorrin) that is present in saliva and gastric juice (see Figure 2.3). The release of cobalamin and its transfer to R factor is optimal at a pH of 1 to 1.3, a level not achieved by achlorhydric individuals.[21] While intrinsic factor (secreted by gastric mucosa) is required for the absorption of at least 60% of oral cobalamin, passive absorption

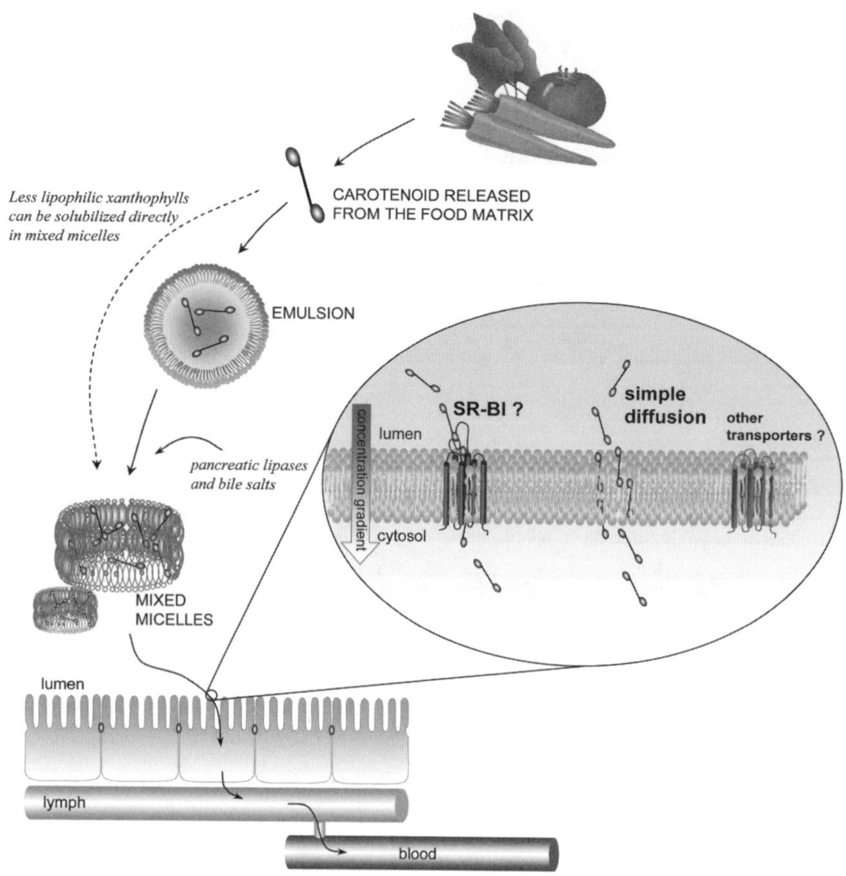

Figure 2.4 Dietary carotenoid absorption. From: ,. Copyright Wiley-VCH Verlag GmbH & Co. KGaA. Reproduced with permission.

captures 1–5% of free cobalamin.[52] This latter route is likely why high doses of oral cobalamin can effectively treat deficiencies, because it bypasses the active absorption process in sufficient amounts.[53,54]

Fat-soluble vitamins

Fat-soluble vitamins require effective lipid digestion as well as bile salts for absorption. For example, dietary retinyl esters (vitamin A) are hydrolyzed in the intestine by the pancreatic triglyceride lipase (a pancreatic enzyme) and by phospholipase B (an intestinal brush border enzyme).[55] The digestion of vitamin E in the small intestine lumen does not differ from that of dietary fats. The presence of bile salts and pancreatic enzymes is required for micelle formation and enzymatic hydrolysis, respectively.[56]

Carotenoids and flavonoids. Carotenoids are also bound to fiber, digestible polysaccharides, and proteins, and require many of the same processes found in fat digestion. They form mixed micelles in the duodenum using bile salts and the hydrolysis of emulsified lipid by pancreatic lipase and colipase. It is unclear if micelles are absorbed by passive diffusion or are receptor mediated. Recent evidence suggests that beta-carotene and lutein are transported into enterocytes through a receptor, possibly a scavenger receptor class B type 1 (SR-BI)[57] (Figure 2.4). In general, carotenoids are more bioavailable when cooked than raw, in some cases up to 6-fold more.[58] For example, 65% of the beta-carotene was absorbed from cooked carrots, versus 41% from raw carrots.[59]

There is very limited research on flavonoid digestion, but current evidence is suggestive that only very small amounts of flavonoids are absorbed. In one model of the GI tract, only 5% of raspberry

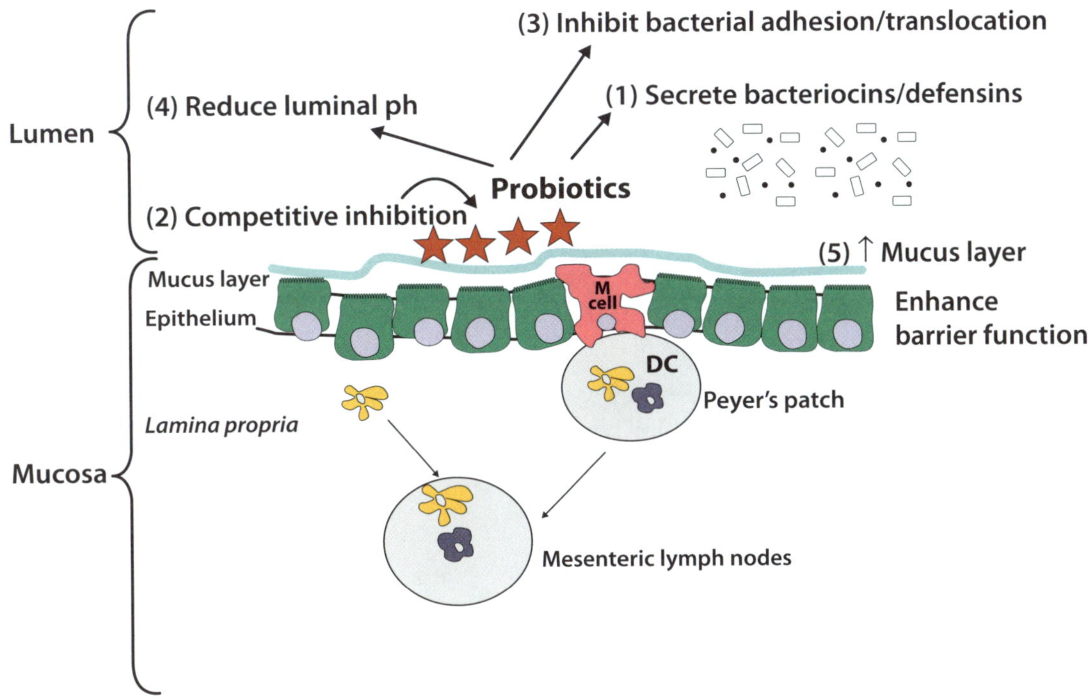

Figure 2.6 Inhibition of enteric bacteria and enhancement of barrier function by probiotics. From: Ng SC, Hart AL, Kamm MA. Mechanisms of action of probiotics: recent advances. *Inflamm Bowel Dis.* 2009 Feb;15(2):300-10 Reproduced with permission of John Wiley & Sons, Inc.

anthocyanidins was absorbed.[60] In another human study, the anthocyanidins found in strawberries were found to have a urine recovery that increased linearly with increasing dose, although only 2% of the initial dose was recovered (see Figure 2.5).[61]

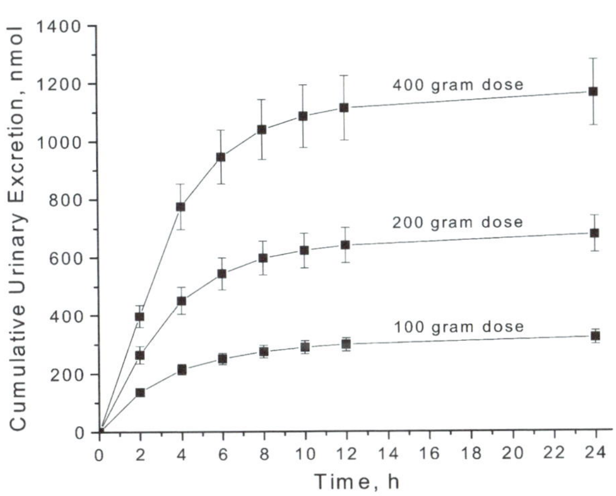

Figure 2.5 Anthocyanin secretion in urine following ingestion of 3 different doses of strawberries. From: Carkeet C, Clevidence BA, Novotny JA. Anthocyanin excretion by humans increases linearly with increasing strawberry dose. *J Nutr.* 2008 May;138(5):897-902. Reproduced with permission of the American Society for Nutrition.

Gut Flora (Microbiota)

The gut microbiota which populates both the lumen and the mucosa of the GI tract is thought to have a number of diverse roles in the maintenance of healthy digestion and in disease prevention. Perhaps the most acknowledged are the conversion of indigestible food components and the production of essential vitamins and co-factors. But many other benefits of microbiota have come to light recently, including the ability to antagonize pathogenic bacteria, enhance intestinal barrier function through modulation of cytoskeletal and tight junctional protein phosphorylation, metabolize toxins, reduce GI inflammation, and help maintain immune homeostasis within the gut-associated lymphoid tissues (GALT) (see Table 2.2 for probiotic mechanism of action, and Figure 2.6 illustrating effect on intestinal barrier).[62]

An unprecedented number of bacterial species are now thought to reside in the GI tract.

While recent estimates place the number of bacterial species at 442, this only accounts for the cultivatable fraction, and appears to be a gross underestimate of the bacterial population (Figure 2.7).[63] Analyses of bacterial rDNA sequences (metagenomics) have revealed our gut microbiota consists of at least 1800 genera and around 15,000–36,000 species of bacteria, depending on whether species are conservatively or liberally classified. This same report estimates that at best only 50% of species-level diversity has yet been sampled.[64] Additionally, the human intestinal microbiota collective genome (microbiome) contains more than 100 times the number of genes found in the human genome.[65] The GI microbiota is distributed along the entire GI tract, with the density and diversity increasing from the stomach to the colon.

Table 2.2 – Mechanisms of action of probiotics

Antimicrobial Activity

- Decrease luminal pH
- Secrete antimicrobial peptides
- Inhibit bacterial invasion
- Block bacterial adhesion to epithelial cells

Enhancement of Barrier Function

- Increase mucus production
- Enhance barrier integrity

Immunomodulation

- Effects on epithelial cells
- Effects on dendritic cells
- Effects on monocytes/macrophage
- Effects on lymphocytes
  - B lymphocytes
  - NK cells
  - T cells
  - T cell redistribution

From: Ng SC, Hart AL, Kamm MA. Mechanisms of action of probiotics: recent advances. *Inflamm Bowel Dis.* 2009 Feb;15(2):300-10. Reproduced with permission of John Wiley & Sons, Inc.

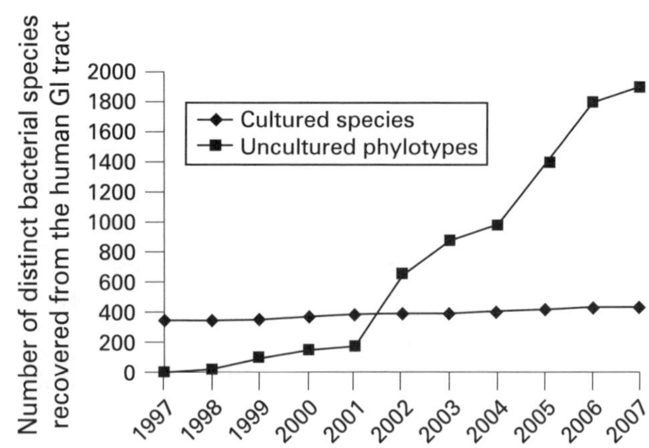

Figure 2.7 Number of distinct bacterial species in the human GI tract. From: Zoetendal EG, Rajilic-Stojanovic M, de Vos WM. High-throughput diversity and functionality analysis of the gastrointestinal tract microbiota. *Gut.* 2008 Nov;57(11):1605-15. Reproduced with permission of BMJ Publishing Group Ltd.

Obesity and microbiota

A trial using culture-independent methods (sequencing of 16S ribosomal RNA genes) found that the relative proportions of two of the dominant bacterial phyla was different between obese and lean individuals. Specifically, the proportion of Bacteroidetes was lower than the proportion of Firmicutes in obese people, but after 52 weeks on either a fat-restricted or carbohydrate-restricted diet, the relative proportions approached those of lean individuals (Figure 2.8).[66] Animal studies have also supported the link between microbial ecology and obesity, perhaps due to the more efficient extraction of calories by some bacterial species.[67]

Small bowel bacterial overgrowth (SBBO) (also called small intestine bacterial overgrowth, or SIBO)

SBBO is characterized by steatorrhea, diarrhea, flatulence, abdominal pain, and bloating. Symptoms of macrocytic anemia, weight loss, malabsorption of nutrients and vitamins, and bone loss are related to severe bacterial overgrowth syndrome.[68] It has been hypothesized that overgrowth of bacteria in the small intestine may be at least partly due to overuse of proton pump inhibitors, and may lead to a diagnosis

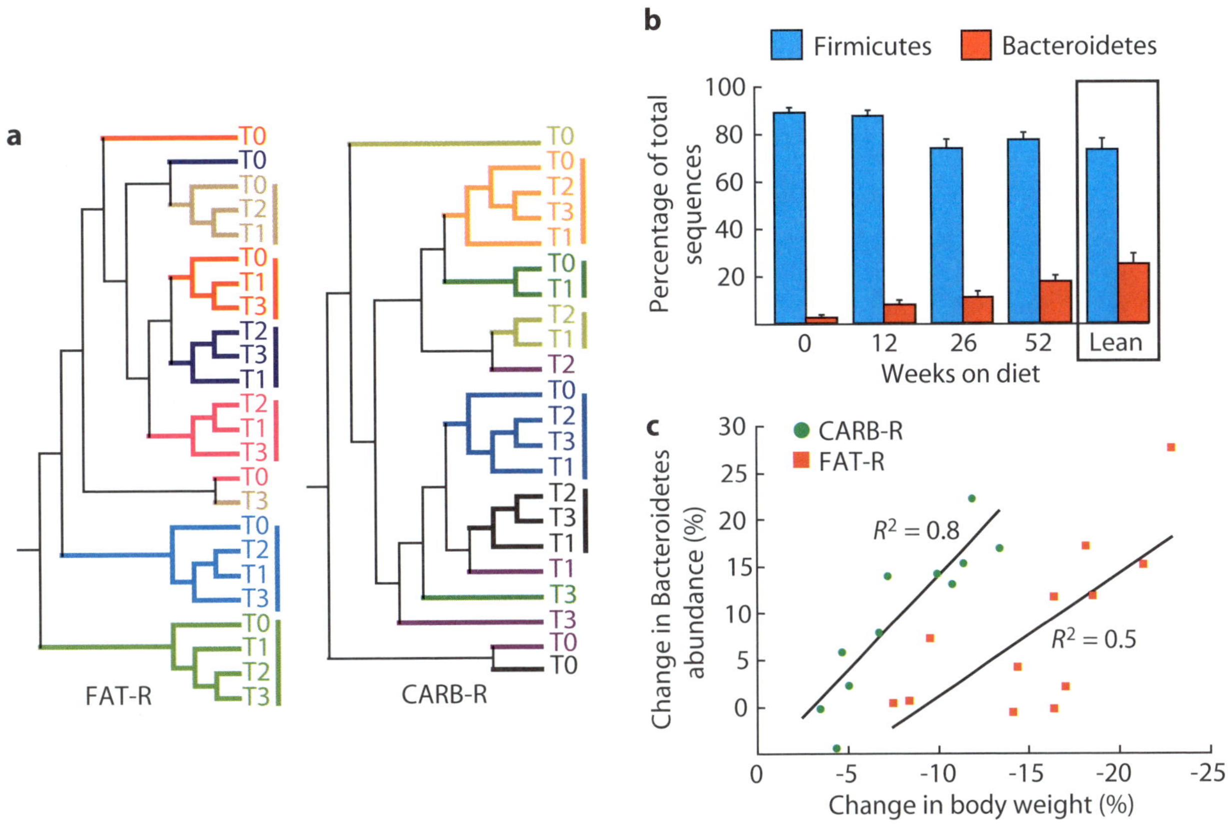

Figure 2.8 Correlation between body-weight loss and gut microbial ecology. From: Ley RE, Turnbaugh PJ, Klein S, et al. Microbial ecology: human gut microbes associated with obesity. *Nature*. 2006 Dec 21;444(7122):1022-3. Reproduced with permission of Macmillan Publishers Ltd.

of IBS.[69] Additionally, SBBO may play a role in acute pancreatitis, bacterial gastroenteritis, irritable bowel syndrome, inflammatory bowel disease, hepatic encephalopathy, fibromyalgia, and burn injury.[70]

Microbiota and immune homeostasis

GI mucosal immune cells have the heroic task of differentiating between pathogens and commensal bacteria. Although the majority of the microbiota in the GI tract is found within the lumen, organisms associated with the mucosa may be of greater importance to the host because of their interaction with the GALT (gut-associated lymphoid tissue). Although stool specimens often are analyzed as a proxy for the entire gastrointestinal microbiota, it is unlikely that they are an accurate representation of mucosal microbiota populations, highlighting the limitations of stool sample cultures.

The mucosal microbiota has been shown to interact with B and T cells, macrophages and monocytes, natural killer cells, and dendritic cells.[62] Mechanisms by which microbiota influence immune signaling include the inhibition of the NF-κB pathway through the stabilization of IκBα, prevention of endothelial apoptosis, and the elicitation of secretory IgA responses at mucosal surfaces.[71] For example, *Lactobacillus casei* has been shown to act by stabilizing IκBα, preventing inflammation induced by *Shigella flexneri*.[72]

Microbiota may also enable epithelial recovery or prevent apoptosis of epithelial cells, which has value in an environment of pro-apoptotic cytokines. This protective ability has been demonstrated with *Lactobacillus rhamnosus* (GG).[73,74] Healthy flora also has direct effects on undesirable species. For example, Lactobacillus has been shown to inhibit biofilms of *Streptococcus mutans*.[75]

Atopy

The composition of the gut microbiota is thought to influence the development and progression of allergic diseases. In the KOALA Birth Cohort Study, it was demonstrated that differences in gut microbiota composition precede the development of atopic sensitization during infancy. Specifically, infants with greater amounts of *E. coli* or *C. difficile* had a greater incidence of eczema, recurrent wheeze, or allergic sensitization.[76] Compared to mothers receiving placebo, pregnant and/or breast-feeding mothers receiving either *Lactobacillus rhamnosus* or *reuteri* significantly reduced the risk of atopic eczema in their infants.[77,78,79] Not all primary prevention trials have shown benefit, however.[80] A recent study found that although probiotics did not lead to a difference in allergy incidence by 5 years of age in children born vaginally, babies born by cesarian did have roughly half the rate of allergic disease if they received probiotics than if they did not.[81]

GI Dysfunction

Hypochlorhydria

Lack of sufficient stomach acid has been associated with reduced vitamin and mineral absorption,[82,83] incomplete protein digestion and subsequent food allergy,[33,35] and bacterial infections of the GI tract. Gastric acidity constitutes a major defense mechanism against ingested pathogens, and loss of the normal stomach acidity has been associated with colonization of the normally sterile upper GI tract.[84]

Acid suppression is a frequent cause of hypochlorhydria. In an examination of nearly 1700 cases of *C. difficile* infection and acid suppression, the

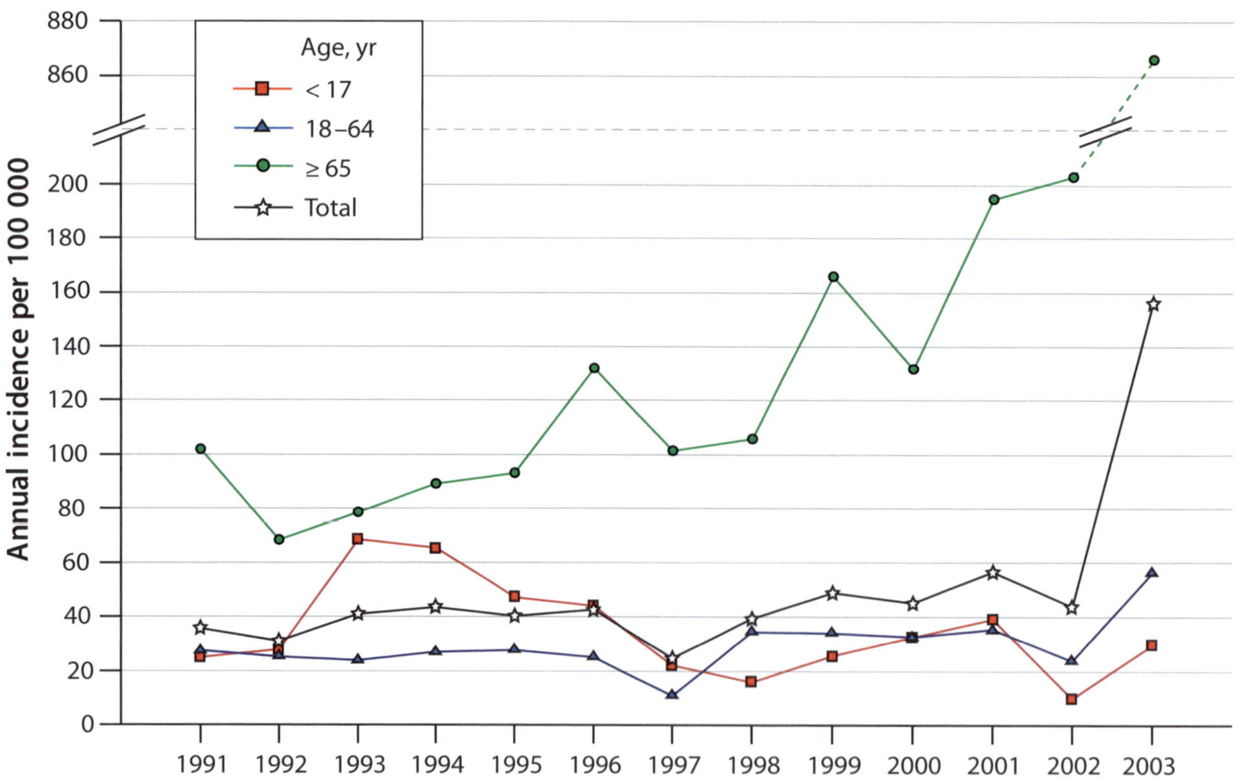

Figure 2.9 Annual incidence (per 100 000 population) of *Clostridium difficile*-associated diarrhea (CDAD) in Sherbrooke, Que., 1991–2003. From: Pépin J, Valiquette L, Alary ME, et al. *Clostridium difficile*-associated diarrhea in a region of Quebec from 1991 to 2003: a changing pattern of disease severity. *CMAJ*. 2004 Aug 31;171(5):466-72.

adjusted rate ratio of infection was 2.9 with the use of proton-pump inhibitors (PPIs), and 2.0 with H_2 receptor antagonists.[84] The frequency of B12 deficiency among long-term users of PPIs was recently found to be 29%, although it is often missed by serum cobalamin evaluation alone.[82] Autoimmune gastritis and *H. pylori* have both been shown to play a significant role in unexplained or refractory iron deficiency anemia.[82]

Advanced age also contributes to reduced gastric acid content, as the acidity of the stomach declines with age. This decline is associated with a greater number of nutrient deficiencies and a greater infection risk (Figure 2.9). In a sample of nearly 250 patients age 65 or greater, only 67% had consistent acid secretion, while 22% had intermittent secretion, and 11% were consistent hyposecretors. Interestingly, a pH less than 3.5 was defined as acidic, largely because of the poor sensitivity of the marker used to monitor gastric acidity.[85]

Increasing age and the use of acid suppression drugs have additive effects. For example, while the incidence of *C. difficile* was found to be fairly steady over a 12-year period in the population of Sherbrooke, Quebec, it was higher among the elderly, who experienced a dramatic rise in incidence in 2003.[86] The increase in *C. difficile* prevalence likely corresponds to the increase in PPIs prescribed over this period, extrapolating from data from a study done in the U.K.[87]

H. pylori is also a significant risk factor for hypochlorhydria. It has been estimated that 30–40% of the U.S. population is infected with *H. pylori*, with an increasing prevalence associated with age.[88] Data from over 7000 adults in the NHANES study (1988–91) found a seroprevalence of 16.7% for persons 20–29 years old and 56.9% for those ≥70 years old.[89]

H. pylori is known to be a primary cause of peptic ulcers, especially duodenal, and it also causes chronic gastritis, leading to atrophy and loss of parietal cells, and therefore to reduced gastric acidity. The pepsinogen I/II ratio is often used as a marker for gastric atrophy, and correlates well with gastric pH (Figure 2.10).[90]

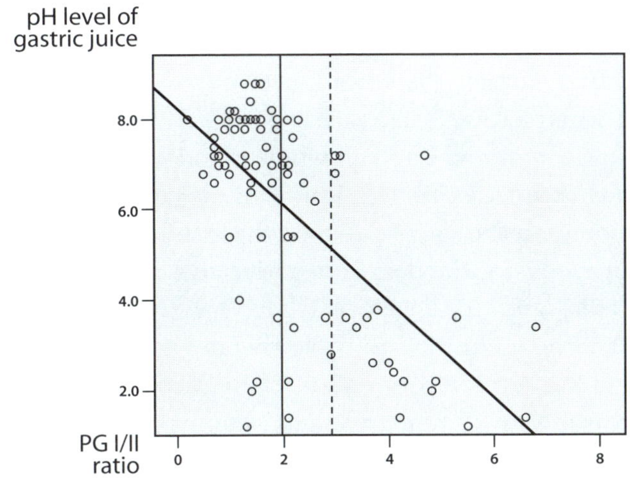

Figure 2.10 Degree of atrophy determined by pepsinogen I/II ratio and gastric juice pH in the *H. pylori* infection-positive stomach. From: Kato S, Matsukura N, Matsuda N, et al. Normalization of pH level and gastric mucosa after eradication of *H. pylori* in the remnant stomach. *J Gastroenterol Hepatol.* 2008 Dec;23 Suppl 2:S258-61. Reproduced with permission of John Wiley & Sons, Inc.

A recent study found that eradication of *H. pylori* was associated with a return to normal gastric acidity and pepsinogen ratio in both intact stomachs and those removed by distal gastrectomy.[90] The benefit of eradicating *H. pylori* was also supported by an earlier study which monitored pepsinogens and gastrin in 172 patients who underwent eradication therapy. At 12–15 months post-treatment, serum pepsinogen I/II ratio and gastrin levels were comparable to those without previous infection.[91]

Antioxidant therapy, particularly vitamin C, and sufficient zinc status have been shown to be important with *H. pylori* infection. An increase in polymorphonuclear (PMN) cell infiltration and augmented inflammation has been associated with low zinc in the gastric mucosa. PMN cells are thought to produce significant amounts of reactive oxygen species, which cause much of the damage to the gastric mucosa, along with the carcinogenic N-nitroso compounds formed.[92] Vitamin C has been shown to block nitrosation, with doses of vitamin C from as low as 9 mg to 1000 mg/d reported to inhibit *in vivo* nitrosamine formation by between 20 and 100%.[94,93]

While vitamin C may help to reduce nitrosamine formation, infection with *H. pylori* causes significantly enhanced consumption of vitamin C, as well as reduced secretion of the vitamin into the gastric lumen.[94] Eradication results in a return to normal levels.[95] An analysis of 452 children found that vitamin C levels in whole blood, plasma, and gastric juice exhibited significant negative correlation with the age of patients, the histologic density of *H. pylori*, the degree of active and chronic gastritis, and the severity of *H. pylori* infection.[96] Adding vitamin C to triple therapy improved the eradication rate from 68–85% in a low-dose clarithromycin group, producing comparable results to the high-dose clarithromycin group.[97]

Pancreatic insufficiency

A number of factors contribute to a decline in pancreatic function, including age, alcohol use, pancreatitis, and diabetes. Fat malabsorption is the most important digestive malfunction caused by pancreatic exocrine insufficiency. Normally, gastric lipase is responsible for only 10% of lipid digestion; however, this percentage increases drastically with pancreatic insufficiency.[98] Steatorrhea is common, as is malabsorption of the lipid-soluble vitamins A, D, E, and K, and other lipid-soluble nutrients.

When the pancreas fails to secrete bicarbonate, it does not neutralize the acidic chyme entering the small intestine. Gastroduodenal and small-intestinal transit is significantly accelerated, and the available time for digestion and absorption is markedly decreased, further contributing to nutrient malabsorption.[98] Amylase deficiency can result in starch malabsorption; the unabsorbed starch may then be metabolized by local flora. The products of this bacterial fermentation of carbohydrates are smaller, osmotically active molecules and organic acids that often produce diarrhea.[98]

Increased intestinal permeability

Abnormal permeability refers to a measurable increase in flux of small water-soluble compounds across the paracellular pathway of the small intestine. Intracellular enterocyte and tight junction proteins regulate the rate of movement and permeability through this pathway (Figure 2.11). Altered intestinal permeability appears to play a role in a number of digestive diseases, including celiac, IBD, and food allergy, and may precede these illnesses.[99]

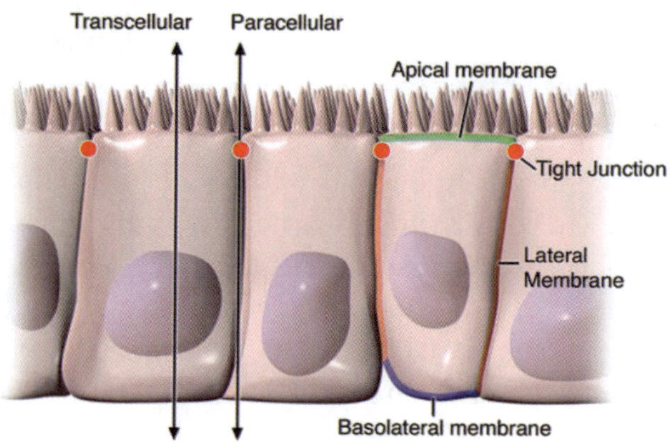

Figure 2.11 Structure of the mucosal barrier with pathways of epithelial permeability. From: Groschwitz KR, Hogan SP. Intestinal barrier function: molecular regulation and disease pathogenesis. *J Allergy Clin Immunol.* 2009 Jul;124(1):3-20; Reproduced with permission from Elsevier.

Factors known to alter normal permeability include infection, inflammatory cytokines, nutrient transporter activation, and noxious environmental toxins. Perhaps the factor most strongly associated with intestinal permeability, however, is the composition of the gut microbiota. Certainly in patients with celiac disease, increased permeability is caused by gluten consumption, but a recent *in vitro* study suggests that wheat germ agglutinin (WGA) may have some ability to damage GI epithelium by unique mechanisms.[100] Exercise, when accompanied by dehydration, may also increase GI permeability. A small study of 20 runners found that 1 hour of exercise increases leaky gut if no fluid is consumed during the activity.[101]

Immune dysfunction is an established component for at least some cases of intestinal damage. In addition to autoimmune disorders, immune dysregulation may lead to increased intestinal inflammation, at least partly mediated by mast cell activation (Figure 2.12). Mast cells have been shown to be key regulators of the integrity and function of the gastrointestinal barrier.

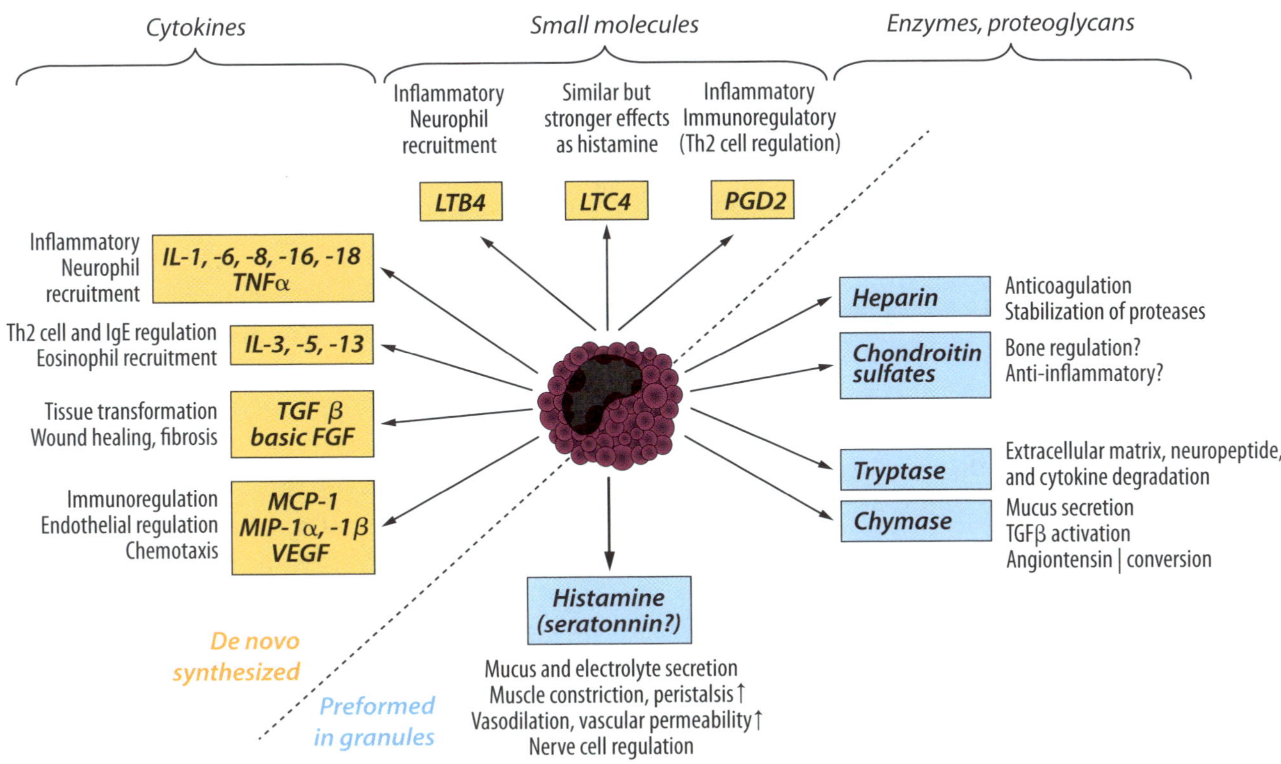

Figure 2.12 Human mast cell mediators. From: Bischoff SC, Krämer S. Human mast cells, bacteria, and intestinal immunity. *Immunol Rev.* 2007 Jun;217:329-37. Reproduced with permission of John Wiley & Sons, Inc.

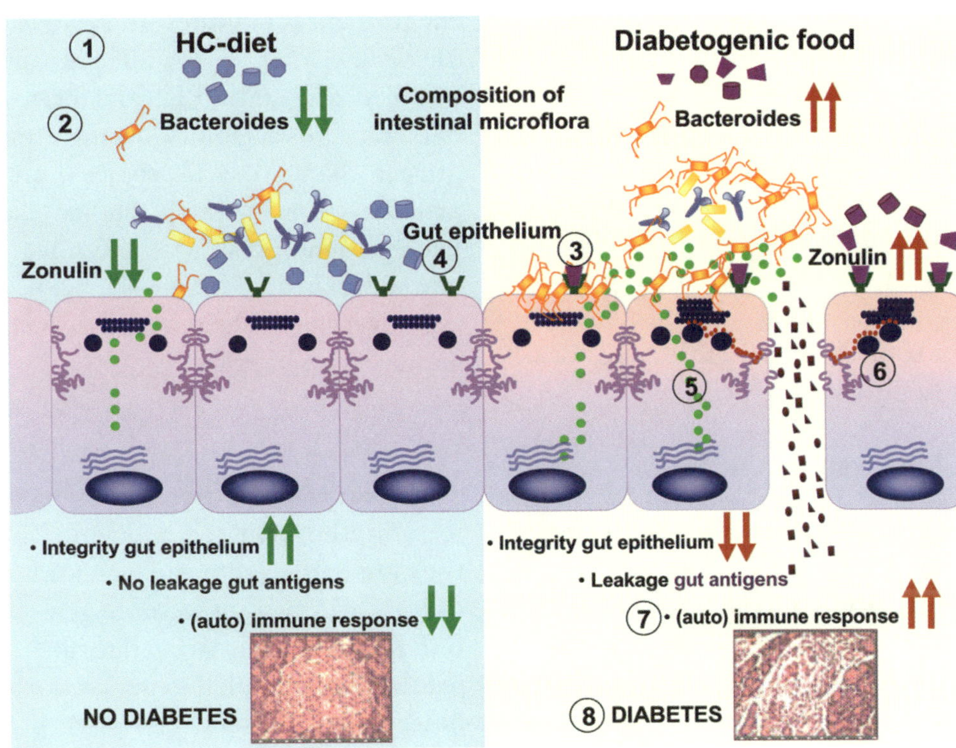

Figure 2.13 Diet affects the composition of the intestinal microflora, and gluten interaction influences diabetes development. From: Visser J, Rozing J, Sapone A, et al. Tight junctions, intestinal permeability, and autoimmunity: celiac disease and type 1 diabetes paradigms. *Ann N Y Acad Sci.* 2009 May;1165:195-205. Reproduced with permission of John Wiley & Sons, Inc.

The effects of gut inflammation associated with altered permeability are not restricted to the gut. For example, animal models of type 1 diabetes have shown that intestinal permeability, with resultant inflammation, plays a role in the autoimmune destruction of pancreatic islet cells. Recent data suggest that the same is true for type 1 diabetes in humans, with diet affecting gut microbiota composition, which in turn affects intestinal integrity (see Figure 2.13). Increased lactulose permeability (with normal mannitol) appeared to precede the detectable clinical onset of disease, suggesting that the small intestine participates in the pathogenesis of the disease.

Given that the intestinal barrier controls the equilibrium between tolerance and immunity to nonself-antigens, loss of intestinal barrier function may also be associated with other autoimmune diseases, such as multiple sclerosis, ankylosing spondylitis, IgA nephropathy, and nonalcoholic steatohepatitis (NASH), as well as digestive autoimmune processes, such as Crohn's and celiac diseases.[102] Inflammation in the gut may also be associated with osteoporosis, as demonstrated with both celiac and Crohn's disease.[103]

NSAIDS are recognized causes of increased intestinal permeability in both the short and long term, causing significant morbidity and mortality.[104] Aspirin was recently shown to increase the susceptibility to "gut leakiness" in patients with NASH. Although lactulose/mannitol was not modified by aspirin, the urinary sucralose increased only in patients with NASH, suggesting a colonic permeability increase.[105]

Food allergy/intolerance

In addition to loss of gastric acidity and incomplete protein digestion (see above), a loss of selective intestinal permeability is also a factor in the development of food allergies. A recent trial found increased intestinal permeability of all subjects with adverse reactions to food, with the severity of the clinical symptoms correlated with the degree of permeability, as measured by lactulose/mannitol.[106]

Assessment and Intervention

Hypochlorhydria

Lack of sufficient stomach acid has been associated with reduced vitamin and mineral absorption,[107,108] incomplete protein digestion and subsequent food allergy,[33,35] bacterial infections of the GI tract, and a large number of chronic diseases. There is disagreement about the incidence of hypochlorhydria, which has been estimated as ranging from 10–50%.[109,110] Much of the controversy may be due to the diversity of testing methodologies and varying age of study participants. Testing only resting pH will provide a much lower incidence than testing the ability to acidify a standard meal or bicarbonate challenge.

Diagnosis

Laboratory diagnosis can be done using Heidelberg pH capsule gastric analysis, gastric tube, serum pepsinogen I (S-PGI), and serum gastrin-17 (S-G-17). For clinical diagnosis, our review of the evidence indicates that high predictability factors include *H. pylori* infection, use of antacids, H_2 blockers, and PPIs, and pernicious anemia. Medium predictability factors include an age greater than 60, acne rosacea, and rheumatoid arthritis. Lower predictability factors include nausea, abdominal gas, belching, constipation, chronic diarrhea, dyspepsia, weak/cracked/peeling fingernails, osteoporosis, asthma, gastric ulcer, and decreased ferritin.

Intervention

The first step in treating hypochlorhydria is to stop the acid-secretion-inhibiting drugs if they are being used; the next step is to treat the causes of any gastroesophageal reflux disease (GERD). Specifically, eradicate *H. pylori* (see below), and stimulate regeneration of the gastric mucosa and parietal cells (see below). If HCl production does not return, initiate oral HCl supplementation. The following patient instructions are often used:

1. Begin by taking one tablet or capsule containing 500–600 mg of hydrochloric acid at your next large meal. If this does not aggravate your symptoms, at every meal after that of the same size take one more tablet or capsule. (One at the next meal, two at the meal after that, then three at the next meal.)
2. Continue to increase the dose until you reach 7 tablets or when you feel a warmth in your stomach whichever occurs first. A feeling of warmth in the stomach means that you have taken too many tablets for that meal, and you need to take one less tablet for that meal size. It is a good idea to try the larger dose again at another meal to make sure that it was the HCl that caused the warmth and not something else.
3. After you have found that the largest dose that you can take at your large meals without feeling any warmth, maintain that dose at all of meals of similar size. You will need to take less at smaller meals.
4. When taking a number of tablets or capsules it is best to take them throughout the meal.
5. As your stomach begins to regain the ability to produce the amount of HCl needed to properly digest your food, you will notice the warm feeling again and will have to cut down the dose level.

To treat *H. pylori*, the standard intervention has been to use triple drug therapy (two antibiotics and an H_2 inhibitor), although this may soon be replaced by sequential therapy. A recent meta-analysis suggests that sequential therapy has >90% efficacy, considerably greater than triple drug therapy.[111] Concurrent *Lactobacillus rhamnosus* supplementation makes standard drug therapy more effective and reduces adverse drug reactions.[112]

Other effective natural therapies include vitamin C, curcumin, and DGL. Vitamin C at 5 grams per day for 4 weeks eliminated *H. pylori* in 30% of study participants, and long-term (5-year) use inhibited *H. pylori* growth and reversed gastric atrophy as measured by pepsinogen secretion.[113,114] *Curcuma longa* has great potential as it is both bactericidal to *H. pylori* and, in an animal model, it decreased the inflammation associated with the infection.[115] Human research, however, is limited. One study concluded that since curcumin only eradicated *H. pylori* in 12% of the participants, it was not successful. However, treatment was only 7 days in duration and was combined with other nutrients. The patients showed significant improvement in dyspeptic symptoms and reduction in serological signs of gastric inflammation 2 months after the end of the short therapy.[116] The inhibition of *H. pylori* and anti-inflammatory effects may help explain curcumin's anti-gastric cancer effects.[117]

Deglycyrrhizinated licorice (DGL) has demonstrated clinical benefit for improving gastric mucosal health. The flavonoids found in *Glycyrrhiza glabra* impair *H. pylori* growth (including antibiotic-resistant strains),[118] and it has also been shown to stimulate regeneration of the gastric mucosa, potentially explaining its long history of use in the successful treatment of gastric ulcers,[119,120] Glycyrrhizin is removed to allow long-term use, because glycyrrhizinic acid can cause pseudohyperaldosteronism.[121]

Increased intestinal permeability

Diagnosis

Laboratory assessment of intestinal permeability is done primarily with the lactulose/mannitol test. After drinking a measured amount of these two sugars, the amount recovered in the urine indicates the degree of absorption of each, and is an index of permeability. Monosaccharides, such as mannitol (or L-rhamnose), are absorbed through the transcellular pathway and reflect the degree of absorption of small molecules. Disaccharides, such as lactulose (or cellobiose), are absorbed through the paracellular junction complex, which corresponds to the permeability of larger molecules.[122] The efficacy of treatment may also be monitored with this same test.

Our research has shown that clinical factors with high predictability for intestinal permeability include IBS, diabetes type 1, migraine, celiac disease, and food allergies. Medium predictability factors include diabetes type 2, inflammatory bowel disease, use of ibuprofen, indomethacin, naproxen, or aspirin, Giardia, *Blastocystis hominis*, *Entamoeba histolytica*, *Candida albicans*, atopic dermatitis, psoriasis, asthma, hypochlorhydria, abdominal bloating, aphthous stomatitis, and chronic stress. Lower probability factors include taking cyclooxygenase (COX) inhibitors and having essential fatty acid deficiency.

Intervention

The strategy to facilitate repair of the damaged intestinal mucosa involves three steps, the first of which is to stop the damage by avoiding known GI toxins; next is to reestablish a healthy microbial flora; and the last step is to stimulate regeneration. As discussed previously, commensal bacteria have a very significant impact on intestinal integrity.

For example, the probiotic species *Bifidobacterium longum* (BB536) has been found to prevent damage to intestinal cells and to increase production of tight junction cell proteins, which improves intestinal integrity. This strain has been used with success in a number of clinical trials, and has proven efficacy for restoring intestinal health in patients with abnormal permeability, such as those with Crohn's disease and ulcerative colitis (UC). For example, in a trial of patients with UC, BB536 was shown to not only induce remission, but it also upregulated gene expression of tight junction molecules (claudin-1 and ZO-1), known to be key to selective permeability.[123] And the combination of prebiotics and probiotics (synbiotic therapy) has been shown to help UC patients achieve greater improvement in quality of life and inflammatory markers than either therapy alone.[124]

Other nutrients have also been shown to stimulate regeneration of intestinal mucosa. L-glutamine, which has long been recognized as the primary amino acid source for intestinal cells, has recently been shown to regulate intercellular junction integrity.[125] N-acetyl glucosamine (NAG) provides a substrate for the glycosaminoglycans that are normally broken down in a leaky gut. A trial in children with IBD showed significant potential for this nutrient.[126] Zinc deficiency has been shown to disrupt tight junctions, alter membrane permeability, impair immune function, and cause intestinal ulceration.[127] Antioxidants, including vitamin C, vitamin E, beta-carotene, grape seed extract, and milk thistle extract both protect the GI from oxidant damage and help with hepatic detoxification of compounds associated with intestinal dysfunction. And the antioxidant quercetin appears to be critical to intestinal integrity. Quercetin acts through a number of mechanisms, including the assembly of a number of tight junction proteins (zonula occludens (ZO)-2, occludin, claudin-1, and claudin-4).[128,129] Quercetin also helps to stabilize mast cells, which (as mentioned above) are important regulators of intestinal function and tight junction integrity.

Exocrine pancreatic insufficiency

Diagnosis

A consequence of cystic fibrosis,[131] chronic pancreatitis,[132] diabetes, and IBD, pancreatic insufficiency is often diagnosed by stool samples. Although most direct tests are generally accurate, they are usually invasive and expensive. For this reason, pancreatic elastase 1 (PE1) is often used in their place. It is a pancreas-specific protease that undergoes minimal changes during intestinal transit, is easily measured in stool samples, and has reasonable accuracy, particularly with more severe insufficiency.[133] A cut-off of 200 mcg/g is often used, with lower levels indicating insufficiency. Fecal chymotrypsin is sometimes used, but is not as sensitive or specific.[134]

Clinically, one of the more obvious, but later, symptoms is the presence of an oily, foul-smelling, and buoyant stool, due to the increased fat content. Lipase activity declines long before proteolytic enzyme activity; thus, steatorrhea is present well before azotorrhea (nitrogen in the stool), at least from insufficiency due to chronic pancreatitis.[135] Other symptoms such as abdominal pain are more likely in acute or chronic pancreatitis, not necessarily due to insufficiency, and gas and bloating are likely but not very specific.

Diabetes, both types 1 and 2, is a frequent cause of pancreatic insufficiency. Overall, 27% of patients with diabetes (n = 2001) had a fecal elastase-1 <100 mcg/g, a marker of severe pancreatic insufficiency, while only 58% had a level >200 mcg/g.[136] Compared to control subjects, patients with Crohn's disease were found to have a greater than 8-fold risk for a FE1 <200 mcg/g, and those with ulcerative colitis had nearly a 13-fold greater risk.[137] Celiac disease has also emerged as a cause of pancreatic insufficiency, with at least 20% of celiac patients estimated to have a deficiency.[138] Although the removal of gluten from the diets of these patients improves pancreatic function in some, those with chronic diarrhea despite gluten avoidance are more likely to have reduced pancreatic function.[139] (See below for celiac diagnosis.)

Intervention

Although the etiology may not always be clear, patients with pancreatic insufficiency should avoid alcohol and smoking, particularly those with chronic pancreatitis. Additionally, avoidance of gluten in those with celiac disease may also improve the pancreatic performance in some cases.[140] Pancreatic enzyme replacement is also essential, and should include proteolytic enzymes for protein digestion, lipase for fat digestion, as well as enzymes that digest carbohydrate. It should be taken during or immediately after meals for the greatest efficacy.[141]

Given the variety of nutrient deficiencies likely to accompany pancreatic insufficiency, fat-soluble vitamins (A, D, E, and K) are likely to be deficient in patients with poor pancreatic function, as are essential fatty acids.[142,143] Supplementation of these nutrients may be indicated.

Although clinical research is lacking, melatonin may have an important role in pancreatic function. The concentration of melatonin in the GI tract is 10–100x higher than in the plasma and the total amount of melatonin is around 400x higher than the amount of melatonin in the pineal gland.[144] It has been shown to have some protective function for the pancreas and to strongly stimulate pancreatic amylase secretion.[145]

Celiac disease

Although it is often thought of as a food sensitivity/allergy, celiac disease is better understood as an autoimmune disease. What sets it apart from other autoimmune diseases is that some of the genes involved, the target autoantigen, and the environmental trigger are all known. In genetically susceptible individuals, consumption of gluten triggers an immune-mediated enteropathy, marked by the production of highly disease-specific IgA and IgG autoantibodies to tissue transglutaminase. This in turn leads to a number of nutrient deficiencies, including iron, folate, B12, and other B vitamins, calcium, magnesium, and fat-soluble vitamins.[156] Celiac disease is also associated with an increased risk for other autoimmune diseases[146] and other digestive disturbances, such as pancreatic insufficiency, lactose intolerance,[147] and increased intestinal permeability.[148]

Diagnosis

As an initial screening test, serological tests are an excellent starting point, and may be followed by a biopsy of the small intestine for a definitive diagnosis. Antitransglutaminase IgA antibodies currently have the highest sensitivity and specificity, ranging from 85–98.5% and 95–99%, respectively,[149] and most reports place both values at or above 95% if the human recombinant-based test is used.[150] Including a total serum IgA is indicated, because individuals who have both a selective IgA deficiency as well as celiac disease will not otherwise be identified.[153] Genetic testing for HLA-DQ2 and DQ8 have poor positive predictive value, but are considered up to 100% sensitive, thus able to assist in ruling out celiac disease.[151]

Clinically, although symptoms of malabsorption, such as a low body mass index, were thought to be common among individuals with celiac disease, it is now thought that only a minority (5%) are underweight, with the majority being of normal BMI or overweight, making these indicators unreliable.[152] Common complaints include non-specific abdominal pain or bloating, symptoms similar to those of irritable bowel syndrome, and even upper gastrointestinal symptoms. At least half have no GI-related symptoms, but present with fatigue, sub-fertility, osteoporosis, joint pain, unexplained iron deficiency, autoimmune disease, or dermatitis herpetiformis, a skin condition found exclusively in celiac patients.[153] It should also be noted that some patients may have "latent" celiac disease, defined as positive serological testing, but a normal biopsy. These individuals are at risk for developing celiac disease. Finally, quite separate from celiac disease, many patients have wheat and/or gluten intolerances. These patients may have antibodies to wheat or gluten (but not autoantibodies), but a therapeutic trial of a gluten-free diet may be necessary to diagnose.

Intervention

Complete gluten-avoidance remains the mainstay of treatment. Most celiac-related symptoms resolve with this approach, although some degree of increased gut permeability may remain.[154] Additionally, at least temporary avoidance of lactose is often helpful, given the relative lactose deficiency which often accompanies the gluten-induced enteropathy.[155]

Even while on a gluten-free diet, stores of several nutrients are known to be lacking. In a recent double-blind trial, a combination of folic acid (0.8 mg), B6 (3 mg), and B12 (0.5 mg) was shown to lower homocysteine as well as improve anxiety and depressed mood, compared to placebo.[156] Other potential nutritional deficiencies include iron, zinc, calcium, copper, fat-soluble vitamins, and dietary fiber.[157,158]

Celiac patients should be assessed and treated for pancreatic insufficiency. Low fecal elastase-1, a marker for pancreatic insufficiency, is fairly common among individuals with celiac disease, even while avoiding gluten, particularly among those with chronic diarrhea (30%).[141] Proteolytic enzyme replacement is likely to provide benefit for these patients.

Inflammatory bowel disease (IBD)

The etiology of IBD is not completely understood, but the commensal microbiota appears to be a critical piece in disease development, specifically the innate immune response to the gut flora, as suggested by the success of both antibiotic and probiotic use, and animal models of IBD.[159] These relationships may provide a clue about the abnormal intestinal permeability found in these patients, which further disrupts immune tolerance to commensal bacteria, as well as tolerance to food antigens, setting the stage for food allergy and continued inflammation.

Diagnosis

Although the diagnosis of IBD requires endoscopy, the value of non-invasive biomarkers for both initial diagnosis and disease monitoring is increasingly becoming recognized. The classic antibodies associated with IBD are anti-*Saccharomyces cerevisiae* antibody (ASCA) for Crohn's disease, and perinuclear antineutrophil cytoplasmic antibody (pANCA) for ulcerative colitis, and although these tests are considered very specific (100% and 90%, respectively), they have very poor sensitivity.[160] Fecal markers such as calprotectin and, more recently, the protein S100A12 have been suggested as screening tests for IBD, and may be the most accurate non-invasive tests. S100A12 was recently shown to have a sensitivity and specificity of 97% in children, while calprotectin had a sensitivity of 100% and specificity of 67%.[161] C-reactive protein (CRP), a marker of inflammation, has been shown in a prospective study to be a predictor of disease extent at diagnosis, as well indicating a risk for surgery.[162]

Symptoms of IBD often include diarrhea, abdominal pain and cramping, and blood in the stool, as well as fatigue due to anemia from blood loss; by themselves, however, these symptoms are not reliable for diagnosis as they are commonly found in too many other conditions as well.

Intervention

Reducing inflammation is a critical part of therapy for IBD. The first step is addressing any food allergy, which may play a role in the pathogenesis of IBD, or it may be a result of the impaired intestinal permeability associated with IBD. Utilizing an elimination diet, or a full or partial elemental diet may be of benefit in reducing intestinal inflammation.[163,164,165]

In an allergy elimination diet commonly eaten foods are eliminated and replaced with either hypoallergenic foods and foods that are rarely eaten, or special hypoallergenic formulas. The fewer the allergenic foods eaten, the greater the ease of establishing a diagnosis using an elimination diet. The standard elimination diet consists of lamb, chicken, potatoes, rice, banana, apple, and a cabbage-family vegetable (cabbage, brussels sprouts, broccoli, etc.). There are variations of the elimination diet that are suitable. However, it is extremely important that no allergenic foods be consumed.

The patient stays on the elimination diet for at least one week, and up to 1 month. If the symptoms are related to food sensitivity, they will typically disappear by the fifth or sixth day of the diet. If the symptoms do not disappear, it is possible that a reaction to a food in the elimination diet is responsible. In that case, an even more restricted diet must be utilized.

After the elimination-diet period, individual foods are reintroduced every two days. Methods range from reintroducing only a single food every two days, to reintroducing a food every one or two meals. Usually, after the one-week "cleansing" period, the patient will develop an increased sensitivity to offending foods.

Reintroduction of allergenic foods will typically produce a more severe or recognizable symptom than before. A careful, detailed record must be maintained, describing when foods were reintroduced and what symptoms appeared upon reintroduction. It can be very useful to track the wrist pulse during reintroduction, as pulse changes may occur when an allergenic food is consumed.

Supplementation may be especially important because deficiencies have been found in patients with IBD, including vitamins D and K, which are both associated with a lower bone mineral density.[166] Other common deficits include vitamins A, C, and E, several B vitamins, calcium, and zinc.[167]

Several studies have shown other probiotic strains as well as prebiotics to be useful in IBD treatment. For example, *Lactobacillus rhamnosus* has been shown to prolong the time between relapse in patients with ulcerative colitis, but not with Crohn's disease.[168] In general, *Saccharomyces boulardii* has shown benefit in early trials for ulcerative colitis and Crohn's disease.[169,170] A probiotic preparation containing four strains of lactobacilli (*L. acidophilus, bulgaricus, casei,* and *plantarum*), three strains of bifidobacteria (*B. breve, infantis,* and *longum*), and *Streptococcus thermophilus* has been shown in several trials to prevent relapse of chronic pouchitis and to be of benefit in the treatment of active ulcerative colitis.[171] The existing data indicate a multi-strain may offer the greatest benefit vs. the use of any single strain.

Since reducing inflammation is a critical part of therapy for IBD, it is important to utilize a high-quality fish oil to provide the omega-3 fatty acids EPA and DHA. Most clinical studies with fish oils in IBD have shown the treatment is able to reduce disease activity and improve endoscopic scores, especially if dosages of at least 3000 mg/d total EPA and DHA combined was used.[172]

If needed, natural anti-inflammatory agents such as curcumin preparations and boswellia extracts may be helpful. Curcumin, known to have anti-inflammatory effects mediated through several pathways,[173] has also shown potential for treating IBD. In a double-blind, placebo-controlled trial, individuals with ulcerative colitis taking 1 g curcumin twice per day had lower relapse rates and better indices of clinical activity and endoscopy, when taken with sulfasalazine or mesalamine.[174] Boswellia extracts (300–350 mg three times daily) have also shown similar efficacy to mesalazine and sulfasalazine, with better tolerability.[175,176]

Mastic is a resin obtained from the mastic tree (*Pistacia lentiscus*). People in the Mediterranean region have used mastic as a medicine for gastrointestinal ailments for several thousand years. Recent studies indicate that it may have benefit in functional dyspepsia, peptic ulcers, and IBD.[177,178,179] For example, in a double-blind clinical trial carried out on 38 patients with symptomatic and endoscopically proven duodenal ulcer patients were given either mastic gum (1 g daily) or a placebo for 2 weeks. Symptomatic relief was obtained in sixteen (80%) patients on mastic and in nine (50%) patients on placebo, while endoscopically proven healing occurred in fourteen (70%) patients on mastic and four (22%) patients on placebo.

Berberine exerts broad-spectrum antimicrobial activity including activity against *C. albicans*. It has shown significant success in the treatment of acute diarrhea in several clinical studies with clinical results comparable to standard medical treatment in most cases. In addition to direct antimicrobial activity, berberine has shown inhibition of microbial attachment to mucous membranes and blocking of the action of toxins produced by several pathogenic bacteria.[180,181]

Chamomile may be helpful due to its antispasmodic properties which help relax smooth muscles, such as those in the intestines and stomach. Historically, chamomile has been used to treat digestive conditions such as colic, gas, diarrhea, stomach cramps, indigestion, and other symptoms now related to IBS. Enteric-coated peppermint oil also has significant clinical benefits (see under IBS intervention).

Irritable bowel syndrome (IBS)

The causes of IBS remain uncertain, partly because it is a diagnosis of exclusion, but several contributory factors are known. Among them are altered gastrointestinal motility, gut hypersensitivity, mucosal inflammation, altered intestinal flora and/or permeability, food allergies, and infection.[182] Additionally, because many patients are diagnosed with IBS without a thorough evaluation, conditions such as celiac disease or sugar malabsorption (lactose or fructose) may be misdiagnosed as IBS. A growing body of evidence suggests that disturbances of the intestinal epithelial barrier, in particular increased gut permeability, may play an important role in the sequence leading to gut dysfunction and onset of IBS symptoms. This pattern was found in all sub-types of IBS patients.[183]

A cause-and-effect relationship between mucosal barrier alterations and visceral hypersensitivity has also been described in a recent animal study, possibly accounting for the pain in IBS.[184] Serum IgG4 antibodies to common allergens (wheat, beef, pork, milk, eggs, and lamb) are elevated in patients with IBS, and an antibody-guided exclusion diet has been shown to significantly improve symptoms.[185,186] Eradication of small intestinal bacterial overgrowth (discussed earlier) has been shown to eliminate IBS by Rome I criteria in nearly 50% of patients, and probiotics improve the symptoms of IBS, suggesting that microbiota composition is likely an important etiology.[187,188]

Diagnosis

No laboratory test rules in IBS, but several may be used to exclude other conditions. For example, the screening tests for IBD may help differentiate between the two conditions. In some patients with IBS, celiac disease may be the underlying cause. A 7-fold increased risk for celiac disease was found among IBS patients, indicating that a screen for celiac is indicated.[189] Also, malabsorption of dietary sugars, such as lactose and fructose, is common among IBS patients, and should be screened for.[190] It has been hypothesized that overgrowth of bacteria in the small intestine may lead to a diagnosis of IBS, and thus evaluation by the lactulose breath test or stool genomic analysis may reveal this underlying etiology.[191] Also, given the frequency of food sensitivities among patients with IBS, either an elimination diet or evaluation of IgG antibodies should be done.[192]

Clinically, the Rome III criteria are used for confirming diagnosis. This model calls for recurrent abdominal pain greater than 3 days per month in the last 3 months, along with two of the following three symptoms: improvement with defecation, onset associated with a change in frequency of stool, or onset associated with a change in the form of stool. Additionally, symptoms must have onset more than 6 months before diagnosis. Abdominal pain is included in most definitions of IBS, because its absence reduces the likelihood of IBS as the cause of symptoms. However, given the number of causes of IBS, the grouping of symptoms often does not clarify the etiology for the individual patient, and a recent review found that existing criteria for distinguishing IBS from organic disease perform only modestly well, and better diagnostic criteria are recommended.[193]

Intervention

One of the mainstays of treatment for IBS is soluble fiber. Especially for those with constipation-predominant IBS, the use of soluble fiber has been shown to produce significant clinical improvement in global IBS symptoms, as well as constipation.[194] Clinicians are advised to increase dietary fiber slowly, adding supplemental soluble fiber at 25–35 g/d. Insoluble fiber, however, may worsen some IBS symptoms and should be avoided.

A small study found that individuals with IBS have an increased response to noxious agents, such as NSAIDs, which increase their intestinal permeability to a greater degree observed in healthy subjects.[195] Food allergy avoidance has also been shown to improve symptoms of IBS.[190,191] Probiotics, including *Bifidobacterium longum* and *Lactobacillus spp* have been shown to reduce overall symptom scores, including flatulence and distention, in a number of clinical trials. Daily dosing of at least 1×10^{10} seems to be most consistently associated with benefit.[192]

Enteric-coated peppermint oil (ECPO) has been shown to be quite helpful in improving IBS, as several double-blind studies have shown ECPO to be effective in relieving all symptoms of IBS in approximately 70–85% of cases within 2–4 weeks.[196,197] In fact, peppermint oil was recently found to be more effective than not only placebo for IBS, but also fiber and conventional anti spasmodics. The relative risk of persistent symptoms was reduced by 57% in a meta-analysis.[198] One of the central findings in IBS is a hypercontractility (excessive contraction) of intestinal smooth muscle. Peppermint oil inhibits the hypercontractility of intestinal smooth muscle, making it useful in IBS as well as esophageal spasm and intestinal colic.

Finally, melatonin has shown benefit in several recent trials for patients with IBS, with one small trial citing a percent response rate of 88%, vs. 47% to placebo. This study and a previous one noted that no changes were seen in sleep, anxiety, or depression, despite the positive changes seen in IBS symptoms.[199,200] The dose used was 3 mg at bedtime.

References

1. Jones, David. *The Textbook of Functional Medicine.* The Institute for Functional Medicine. Copyright 2006, Gig Harbor WA. Quote in Chapter 28, Thomas Sult.
2. Kappelman MD, Rifas-Shiman SL, Kleinman K, et al. The prevalence and geographic distribution of Crohn's disease and ulcerative colitis in the United States. *Clin Gastroenterol Hepatol.* 2007 Dec;5(12):1424-9.
3. Camilleri M, Dubois D, Coulie B, et al. Prevalence and socioeconomic impact of upper gastrointestinal disorders in the United States: results of the U.S. Upper Gastrointestinal Study. *Clin Gastroenterol Hepatol.* 2005 Jun;3(6):543-52.
4. Jiang X, Locke GR 3rd, Choung RS, et al. Prevalence and risk factors for abdominal bloating and visible distention: a population-based study. *Gut.* 2008 Jun;57(6):756-63.
5. Tuteja AK, Talley NJ, Joos SK, et al. Abdominal bloating in employed adults: prevalence, risk factors, and association with other bowel disorders. *Am J Gastroenterol.* 2008 May;103(5):1241-8.
6. Geeraerts B, Tack J. Functional dyspepsia: past, present, and future. *J Gastroenterol.* 2008;43(4):251-5.
7. van Heel DA, West J. Recent advances in coeliac disease. *Gut.* 2006 Jul;55(7):1037-46.
8. Hopper AD, Hadjivassiliou M, Butt S, et al. Adult coeliac disease. *BMJ.* 2007 Sep 15;335(7619):558-62.
9. Sanders DS, Carter MJ, Hurlstone DP, et al. Association of adult coeliac disease with irritable bowel syndrome: a case-control study in patients fulfilling ROME II criteria referred to secondary care. *Lancet.* 2001 Nov 3;358(9292):1504-8.
10. Fasano A, Berti I, Gerarduzzi T, et al. Prevalence of celiac disease in at-risk and not-at-risk groups in the United States: a large multicenter study. *Arch Intern Med.* 2003 Feb 10;163(3):286-92.
11. Kellett GL, Brot-Laroche E, Mace OJ, et al. Sugar absorption in the intestine: the role of GLUT2. *Annu Rev Nutr.* 2008;28:35-54.
12. Eny KM, Wolever TM, Fontaine-Bisson B, et al. Genetic variant in the glucose transporter type 2 is associated with higher intakes of sugars in two distinct populations. *Physiol Genomics.* 2008 May 13;33(3):355-60.
13. Kwon O, Eck P, Chen S, et al. Inhibition of the intestinal glucose transporter GLUT2 by flavonoids. *FASEB J.* 2007 Feb;21(2):366-77.
14. Robayo-Torres CC, Quezada-Calvillo R, Nichols BL. Disaccharide digestion: clinical and molecular aspects. *Clin Gastroenterol Hepatol.* 2006 Mar;4(3):276-87.
15. Ojetti V, Nucera G, Migneco A, et al. High prevalence of celiac disease in patients with lactose intolerance. *Digestion.* 2005;71(2):106-10.
16. Choi YK, Kraft N, Zimmerman B, et al. Fructose intolerance in IBS and utility of fructose-restricted diet. *J Clin Gastroenterol.* 2008 Mar;42(3):233-8.
17. Choi YK, Johlin FC Jr, Summers RW, et al. Fructose intolerance: an under-recognized problem. *Am J Gastroenterol.* 2003 Jun;98(6):1348-53.
18. Lomer MC, Parkes GC, Sanderson JD. Review article: lactose intolerance in clinical practice—myths and realities. *Aliment Pharmacol Ther.* 2008 Jan 15;27(2):93-103.
19. Almeida JA, Kim R, Stoita A, et al. Lactose malabsorption in the elderly: role of small intestinal bacterial overgrowth. *Scand J Gastroenterol.* 2008;43(2):146-54.
20. Fernández-Bañares F, Rosinach M, Esteve M, et al. Sugar malabsorption in functional abdominal bloating: a pilot study on the long-term effect of dietary treatment. *Clin Nutr.* 2006 Oct;25(5):824-31.
21. Tadataka Yamada. *Yamada's Textbook of Gastroenterology.* 4th edition, May 2003. Lippincott Williams & Wilkins.
22. Pafumi Y, Lairon D, de la Porte PL, et al. Mechanisms of inhibition of triacylglycerol hydrolysis by human gastric lipase. *J Biol Chem.* 2002 Aug 2;277(31):28070-9.
23. Mu H, Høy CE. The digestion of dietary triacylglycerols. *Prog Lipid Res.* 2004 Mar;43(2):105-33.
24. Lowe ME. Structure and function of pancreatic lipase and colipase. *Annu Rev Nutr.* 1997;17:141-58.
25. Houten SM, Auwerx J. The enterohepatic nuclear receptors are major regulators of the enterohepatic circulation of bile salts. *Ann Med.* 2004;36(7):482-91.
26. Thomas C, Pellicciari R, Pruzanski M, et al. Targeting bile-acid signalling for metabolic diseases. *Nat Rev Drug Discov.* 2008 Aug;7(8):678-93.
27. Watanabe M, Houten SM, Mataki C, et al. Bile acids induce energy expenditure by promoting intracellular thyroid hormone activation. *Nature.* 2006 Jan 26;439 (7075):484-9.
28. Thomas C, Auwerx J, Schoonjans K. Bile acids and the membrane bile acid receptor TGR5—connecting nutrition and metabolism. *Thyroid.* 2008 Feb;18(2):167-74.
29. Mann ST, Mann V, Stracke H, et al. Fecal elastase 1 and vitamin D3 in patients with osteoporotic bone fractures. *Eur J Med Res.* 2008 Feb 25;13(2):68-72.
30. Hardt PD, Hauenschild A, Nalop J, et al. High prevalence of exocrine pancreatic insufficiency in diabetes mellitus. A multicenter study screening fecal elastase 1 concentrations in 1,021 diabetic patients. *Pancreatology.* 2003;3(5):395-402. Epub 2003 Sep 24.
31. Hardt PD, Brendel MD, Kloer HU, et al. Is pancreatic diabetes (type 3c diabetes) underdiagnosed and misdiagnosed? *Diabetes Care.* 2008 Feb;31 Suppl 2:S165-9.
32. Leeds JS, Hopper AD, Hurlstone DP, et al. Is exocrine pancreatic insufficiency in adult coeliac disease a cause of persisting symptoms? *Aliment Pharmacol Ther.* 2007 Feb 1;25(3):265-71.
33. Untersmayr E, Jensen-Jarolim E. The role of protein digestibility and antacids on food allergy outcomes. *J Allergy Clin Immunol.* 2008 Jun;121(6):1301-8.

34. Pohl D, Fox M, Fried M, et al. Do we need gastric acid? *Digestion*. 2008;77(3-4):184-97.

35. Untersmayr E, Jensen-Jarolim E. The effect of gastric digestion on food allergy. *Curr Opin Allergy Clin Immunol*. 2006 Jun;6(3):214-9.

36. Radimer K, Bindewald B, Hughes J, et al. Dietary supplement use by U.S. adults: data from the National Health and Nutrition Examination Survey, 1999-2000. *Am J Epidemiol*. 2004 Aug 15;160(4):339-49.

37. Gass J, Vora H, Hofmann AF, et al. Enhancement of dietary protein digestion by conjugated bile acids. *Gastroenterology*. 2007 Jul;133(1):16-23.

38. Basivireddy J, Jacob M, Ramamoorthy P, et al. Indomethacin-induced free radical-mediated changes in the intestinal brush border membranes. *Biochem Pharmacol*. 2003 Feb 15;65(4):683-95.

39. Sivalingam N, Basivireddy J, Balasubramanian KA, et al. Curcumin attenuates indomethacin-induced oxidative stress and mitochondrial dysfunction. *Arch Toxicol*. 2008 Jul;82(7):471-81.

40. Basivireddy J, Jacob M, Balasubramanian KA. Oral glutamine attenuates indomethacin-induced small intestinal damage. *Clin Sci* (Lond). 2004 Sep;107(3):281-9.

41. Watanabe T, Higuchi K, Kobata A, et al. Non-steroidal anti-inflammatory drug-induced small intestinal damage is Toll-like receptor 4 dependent. *Gut*. 2008 Feb; 57(2):181-7.

42. Kessel A, Toubi E, Pavlotzky E, et al. Treatment with glutamine is associated with down-regulation of Toll-like receptor-4 and myeloid differentiation factor 88 expression and decrease in intestinal mucosal injury caused by lipopolysaccharide endotoxaemia in a rat. *Clin Exp Immunol*. 2008 Feb;151(2):341-7.

43. Mowat AM. Coeliac disease—a meeting point for genetics, immunology, and protein chemistry. *Lancet*. 2003 Apr 12;361(9365):1290-2.

44. Guéguen L, Pointillart A. The bioavailability of dietary calcium. *J Am Coll Nutr*. 2000 Apr;19(2 Suppl):119S-136S.

45. Walters JR, Balesaria S, Chavele KM, et al. Calcium channel TRPV6 expression in human duodenum: different relationships to the vitamin D system and aging in men and women. *J Bone Miner Res*. 2006 Nov;21(11):1770-7.

46. Thankachan P, Walczyk T, Muthayya S, et al. Iron absorption in young Indian women: the interaction of iron status with the influence of tea and ascorbic acid. *Am J Clin Nutr*. 2008 Apr;87(4):881-6.

47. Muhammad A, Pitchumoni CS. Newly detected celiac disease by wireless capsule endoscopy in older adults with iron deficiency anemia. *J Clin Gastroenterol*. 2008 Oct;42(9):980-3.

48. Zamani F, Mohamadnejad M, Shakeri R, et al. Gluten sensitive enteropathy in patients with iron deficiency anemia of unknown origin. *World J Gastroenterol*. 2008 Dec 28;14(48):7381-5.

49. Hunt JR, Beiseigel JM, Johnson LK. Adaptation in human zinc absorption as influenced by dietary zinc and bioavailability. *Am J Clin Nutr*. 2008 May;87(5):1336-45.

50. Greger JL. Nondigestible carbohydrates and mineral bioavailability. *J Nutr*. 1999 Jul;129(7 Suppl):1434S-5S.

51. Hurrell RF, Reddy MB, Juillerat MA, et al. Degradation of phytic acid in cereal porridges improves iron absorption by human subjects. *Am J Clin Nutr*. 2003 May;77(5):1213-9.

52. Dali-Youcef N, Andrès E. An update on cobalamin deficiency in adults. *QJM*. 2009 Jan;102(1):17-28.

53. Bolaman Z, Kadikoylu G, Yukselen V, et al. Oral versus intramuscular cobalamin treatment in megaloblastic anemia: a single-center, prospective, randomized, open-label study. *Clin Ther*. 2003 Dec;25(12):3124-34.

54. Andrès E, Dali-Youcef N, Vogel T, et al. Oral cobalamin (vitamin B) treatment. An update. *Int J Lab Hematol*. 2009 Feb;31(1):1-8.

55. Harrison EH. Mechanisms of digestion and absorption of dietary vitamin A. *Annu Rev Nutr*. 2005;25:87-103.

56. Hacquebard M, Carpentier YA. Vitamin E: absorption, plasma transport and cell uptake. *Curr Opin Clin Nutr Metab Care*. 2005 Mar;8(2):133-8.

57. Yonekura L, Nagao A. Intestinal absorption of dietary carotenoids. *Mol Nutr Food Res*. 2007 Jan;51(1):107-15.

58. van Het Hof KH, West CE, Weststrate JA, et al. Dietary factors that affect the bioavailability of carotenoids. *J Nutr*. 2000 Mar;130(3):503-6.

59. Livny O, Reifen R, Levy I, et al. Beta-carotene bioavailability from differently processed carrot meals in human ileostomy volunteers. *Eur J Nutr*. 2003 Dec;42(6):338-45.

60. McDougall GJ, Dobson P, Smith P, et al. Assessing potential bioavailability of raspberry anthocyanins using an *in vitro* digestion system. *J Agric Food Chem*. 2005 Jul 27;53(15):5896-904.

61. Carkeet C, Clevidence BA, Novotny JA. Anthocyanin excretion by humans increases linearly with increasing strawberry dose. *J Nutr*. 2008 May;138(5):897-902.

62. Ng SC, Hart AL, Kamm MA. Mechanisms of action of probiotics: recent advances. *Inflamm Bowel Dis*. 2009 Feb;15(2):300-10.

63. Zoetendal EG, Rajilic-Stojanovic M, de Vos WM. High-throughput diversity and functionality analysis of the gastrointestinal tract microbiota. *Gut*. 2008 Nov;57(11):1605-15.

64. Frank DN, Pace NR. Gastrointestinal microbiology enters the metagenomics era. *Curr Opin Gastroenterol*. 2008 Jan;24(1):4-10.

65. Magalhaes JG, Tattoli I, Girardin SE. The intestinal epithelial barrier: how to distinguish between the microbial flora and pathogens. *Semin Immunol*. 2007 Apr;19(2):106-15.

66. Ley RE, Turnbaugh PJ, Klein S, et al. Microbial ecology: human gut microbes associated with obesity. *Nature*. 2006 Dec 21;444(7122):1022-3.

67. Turnbaugh PJ, Ley RE, Mahowald MA, et al. An obesity-associated gut microbiome with increased capacity for energy harvest. *Nature.* 2006 Dec 21;444(7122):1027-31.

68. Kerckhoffs AP, Visser MR, Samsom M, et al. Critical evaluation of diagnosing bacterial overgrowth in the proximal small intestine. *J Clin Gastroenterol.* 2008 Nov-Dec; 42(10):1095-102.

69. Spiegel BM, Chey WD, Chang L. Bacterial overgrowth and irritable bowel syndrome: unifying hypothesis or a spurious consequence of proton pump inhibitors? *Am J Gastroenterol.* 2008 Dec;103(12):2972-6.

70. Othman M, Agüero R, Lin HC. Alterations in intestinal microbial flora and human disease. *Curr Opin Gastroenterol.* 2008 Jan;24(1):11-6.

71. Tsuji M, Suzuki K, Kinoshita K, et al. Dynamic interactions between bacteria and immune cells leading to intestinal IgA synthesis. *Semin Immunol.* 2008 Feb;20(1):59-66.

72. Tien MT, Girardin SE, Regnault B, et al. Anti-inflammatory effect of *Lactobacillus casei* on Shigella-infected human intestinal epithelial cells. *J Immunol.* 2006 Jan 15;176(2): 1228-37.

73. Yan F, Polk DB. Probiotic bacterium prevents cytokine-induced apoptosis in intestinal epithelial cells. *J Biol Chem.* 2002 Dec 27;277(52):50959-65.

74. Lin PW, Nasr TR, Berardinelli AJ, et al. The probiotic Lactobacillus GG may augment intestinal host defense by regulating apoptosis and promoting cytoprotective responses in the developing murine gut. *Pediatr Res.* 2008 Nov;64(5):511-6.

75. Chung J, Ha ES, Park HR, et al. Isolation and characterization of Lactobacillus species inhibiting the formation of Streptococcus mutans biofilm. *Oral Microbiol Immunol.* 2004 Jun;19(3):214-6.

76. Penders J, Thijs C, van den Brandt PA, et al. Gut microbiota composition and development of atopic manifestations in infancy: the KOALA Birth Cohort Study. *Gut.* 2007 May;56(5):661-7. Epub 2006 Oct 17.

77. Rautava S, Kalliomäki M, Isolauri E. Probiotics during pregnancy and breast-feeding might confer immunomodulatory protection against atopic disease in the infant. *J Allergy Clin Immunol.* 2002 Jan;109(1):119-21.

78. Böttcher MF, Abrahamsson TR, Fredriksson M, et al. Low breast milk TGF-beta2 is induced by *Lactobacillus reuteri* supplementation and associates with reduced risk of sensitization during infancy. *Pediatr Allergy Immunol.* 2008 Sep;19(6):497-504.

79. Wickens K, Black PN, Stanley TV, et al. A differential effect of 2 probiotics in the prevention of eczema and atopy: a double-blind, randomized, placebo-controlled trial. *J Allergy Clin Immunol.* 2008 Oct;122(4):788-94.

80. Kopp MV, Hennemuth I, Heinzmann A, et al. Randomized, double-blind, placebo-controlled trial of probiotics for primary prevention: no clinical effects of *Lactobacillus GG* supplementation. *Pediatrics.* 2008 Apr;121(4):e850-6.

81. Kuitunen M, Kukkonen K, Juntunen-Backman K, et al. Probiotics prevent IgE-associated allergy until age 5 years in cesarean-delivered children but not in the total cohort. *J Allergy Clin Immunol.* 2009 Feb;123(2): 335-41.

82. Hershko C, Hoffbrand AV, Keret D, et al. Role of autoimmune gastritis, *Helicobacter pylori* and celiac disease in refractory or unexplained iron deficiency anemia. *Haematologica.* 2005 May;90(5):585-95.

83. Hirschowitz BI, Worthington J, Mohnen J. Vitamin B12 deficiency in hypersecretors during long-term acid suppression with proton pump inhibitors. *Aliment Pharmacol Ther.* 2008 Jun 1;27(11):1110-21.

84. Dial S, Delaney JA, Barkun AN, et al. Use of gastric acid-suppressive agents and the risk of community-acquired *Clostridium difficile*-associated disease. *JAMA.* 2005 Dec 21;294(23):2989-95.

85. Hurwitz A, Brady DA, Schaal SE, Gastric acidity in older adults. *JAMA.* 1997 Aug 27;278(8):659-62.

86. Kelly CP, LaMont JT. *Clostridium difficile*—more difficult than ever. *N Engl J Med.* 2008 Oct 30;359(18):1932-40.

87. Dial S, Delaney JA, Barkun AN, et al. Use of gastric acid-suppressive agents and the risk of community-acquired *Clostridium difficile*-associated disease. *JAMA.* 2005 Dec 21;294(23):2989-95

88. Chey WD, Wong BC. Practice Parameters Committee of the American College of Gastroenterology. American College of Gastroenterology guideline on the management of *Helicobacter pylori* infection. *Am J Gastroenterol.* 2007 Aug;102(8):1808-25.

89. Everhart JE, Kruszon-Moran D, Perez-Perez GI, et al. Seroprevalence and ethnic differences in *Helicobacter pylori* infection among adults in the United States. *J Infect Dis.* 2000 Apr;181(4):1359-63.

90. Kato S, Matsukura N, Matsuda N, et al. Normalization of pH level and gastric mucosa after eradication of *H. pylori* in the remnant stomach. *J Gastroenterol Hepatol.* 2008 Dec;23 Suppl 2:S258-61.

91. Ohkusa T, Miwa H, Nomura T, et al. Improvement in serum pepsinogens and gastrin in long-term monitoring after eradication of *Helicobacter pylori*: comparison with *H. pylori*-negative patients. *Aliment Pharmacol Ther.* 2004 Jul;20 Suppl 1:25-32.

92. Sempértegui F, Díaz M, Mejía R, et al. Low concentrations of zinc in gastric mucosa are associated with increased severity of *Helicobacter pylori*-induced inflammation. *Helicobacter.* 2007 Feb;12(1):43-8.

93. Mirvish SS, Grandjean AC, Reimers KJ, et al. Effect of ascorbic acid dose taken with a meal on nitrosoproline excretion in subjects ingesting nitrate and proline. *Nutr Cancer.* 1998;31(2):106-10.

94. Zhang ZW, Farthing MJ. The roles of vitamin C in *Helicobacter pylori* associated gastric carcinogenesis. *Chin J Dig Dis.* 2005;6(2):53-8.

95. Rokkas T, Papatheodorou G, Karameris A, et al. *Helicobacter pylori* infection and gastric juice vitamin C levels. Impact of eradication. *Dig Dis Sci.* 1995 Mar;40(3):615-21.
96. Park JH, Kim SY, Kim DW, et al. Correlation between *Helicobacter pylori* infection and vitamin C levels in whole blood, plasma, and gastric juice, and the pH of gastric juice in Korean children. *J Pediatr Gastroenterol Nutr.* 2003 Jul;37(1):53-62.
97. Chuang CH, Sheu BS, Kao AW, et al. Adjuvant effect of vitamin C on omeprazole-amoxicillin-clarithromycin triple therapy for *Helicobacter pylori* eradication. *Hepatogastroenterology.* 2007 Jan-Feb;54(73):320
98. Ferrone M, Raimondo M, Scolapio JS. Pancreatic enzyme pharmacotherapy. *Pharmacotherapy.* 2007 Jun;27(6):910-20.
99. Meddings J. The significance of the gut barrier in disease. *Gut.* 2008 Apr;57(4):438-40.
100. Dalla Pellegrina C, Perbellini O, Scupoli MT, et al. Effects of wheat germ agglutinin on human gastrointestinal epithelium: insights from an experimental model of immune/epithelial cell interaction. *Toxicol Appl Pharmacol.* 2009 Jun 1;237(2):146-53. Epub 2009 Mar 28.
101. Lambert GP, Lang J, Bull A, et al. Fluid restriction during running increases GI permeability. *Int J Sports Med.* 2008 Mar;29(3):194-8.
102. Fasano A, Shea-Donohue T. Mechanisms of disease: the role of intestinal barrier function in the pathogenesis of gastrointestinal autoimmune diseases. *Nat Clin Pract Gastroenterol Hepatol.* 2005 Sep;2(9):416-22.
103. Tilg H, Moschen AR, Kaser A. Gut, inflammation and osteoporosis: basic and clinical concepts. *Gut.* 2008 May;57(5):684-94.
104. Bjarnason I, Takeuchi K. Intestinal permeability in the pathogenesis of NSAID-induced enteropathy. *J Gastroenterol.* 2009;44 Suppl 19:23-9.
105. Farhadi A, Gundlapalli S, Shaikh M. Susceptibility to gut leakiness: a possible mechanism for endotoxaemia in non alcoholic steatohepatitis. *Liver Int.* 2008 Aug;28(7):1026-33.
106. Ventura MT, Polimeno L, Amoruso AC. Intestinal permeability in patients with adverse reactions to food. *Dig Liver Dis.* 2006 Oct;38(10):732-6.
107. Hershko C, Hoffbrand AV, Keret D, et al. Role of autoimmune gastritis, *Helicobacter pylori* and celiac disease in refractory or unexplained iron deficiency anemia. *Haematologica.* 2005 May;90(5):585-95.
108. Hirschowitz BI, Worthington J, Mohnen J. Vitamin B12 deficiency in hypersecretors during long-term acid suppression with proton pump inhibitors. *Aliment Pharmacol Ther.* 2008 Jun 1;27(11):1110-21.
109. Hurwitz A, Brady DA, Schaal SE, et al. Gastric acidity in older adults. *JAMA* 1997;278:659-662.
110. Rafsky HA, Weingarten M. A study of the gastric secretory response in the aged. *Gastroent* 1946; May:348-352.
111. Tong JL, Ran ZH, Shen J, et al. Sequential therapy vs. standard triple therapies for *Helicobacter pylori* infection: a meta-analysis. *J Clin Pharm Ther.* 2009 Feb;34(1):41-53.
112. Armuzzi A, Cremonini F, Ojetti V, et al. Effect of *Lactobacillus GG* supplementation on antibiotic-associated gastrointestinal side effects during *Helicobacter pylori* eradication therapy: a pilot study. *Digestion.* 2001;63(1):1-7.
113. Zhang HM, Wakisaka N, Maeda O, et al. Vitamin C inhibits the growth of a bacterial risk factor for gastric carcinoma: *Helicobacter pylori. Cancer* 1997;80:1897-1903
114. Sasazuki S, Sasaki S, Tsubono Y, et al. The effect of 5-year vitamin C supplementation on serum pepsinogen level and *Helicobacter pylori* infection. *Cancer Sci* 2003;94:378-82.
115. De R, Kundu P, Swarnakar S, et al. Antimicrobial activity of curcumin against Indian *Helicobacter pylori* and also during mice infection. *Antimicrob Agents Chemother.* 2009 Feb 9. Epub ahead of print.
116. Di Mario F, Cavallaro LG, Nouvenne A, et al. A curcumin-based 1-week triple therapy for eradication of *Helicobacter pylori* infection: something to learn from failure? *Helicobacter.* 2007 Jun;12(3):238-43.
117. Cheng AL, Hsu CH, Lin JK, et al. Phase I clinical trial of curcumin, a chemopreventive agent, in patients with high-risk or pre-malignant lesions. *Anticancer Res.* 2001 Jul-Aug;21(4B):2895-900.
118. Fukai T, Marumo A, Kaitou K, et al. Anti-*Helicobacter pylori* flavonoids from licorice extract. *Life Sci.* 2002 71:1449-63.
119. Doll R, Hill ID, Hutton CF, et al. Clinical trial of a triterpenoid liquorice compound in gastric and duodenal ulcer. *Lancet* 1962;793-6.
120. van Marle J, Aarsen PN, Lind A, et al. Deglycyrrhizinised liquorice (DGL) and the renewal of rat stomach epithelium. *Eur J Pharmacol.* 1981; 72: 219-225.
121. Armanini D, Lewicka S, Pratesi C, et al. Further studies on the mechanism of the mineralocorticoid action of licorice in humans. *J Endocrinol Invest.* 1996 Oct;19(9):624-9.
122. Dastych M, Dastych M Jr, Novotná H, et al. Lactulose/mannitol test and specificity, sensitivity, and area under curve of intestinal permeability parameters in patients with liver cirrhosis and Crohn's disease. *Dig Dis Sci.* 2008 Oct;53(10):2789-92.
123. Takeda Y, Nakase H, Namba K, et al. Upregulation of T-bet and tight junction molecules by *Bifidobactrium longum* improves colonic inflammation of ulcerative colitis. *Inflamm Bowel Dis.* 2009 Nov;15(11):1617-8.
124. Fujimori S, Gudis K, Mitsui K, et al. A randomized controlled trial on the efficacy of synbiotic versus probiotic or prebiotic treatment to improve the quality of life in patients with ulcerative colitis. *Nutrition.* 2009 May;25(5):520-5. Epub 2009 Feb 8.

125. Li N, Neu J. Glutamine deprivation alters intestinal tight junctions via a PI3-K/Akt mediated pathway in Caco-2 cells. *J Nutr.* 2009 Apr;139(4):710-4.

126. Salvatore S, Heuschkel R, Tomlin S, et al. A pilot study of N-acetyl glucosamine, a nutritional substrate for glycosaminoglycan synthesis, in paediatric chronic inflammatory bowel disease. *Aliment Pharmacol Ther.* 2000 Dec;14(12):1567-79.

127. Amasheh M, Andres S, Amasheh S, et al. Barrier effects of nutritional factors. *Ann N Y Acad Sci.* 2009 May;1165:267-73.

128. Suzuki T, Hara H. Quercetin enhances intestinal barrier function through the assembly of zonula [corrected] occludens-2, occludin, and claudin-1 and the expression of claudin-4 in Caco-2 cells. *J Nutr.* 2009 May;139(5):965-74.

129. Amasheh M, Schlichter S, Amasheh S, et al. Quercetin enhances epithelial barrier function and increases claudin-4 expression in Caco-2 cells. *J Nutr.* 2008 Jun;138(6):1067-73.

130. Bischoff SC, Krämer S. Human mast cells, bacteria, and intestinal immunity. *Immunol Rev.* 2007 Jun;217:329-37.

131. Rovner AJ, Stallings VA, Schall JI, et al. Vitamin D insufficiency in children, adolescents, and young adults with cystic fibrosis despite routine oral supplementation. *Am J Clin Nutr.* 2007 Dec;86(6):1694-9.

132. Lin Y, Tamakoshi A, Hayakawa T, et al. Cigarette smoking as a risk factor for chronic pancreatitis: a case-control study in Japan. Research Committee on Intractable Pancreatic Diseases. *Pancreas.* 2000 Aug;21(2):109-14.

133. Naruse S, Ishiguro H, Ko SB, et al. Fecal pancreatic elastase: a reproducible marker for severe exocrine pancreatic insufficiency. *J Gastroenterol.* 2006 Sep;41(9):901-8.

134. Siegmund E, Löhr JM, Schuff-Werner P. The diagnostic validity of non invasive pancreatic function tests—a meta-analysis. *Z Gastroenterol.* 2004 Oct;42(10):1117-28.

135. Yamada T. *Yamada's Textbook of Gastroenterology.* 4th edition, May 2003. Lippincott Williams & Wilkins.

136. Hardt PD, Brendel MD, Kloer HU, et al. Is pancreatic diabetes (type 3c diabetes) underdiagnosed and misdiagnosed? *Diabetes Care.* 2008 Feb;31 Suppl 2:S165-

137. Maconi G, Dominici R, Molteni M, et al. Prevalence of pancreatic insufficiency in inflammatory bowel diseases. Assessment by fecal elastase-1. *Dig Dis Sci.* 2008 Jan;53(1):262-70. Epub 2007 May 26.

138. Freeman HJ. Pancreatic endocrine and exocrine changes in celiac disease. *World J Gastroenterol.* 2007 Dec 21; 13(47):6344-6.

139. Leeds JS, Hopper AD, Hurlstone DP, et al. Is exocrine pancreatic insufficiency in adult coeliac disease a cause of persisting symptoms? *Aliment Pharmacol Ther.* 2007 Feb 1;25(3):265-71.

140. Carroccio A, Iacono G, Montalto G, et al. Exocrine pancreatic function in children with coeliac disease before and after a gluten free diet. *Gut.* 1991 Jul;32(7):796-9.

141. Domínguez-Muñoz JE, Iglesias-García J, Iglesias-Rey M, et al. Effect of the administration schedule on the therapeutic efficacy of oral pancreatic enzyme supplements in patients with exocrine pancreatic insufficiency: a randomized, three-way crossover study. *Aliment Pharmacol Ther.* 2005 Apr 15;21(8):993-1000.

142. Peretti N, Marcil V, Drouin E, et al. Mechanisms of lipid malabsorption in Cystic Fibrosis: the impact of essential fatty acids deficiency. *Nutr Metab* (Lond). 2005 May 3;2(1):11.

143. Dodge JA, Turck D. Cystic fibrosis: nutritional consequences and management. *Best Pract Res Clin Gastroenterol.* 2006;20(3):531-46.

144. Bubenik GA. Thirty four years since the discovery of gastrointestinal melatonin. *J Physiol Pharmacol.* 2008 Aug;59 Suppl 2:33-51.

145. Jaworek J, Nawrot-Porabka K, Leja-Szpak A, et al. Melatonin as modulator of pancreatic enzyme secretion and pancreatoprotector. *J Physiol Pharmacol.* 2007 Dec;58 Suppl 6:65-80.

146. Fasano A. Systemic autoimmune disorders in celiac disease. *Curr Opin Gastroenterol.* 2006 Nov;22(6):674-9.

147. Ojetti V, Nucera G, Migneco A, et al. High prevalence of celiac disease in patients with lactose intolerance. *Digestion.* 2005;71(2):106-10.

148. Vilela EG, Torres HO, Ferrari ML, et al. Gut permeability to lactulose and mannitol differs in treated Crohn's disease and celiac disease patients and healthy subjects. *Braz J Med Biol Res.* 2008 Dec;41(12):1105-9.

149. Mikesh LM, Crowe SE, Bullock GC, et al. Celiac disease refractory to a gluten-free diet? *Clin Chem.* 2008 Feb;54(2):441-4.

150. Hill ID. What are the sensitivity and specificity of serologic tests for celiac disease? Do sensitivity and specificity vary in different populations? *Gastroenterology.* 2005 Apr;128(4 Suppl 1):S25-32.

151. Hadithi M, von Blomberg BM, Crusius JB, et al. Accuracy of serologic tests and HLA-DQ typing for diagnosing celiac disease. *Ann Intern Med.* 2007 Sep 4;147(5):294-302.

152. Hopper AD, Hadjivassiliou M, Butt S, et al. Adult coeliac disease. *BMJ.* 2007 Sep 15;335(7619):558-62.

153. Harrison MS, Wehbi M, Obideen K. Celiac disease: more common than you think. *Cleve Clin J Med.* 2007 Mar;74(3):209-15.

154. Vilela EG, Torres HO, Ferrari ML, et al. Gut permeability to lactulose and mannitol differs in treated Crohn's disease and celiac disease patients and healthy subjects. *Braz J Med Biol Res.* 2008 Dec;41(12):1105-9.

155. Ojetti V, Gabrielli M, Migneco A, et al. Regression of lactose malabsorption in coeliac patients after receiving a gluten-free diet. *Scand J Gastroenterol.* 2008;43(2):174-7.

156. Hallert C, Svensson M, Tholstrup J, et al. Clinical trial: B Vitamins improve health in coeliac patients living on a

gluten-free diet. *Aliment Pharmacol Ther.* 2009 Jan 20. Epub ahead of print.

157. Henri-Bhargava A, Melmed C, et al. Neurologic impairment due to vitamin E and copper deficiencies in celiac disease. *Neurology.* 2008 Sep 9;71(11):860-1.
158. Kupper C. Dietary guidelines and implementation for celiac disease. *Gastroenterology.* 2005 Apr;128(4 Suppl 1):S121-7.
159. Xavier RJ, Podolsky DK. Unravelling the pathogenesis of inflammatory bowel disease. *Nature.* 2007 Jul 26;448(7152):427-34.
160. Wong A, Bass D. Laboratory evaluation of inflammatory bowel disease. *Curr Opin Pediatr.* 2008 Oct;20(5):566-70.
161. Sidler MA, Leach ST, Day AS. Fecal S100A12 and fecal calprotectin as noninvasive markers for inflammatory bowel disease in children. *Inflamm Bowel Dis.* 2008 Mar;14(3):359-66.
162. Henriksen M, Jahnsen J, Lygren I, et al. C-reactive protein: a predictive factor and marker of inflammation in inflammatory bowel disease. Results from a prospective population-based study. *Gut.* 2008 Nov;57(11):1518-23.
163. Jones VA, Dickinson RJ, Workman E, et al. Crohn's disease: maintenance of remission by diet. *Lancet.* 1985 Jul 27;2(8448):177-80.
164. Takagi S, Utsunomiya K, Kuriyama S, et al. Effectiveness of an 'half elemental diet' as maintenance therapy for Crohn's disease: A randomized-controlled trial. *Aliment Pharmacol Ther.* 2006 Nov 1;24(9):1333-40.
165. Yamamoto T, Nakahigashi M, Umegae S. Impact of long-term enteral nutrition on clinical and endoscopic recurrence after resection for Crohn's disease: A prospective, non-randomized, parallel, controlled study. *Aliment Pharmacol Ther.* 2007 Jan 1;25(1):67-72.
166. Kuwabara A, Tanaka K, Tsugawa N, et al. High prevalence of vitamin K and D deficiency and decreased BMD in inflammatory bowel disease. *Osteoporos Int.* 2008 Sep 30. Epub ahead of print.
167. Vagianos K, Bector S, McConnell J, et al. Nutrition assessment of patients with inflammatory bowel disease. *JPEN J Parenter Enteral Nutr.* 2007 Jul-Aug;31(4):311-9.
168. Zocco MA, dal Verme LZ, Cremonini F, et al. Efficacy of *Lactobacillus GG* in maintaining remission of ulcerative colitis. *Aliment Pharmacol Ther.* 2006 Jun 1;23(11):1567-74.
169. Guslandi M, Mezzi G, Sorghi M, et al. *Saccharomyces boulardii* in maintenance treatment of Crohn's disease. *Dig Dis Sci.* 2000 Jul;45(7):1462-4.
170. Guslandi M, Giollo P, Testoni PA. A pilot trial of *Saccharomyces boulardii* in ulcerative colitis. *Eur J Gastroenterol Hepatol.* 2003 Jun;15(6):697-8.
171. Damaskos D, Kolios G. Probiotics and prebiotics in inflammatory bowel disease: microflora 'on the scope' *Br J Clin Pharmacol.* 2008 Apr;65(4):453-67. Epub 2008 Feb 12.
172. Head KA, Jurenka JS. Inflammatory bowel disease Part 1: ulcerative colitis—pathophysiology and conventional and alternative treatment options. *Altern Med Rev.* 2003 Aug;8(3):247-83.
173. Aggarwal BB, Sung B. Pharmacological basis for the role of curcumin in chronic diseases: an age-old spice with modern targets. *Trends Pharmacol Sci.* 2009 Feb;30(2):85-94.
174. Hanai H, Iida T, Takeuchi K, et al. Curcumin maintenance therapy for ulcerative colitis: randomized, multicenter, double-blind, placebo-controlled trial. *Clin Gastroenterol Hepatol.* 2006 Dec;4(12):1502-6.
175. Gupta I, Parihar A, Malhotra P, et al. Effects of *Boswellia serrata* gum resin in patients with ulcerative colitis. *Eur J Med Res.* 1997 Jan;2(1):37-43.
176. Gerhardt H, Seifert F, Buvari P, et al. Therapy of active Crohn disease with *Boswellia serrata* extract H 15. *Z Gastroenterol.* 2001 Jan;39(1):11-7.
177. Dabos KJ, Sfika E, Vlatta LJ, et al. Is Chios mastic gum effective in the treatment of functional dyspepsia? A prospective randomised double-blind placebo controlled trial. *J Ethnopharmacol.* 2010 Feb 3;127(2):205-9.
178. Al-Habbal MJ, Al-Habbal Z, Huwez FU. A double-blind controlled clinical trial of mastic and placebo in the treatment of duodenal ulcer. *Clin Exp Pharmacol Physiol.* 1984 Sep-Oct;11(5):541-4.
179. Kaliora AC, Stathopoulou MG, Triantafillidis JK, et al. Chios mastic treatment of patients with active Crohn's disease. *World J Gastroenterol.* 2007 Feb 7;13(5):748-53.
180. Maung-U K, Khin M, Nyunt-Wai N, et al. Clinical trial of berberine in acute watery diarrhea. *Br Med J* 1985;291:1601-1605.
181. Kamath SA. Clinical trial of berberine hydrochloride for the control of acute diarrhea in gastroenteritis. *J Assoc Phys Ind.* 1967; 15: 55-59.
182. Clark C, DeLegge M. Irritable bowel syndrome: a practical approach. *Nutr Clin Pract.* 2008 Jun-Jul;23(3):263-7.
183. Piche T, Barbara G, Aubert P, et al. Impaired intestinal barrier integrity in the colon of patients with irritable bowel syndrome: involvement of soluble mediators. *Gut.* 2009 Feb;58(2):196-201. Epub 2008 Sep 29.
184. Ait-Belgnaoui A, Bradesi S, Fioramonti J, et al. Acute stress-induced hypersensitivity to colonic distension depends upon increase in paracellular permeability: role of myosin light chain kinase. *Pain.* 2005 Jan;113(1-2): 141-7.
185. Zar S, Mincher L, Benson MJ, et al. Food-specific IgG4 antibody-guided exclusion diet improves symptoms and rectal compliance in irritable bowel syndrome. *Scand J Gastroenterol.* 2005 Jul;40(7):800-7.
186. Zar S, Benson MJ, Kumar D. Food-specific serum IgG4 and IgE titers to common food antigens in irritable bowel syndrome. *Am J Gastroenterol.* 2005 Jul;100(7):1550-7.
187. Spiller R. Review article: probiotics and prebiotics in irritable bowel syndrome. *Aliment Pharmacol Ther.* 2008 Aug 15;28(4):385-96. Epub 2008 Jun 4.

188. Pimentel M, Chow EJ, Lin HC. Eradication of small intestinal bacterial overgrowth reduces symptoms of irritable bowel syndrome. *Am J Gastroenterol.* 2000 Dec; 95(12):3503-6.

189. Sanders DS, Carter MJ, Hurlstone DP, et al. Association of adult coeliac disease with irritable bowel syndrome: a case-control study in patients fulfilling ROME II criteria referred to secondary care. *Lancet.* 2001 Nov 3;358(9292):1504-8.

190. Choi YK, Kraft N, Zimmerman B, et al. Fructose intolerance in IBS and utility of fructose-restricted diet. *J Clin Gastroenterol.* 2008 Mar;42(3):233-8.

191. Spiegel BM, Chey WD, Chang L. Bacterial overgrowth and irritable bowel syndrome: unifying hypothesis or a spurious consequence of proton pump inhibitors? *Am J Gastroenterol.* 2008 Dec;103(12):2972-6.

192. Zar S, Benson MJ, Kumar D. Food-specific serum IgG4 and IgE titers to common food antigens in irritable bowel syndrome. *Am J Gastroenterol.* 2005 Jul;100(7):1550-7.

193. Ford AC, Talley NJ, Veldhuyzen van Zanten SJ, et al. Will the history and physical examination help establish that irritable bowel syndrome is causing this patient's lower gastrointestinal tract symptoms? *JAMA.* 2008 Oct 15; 300(15):1793-805.

194. Bijkerk CJ, Muris JW, Knottnerus JA, et al. Systematic review: the role of different types of fibre in the treatment of irritable bowel syndrome. *Aliment Pharmacol Ther.* 2004 Feb 1;19(3):245-51.

195. Kerckhoffs AP, Akkermans LM, de Smet MB, et al. Intestinal Permeability in Irritable Bowel Syndrome Patients: Effects of NSAIDs. *Dig Dis Sci.* 2009 Mar 3. Epub ahead of print.

196. Cappello G, Spezzaferro M, Grossi L, et al. Peppermint oil (Mintoil) in the treatment of irritable bowel syndrome: a prospective double blind placebo-controlled randomized trial. *Dig Liver Dis.* 2007 Jun;39(6):530-6.

197. Merat S, Khalili S, Mostajabi P, et al. The effect of enteric-coated, delayed-release peppermint oil on irritable bowel syndrome. *Dig Dis Sci.* 2010 May;55(5):1385-90.

198. Ford AC, Talley NJ, Spiegel BM, et al. Effect of fibre, antispasmodics, and peppermint oil in the treatment of irritable bowel syndrome: systematic review and meta-analysis. *BMJ.* 2008 Nov 13;337:a2313.

199. Lu WZ, Gwee KA, Moochhalla S, et al. Melatonin improves bowel symptoms in female patients with irritable bowel syndrome: a double-blind placebo-controlled study. *Aliment Pharmacol Ther.* 2005 Nov 15;22(10):927-34.

200. Song GH, Leng PH, Gwee KA, et al. Melatonin improves abdominal pain in irritable bowel syndrome patients who have sleep disturbances: a randomised, double blind, placebo controlled study. *Gut.* 2005 Oct;54(10):1402-7. Epub 2005 May 24.

Advanced Detoxification Support

Overview

Given the extraordinary demands placed upon our detoxification systems, it is remarkable that we are not more frequently overwhelmed by the burden. The "chemical soup" we find ourselves in is made up of an ever-increasing number and variety of synthetic substances, for most of which we have minimal monitoring or health effects data. As many as 80,000 commercial and industrial chemicals are now in use in the United States, with approximately 6.5 billion pounds of chemicals released into the air each year.[1]

Unfortunately, although significant gains have been made in our understanding of genetic influences on detoxification, the contribution of environmental exposures to disease remains poorly understood. The effects of low-level, virtually continuous exposure to multiple chemicals simultaneously, now a ubiquitous scenario, are for the most part unknown.[2] It has been estimated that at current funding levels, it would take 1,000 years to adequately document the health effects of the chemicals commonly encountered in commerce and industry.[3]

Of course we have always been exposed to a wide variety of natural toxins in our air, food, and water, though it could be argued that our detoxification systems have evolved to handle these natural toxins, at least to some degree. For example, the cytochrome enzyme CYP2D6, which is thought to metabolize 20–25% of all drugs at least partially, has a wide range of function, ranging from "poor" to "ultra-rapid" metabolic activity. Although mice have nine active genes at this locus (CYP2D), data from the human genome project has determined that humans have just one polymorphic gene. Because this enzyme has a high affinity for alkaloids, the loss of CYP2D activity is thought to reflect a loss of evolutionary pressure to metabolize alkaloids. This may explain why in some regions, particularly Northeast Africa, a much higher prevalence of the ultra-rapid genotype is still found, giving those individuals a greater capacity for detoxification of plant toxins and providing an adaptive benefit during periods of starvation.[4]

Overview (continued)

Thus, the toxicity of a substance is determined both by its inherent properties and by how it is metabolized in the body. Not only do genetic factors influence detoxification capacity, but virtually all chemical exposures occur in a context of diverse other factors, including nutritional status, underlying disease states, smoking, digestive function, alcohol consumption, lifestyle, etc. There are many uncertainties in the field of toxicology and detoxification. Much of the exposure we receive is not controllable, and we may have genetic predispositions that increase the vulnerability to damage. Using a corollary of the precautionary principle as a guide, we can work to avoid exposure, and also to recognize how toxins cause damage and how our detoxification systems may be optimized to prevent it.

Clinical Consequences of Toxin Exposure

As mentioned above, many effects of exposure to toxins are not clearly understood, particularly the interactions of the numerous toxins within the human body. However, a number of examples indicate the severity of toxin exposure, how common such exposure is, and the significant degree of clinical impact.

To illustrate this point, consider that, according to NHANES data, 73% of U.S. women age 50+ have levels of cadmium between 0.50 and 1.00 mcg/g creatinine. This level of exposure has been associated with a 43% greater risk for osteoporosis, and may account for 21% of the osteoporosis prevalence in this age group.[5] Additionally, this same level of exposure has been associated with an 80% increase in risk for myocardial infarction, a clear example of a toxin that we are commonly exposed to having significant health consequences.[6] The many health effects of cadmium exposure in humans are depicted in Figure 3.1.

Other heavy metals are also relevant to common clinical conditions. For example, arsenic has been shown to increase the risk of diabetes nearly 4-fold, and nearly 92% of children born

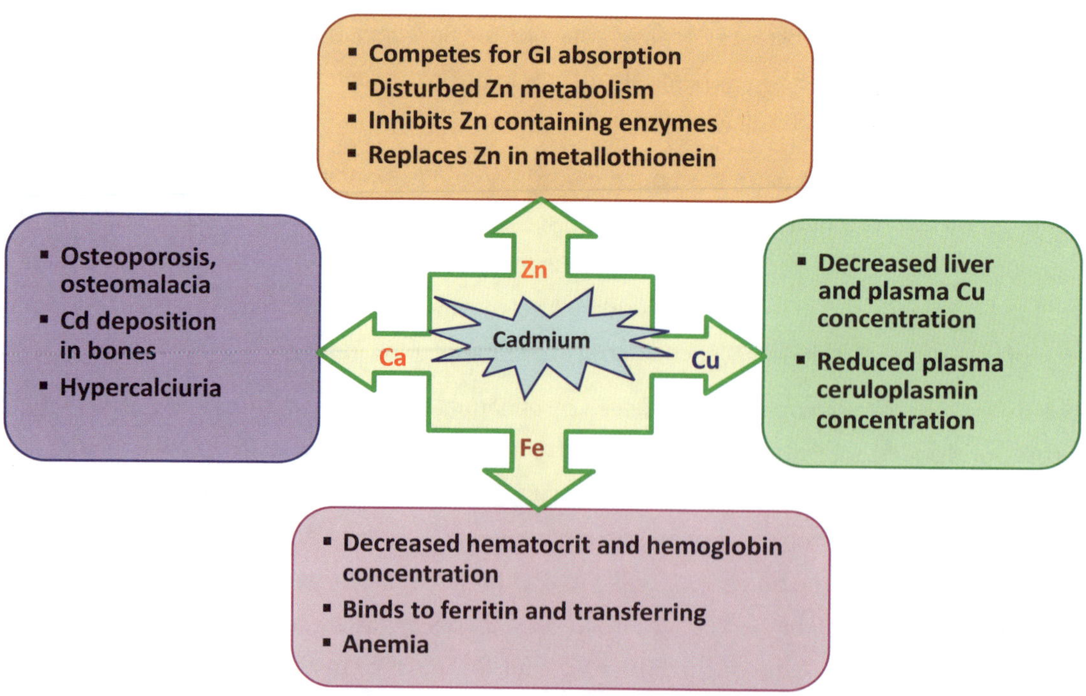

Figure 3.1 Interaction of cadmium with essential nutrients by which it causes toxicity. From: Flora SJ, Mittal M, Mehta A. Heavy metal induced oxidative stress and its possible reversal by chelation therapy. *Indian J Med Res.* 2008 Oct;128(4):501-23. Reprinted with permission from the *Indian Journal of Medical Research (IJMR).*

in the U.S. still have an increased risk of neurodevelopmental damage from lead toxicity.[7,8] Along with heavy metals, other toxins are also associated with significant harm. For example, a strong dose-response relationship between diabetes and persistent organic pollutants (POPs) was observed in the NHANES data, with an astounding increased risk of up to 38-fold for those with the highest levels.[9] Organochlorine pesticides specifically increased the risk of insulin resistance and abdominal obesity,[10] and they have also been shown to increase the risk of peripheral neuropathy in those with glucose abnormalities, beyond the effects of diabetes itself.[11]

Along with metabolic abnormalities, toxin exposure has been associated with arthritis risk. In a recent trial, PCBs were shown to increase the risk of rheumatoid arthritis by 8.5-fold, while organochlorine pesticides increased the risk 3.5-fold. The risk of osteoarthritis was also raised nearly 3-fold by some types of PCBs.[12] POPs were found to increase the risk of cardiovascular disease up to 5-fold, particularly in women, while pesticides increase neurodegenerative disease risk more than 2-fold.[13,14] Understanding how toxins cause damage may help to clarify how they have such widespread effects over numerous body systems.

How Toxins Cause Damage

Toxins cause damage by a variety of mechanisms, including an increase in reactive oxygen species (ROS) formation, direct damage to DNA and cell membranes, enzyme inhibition, and endocrine disruption.[15]

Oxidative damage

Many toxins cause oxidative damage through diverse mechanisms. For example, cadmium has been shown to increase a variety of ROS, including H_2O_2, $O_2^{\bullet-}$, and $^{\bullet}OH$, but it also interferes with cellular defenses by targeting the antioxidant enzymes catalase and glutathione reductase, and the cellular antioxidant glutathione. The resultant oxidation leads to DNA damage, abnormal protein folding, and lipid peroxidation, including mitochondrial membrane damage.[16] Figures 3.2 and 3.3 depict mechanisms and target tissues of

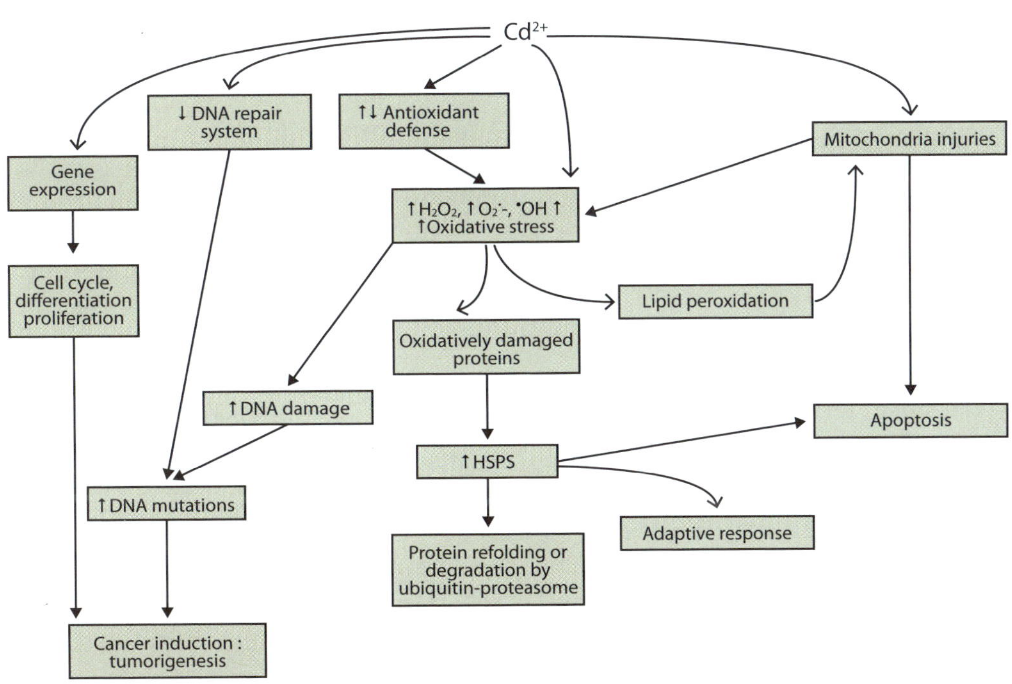

Figure 3.2 Biological consequences of cadmium intoxication in cells. From: Bertin G, Averbeck D. Cadmium: cellular effects, modifications of biomolecules, modulation of DNA repair and genotoxic consequences (a review). Biochimie. 2006 Nov;88(11):1549-59. Used with permission from Elsevier.

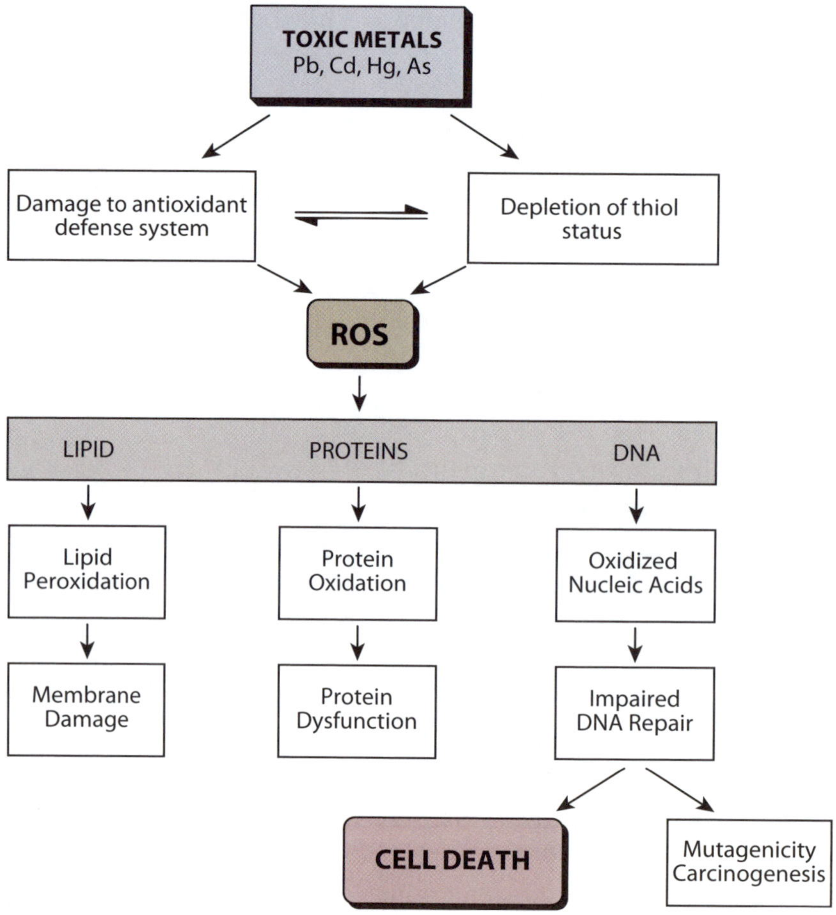

Figure 3.3 Potential mechanisms of heavy metal induced oxidative stress. From: Ercal N, Gurer-Orhan H, Aykin-Burns N. Toxic metals and oxidative stress part I: mechanisms involved in metal-induced oxidative damage. *Curr Top Med Chem.* 2001 Dec;1(6):529-39. Used with permission from Bentham Science Publishers Ltd.

toxin oxidative damage. These are common mechanisms of toxicity for heavy metals.[17,18] Fortunately, antioxidants play an important role in reducing heavy metal toxicity. For example, in a recent animal based study, N-acetylcysteine reduced cadmium-induced ototoxicity, likely through its antioxidant effects.[19]

Other toxins known to cause oxidative damage are pesticides. Malathion, one of the most widely used organophosphate (OP) pesticides, has been shown to induce oxidative stress in human erythrocytes, an effect attributed to inhibition of catalase, glutathione peroxidase, and superoxide dismutase. This effect can, in part, be prevented by vitamins C and E.[20] Oxidative stress from Malathion may also be a result of damage to mitochondrial complexes, as it appears to significantly inhibit the activity of complex IV.[21]

Neurodegenerative disease and oxidative damage

Oxidative damage combined with an inhibition of antioxidant enzymes is hypothesized to play a significant role in neurodegenerative disease. For example, the "multi-hit hypothesis" of Parkinson's disease suggests that, while the brain may be capable of withstanding the effects of an individual chemical toxic to the dopaminergic system, multiple chemicals targeting numerous sites compromise oxidative defense mechanisms and result in neuronal death. A number of pesticides that increase mitochondrial oxidative damage have also been implicated, with synergistic effects that may more closely represent actual exposure.[22] Oxidative stress from pesticides, air pollution, smoke, radiation, heavy metals, and dietary intake have all been associated with other neurodegenerative diseases.[23]

Enzyme inhibition

One of the best examples of toxin-based enzyme poisoning is lead's inhibition of delta aminolevulinic acid dehydratase (ALAD, aka porphobilinogen synthase). Lead effectively displaces zinc, which is normally found in the active site of this enzyme, severely inhibiting enzyme activity and interfering with the synthesis of heme (Figure 3.4).[24,25] A build-up of ALA increases oxidative stress, which causes widespread damage to cardiovascular and neurological tissue, as well as to the kidney, liver, and reproductive organs.

Damage to DNA

Various toxins directly damage DNA or interfere with DNA repair enzymes. These include air pollution (particulate matter), benzene, pesticides, insecticides, and phthalates. For example, particulates have been shown to inhibit DNA repair as well as increase DNA replication errors.[26] Benzene is known to cause direct DNA damage, chromosomal alterations, and impairment of DNA repair processes, but its toxicity is strongly influenced by detoxification enzyme polymorphisms.[27] In a recent study of over 200 workers with occupational benzene exposure, a combination of genetic polymorphisms in 3 detoxification enzymes (NAD(P)H: quinone oxidoreductase 1 [NQO1]; microsomal epoxide hydrolase [EPHX]; glutathione S-transferase T1 [GSTT1]) predicted a 5.5-fold greater incidence of single strand DNA breaks.[27]

Pesticides also cause DNA damage and, like benzene, their interactions with genetic predispositions influence the degree of harm. Many studies have been done involving fruit growers, because they have a high exposure level and a higher risk of cancer, specifically leukemia and multiple myeloma. They also have a higher risk for DNA damage, an effect modified by GSTP1 and XRCC1 genotypes, enzymes involved in DNA repair and pesticide detoxification.[28,29]

Insecticides also cause DNA damage. Metabolites of pyrethroid insecticides in urine have been associated not only with decreased semen quality but also with sperm DNA damage. Pyrethroid insecticides are in widespread use, and the level associated with these abnormalities is similar to that found in most U.S. men, per the 3rd National Report on Human Exposure to Environmental Chemicals.[30]

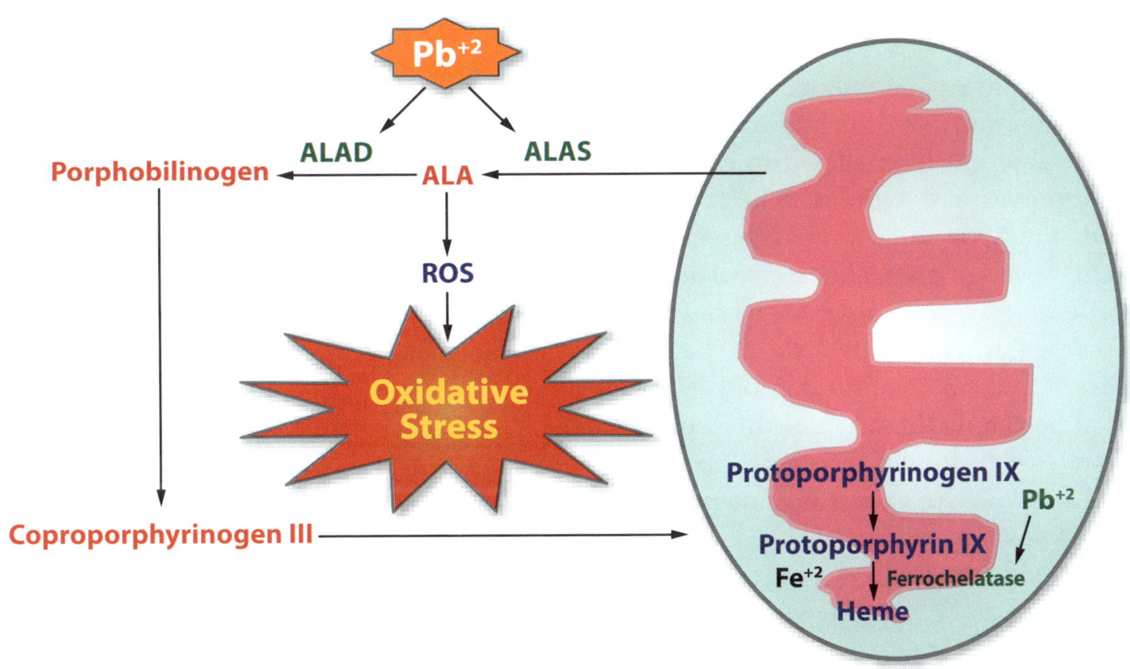

Figure 3.4 Effect of lead on heme biosynthesis. From: Flora SJ, Mittal M, Mehta A. Heavy metal induced oxidative stress and its possible reversal by chelation therapy. *Indian J Med Res.* 2008 Oct;128(4):501-23. Reprinted with permission from the *Indian Journal of Medical Research* (IJMR).

Phthalates, which are found in plastics, personal care products, and food packaging materials, have been shown to damage sperm DNA at levels commonly found in U.S. men.[31]

Damage to cell membranes

Yet another mechanism of damage is mediated via direct toxicity to cell membranes. This common mechanism results in loss of cellular function through the inactivation of membrane enzymes, ion channels, and pumps.[32,33,34] Indirect effects, such as peroxidation of the lipids that comprise cell membranes, impair cellular function as well as membrane function. Membrane damage has been implicated in ischemia/reperfusion injury, inflammation, as well as the pathogenesis of various degenerative diseases, including arteriosclerosis, diabetes, and neurodegenerative disorders.[35]

Endocrine disruption

Perhaps one of the most important effects of exogenous toxins is interference with or mimicking of hormonal action. We now know that many substances act as estrogens and antiestrogens, androgens and antiandrogens, thyroid disruptors, inhibitors of steroid hormone synthesis,[36] and retinoid agonists, through both direct and epigenetic mechanisms.

Arsenic, persistent organic pollutants, and phthalates provide a few examples of this mechanism of toxicity. Arsenic has been shown to disrupt the thyroid hormone and retinoic acid receptors.[37] Data from the 2003–2004 NHANES indicated that urinary levels of arsenic were associated with the prevalence of type 2 diabetes, with a nearly 4-fold increase in risk between the 80th and 20th percentiles.[38] One mechanism for this effect is thought to be the modification of the expression of genes related to insulin resistance.[39] Similarly, the toxins known as persistent organic pollutants (POPs) are known to concentrate in white adipose tissue, with endocrine effects that contribute to diabetes as well as obesity (known as the "environmental obesogen hypothesis").[40,41]

The nearly ubiquitous phthalates have been associated with insulin resistance and waist circumference in NHANES analysis.[42] Metabolism of phthalates involves a phase I hydrolysis, which creates more biologically active intermediates, followed by phase II conjugation, suggesting that those with rapid phase I and impaired phase II functions have an even greater risk with exposure. This effect has been documented for a heightened risk of adenomyosis and leiomyoma in those with phthalate exposure and glutathione transferase polymorphisms. In a case-control study, those with a null GST genotype had a greater than 5-fold increased risk for adenomyosis, but if they also had high urinary phthalate levels the risk increased to more than 10-fold.[43,44,45]

Types of Toxin Exposure: Exogenous and Endogenous

Exogenous toxins

Exogenous toxins (heavy metals, persistent organic pollutants, and prescription medications) are ubiquitous in our environment, with physiological effects and interactions with one another that are not yet understood. Lead and mercury are heavy metals with far-reaching consequences. Lead, for example, is found in 1.6% of children aged 1–5 in the U.S. at a blood lead level (BLL) ≥10 mcg/dl, a tremendous decline from 77.8% in the late 1970s. However, an estimated 91.7% still have detectable levels in the blood, with 2.4 million at levels between 5 and 9.9 mcg/dl.[46] Among adults from the NHANES population, this level of lead toxicity (BLL of 5–9 mcg/dl) has been associated with an increased risk of death from all causes, cardiovascular disease, and cancer.[47]

Mercury is commonly found in the environment, as elemental, organic, or inorganic mercury. Eight percent of women enrolled in the NHANES 1999–2000 study had concentrations higher than the U.S. Environmental Protection Agency's recommended reference dose (5.8 mcg/l) for women of reproductive age.[48] Based on these data, it is estimated that >300,000 newborns each year in the United States may have been exposed *in utero* to concentrations that may not be safe: that is, the levels were higher than those considered to be without increased risk of adverse neurodevelopmental effects.[49] Blood mercury concentrations up to 7 times greater have been found among women consuming fish and shellfish more frequently.[50] Unfortunately, as more fish meal is used in animal feed, mercury exposure is expected to rise among those consuming other animal products as well.[51]

Along with heavy metals such as lead, mercury, arsenic, and cadmium, persistent organic pollutant exposure is widespread. Individually and collectively, POPs have been associated with increased risk of cardiovascular disease,[52] diabetes and insulin resistance, impaired neurological development, learning disorders and attention deficit, endometriosis, and deficits in the hypothalamic-pituitary-thyroid axis.[53,54,55,56]

In addition to heavy metals and industrial toxins, exposure to prescription medication is common, and not limited to drugs intentionally consumed. For example, a study conducted by the Environmental Working Group released in 2008 found that at least 40 million Americans drink tap water with detectable levels of prescription medications such as antibiotics, hormones, and drugs used to treat epilepsy and depression.[57]

Our exposure to a great number of toxins simultaneously, with multiple harmful effects and varying mechanisms of damage, and with unknown and virtually unexamined interactions, may be the greatest risk of all—and one that we have the least data for. To highlight this problem, a study led by the Mount Sinai School of Medicine in New York found an average of 91 industrial compounds, pollutants, and other chemicals in the blood and urine of nine volunteers, with a total of 167 chemicals found in the group. Many of these compounds are known to be carcinogenic, neurotoxic, or teratogenic.[58] We already know that, in some cases, chemicals have synergistic effects rather than just additive. Such an effect has been observed in Parkinson's disease, where metals and pesticides have a synergistic effect on alpha-synuclein fibrillation.[59]

Endogenous toxins

Endogenous toxins, such as metabolites not detoxified properly, non-end-product metabolites, and bowel microbial toxins, can cause damage and also place a strain on the detoxification system. For example, estrogen metabolism involves close interaction between oxidizing phase I and conjugating phase II enzymes. Catechol estrogens and estrogen quinones are byproducts of phase I estradiol metabolism, and are associated with reproductive tissue cancers and oxidative damage. A combination of increased phase I activity, particularly of CYP1B1, and low phase II activity, primarily catechol-O-methyltransferase and glutathione S-transferase, increases the production of these reactive and toxic intermediates.[60,61]

Non-end-product metabolites include homocysteine and methylmalonic acid, the former being a known risk factor for ischemic heart disease and stroke, neural tube defects, and neurodegenerative diseases.[63] Homocysteine metabolism depends on a number of vitamin cofactors, including vitamin B12, folic acid, and vitamin B6. Elevated levels of homocysteine cause damage through several mechanisms, including the generation of reactive oxygen species, hypomethylation, modification of other proteins by N-homocysteinylation, and inducing endothelial dysfunction and vascular inflammation.[62,63] Methylmalonic acid, a metabolic byproduct that builds up in several inborn errors of metabolism, as well as via a B12 deficiency, may be directly toxic to neurological and renal tissues, possibly by itself or through synergistic action with other metabolic toxins, such as propionyl-CoA.[64,65]

Bowel microbial toxins are another example of endogenously produced toxins. Endotoxins from bowel flora have been associated with depression, chronic fatigue, inflammatory bowel disease, diabetes, and atherosclerosis, at least in part through inflammatory pathways.[66,67,68,69] This effect is influenced by both bacterial species and intestinal permeability.[70]

An overview of how the detoxification process works may help explain not only how both endogenous and exogenous toxins cause damage, but

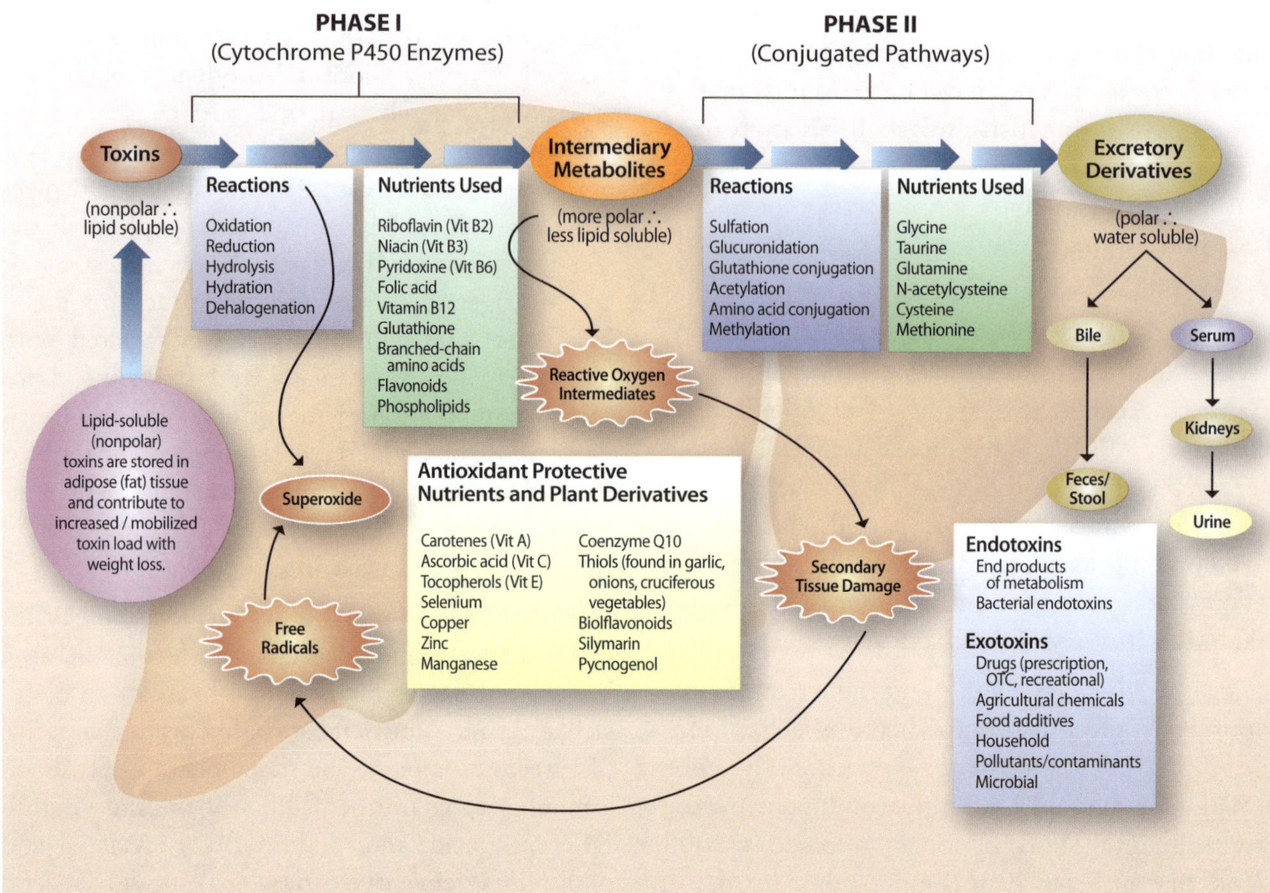

Figure 3.5 Liver detoxification pathways, activities, influences, and effects. (c) 2005 The Institute for Functional Medicine. Used with permission granted by The Institute for Functional Medicine, www.functionalmedicine.org. No part of this content may be reproduced or transmitted in any form or by any means without the express written consent of The Institute for Functional Medicine, except as permitted by applicable law.

how we can adequately support detoxification processes and help to ensure safe toxin elimination.

Detoxification Overview

Endogenous substrates as well as xenobiotics are mostly metabolized by phase I and/or phase II detoxification processes, often both, and by multiple enzymes of each phase. Both phases typically render a substance more water-soluble, and thus able to be excreted more easily; however, in the process, many substances are made more biologically active and potentially toxic. Phase I reactions modify a substance through oxidation, reduction, or hydrolysis, while phase II conjugates the modified substance (the intermediary metabolites). These steps do not always require one another, and, although phase I usually occurs first, it does not always, and there are many diet/genomic/exposure interactions and influences (Figure 3.5).

Considerable variation in detoxification capacity exists. Although dependent on a number of factors, including nutrition, age, gender, drug use, and environmental exposures, it has been estimated that 20–95% of the variability in drug response is due to genetic factors.[71] For example, 1% of Asians and 10% of Caucasians have completely absent CYP2D6 activity; yet 20–25% of all drugs are metabolized at least in part by this enzyme.[72] Approximately 66% of Caucasians and 40% of African-Americans do not possess any CYP3A5 activity,[73] although CYP3A4 may compensate at least partially for this.

In addition to genetic variability, we are exposed to numerous inducers and inhibitors of activity. For example, grapefruit juice has been shown to increase the AUC (area under the concentration-time curve) for some drugs by 100-fold![74] At least 56% of adverse drug reactions are due to drugs metabolized by polymorphic phase I enzymes.[75]

Cytochrome P450 enzymes are found in practically all tissues, with the highest abundance and largest number of individual CYP forms present in the liver.[76] However, many cytochrome enzymes are found in the lungs, adrenals, kidneys, and small intestine, which metabolize a wide variety of endogenous substrates, including vitamins, eicosanoids, fatty acids, and steroids.[77] Although there are 57 genes for cytochrome enzymes, 10–15 carry out the metabolism for almost all xenobiotics (Table 3.1).

Table 3.1 Human cytochromes P450 grouped according to their major substrate class

sterols	xenobiotics	fatty acids	eicosanoids	vitamins	unknown
1B1	1A1	2J2	4F2	2R1	2A7
7A1	1A2	4A11	4F3	24A1	2S1
7B1	2A6	4B1	4F8	26A1	2U1
8B1	2A13	4F12	5A1	26B1	2W1
11A1	2B6		8A1	26C1	3A43
11B1	2C8			27B1	4A22
11B2	2C9				4F11
17A1	2C18				4F22
19A1	2C19				4V2
21A2	2D6				4 x 1
27A1	2E1				4Z1
39A1	2F1				20A1
46A1	3A4				27C1
51A1	3A5				
	3A7				

Reprinted with permission. From Guengerich FP. Cytochrome p450 and chemical toxicology. *Chem Res Toxicol.* 2008 Jan;21(1):70-83. Copyright 2010 American Chemical Society.

CYP3 family members are the most abundant family in the liver, with the principal protein being CYP3A4. This family is also the most prominent in the intestine, which is likely the most important non-hepatic site for drug metabolism, i.e., first-pass metabolism. CYP3A4 accounts for 80% of intestinal P450.[78] Although the total content of CYP3A in the entire human small intestine is only 1% of that found in the liver, intestinal extraction of 3A substrates equals or exceeds that of the liver for some substances, while for others it is less.[78] This may be because first-pass exposure to the enterocyte enzymes is likely to be greater, due to a slower flux though the cell, whereas hepatic biotransformation has a much faster flow, and metabolism is also impaired by substrate binding to blood components.[79]

Phase I detoxification

Types of phase I enzyme actions

Phase I enzymes fall into one of three cytochrome P450 families, CYP 1, 2, or 3. All enzymes catalyze reactions largely through one of three processes, oxidation, reduction, or hydrolysis. In general, CYP1 family members are predominantly responsible for the bioactivation of polycyclic aromatic hydrocarbons, aromatic amines, and other carcinogens. Enzymes in this family are also involved in estrogen metabolism. Some enzymes in this family illustrate that it is not always beneficial to have rapid phase I activity. For example, elevated activity of CYP1A1 has been associated with increased lung cancer risk, especially when combined with the GSTM1 null genotype and toxin exposure.[80] Essentially, the bioactive intermediates are not removed quickly enough, and the resulting bottleneck of more toxic molecules causes greater damage. Similarly, CYP1A2 hydroxylates estradiol at carbon 2, creating a less reactive intermediate, while CYP1B1 hydroxylates it at C4, creating a more genotoxic intermediate. As might be expected, variants in these genes have been associated with both breast and prostate cancer,[81,82] while interventions such as quercetin and cruciferous vegetables, which increase 1A1 activity relative to 1B1, reduce the production of genotoxic intermediates, potentially reducing

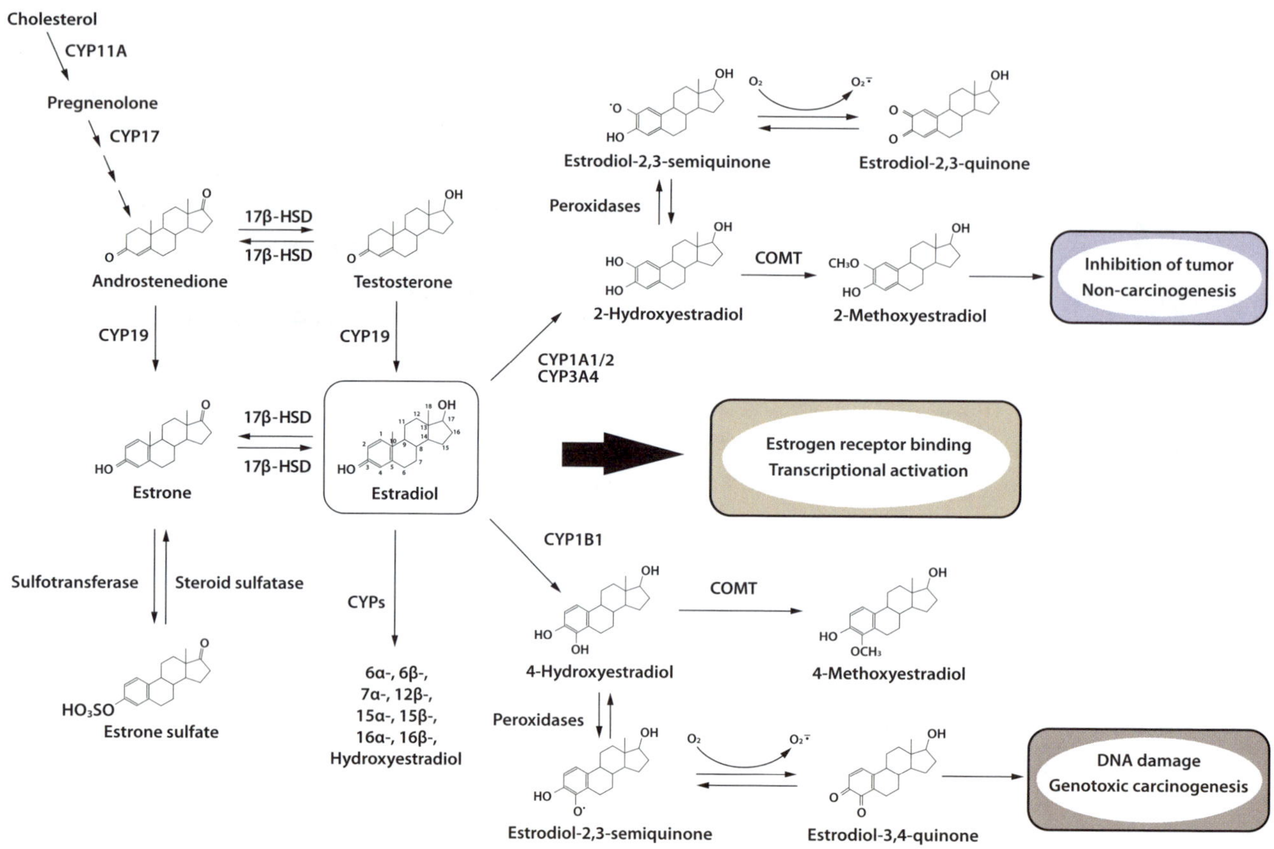

Figure 3.6 Cytochrome P450-mediated detoxification pathways of estradiol. From: Tsuchiya Y, Nakajima M, Yokoi T. Cytochrome P450-mediated metabolism of estrogens and its regulation in human. *Cancer Lett.* 2005 Sep 28;227(2):115-24. Used with permission from Elsevier.

risk.[83] Figure 3.6 displays the metabolic pathways of estradiol, and shows the consequences of either 1A1 or 1B1 induction.

CYP2 is a very diverse family containing the largest number of enzymes, numbering at least 12, of which 7 are known to be clinically important. Two important points may be illustrated through members of the CYP2 family—namely, that there is tremendous variation in activity between people, and that there is a significant interaction between genetic predisposition and environmental exposure.

Wide variability in activity

The enzymes CYP2C9, CYP2C19, and CYP2D6 are all known to have genetic variations that impact their catalytic efficacy. For example, 2C9 catalyzes S-warfarin metabolism, and at least 16 NSAIDs are partly metabolized by this enzyme.[84] Yet, the **2* and **3* alleles code for a less active enzyme, with allele frequencies of 10.5% and 8.4%, respectively, in a Caucasian population.[85] East Asians and African Americans were found to have allele frequencies of 0% and 3.2% for **2*, and 1–3% and 1.3% for **3*, respectively.[86] Similarly, 2C19 metabolizes amides and weak bases, and is the primary enzyme for proton pump inhibitor metabolism and some antidepressants. Yet, there is substantial variation in activity of this enzyme. Among the Asian population, up to 20% are considered poor metabolizers,[76] with a 5-fold difference in activity between poor metabolizers and extensive metabolizers (more so if CYP3A4 is also inhibited).[87] Additionally, there is an ultrapid allele found with a frequency of 18% in both Swedes and Ethiopians, and 4% in Chinese subjects,[88] emphasizing that one dose fits all is an unrealistic assumption for drugs metabolized by this enzyme.

The impact of genetic variation on clinical outcomes may be seen most clearly when considering CYP2D6 activity, perhaps the most well studied of all cytochrome enzymes. CYP2D6 metabolizes a large number of drugs (~25% of all), yet approximately 7% and 5.5% of Caucasians have been genotyped as either poor (PM) or ultrarapid metabolizers (UM), respectively. More adverse drug effects are seen in poor metabolizers, because they are essentially receiving at higher dose than someone with more rapid activity. Similarly, ineffective dosing is more common among ultrarapid metabolizers.[89,90] PM is nearly nonexistent among Asian populations, and UM is found with much higher frequency in Arabian and Eastern African populations (~30%).[91]

Polymorphisms and environmental interactions

CYP2D6 illustrates how important genetic predisposition is in determining the toxicity of exposures. In a study of Caucasian women with multiple chemical sensitivities (MCS), those with more active alleles had an OR of 3.36 compared to controls. When this was combined with high activity of N-acetyltransferase 2 (NAT2), the OR jumped to 18.7.[92] CYP2D6 involvement in Parkinson's disease risk is even more illustrative. A case-control study (with 247 cases and 676 controls) found that, in the absence of pesticides, those with low CYP2D6 activity are not at increased risk. However, when low CYP2D6 activity is combined with pesticide exposure, the risk increases to an OR of 2.0.[93] These results were supported by a second study, which found an OR of 2.09 for those with occasional pesticide exposure and low activity, and 8.41 for those with regular exposure and low activity.[94]

CYP2E1 is also a good example of how exposure interacts with enzymatic activity to determine outcome. This enzyme has a dominant role in metabolizing small molecular weight carcinogens, such as benzene, carbon tetrachloride, and vinyl chloride, but it is most studied for its role in determining acetaminophen (APAP) toxicity. It is a very inducible enzyme, particularly by alcohol, with induction resulting in the bioactivation of many toxins and drugs, as well as increased ROS production. Thus, induction combined with exposure to APAP results in the production of the more toxic metabolite (N-acetyl-p-benzoquinone imine [NAPQI]), which causes an increase in reactive oxygen species and nitrosamines, mitochondrial poisoning, lipid peroxidation, and covalent binding to proteins, with eventual necrosis.[95] This toxicity is amplified if glutathione is low (another effect of alcohol), because glutathione rapidly detoxifies NAPQI. APAP toxicity is by far the leading cause of acute liver failure in the U.S.[96] N-acetylcysteine restores hepatic glutathione, preventing liver damage and cerebral edema.[97]

Induction/inhibition by exogenous compounds affects activity

CYP3A4 is also a good example of an enzyme very susceptible to induction or inhibition by exposure, partly because it has very broad substrate specificity, accepting large and small substrates of various structures. Thus, grapefruit juice, azole antifungals, HIV antivirals, and zingiber compounds inhibit it significantly,[76,98] while St. John's wort induces its production.[99] This is quite clinically relevant because ~50% of drugs in clinical practice are metabolized by CYP3A4,[76] and the difference between induced and inhibited activity may be 400-fold.[91] For example, grapefruit juice reduces levels of CYP3A4 in intestinal cells by as much as 47% within 4 hours of ingestion, with an effect still present 24 hours later. Hypertensive medications may have their oral bioavailability increased over 100% by such an effect, as well as drugs such as benzodiazepines, antihistamines, statins, etc. CYP3A4 is also known to have associations with breast and prostate cancer, likely due to hydroxylation of estradiol at C2 and C16. It is inducible by many xenobiotics that target the pregnane X receptor, including glucocorticoids and phthalates.[100,101,102]

The other significant enzyme in this family is CYP3A5, which is detectable in only 10–30%

of adult Caucasians and Asians, whereas 60% of African Americans express the protein.[103] The frequency of the **3* allele, which is thought to have no activity, was found to be 85% in Caucasians, 76% in the Chinese population and about 60% in Malays and Indians, but only 48% among African-Americans. This has led to the hypothesis that CYP3A5 may be the most important genetic contributor to interindividual as well as interethnic differences in clearance of CYP3A substrates.[104] Updated references for all substrates, inducers, and inhibitors of CYP enzymes can be found at http://medicine.iupui.edu/flockhart/table.htm.

Phase II detoxification

Phase II enzymes generally increase the water solubility and molecular weight of a substrate, allowing for easier excretion from the body. In some cases, this is made easier by a phase I oxidation reaction that creates or exposes the conjugation site. Once conjugated, substrates of phase II become more hydrophilic and generally require a transporter to enter the bile or sinusoidal blood supply.[105] In general, phase II enzymes are much less inducible than phase I, but wide variation still exists in inter-individual activity levels. Additionally, several common polymorphisms have significant clinical impact.

Types of phase II reactions

Phase II reactions fall into several categories, including glucuronidation (UGT), sulfation, glutathione conjugation, glutathione S-transferase, acetylation (NAT), quinone reductase, epoxide hydrolase, N-, O-, or S-methylation, and amino acid conjugation. Many nutritional interventions can target support for phase II reactions, because they often rely on substrates which can be supplied. Usually, a deficit in phase II is in large part responsible for the accumulation of reactive intermediates.

Glucuronidation is the process of adding a sugar (uridine diphosphate-glucuronic acid, or UDP-GA) to a site often created by a phase I reaction. This usually results in inactivated detoxification products ready for biliary or urinary excretion (with some exceptions, such as morphine-6-glucuronide, which is more reactive). It typically works with sulfation, because although it is overwhelmed by high toxin exposure (e.g., acetaminophen), it has a much greater capacity (i.e., UDP-GA concentration is ~300–400 nmol/g liver vs. ~23 nmol/g liver PAPS).[105] Glucuronidation is reversible, often by enzymatic cleavage by beta-glucuronidase. While this enzyme has low activity in the liver, high activity in the gut microflora may result in enterohepatic recycling of parent compounds after cleavage.

Clinically, it is associated with Gilbert's syndrome, i.e., unconjugated hyperbilirubinemia caused by low activity of UGT1A1, characterized by mild jaundice and elevated serum total bilirubin. Gilbert's syndrome affects 5–11% of U.S., 4–12% of German,[106] 3–5% of Singapore,[107] and up to 36% of African populations.[108] Also, low activity genotypes are associated with increased rates of colon cancer in Caucasians, and may modify risk of exposure to heterocyclic amines.[109]

Sulfation has high affinity and low capacity for substrates; as mentioned above, it often works in conjunction with glucuronidation, especially when the sulfation pathway is saturated or limited by the sulfur pool. The sulfate donor, PAPS (3-phosphoadenosine-5-phosphosulfate), is dependent upon ATP sulfurylase and APS kinase, but most importantly the supply of inorganic sulfate. Thus sulfation is a cofactor, not a rate-limited enzyme.[105]

It has the highest activity in the periportal region of the liver (i.e., first catch), and is more active than glucuronidation when low amounts of substrate are present. Clinically, it is associated with intestinal toxicity, Alzheimer's disease, Parkinson's disease, motor neuron disease, rheumatoid arthritis, delayed food sensitivity, multiple chemical sensitivities, and diet-responsive autism.

Glutathione conjugation is a very important reaction, because many potent electrophiles which would otherwise covalently bind to intracellular macromolecules are instead conjugated to glutathione and eliminated. Although this reaction may occur spontaneously if hepatic glutathione levels are sufficient, it is much faster if catalyzed by glutathione S-transferase (GST). Clinically, polymorphisms in conjugation enzymes have been linked to a number of cancers. For example, lung cancer has shown mixed findings, but is probably associated with an increased risk with GST null polymorphisms.[110,111] For breast cancer, an analysis of over 3000 cases and 3000 controls participating in the Shanghai Breast Cancer Study found that women with a low activity genotype had a greater risk. This increased risk was somewhat modified by high cruciferous vegetable intake, as cruciferous vegetables are known to induce GST activity.[112] Similar results have been found for other cancers, highlighting the relationship between cruciferous intake and GST polymorphisms for kidney, bladder, and colorectal cancer.[113,114,119] Upregulation of GSTs may also protect against adverse effects of diesel exhaust,[115] and sulforaphane from cruciferous vegetables is a potent inducer of this benefit.[116] Low levels of glutathione and/or transferase activity are also associated with chronic exposure to chemical toxins and alcohol, cadmium exposure, AIDS/HIV, macular degeneration, Parkinson's disease, and other neurodegenerative disorders.[117]

Acetylation (NAT) generally reduces the toxicity of a substrate, but it may also increase toxicity. It is also a good example of the wide individual variability in phase II detoxification activity. For example, the slow acetylator phenotype is found in 52–68% of Caucasians and only 10–15% of Japanese.[118] Fast acetylation can be up to 4 times faster than slow acetylation. Clinically, a 40% increase in bladder cancer has been shown for those with the low activity genotype for NAT2, especially when exposed to carcinogens such as cigarette smoke.[119] Additionally, an increased risk of breast cancer in smokers has been shown, with an OR of 1.49 for slow genotypes and smokers.[120] There have been inconsistent findings in neurodegenerative disease.

Quinone reductase detoxifies quinones produced by phase I enzymes, auto exhaust, cigarette smoke, and any burned organic materials. Generally quinone reductases produce hydroxyquinones, which are more easily excreted. NQO2 has been shown to be highly polymorphic, but not NQO1. A number of inhibitors exist, including benzo(a) pyrene, quercetin,[122] and resveratrol.[123] Clinically, high activity has been associated with Parkinson's disease,[124] but greater activity may be protective against benzene toxicity.[125] Quinone reductase is also involved in reduction of Vitamin K.[126]

Epoxide hydrolases. Generally considered protective enzymes, they are involved in oxidative defense, with a role in the activation and detoxification of polycyclic aromatic hydrocarbons and aromatic amines. While most xenobiotics are made less reactive by phase I detoxification, some (such as benzo(a)pyrene), are made more toxic. Clinically, activity is determined by polymorphisms at 2 sites, with low activity associated with a 35% decrease in lung cancer risk.[127] Variations may also be involved in blood pressure regulation, inflammation, and cancer progression.[128]

N-, O-, S-methylation. Methylation has a number of biological roles. Methylation of sulfur atoms is required to generate methionine from homocysteine. Methylation of oxygen atoms often inactivates bioactive carboxylates, phenols, or alcohols. Methylation of aliphatic amines occurs on lysine residues in proteins, on phosphatidylethanolamine to yield phosphatidylcholine, and on epinephrine to produce norepinephrine. Methylation of nucleotide bases is an important mechanism by which the functions of DNA, nucleosomes, and transcription are influenced.[129]

Methylation is also significantly affected by nutrient status, with an upregulation caused by several lipotropic nutrients (choline, methionine, betaine, folic acid, and vitamin B12), as well as ellagic acid. It is also known to be inhibited by homocysteine, S-adenosyl-l-homocysteine (SAH), and a deficiency of folate, B6, or B12. COMT also has magnesium as a cofactor. As shown in Figure 3.7, SAH excess inhibits COMT, leading to a buildup of intermediates and radicals which cause damage to the cardiovascular and central nervous systems, an effect minimized by sufficient B vitamins.[130]

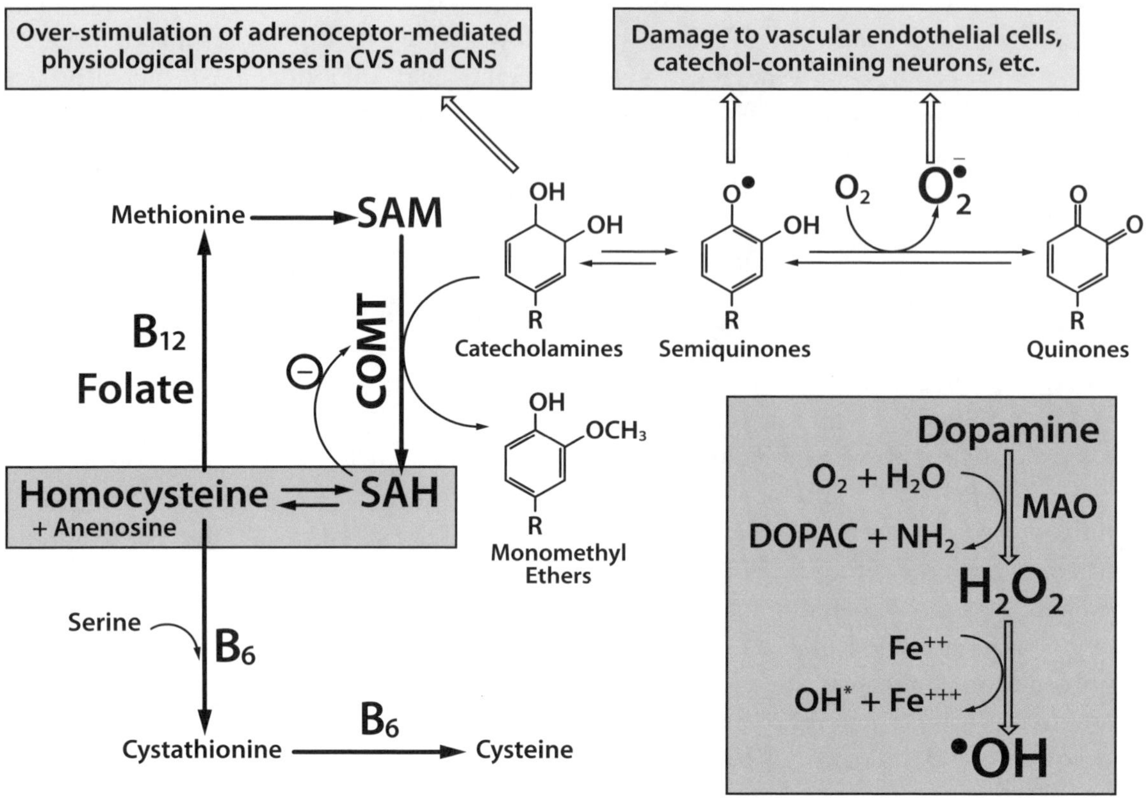

Figure 3.7 Proposed mechanism of homocysteine pathophysiology and pathogenesis based on accumulation of intracellular SAH. From: Zhu BT. Catechol-O-Methyltransferase (COMT)-mediated methylation metabolism of endogenous bioactive catechols and modulation by endobiotics and xenobiotics: importance in pathophysiology and pathogenesis. *Curr Drug Metab.* 2002 Jun;3(3):321-49. Used with permission from Bentham Science Publishers Ltd.

Clinically, the effects of inadequate methylation are most likely related to inappropriately detoxified steroidal hormones (breast cancer, PMS). Higher activity COMT polymorphisms have been associated with an approximate reduction in breast cancer risk of 30%.[131] Additionally, methylation activity also has been shown to affect the risk of atherosclerosis and neurological diseases (e.g., Alzheimer's, Parkinson's, and cognitive decline with aging).[132,133,134]

Amino acid conjugation involves initial formation of a xenobiotic acyl-CoA thioester, which in turn is conjugated to glycine or, to a lesser extent, taurine. This pathway is not as well characterized, mostly because it primarily metabolizes small compounds, and is not of significant drug-manufacturer interest. Clinically it is important in heavy alcohol consumption, intestinal toxicity, and toxemia of pregnancy.[135]

Dysfunctional detoxification patterns

Because most toxins are metabolized through a combination of phase I and phase II activities, the relationship between the phases is important in determining toxicity. For example, one of the imbalances most associated with harm is phase I in excess of phase II, i.e., fast bioactivation followed by slow removal. One example of this is the interaction between smoking and polymorphisms in acetylation genes (NAT2 genetic polymorphisms). Many of the toxins in smoke are activated to more reactive compounds by phase I; thus, a very active phase I combined with a low phase II is likely to increase the risk of harm. And, indeed, this is what we find, at least in regard to breast cancer. Numerous studies over the years have found that women with a genotype for slow acetylation have an increased risk for breast cancer, between

2–4-fold. Those with rapid acetylation do not appear to have any increased risk.[136,137]

Bowel detoxification

In addition to hepatic phase I and II detoxification, the bowel has recently been recognized as playing an important role in overall detoxification. A substantial portion of the toxic load on the liver comes from the bowel. Unique among the veins, the portal vein draining the bowel goes directly to the liver (Figure 3.8). There, when functioning properly, the Kupffer cells (imbedded white cells) filter and detoxify 99% of the toxins coming from the portal vein. These toxins include whole and parts of bacteria, undigested proteins, immune complexes, bacterial metabolic products, etc.

A bowel with anaerobic dysbiosis, increased permeability, and enterocyte inflammation increases the load on the liver and the risk of systemic effects. Fortunately, a bowel with healthy flora may do just the opposite. Animal studies have shown that *Lactobacillus acidophilus* reduces the load on the liver by increasing first-pass metabolism, and protecting the liver and stomach from injury.[138] And bifidobacteria, by reducing the level of endotoxin, may be able to reduce the rate of diabetes and obesity.[139] Additionally, gut flora may play an important role in detoxifying a number of chemicals, including heterocyclic aromatic amines.[140,141] Unfortunately, the antibiotic use that leads to dysbiosis is widespread, and in some cases unintentional; the NHANES 2003–2004 data found that 75% of the U.S. population age 6 or higher had detectable concentrations of triclosan, a broad antimicrobial, in their urine.[142]

Assessment

A comprehensive assessment of the detoxification system involves an evaluation of exposure to

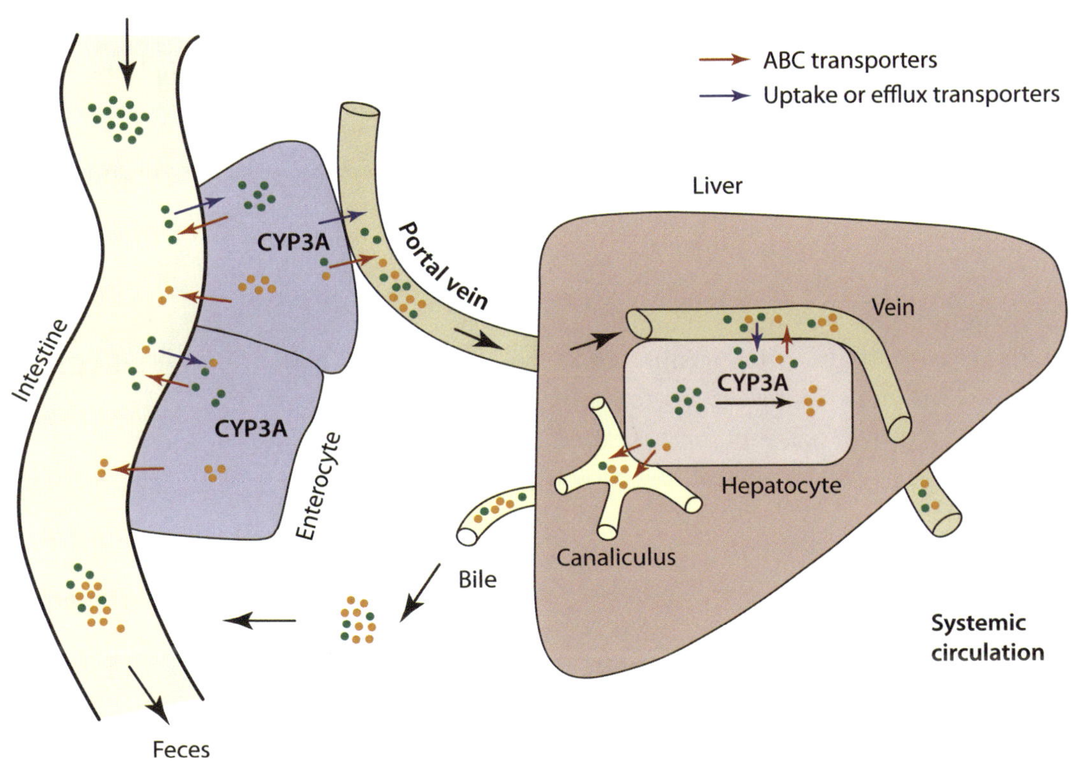

Figure 3.8 First-pass metabolism after oral administration of a drug and interaction with grapefruit juice. From: van Herwaarden AE. How important is intestinal cytochrome P450 3A metabolism? *Trends Pharmacol Sci.* 2009 May;30(5):223-7. Used with permission from Elsevier.

various toxins, as well as analysis of the detoxification systems themselves. Ideally, this would include evaluation of hepatic detoxification as well as bowel detoxification, given that the greatest portion of the toxic load on the liver comes from the bowel. Evaluation of increased intestinal permeability is an important determination in patients exhibiting signs and symptoms of poor detoxification. See page 2.17 on the lactulose/mannitol test to evaluate small intestine permeability.

Evaluation of exposure

Unfortunately, no gold standard exists for the evaluation of many environmental toxins, although many tests are clinically available to measure toxin levels in the serum, urine, feces, and adipose tissue. In general, serum and urine levels represent acute exposure, but often do not represent chronic exposure. For example, blood lead levels are quite accurate for detecting current exposure, but very poor in determining chronic exposure, or body burden.[143] The body burden of lead (determined by bone lead levels) is quite significant in predicting disease risk. In a prospective trial of nearly 1000 men, bone lead was found to be associated with all cause (HR 2.52) and cardiovascular (HR 5.63) mortality. It should be emphasized that this population of men had low blood lead levels, i.e., they did not currently have significant exposure.[144] Clinicians should recognize both that urine, serum, and fecal levels of toxins only represent acute exposure, and that exposure does not necessarily reflect the toxicity of a substance. Keeping this in mind, practitioners now have a new tool to at least assess the exposure level of their patients compared to national standards. The CDC has published national exposure data for serum or tissue levels for many heavy metals and POPs, and although reference ranges are not available for toxicity, they are for exposure (http://www.cdc.gov/exposurereport/). Lastly, for fat-soluble substances, it may be assumed that toxin distribution is equal in all adipose tissue, and represented by lipid-adjusted serum values.[145]

Evaluation of heavy metal exposure

While many POPs and solvents may be assessed through serum or urine for acute exposure, and adipose tissue for body burden, heavy metals may also be assessed through chelation (i.e., urinary provocation or challenge). Metallic mercury, for example, has a short half-life in the blood; therefore, a 24-hour urine is the preferred assessment method, unless testing within 3 days of exposure, while whole blood is the primary indicator for acute ethyl/methyl exposure.[146] Hair Hg >5 ppm is sometimes used to indicate mercury intoxication, but poor detoxifiers have false negatives, and it is not a good estimate of inorganic mercury, (although it is better for acute methylmercury exposure). For example, an EPA study found a decrease in IQ of 0.18 points for each ppm increase in maternal hair mercury.[147]

In addition to laboratory evaluation, many clinicians use symptom/exposure questionnaires to evaluate risk. The following is a short questionnaire which may indicate heavy metal exposure.[148]

- Has the patient knowingly been exposed to metals?
- What is the patient's occupation (dentist, welder, ship builder, etc.)?
- How frequently does the patient eat tuna, swordfish or shark?
- Does the patient have mercury amalgam fillings?
- If the patient is taking any dietary supplements, do they have certificates of analysis that they are free of contaminants?
- Is the patient taking any Ayurvedic or traditional Chinese medicine dietary supplements?
- Does the patient experience a metallic taste in their mouth, and has not recently been taking medications documented to cause metallic taste?
- Does the patient have a history of smoking (particularly high in cadmium)?

Urinary provocation with a chelating agent

Unprovoked urine, representing acute exposure, has reference ranges established for the U.S. population for various toxins, but many clinicians use a chelating agent to determine chronic exposure. There are limitations to this procedure. Specifically, there are no reference ranges for provoked urine, and most chelating agents do not extract metals from all tissues, and thus do not necessarily represent an accurate body burden. For example, the brain is one of the main target organs for both elemental and organic mercury, yet no chelating agents are able to extract brain mercury.[149] Despite these limitations, provocation tests are widely used and advocated by clinicians based on empirical evidence; pre- and post-treatment provocation tests can help to determine the efficacy of a particular chelating agent, offering a guide for future treatment.

The value of chelating agents may vary from one metal to another. For example, use of a chelating agent may be superior to blood for evaluating chronic lead exposure. Because more than 90% of body lead is stored in bones and not detected in blood, provoked lead reflects the toxicologically active fraction of the total lead body burden. In individuals with previous lead exposure but low recent exposure, blood lead may be only slightly increased, whereas the mobilizable pool is significantly increased.[150]

Evaluation of detoxification capacity

While laboratory evaluations are not available for every enzyme and phase II reaction, there are several standard assessments that may be clinically useful. For example, caffeine is often used as a probe to determine CYP1A2 activity and glucuronidation may be assessed by acetaminophen clearance, i.e., low activity results in low urine acetaminophen glucuronides. More specific probes for glucuronidation include estradiol (3OH-glucuronidation; UGT1A1), trifluoperazine (UGT1A4) serotonin (UGT1A6), propofol (UGT1A9), 3'-azidothymidine (UGT2B7), and S-oxazepam (UGT2B15).[151]

Sulfation can also be assessed with acetaminophen, with low activity showing low urinary acetaminophen sulfates. Glutathione conjugation can be assessed with both genomic testing, as well as acetaminophen clearance (low urine acetaminophen mercapturates). Methyl bromide or ethylene oxide may also be used as probes.[152] Methylation is often roughly approximated with homocysteine levels, while amino acid conjugation may be determined by measuring the level of urinary salicyluric acid following acetylsalicylic acid administration.[153]

Examples of phase I enzymes with reliable genomic tests include CYP2C9 (**2* and **3* alleles have low activity); CYP2C19 (ultrarapid alleles and those with low activity); and CYP2D6 (poor and extensive metabolizer genotype). Phase II pathways with good genomic predictability include acetylation, methylation, and glucuronidation.

Treatment

General

The most important dietary guidelines for supporting detoxification process are also those that support good general health: eat a health promoting diet; consume plenty of organic vegetables and legumes for their high fiber and nutrient content; and drink at least 48 ounces of water each day. Eating a mostly plant-based diet has the benefit of reducing toxin exposure, providing nutrients for phase II support, and ensuring higher antioxidant intake. Certain foods are particularly helpful because they contain the nutrients needed to produce and activate the dozens of enzymes involved in the various phases of detoxification.

Such foods include:

- Garlic, legumes, onions, eggs, and other foods with a high sulfur content.
- Good sources of water-soluble fibers, such as pears, oat bran, apples, and legumes.
- Cabbage-family vegetables, especially broccoli, Brussels sprouts, and cabbage.

- Artichokes, beets, carrots, dandelion greens, and many herbs and spices such as turmeric, cinnamon, and licorice.
- Green foods like green leafy vegetables, green tea, wheat grass juice, dehydrated barley grass juice, chlorella, and spirulina.

Additionally, any therapeutic program should include an evaluation for acute exposure and, if present, should identify the source and remove it. Chelation is often used to treat heavy metal intoxication, along with supportive therapies that include replacing minerals depleted by chelation, providing antioxidant support, and supporting the detoxification systems, including liver and bowel detoxification. For general support of detoxification process, the principles that were described in Clinical Focus 1—A Cellular Approach to Health are applicable here.

Antioxidant support

Nutrients that boost cellular glutathione and antioxidant levels are of critical importance. Stimulating glutathione production is perhaps the most important goal in cellular protection because so much of the damage induced by toxins is due to reactive oxygen species. Additionally, some antioxidants also have the potential to reduce the burden of toxins, including heavy metals. For example, vitamins C and E have been shown to be protective against oxidative damage, and in one human study they also showed a small reduction in lead retention.[154] N-acetylcysteine (NAC) and alpha-lipoic acid both increase cellular levels of glutathione, which binds to mercury and reactive oxygen species and participates in the detoxification of many xenobiotics via conjugation reactions. They are also powerful antioxidants and have been found to reduce toxicity to multiple organs from lead, arsenic, mercury, and cadmium.[155,156] Lipoic acid not only protects against mercury damage to the nervous system, but it also reduces the hepatotoxicity and ototoxicity of cadmium.[157]

Other antioxidants that may have particular benefit during detoxification are melatonin and carotenoids. Melatonin, a powerful antioxidant, has shown a protective benefit in animal studies of lead, cadmium, and arsenic toxicity. And serum levels of alpha and beta carotene had a significant dose-response relationship for arsenic-related ischemic heart disease.[158,159,160,161]

Detoxification pathway and hepatic support

Other nutrients which support detoxification include sodium glucuronate, shown to support the phase II pathway of detoxification by providing the precursor for glucuronidation. Conjugation of glucuronic acid with a wide variety of functional groups, including hydroxyls, phenols, and carboxyls, is mediated in the liver as well as the intestine. Green tea has been shown to protect the liver from CYP2E1-dependent alcoholic liver damage, as well as to inhibit the proliferation of breast cancer cells *in vitro* and *in vivo*.[162,163] Alpha-lipoic acid is a water- and fat-soluble antioxidant, involved in hepatoprotection and cell damage prevention. It has the ability to alter the redox status of cells and interact with thiols, increasing hepatic glutathione content. Silybin is the most active flavonolignan isomer of silymarin, acting through a number of pathways, including antioxidative, anti-lipid peroxidative, antifibrotic, anti-inflammatory, and liver regenerating mechanisms. It also enhances glucuronidation and protects against glutathione depletion. The amino acid taurine supports amino acid conjugation, with animal studies suggesting a protective effect against cadmium toxicity.[164,165]

The use of curcumin is also recommended. Curcumin upregulates a number of phase II enzymes, including GST and NAD(P)H:quinone oxidoreductase-1, and it also downregulates some phase I enzymes associated with carcinogenic toxicity.[166] It has been shown to protect against arsenic toxicity, prevent DNA damage, and enhance DNA repair enzymes against arsenic-induced damage.[167] Among the numerous other benefits of curcumin is the prevention of mitochondrial oxidative damage, suggesting a role in neurodegenerative disease.[168]

Heavy metal detoxification

With higher body heavy metal burden it may be necessary to use one of the many chelating agents now available for removing heavy metals from the body, including DMPS, DMSA, EDTA, BAL, d-penicillamine (DPA), and newer esters of DMSA. Although not intended as a complete guide, the following suggestions as to which agent is best suited for each of the more common heavy metals should be useful.

Mercury is often chelated with either DMSA or DMPS. Of the two, DMSA is certainly the least toxic, and may be given orally.[169] Unfortunately, neither removes CNS mercury, and both also chelate copper, zinc, and chromium (DMPS), which should be supplemented between treatments. Along with traditional chelating agents, lipoic acid has been shown to prevent neuronal damage from mercury, as well as increase its excretion.[170]

Lead chelation with EDTA has a long history, and it is still the agent most often used. Despite this, oral DMSA has been shown to be as effective, although it may mobilize different sites of lead deposition. EDTA also depletes Zn, Cu, Fe, Co, and Mn. Although DMSA may not remove bone lead, it has been shown to reduce hippocampal lead. Lastly, a combination of both EDTA and DMSA may be more effective than either alone. In a study of lead-exposed workers, an initial dose of EDTA increased the amount excreted by subsequent DMSA.[171,172]

For both **arsenic** and **cadmium** chelation, DMSA is quite useful for acute exposure, but is unlikely to remove intracellular levels of these heavy metals. The DMSA derivative monoisoamyl dimercaptosuccinic acid (MiADMSA) has been shown to remove arsenic from blood and soft tissue when given with DMSA, but in animal studies only. Similarly, the DMSA derivatives (monomethyl DMSA [MmDMSA] and monocyclohexyl DMSA [MchDMSA]) have been shown to reduce total body cadmium with no redistribution of brain calcium, but in animal studies only.[173,174,175]

As mentioned above, two of the most potent antioxidants with particular benefit for treating heavy metal toxicity are N-acetylcysteine (NAC) and alpha-lipoic acid. NAC, for example, has shown benefit as an antioxidant for lead, arsenic, and cadmium toxicity, and it may also assist in mercury removal. *Spirulina platensis* has also been found to protect against heavy metal induced organ damage as well as to prevent anemia, leukopenia and the deposition of heavy metals in the brain. Spirulina also contains significant amounts of alkaline phosphatase activity, which may assist in the detoxification of organophosphorus pesticides. Forty-one patients of chronic arsenic poisoning were randomly treated orally by either placebo or spirulina extract (250 mg) plus zinc (2 mg) twice daily for 16 weeks. There was a sharp increase in urinary excretion of arsenic (138 mcg/l) at 4 weeks following spirulina plus zinc administration and the effect was continued for another 2 weeks. Spirulina extract plus zinc removed 47.1% arsenic from scalp hair. In spirulina extract plus zinc-treated group, the clinical scores for keratosis before and after treatment was statistically significant.[176]

Treatment of bowel intoxication

Because many toxins originate in the GI tract —e.g., bacteria, undigested proteins, immune complexes, and metabolic products—and because increased intestinal permeability and enterocyte inflammation increase the load on hepatic detoxification, a basic program for eliminating unhealthy bacteria, reseeding and supporting healthy flora, and restoring intestinal membrane integrity is recommended as part of any detoxification program.

Nutrients such as L-glutamine can help restore GI integrity; it is the primary amino acid source for intestinal cells, and an important regulator of intercellular junction integrity.[177,178] Probiotics may be particularly beneficial for assisting in detoxification. As mentioned earlier, many toxins increase the risk for diabetes and metabolic syndrome via endocrine disruption. Bifidobacterium has been shown to reduce the rate of diabetes and obesity by lowering endotoxin levels.[179]

Additional considerations

Fasting, sauna, and hydrotherapy have all shown benefit for reducing the body burden of toxins; they are often used in combination. The use of a sauna, for example, helps to eliminate cadmium, lead, PCBs, PBBs, and HCBs, as well as increase the rate of lipolysis.[180] Similarly, fasting has been shown to help eliminate PCBs, DDT, and circulating immune complexes from food allergies.[181,182] Certainly any fasting, particularly long-term, should be done with caution and under physician supervision.

Summary

Toxin exposure is widespread, with diverse chemical and environmental toxins proven to have damaging health consequences, and minimal research documenting their interactions within living organisms. In addition to toxin avoidance, enhancing a patient's detoxification and elimination capacity helps to both minimize their total load of toxins, and reduce the harm caused by their current exposure. This chapter provides the latest research related to environmental toxicity, and suggests optimal treatment plans for restoring a healthy detoxification system.

References

1. De Rosa CT, Hicks HE, Ashizawa AE, et al. A regional approach to assess the impact of living in a chemical world. *Ann N Y Acad Sci*. 2006 Sep;1076:829-38.
2. Cory-Slechta DA. Studying toxicants as single chemicals: does this strategy adequately identify neurotoxic risk? *Neurotoxicology*. 2005 Aug;26(4):491-510.
3. De Rosa CT. Restoring the foundation: Tracking chemical exposures and human health. *Environ Health Perspect*. 2003 Jun;111(7):A374-5.
4. Ingelman-Sundberg M. The human genome project and novel aspects of cytochrome P450 research. *Toxicol Appl Pharmacol*. 2005 Sep 1;207(2 Suppl):52-6.
5. Gallagher CM, Kovach JS, Meliker JR. Urinary cadmium and osteoporosis in U.S. Women >or= 50 years of age: NHANES 1988-1994 and 1999-2004. *Environ Health Perspect*. 2008.
6. Everett CJ, Frithsen IL. Association of urinary cadmium and myocardial infarction. *Environ Res*. 2008.
7. Navas-Acien A, Silbergeld EK, Pastor-Barriuso R, et al. Arsenic exposure and prevalence of type 2 diabetes in U.S. adults. *JAMA*. 2008.
8. Iqbal S, et al. Estimated burden of blood lead levels 5 microg/dl in 1999-2002 and declines from 1988 to 1994. *Environ Res*. 2008.
9. Lee DH. A strong dose-response relation between serum concentrations of persistent organic pollutants and diabetes: results from the National Health and Examination Survey 1999-2002. *Diabetes Care*. 2006.
10. Lee DH, et al. Relationship between serum concentrations of persistent organic pollutants and the prevalence of metabolic syndrome among non diabetic adults: results from the National Health and Nutrition Examination Survey 1999-2002. *Diabetologia*. 2007.
11. Lee DH, et al. Association of organochlorine pesticides with peripheral neuropathy in patients with diabetes or impaired fasting glucose. *Diabetes*. 2008 Nov;57(11):3108-11. Epub 2008 Jul 22.
12. Lee DH. Positive associations of serum concentration of polychlorinated biphenyls or organochlorine pesticides with self-reported arthritis, especially rheumatoid type, in women. *Environ Health Perspect*. 2007.
13. Ha MH, et al. Association between serum concentrations of persistent organic pollutants and self-reported cardiovascular disease prevalence: results from the National Health and Nutrition Examination Survey, 1999-2002. *Environ Health Perspect*. 2007.
14. Priyadarshi A, Khuder SA, Schaub EA, et al. Environmental risk factors and Parkinson's disease: a metaanalysis. *Environ Res*. 2001.
15. Limón-Pacheco J, Gonsebatt ME. The role of antioxidants and antioxidant-related enzymes in protective responses to environmentally induced oxidative stress. *Mutat Res*. 2008 Oct 8. Epub ahead of print.
16. Bertin G, Averbeck D. Cadmium: cellular effects, modifications of biomolecules, modulation of DNA repair and genotoxic consequences (a review). *Biochimie*. 2006 Nov;88(11):1549-59.
17. Ercal N, Gurer-Orhan H, Aykin-Burns N. Toxic metals and oxidative stress part I: mechanisms involved in metal-induced oxidative damage. *Curr Top Med Chem*. 2001 Dec;1(6):529-39.
18. Kawata K, Yokoo H, Shimazaki R, et al. Classification of heavy-metal toxicity by human DNA microarray analysis. *Environ Sci Technol*. 2007 May 15;41(10):3769-74.
19. Kim SJ, Jeong HJ, Myung NY, et al. The protective mechanism of antioxidants in cadmium-induced ototoxicity *in vitro* and *in vivo*. *Environ Health Perspect*. 2008 Jul;116(7):854-62.
20. Durak D, Uzun FG, Kalender S, et al. Malathion-induced oxidative stress in human erythrocytes and the protective effect of vitamins C and E *in vitro*. *Environ Toxicol*. 2008 Jul 24. Epub ahead of print.
21. Delgado EH, Streck EL, Quevedo JL, et al. Mitochondrial respiratory dysfunction and oxidative stress after chronic malathion exposure. *Neurochem Res*. 2006 Aug;31(8):1021-5.
22. Drechsel DA, Patel M. Role of reactive oxygen species in the neurotoxicity of environmental agents implicated in Parkinson's disease. *Free Radic Biol Med*. 2008 Jun 1;44(11):1873-86.
23. Migliore L, Coppedè F. Environmental-induced oxidative stress in neurodegenerative disorders and aging. *Mutat Res*. 2008 Oct 5. Epub ahead of print.
24. Warren MJ, Cooper JB, Wood SP, et al. Lead poisoning, haem synthesis and 5-aminolaevulinic acid dehydratase. *Trends Biochem Sci*. 1998 Jun;23(6):217-21.
25. Jaffe EK, Martins J, Li J, et al. The molecular mechanism of lead inhibition of human porphobilinogen synthase. *J Biol Chem*. 2001 Jan 12;276(2):1531-7.
26. Mehta M, Chen LC, Gordon T, et al. Particulate matter inhibits DNA repair and enhances mutagenesis. *Mutat Res*. 2008 Aug 29. Epub ahead of print.
27. Garte S, Taioli E, Popov T, et al. Genetic susceptibility to benzene toxicity in humans. *J Toxicol Environ Health A*. 2008;71(22):1482-9.
28. Wong RH, Chang SY, Ho SW, et al. Polymorphisms in metabolic GSTP1 and DNA-repair XRCC1 genes with an increased risk of DNA damage in pesticide-exposed fruit growers. *Mutat Res*. 2008 Jul 31;654(2):168-75.
29. Liu YJ, Huang PL, Chang YF, et al. GSTP1 genetic polymorphism is associated with a higher risk of DNA damage in pesticide-exposed fruit growers. *Cancer Epidemiol Biomarkers Prev*. 2006 Apr;15(4):659-66.
30. Meeker JD, Barr DB, Hauser R. Human semen quality and sperm DNA damage in relation to urinary metabolites of pyrethroid insecticides. *Hum Reprod*. 2008 Aug;23(8):1932-40.

31. Hauser R, Meeker JD, Singh NP, et al. DNA damage in human sperm is related to urinary levels of phthalate monoester and oxidative metabolites. *Hum Reprod.* 2007 Mar;22(3):688-95.
32. Babu KR, Rajmohan HR, Rajan BK, et al. Plasma lipid peroxidation and erythrocyte antioxidant enzymes status in workers exposed to cadmium. *Toxicol Ind Health.* 2006 Sep;22(8):329-35.
33. Stark G. Functional consequences of oxidative membrane damage. *J Membr Biol.* 2005 May;205(1):1-16.
34. Yücebilgiç G, Bilgin R, Tamer L, et al. Effects of lead on Na(+)-K(+) ATPase and Ca(+2) ATPase activities and lipid peroxidation in blood of workers. *Int J Toxicol.* 2003 Mar-Apr;22(2):95-7.
35. Mattson MP. Roles of the lipid peroxidation product 4-hydroxynonenal in obesity, the metabolic syndrome, and associated vascular and neurodegenerative disorders. *Exp Gerontol.* 2009 Oct;44(10):625-33.
36. Sanderson JT. The steroid hormone biosynthesis pathway as a target for endocrine-disrupting chemicals. *Toxicol Sci.* 2006 Nov;94(1):3-21.
37. Davey JC, Nomikos AP, Wungjiranirun M, et al. Arsenic as an endocrine disruptor: arsenic disrupts retinoic acid receptor-and thyroid hormone receptor-mediated gene regulation and thyroid hormone-mediated amphibian tail metamorphosis. *Environ Health Perspect.* 2008 Feb;116(2):165-72.
38. Navas-Acien A, Silbergeld EK, Pastor-Barriuso R, et al. Arsenic exposure and prevalence of type 2 diabetes in U.S. adults. *JAMA.* 2008 Aug 20;300(7):814-22.
39. Díaz-Villaseñor A, Burns AL, Hiriart M, et al. Arsenic-induced alteration in the expression of genes related to type 2 diabetes mellitus. *Toxicol Appl Pharmacol.* 2007 Dec 1;225(2):123-33.
40. Müllerová D, Kopecký J. White adipose tissue: storage and effector site for environmental pollutants. *Physiol Res.* 2007;56(4):375-81.
41. Grün F, Blumberg B. Environmental obesogens: organotins and endocrine disruption via nuclear receptor signaling. *Endocrinology.* 2006 Jun;147(6 Suppl):S50-5.
42. Hatch EE, Nelson JW, Qureshi MM, et al. Association of urinary phthalate metabolite concentrations with body mass index and waist circumference: a cross-sectional study of NHANES data, 1999-2002. *Environ Health.* 2008 Jun 3;7:27.
43. Frederiksen H, Skakkebaek NE, Andersson AM. Metabolism of phthalates in humans. *Mol Nutr Food Res.* 2007 Jul;51(7):899-911.
44. Silva MJ, Barr DB, Reidy JA, et al. Glucuronidation patterns of common urinary and serum monoester phthalate metabolites. *Arch Toxicol.* 2003 Oct;77(10):561-7.
45. Huang PC, Tsai EM, Li WF, et al. Association between phthalate exposure and glutathione S-transferase M1 polymorphism in adenomyosis, leiomyoma and endometriosis. *Hum Reprod.* 2010 Apr;25(4):986-94. Epub 2010.
46. Iqbal S, Muntner P, Batuman V, et al. Estimated burden of blood lead levels 5 microg/dl in 1999-2002 and declines from 1988 to 1994. *Environ Res.* 2008 Jul;107(3):305-11.
47. Schober SE, Mirel LB, Graubard BI, et al. Blood lead levels and death from all causes, cardiovascular disease, and cancer: results from the NHANES III mortality study. *Environ Health Perspect.* 2006 Oct;114(10):1538-41.
48. Schober SE, Sinks TH, Jones RL, et al. Blood mercury levels in U.S. children and women of childbearing age, 1999-2000. *JAMA.* 2003 Apr 2;289(13):1667-74.
49. Mahaffey KR, Clickner RP, Bodurow CC. Blood organic mercury and dietary mercury intake: National Health and Nutrition Examination Survey, 1999 and 2000. *Environ Health Perspect.* 2004 Apr;112(5):562-70.
50. Mahaffey KR, Clickner RP, Bodurow CC. Blood organic mercury and dietary mercury intake: National Health and Nutrition Examination Survey, 1999 and 2000. *Environ Health Perspect.* 2004 Apr;112(5):562-70.
51. Dórea JG. Studies of fish consumption as source of methylmercury should consider fish-meal-fed farmed fish and other animal foods. *Environ Res.* 2009.
52. Ha MH, Lee DH, Jacobs DR. Association between serum concentrations of persistent organic pollutants and self-reported cardiovascular disease prevalence: results from the National Health and Nutrition Examination Survey, 1999-2002. *Environ Health Perspect.* 2007 Aug;115(8):1204-9.
53. Darras VM. Endocrine disrupting polyhalogenated organic pollutants interfere with thyroid hormone signalling in the developing brain. *Cerebellum.* 2008;7(1):26-37.
54. Boersma ER, Lanting CI. Environmental exposure to polychlorinated biphenyls (PCBs) and dioxins. Consequences for longterm neurological and cognitive development of the child lactation. *Adv Exp Med Biol.* 2000;478:271-87.
55. Lee DH, Jacobs DR, Porta M. Association of serum concentrations of persistent organic pollutants with the prevalence of learning disability and attention deficit disorder. *J Epidemiol Community Health.* 2007 Jul;61(7):591-6.
56. Lee DH, Lee IK, Jin SH, et al. Association between serum concentrations of persistent organic pollutants and insulin resistance among nondiabetic adults: results from the National Health and Nutrition Examination Survey 1999-2002. *Diabetes Care.* 2007 Mar;30(3):622-8.
57. http://www.ewg.org/node/26128 Accessed 3-28-10.
58. http://archive.ewg.org/reports/bodyburden1/es.php Accessed 3-30-10.
59. Uversky VN. Synergistic effects of pesticides and metals on the fibrillation of alpha-synuclein: implications for Parkinson's disease. *Neurotoxicology.* 2002.
60. Crooke PS, Ritchie MD, Hachey DL, et al. Estrogens, enzyme variants, and breast cancer: a risk model. *Cancer Epidemiol Biomarkers Prev.* 2006 Sep;15(9):1620-9.

61. Dawling S, Hachey DL, Roodi N, et al. *In vitro* model of mammary estrogen metabolism: structural and kinetic differences between catechol estrogens 2- and 4-hydroxyestradiol. *Chem Res Toxicol.* 2004 Sep;17(9):1258-64.

62. Perła-Kaján J, Twardowski T, Jakubowski H. Mechanisms of homocysteine toxicity in humans. *Amino Acids.* 2007;32(4):561-72.

63. Jakubowski H. Pathophysiological consequences of homocysteine excess. *J Nutr.* 2006 Jun;136(6 Suppl):1741S-1749S.

64. Kölker S, Okun JG. Methylmalonic acid—an endogenous toxin? *Cell Mol Life Sci.* 2005 Mar;62(6):621-4.

65. Morath MA, Okun JG, Müller IB, et al. Neurodegeneration and chronic renal failure in methylmalonic aciduria—a pathophysiological approach. *J Inherit Metab Dis.* 2008 Feb;31(1):35-43.

66. Maes M, Kubera M, Leunis JC. The gut-brain barrier in major depression: intestinal mucosal dysfunction with an increased translocation of LPS from gram negative enterobacteria (leaky gut) plays a role in the inflammatory pathophysiology of depression. *Neuro Endocrinol Lett.* 2008 Feb;29(1):117-24.

67. Maes M, Coucke F, Leunis JC. Normalization of the increased translocation of endotoxin from gram negative enterobacteria (leaky gut) is accompanied by a remission of chronic fatigue syndrome. *Neuro Endocrinol Lett.* 2007 Dec;28(6):739-44.

68. Caradonna L, Amati L, Magrone T, et al. Enteric bacteria, lipopolysaccharides and related cytokines in inflammatory bowel disease: biological and clinical significance. *J Endotoxin Res.* 2000;6(3):205-14.

69. Erridge C, Attina T, Spickett CM, et al. A high-fat meal induces low-grade endotoxemia: evidence of a novel mechanism of postprandial inflammation. *Am J Clin Nutr.* 2007 Nov;86(5):1286-92.

70. Purohit V, Bode JC, Bode C, et al. Alcohol, intestinal bacterial growth, intestinal permeability to endotoxin, and medical consequences: summary of a symposium. *Alcohol.* 2008 Aug;42(5):349-61.

71. Belle DJ, Singh H. Genetic factors in drug metabolism. *Am Fam Physician.* 2008 Jun 1;77(11):1553-60.

72. Zanger UM, Raimundo S, Eichelbaum M. Cytochrome P450 2D6: overview and update on pharmacology, genetics, biochemistry. *Naunyn Schmiedebergs Arch Pharmacol.* 2004 Jan;369(1):23-37.

73. Kuehl P, Zhang J, Lin Y, et al. Sequence diversity in CYP3A promoters and characterization of the genetic basis of polymorphic CYP3A5 expression. *Nat Genet.* 2001 Apr;27(4):383-91.

74. Lin JH, Lu AY. Interindividual variability in inhibition and induction of cytochrome P450 enzymes. *Annu Rev Pharmacol Toxicol.* 2001;41:535-67.

75. Ingelman-Sundberg M. The human genome project and novel aspects of cytochrome P450 research. *Toxicol Appl Pharmacol.* 2005 Sep 1;207(2 Suppl):52-6.

76. Pelkonen O, Turpeinen M, Hakkola J, et al. Inhibition and induction of human cytochrome P450 enzymes: current status. *Arch Toxicol.* 2008 Oct;82(10):667-715.

77. Seliskar M, Rozman D. Mammalian cytochromes P450—importance of tissue specificity. *Biochim Biophys Acta.* 2007 Mar;1770(3):458-66.

78. Galetin A, Houston JB. Intestinal and hepatic metabolic activity of five cytochrome P450 enzymes: impact on prediction of first-pass metabolism. *J Pharmacol Exp Ther.* 2006 Sep;318(3):1220-9.

79. Yang J, Jamei M, Yeo KR, et al. Prediction of intestinal first-pass drug metabolism. *Curr Drug Metab.* 2007 Oct;8(7):676-84.

80. Hung RJ, Boffetta P, Brockmöller J, et al. CYP1A1 and GSTM1 genetic polymorphisms and lung cancer risk in Caucasian non-smokers: a pooled analysis. *Carcinogenesis.* 2003 May;24(5):875-82.

81. Wen W, Ren Z, Shu XO, et al. Expression of cytochrome P450 1B1 and catechol-O-methyltransferase in breast tissue and their associations with breast cancer risk. *Cancer Epidemiol Biomarkers Prev.* 2007 May;16(5):917-20.

82. Beuten J, Gelfond JA, Byrne JJ, et al. CYP1B1 variants are associated with prostate cancer in non-Hispanic and Hispanic Caucasians. *Carcinogenesis.* 2008 Sep;29(9):1751-7.

83. Mense SM, Chhabra J, Bhat HK. Preferential induction of cytochrome P450 1A1 over cytochrome P450 1B1 in human breast epithelial cells following exposure to quercetin. *J Steroid Biochem Mol Biol.* 2008 May;110(1-2):157-62.

84. Kirchheiner J, Brockmöller J. Clinical consequences of cytochrome P450 2C9 polymorphisms. *Clin Pharmacol Ther.* 2005 Jan;77(1):1-16.

85. Higashi MK, Veenstra DL, Kondo LM, et al. Association between CYP2C9 genetic variants and anticoagulation-related outcomes during warfarin therapy. *JAMA.* 2002 Apr 3;287(13):1690-8.

86. Xie HG, Prasad HC, Kim RB, et al. CYP2C9 allelic variants: ethnic distribution and functional significance. *Adv Drug Deliv Rev.* 2002 Nov 18;54(10):1257-70.

87. Desta Z, Zhao X, Shin JG, et al. Clinical significance of the cytochrome P450 2C19 genetic polymorphism. *Clin Pharmacokinet.* 2002;41(12):913-58.

88. Sim SC, Risinger C, Dahl ML, et al. A common novel CYP2C19 gene variant causes ultrarapid drug metabolism relevant for the drug response to proton pump inhibitors and antidepressants. *Clin Pharmacol Ther.* 2006 Jan;79(1):103-13.

89. Kirchheiner J, Schmidt H, Tzvetkov M, et al. Pharmacokinetics of codeine and its metabolite morphine in ultra-rapid metabolizers due to CYP2D6 duplication. *Pharmacogenomics J.* 2007 Aug;7(4):257-65.

90. Koski A, Ojanperä I, Sistonen J, et al. A fatal doxepin poisoning associated with a defective CYP2D6 genotype. *Am J Forensic Med Pathol.* 2007 Sep;28(3):259-61.

91. Wilkinson GR. Drug metabolism and variability among patients in drug response. *N Engl J Med.* 2005 May 26;352(21):2211-21.

92. McKeown-Eyssen G, Baines C, Cole DE, et al. Case-control study of genotypes in multiple chemical sensitivity: CYP2D6, NAT1, NAT2, PON1, PON2 and MTHFR. *Int J Epidemiol.* 2004 Oct;33(5):971-8.

93. Elbaz A, Levecque C, Clavel J, et al. CYP2D6 polymorphism, pesticide exposure, and Parkinson's disease. *Ann Neurol.* 2004 Mar;55(3):430-4.

94. Deng Y, Newman B, Dunne MP, et al. Further evidence that interactions between CYP2D6 and pesticide exposure increase risk for Parkinson's disease. *Ann Neurol.* 2004 Jun;55(6):897.

95. Larson AM. Acetaminophen hepatotoxicity. *Clin Liver Dis.* 2007 Aug;11(3):525-48, vi.

96. Larson AM, Polson J, Fontana RJ, et al. Acetaminophen-induced acute liver failure: results of a United States multicenter, prospective study. *Hepatology.* 2005 Dec; 42(6):1364-72.

97. Heard KJ. Acetylcysteine for acetaminophen poisoning. *N Engl J Med.* 2008 Jul 17;359(3):285-92.

98. Subehan S, Usia T, Kadota S, et al. Constituents of *Zingiber aromaticum* and their CYP3A4 and CYP2D6 inhibitory activity. *Chem Pharm Bull* (Tokyo). 2005 Mar;53(3):333-5.

99. Di YM, Li CG, Xue CC, et al. Clinical drugs that interact with St. John's wort and implication in drug development. *Curr Pharm Des.* 2008;14(17):1723-42.

100. Cooper BW, Cho TM, Thompson PM, et al. Phthalate induction of CYP3A4 is dependent on glucocorticoid regulation of PXR expression. *Toxicol Sci.* 2008 Jun;103(2):268-77.

101. Bangsi D, Zhou J, Sun Y, et al. Impact of a genetic variant in CYP3A4 on risk and clinical presentation of prostate cancer among white and African-American men. *Urol Oncol.* 2006 Jan-Feb;24(1):21-7.

102. Haas S, Pierl C, Harth V, et al. Expression of xenobiotic and steroid hormone metabolizing enzymes in human breast carcinomas. *Int J Cancer.* 2006 Oct 15;119(8):1785-91.

103. Roy JN, Lajoie J, Zijenah LS, et al. CYP3A5 genetic polymorphisms in different ethnic populations. *Drug Metab Dispos.* 2005 Jul;33(7):884-7.

104. Balram C, Zhou Q, Cheung YB, et al. CYP3A5 *3 and *6 single nucleotide polymorphisms in three distinct Asian populations. *Eur J Clin Pharmacol.* 2003 Jun;59(2):123-6.

105. Zamek-Gliszczynski MJ, Hoffmaster KA, Nezasa K, et al. Integration of hepatic drug transporters and phase II metabolizing enzymes: mechanisms of hepatic excretion of sulfate, glucuronide, and glutathione metabolites. *Eur J Pharm Sci.* 2006 Apr;27(5):447-86.

106. Sieg A, Arab L, Schlierf G, et al. Prevalence of Gilbert's syndrome in Germany. *Dtsch Med Wochenschr.* 1987 Jul 31;112(31-32):1206-8.

107. Gwee KA, Koay ES, Kang JY. The prevalence of isolated unconjugated hyperbilirubinaemia (Gilbert's syndrome) in subjects attending a health screening programme in Singapore. *Singapore Med J.* 1992 Dec;33(6):588-9.

108. Burchell B, Hume R. Molecular genetic basis of Gilbert's syndrome. *J Gastroenterol Hepatol.* 1999 Oct;14(10):960-6.

109. Girard H, Butler LM, Villeneuve L, et al. UGT1A1 and UGT1A9 functional variants, meat intake, and colon cancer, among Caucasians and African-Americans. *Mutat Res.* 2008 Sep 26;644(1-2):56-63.

110. Carlsten C, Sagoo GS, Frodsham AJ, et al. Glutathione S-transferase M1 (GSTM1) polymorphisms and lung cancer: a literature-based systematic HuGE review and meta-analysis. *Am J Epidemiol.* 2008 Apr 1;167(7):759-74.

111. Shi X, Zhou S, Wang Z, et al. CYP1A1 and GSTM1 polymorphisms and lung cancer risk in Chinese populations: a meta-analysis. *Lung Cancer.* 2008 Feb;59(2): 155-63.

112. Lee SA, Fowke JH, Lu W, et al. Cruciferous vegetables, the GSTP1 Ile105Val genetic polymorphism, and breast cancer risk. *Am J Clin Nutr.* 2008 Mar;87(3):753-60.

113. Moore LE, Brennan P, Karami S, et al. Glutathione S-transferase polymorphisms, cruciferous vegetable intake and cancer risk in the Central and Eastern European Kidney Cancer Study. *Carcinogenesis.* 2007 Sep;28(9): 1960-4.

114. Seow A, Vainio H, Yu MC. Effect of glutathione-S-transferase polymorphisms on the cancer preventive potential of isothiocyanates: an epidemiological perspective. *Mutat Res.* 2005 Dec 30;592(1-2):58-67.

115. Wan J, Diaz-Sanchez D. Antioxidant enzyme induction: a new protective approach against the adverse effects of diesel exhaust particles. *Inhal Toxicol.* 2007;19 Suppl 1:177-82.

116. Ritz SA, Wan J, Diaz-Sanchez D. Sulforaphane-stimulated phase II enzyme induction inhibits cytokine production by airway epithelial cells stimulated with diesel extract. *Am J Physiol Lung Cell Mol Physiol.* 2007 Jan;292(1):L33-9.

117. Townsend DM, Tew KD, Tapiero H. The importance of glutathione in human disease. *Biomed Pharmacother.* 2003 May-Jun;57(3-4):145-55.

118. Boukouvala S, Fakis G. Arylamine N-acetyltransferases: what we learn from genes and genomes. *Drug Metab Rev.* 2005;37(3):511-64.

119. García-Closas M, Malats N, Silverman D. NAT2 slow acetylation, GSTM1 null genotype, and risk of bladder cancer: results from the Spanish Bladder Cancer Study and meta-analyses. *Lancet.* 2005 Aug 20-26;366(9486):649-59.

120. Ambrosone CB, Kropp S, Yang J, et al. Cigarette smoking, N-acetyltransferase 2 genotypes, and breast cancer risk: pooled analysis and meta-analysis. *Cancer Epidemiol Biomarkers Prev.* 2008 Jan;17(1):15-26.

121. Nicholl DJ, Bennett P, Hiller L, et al. A study of five candidate genes in Parkinson's disease and related neurodegenerative disorders. European Study Group on Atypical Parkinsonism. *Neurology.* 1999 Oct 22;53(7): 1415-21.

122. Vella F, Ferry G, Delagrange P, et al. NRH:quinone reductase 2: an enzyme of surprises and mysteries. *Biochem Pharmacol.* 2005 Dec 19;71(1-2):1-12.

123. Cai JB, Zhang ZH, Xu DJ, et al. Negative regulation of quinone reductase 2 by resveratrol in cultured vascular smooth muscle cells. *Clin Exp Pharmacol Physiol.* 2008 Dec;35(12):1419-25.

124. Wang W, Le WD, Pan T, et al. Association of NRH:quinone oxidoreductase 2 gene promoter polymorphism with higher gene expression and increased susceptibility to Parkinson's disease. *J Gerontol A Biol Sci Med Sci.* 2008 Feb;63(2):127-34.

125. Iskander K, Jaiswal AK. Quinone oxidoreductases in protection against myelogenous hyperplasia and benzene toxicity. *Chem Biol Interact.* 2005 May 30;153-154:147-57.

126. Gong X, Gutala R, Jaiswal AK. Quinone oxidoreductases and vitamin K metabolism. *Vitam Horm.* 2008;78:85-101.

127. Kiyohara C, Yoshimasu K, Takayama K, et al. EPHX1 polymorphisms and the risk of lung cancer: a HuGE review. *Epidemiology.* 2006 Jan;17(1):89-99.

128. Morisseau C, Hammock BD. Epoxide hydrolases: mechanisms, inhibitor designs, and biological roles. *Annu Rev Pharmacol Toxicol.* 2005;45:311-33.

129. Krause CD, Yang ZH, Kim YS, et al. Protein arginine methyltransferases: evolution and assessment of their pharmacological and therapeutic potential. *Pharmacol Ther.* 2007 Jan;113(1):50-87.

130. Zhu BT. Catechol-O-Methyltransferase (COMT)-mediated methylation metabolism of endogenous bioactive catechols and modulation by endobiotics and xenobiotics: importance in pathophysiology and pathogenesis. *Curr Drug Metab.* 2002 Jun;3(3):321-49.

131. Ji Y, Olson J, Zhang J, et al. Breast cancer risk reduction and membrane-bound catechol O-methyltransferase genetic polymorphisms. *Cancer Res.* 2008 Jul 15;68(14): 5997-6005.

132. de Frias CM, Annerbrink K, Westberg L, et al. Catechol O-methyltransferase Val158Met polymorphism is associated with cognitive performance in nondemented adults. *J Cogn Neurosci.* 2005 Jul;17(7):1018-25.

133. Serretti A, Olgiati P, De Ronchi D. Genetics of Alzheimer's disease. A rapidly evolving field. *J Alzheimers Dis.* 2007 Aug;12(1):73-92.

134. Hintsanen M, Elovainio M, Puttonen S, et al. Val/Met polymorphism of the COMT gene moderates the association between job strain and early atherosclerosis in young men. *J Occup Environ Med.* 2008 Jun;50(6):649-57.

135. Glew RH, Melah G, El-Nafaty AI, et al. Plasma and urinary free amino acid concentrations in preeclamptic women in northern Nigeria. *Clin Chim Acta.* 2004 Apr;342(1-2):179-85.

136. Ambrosone CB, et al. Cigarette smoking, N-acetyltransferase 2 genetic polymorphisms, and breast cancer risk. *JAMA.* 1996.

137. Baumgartner KB, et al. N-acetyltransferase 2 genotype modification of active cigarette smoking on breast cancer risk among hispanic and non-hispanic white women. *Toxicol Sci.* 2009 Nov;112(1):211-20. Epub 2009 Aug 19.

138. Qing L, Wang T. Lactic acid bacteria prevent alcohol-induced steatohepatitis in rats by acting on the pathways of alcohol metabolism. *Clin Exp Med.* 2008 Dec;8(4):187-91.

139. Cani PD, Neyrinck AM, Fava F, et al. Selective increases of bifidobacteria in gut microflora improve high-fat-diet-induced diabetes in mice through a mechanism associated with endotoxaemia. *Diabetologia.* 2007 Nov;50(11):2374-83.

140. Knasmüller S, Steinkellner H, Hirschl AM. Impact of bacteria in dairy products and of the intestinal microflora on the genotoxic and carcinogenic effects of heterocyclic aromatic amines. *Mutat Res.* 2001 Sep 1;480-481:129-38.

141. Stidl R, Sontag G, Koller V, et al. Binding of heterocyclic aromatic amines by lactic acid bacteria: results of a comprehensive screening trial. *Mol Nutr Food Res.* 2008 Mar;52(3):322-9.

142. Calafat AM, Ye X, Wong LY, et al. Urinary concentrations of triclosan in the U.S. population: 2003-2004. *Environ Health Perspect.* 2008 Mar;116(3):303-7.

143. Hu H, Shih R, Rothenberg S, et al. The epidemiology of lead toxicity in adults: measuring dose and consideration of other methodologic issues. *Environ Health Perspect.* 2007 Mar;115(3):455-62.

144. Weisskopf MG. A prospective study of bone lead concentration and death from all causes, cardiovascular diseases, and cancer in the Department of Veterans Affairs Normative Aging Study. *Circulation.* 2009.

145. DeVito MJ. Comparisons of estimated human body burdens of dioxinlike chemicals and TCDD body burdens in experimentally exposed animals. *Environ Health Perspect.* 1995.

146. Risher JF, Amler SN. Mercury exposure: evaluation and intervention the inappropriate use of chelating agents in the diagnosis and treatment of putative mercury poisoning, *Neurotoxicology.* 2005.

147. Axelrad DA, Bellinger DC, Ryan LM, et al. Dose-response relationship of prenatal mercury exposure and IQ: an integrative analysis of epidemiologic data. *Environ Health Perspect.* 2007.

148. Neustadt J, Pieczenik S. Mercury—an example of heavy metal toxicity. *IMCJ.* 2007;6:1.

149. Rooney JP. The role of thiols, dithiols, nutritional factors and interacting ligands in the toxicology of mercury. *Toxicology*. 2007.

150. Hoet P. Clinical evaluation of a lead mobilization test using the chelating agent dimercaptosuccinic acid. *Clin Chem*. 2006.

151. Court MH. Isoform-selective probe substrates for *in vitro* studies of human UDP-glucuronosyltransferases. *Methods Enzymol*. 2005;400:104-16.

152. Thier R, Brüning T, Roos PH, et al. Markers of genetic susceptibility in human environmental hygiene and toxicology: the role of selected CYP, NAT and GST genes. *Int J Hyg Environ Health*. 2003 Jun;206(3):149-71.

153. Needs CJ, Brooks PM. Clinical pharmacokinetics of the salicylates. *Clin Pharmacokinet*. 1985 Mar-Apr;10(2):164-77.

154. Flora SJ. Heavy metal induced oxidative stress and its possible reversal by chelation therapy. *Indian J Med Res*. 2008.

155. Wang L, Wang Z, Liu J, et al. Protective effect of N-acetylcysteine on experimental chronic cadmium nephrotoxicity in immature female rats. *Hum Exp Toxicol*. 2009.

156. Kim SJ, Jeong HJ, Myung HY, et al. The protective mechanism of antioxidants in cadmium-induced ototoxicity *in vitro* and *in vivo*. *Environ Health Perspect*. 2008.

157. Kim SJ, Jeong HJ, Myung HY, et al. The protective mechanism of antioxidants in cadmium-induced ototoxicity *in vitro* and *in vivo*. *Environ Health Perspect*. 2008.

158. Pal S, Chatterjee AK. Possible Benefcial Effects of Melatonin Supplementation on Arsenic-Induced Oxidative Stress in Wistar Rats. *Drug Chem Toxicol*. 2006.

159. Hsueh YM. Low serum carotene level and increased risk of ischemic heart disease related to long-term arsenic exposure. *Atherosclerosis*. 1998.

160. Kim YO, Pyo MY, Kim JH. Infuence of melatonin on immunotoxicity of lead. *Int J Immunopharmacol*. 2000.

161. Kotler M, Rodríguez C, Sáinz R, et al. Melatonin increases gene expression for antioxidant enzymes in rat brain cortex. *J Pineal Res*. 1998.

162. Yun JW, Kim YK, Lee BS, et al. Effect of dietary epigallocatechin-3-gallate on cytochrome P450 2E1-dependent alcoholic liver damage: enhancement of fatty acid oxidation. *Biosci Biotechnol Biochem*. 2007 Dec;71(12):2999-3006.

163. Thangapazham RL, Singh AK, Sharma A. Green tea polyphenols and its constituent epigallocatechin gallate inhibits proliferation of human breast cancer cells *in vitro* and *in vivo*. *Cancer Lett*. 2007 Jan 8;245(1-2):232-41.

164. Sinha M, Manna P, Sil PC. Taurine protects the antioxidant defense system in the erythrocytes of cadmium treated mice. *BMB Rep*. 2008 Sep 30;41(9):657-63.

165. Manna P, Sinha M, Sil PC. Amelioration of cadmium-induced cardiac impairment by taurine. *Chem Biol Interact*. 2008 Jul 30;174(2):88-97.

166. Garg R, Gupta S, Maru GB. Dietary curcumin modulates transcriptional regulators of phase I and phase II enzymes in benzo[a]pyrene-treated mice: mechanism of its anti-initiating action. *Carcinogenesis*. 2008 May;29(5):1022-32.

167. Mukherjee S, Roy M, Dey S, et al. A Mechanistic Approach for Modulation of Arsenic Toxicity in Human Lymphocytes by Curcumin, an Active Constituent of Medicinal Herb Curcuma longa Linn. *J Clin Biochem Nutr*. 2007 Jul;41(1):32-42.

168. Mythri RB, Jagatha B, Pradhan N, et al. Mitochondrial complex I inhibition in Parkinson's disease: how can curcumin protect mitochondria? *Antioxid Redox Signal*. 2007 Mar;9(3):399-408.

169. Flora SJ, Mittal M, Mehta A. Heavy metal induced oxidative stress & its possible reversal by chelation therapy. *Indian J Med Res*. 2008 Oct;128(4):501-23.

170. Lee BK. Provocative chelation with DMSA and EDTA: evidence for differential access to lead storage sites. *Occup Environ Med*. 1995.

171. Bradberry S, Vale A. A comparison of sodium calcium edetate (edetate calcium disodium) and succimer (DMSA) in the treatment of inorganic lead poisoning. *Clinical Toxicology*. 2009.

172. Bradberry S. Use of oral dimercaptosuccinic acid (succimer) in adult patients with inorganic lead poisoning. *QJM*. 2009.

173. Flora SJ, Flora G, Saxena G, et al. Arsenic and lead induced free radical generation and their reversibility following chelation. *Cell Mol Biol* (Noisy-le-grand). 2007.

174. Bhadauria S, Flora SJS. Response of arsenic-induced oxidative stress, DNA damage, and metal imbalance to combined administration of DMSA and monoisoamyl-DMSA during chronic arsenic poisoning in rats. *Cell Biol Toxicol*. 2007.

175. Jones MM, Singh PK, Gale GR, et al. Cadmium mobilization *in vivo* by intraperitoneal or oral administration of mono alkyl esters of meso 2, 3-dimercaptosuccinic acid. *Pharmacol Toxicol*. 1992.

176. Misbahuddin M, Islam AZ, Khandker S, et al. Efficacy of spirulina extract plus zinc in patients of chronic arsenic poisoning: a randomized placebo-controlled study. *Clin Toxicol*. (Phila). 2006;44(2):135-41.

177. Li N, Neu J. Glutamine deprivation alters intestinal tight junctions via a PI3-K/Akt mediated pathway in Caco-2 cells. *J Nutr*. 2009 Apr;139(4):710-4.

178. Salvatore S, Heuschkel R, Tomlin S, et al. A pilot study of N-acetyl glucosamine, a nutritional substrate for glycosaminoglycan synthesis, in paediatric chronic inflammatory bowel disease. *Aliment Pharmacol Ther*. 2000 Dec;14(12):1567-79.

179. Cani PD, Neyrinck AM, Fava F, et al. Selective increases of bifidobacteria in gut microflora improve high-fat-diet-induced diabetes in mice through a mechanism associated with endotoxaemia. *Diabetologia*. 2007.

180. Schnare DW, Ben M, Shields MG. Body burden reductions of PCBs, PBBs, and chlorinated pesticides in human subjects. *Ambio*. 1984.

181. Imamura M, Tung T: A trial of fasting cure for PCB poisoned patients in Taiwan. *Am J Ind Med*. 5:147-53, 1984

182. Shakman RA. Nutritional influences on the toxicity of environmental pollutants: A review. *Arch Env Health*. 28:105-33, 1974.

The Spectrum of Insulin Resistance

Overview

Insulin resistance was initially proposed as a concept in the 1930s to describe the escalating insulin requirements seen in diabetic patients.[1] Today this metabolic abnormality is thought to have a major physiological role not only in type 2 diabetes mellitus, but also in conditions ranging from impaired glucose tolerance to coronary artery disease and polycystic ovary syndrome. Insulin resistance is often defined as a decreased sensitivity or responsiveness of target tissues to the metabolic actions of insulin, including decreased insulin-mediated glucose disposal into skeletal muscle, impaired inhibition of hepatic gluconeogenesis, and a reduced ability of insulin to inhibit lipolysis in adipose tissue. One consequence of insulin resistance is that higher than normal blood insulin concentrations are required to produce normal physiologic responses to glucose. At least initially, this results in a long period of compensatory increases in insulin production by pancreatic beta-cells. As resistance progresses, however, it is often accompanied by a gradual decline in beta-cell activity and decreasing beta-cell mass; and, when the pancreas can no longer sustain the overproduction of insulin, diabetes is the result.[2,3]

The prevalence of insulin resistance is hard to assess, partly because there are several techniques for assessment that do not overlap completely, but perhaps more so because insulin sensitivity is a continuous variable—it manifests along a spectrum, rather than simply being present or absent. Indeed, a model of diabetes as a continuous progression of definable stages, apparently beginning with insulin resistance, is emerging (Figure 4.1).

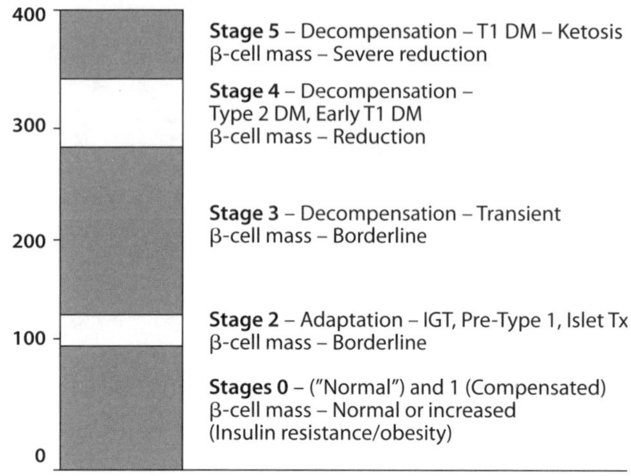

Figure 4.1 Five stages of diabetes progression. From: Weir GC, Bonner-Weir S. Five stages of evolving beta-cell dysfunction during progression to diabetes *Diabetes*. 2004 Dec;53 Suppl 3:S16-21. Copyright 2004 American Diabetes Association. Reprinted with permission from The American Diabetes Association.

We do know that the prevalence of insulin resistance is increasing. A study released in 2007 using National Health and Nutrition Examination Survey (NHANES) data[4] found that approximately 36% of adults in the U.S. had either previously diagnosed diabetes mellitus (6.7%), undiagnosed diabetes (2.9%), or impaired fasting glucose (26.6%) in the period 1999–2002. Percentages were based on fasting plasma glucose levels, using the most recent American Diabetes Association (ADA) diagnostic criteria. This same study found that among normoglycemic persons, standardized mean insulin resistance, calculated by homeostasis model assessment (HOMA), increased from 2.0 in 1988–1994 to 2.2, and the proportion of persons in the top quartile of insulin resistance increased from 26.2–32.2%. Among persons with impaired fasting glucose or undiagnosed diabetes, standardized mean insulin resistance increased from 4.0–4.5, and the proportion of persons in the top quartile of insulin resistance (>4.4) increased from 24.8–31.1%. Paralleling this increase is the widely described rise in overweight and obesity prevalence, a driving force for insulin resistance.

Obesity

In 2003–2004, 17.1% of U.S. children and adolescents were overweight and 66.3% of adults were either overweight or obese.[5] Additionally, the prevalence of extreme obesity was found to be rising, and with it a disproportional rate of extreme obesity among those with diabetes.[6] Although a benign obesity can exist in regard to metabolic abnormalities, the majority of overweight and obese individuals have some degree of insulin resistance.[7] Obesity is associated with a low-grade inflammation of white adipose tissue (WAT). In the past, adipose tissue was viewed as an inactive storage depot for fat; now, it is increasingly being recognized as an active endocrine organ that appears to play a key role in the pathogenesis of insulin resistance through several released metabolites, hormones, and adipocytokines.[8]

Adiponectin is one of the most common cytokines produced by adipose tissue (solely in WAT). Although it sounds counterintuitive, the more adipose tissue people have, the less adiponectin they produce, which is problematic because it has many metabolic actions involving peripheral tissue and the regulation of energy homeostasis, particularly energy expenditure. Adiponectin inhibits liver neoglucogenesis and promotes fatty acid oxidation in skeletal muscle. In addition, it counteracts the pro-inflammatory effects of TNF-alpha on the arterial wall and may protect against the development of arteriosclerosis. It has been clearly shown to be strongly and inversely related to central adiposity, diabetes, blood glucose levels in oral glucose tolerance testing, the insulin sensitivity indices HOMA and QUICKI, and insulin sensitivity markers in frequently sampled intravenous glucose tolerance testing and clamp studies. The relationship appears to exist independent of adiposity, BMI, and hyperglycemia.

Resistin is a plasma protein produced by macrophages. It has had inconsistent associations with insulin resistance in humans, but does appear to increase with body weight. It has been associated more directly with inflammation and atherosclerosis, and may inhibit the function of polymorphonuclear leukocytes (PMNL), an abnormality seen in diabetic patients.[9] TNF-alpha, which is secreted from both macrophages and adipocytes, has been shown to be significantly associated with insulin resistance even when adjusted for adiponectin, resistin, and BMI.[10]

Insulin resistance is multifactorial, and provides a good example of the interaction between genetic predisposition and environmental/lifestyle factors. Dietary factors, environmental toxins, physical activity, mitochondrial function, and genetic polymorphisms all influence the development and progression of insulin resistance and the associated diseases such as diabetes and metabolic syndrome. Adiponectin gene variants have been shown to predict insulin resistance associated with particular macronutrient intake, at least in men.[11] Men with a homozygous polymorphism of the adipoQ gene were significantly less insulin resistant after consumption of diets rich in monounsaturated fats and carbohydrates than diets rich in saturated fats. Similar results have been found for carriers of an apolipoprotein E gene promoter polymorphism,[12] and for carriers of a specific hepatic lipase gene promoter polymorphism.[13] A solid foundation of lifestyle interventions to prevent and treat insulin resistance may soon be combined with targeted interventions for an individual's genetic background.

Metabolic Syndrome

Epidemiology and etiology

The metabolic syndrome (MetS) is a cluster of factors that, together, appear to predict outcomes such as coronary artery disease or diabetes more successfully than the individual factors used separately. The precise definition over the years has not stayed consistent, although most emphasize the core components of obesity (waist circumference), insulin resistance, dyslipidemia, and hypertension. The most recently proposed definition, by the International Diabetes Federation,[14] includes:

- Ethnic/racial specific waist circumference cutoffs, i.e., ≥94 cm for men of European origin, and ≥80 cm for women of European origin

Two of the following:

- Triglycerides >150 mg/dl
- HDL-C <40 mg/dl for men, <50 mg/dl for women
- BP ≥130/85 mmHg
- Fasting plasma glucose (FPG) ≥100 mg/dl

By this definition and using date from the NHANES 1999–2002 study, the prevalence of MetS in the United States is 39% among men and women aged ≥20.[15] Among adolescents, and using a similar definition, approximately 5.8% meet the established criteria.[16] In addition to an elevated risk for cardiovascular disease and diabetes, individuals with MetS report poorer health-related quality of life, both physically and mentally.[17]

While insulin resistance may be the link between the various components of MetS, it is unclear whether lipid alterations precede insulin resistance and impaired glucose metabolism, or whether genetic and behavioral factors come first. The latter may induce insulin resistance, which in turn results in impaired glucose metabolism and dyslipidemia. Lifestyle, molecular, and genetic factors—including obesity, physical inactivity, diet, insulin receptor and signaling anomalies, inflammation, mitochondrial dysfunction, and other genetic predispositions—are certainly involved to some degree.

Metabolic syndrome as a risk factor for other diseases

Type 2 diabetes mellitus

Most patients with type 2 diabetes mellitus (T2D) have insulin resistance and MetS before the onset of diabetes. In a population-based study of more than 4000 individuals without diabetes, a progressive increase in the risk of developing diabetes was associated with the number of components present, defined by these authors as hyperglycemia, hypertension, elevated BMI, abnormal total or HDL cholesterol, proteinuria, and hyperuricemia. A 9-fold increase was seen with 3 components present, up to an astounding 33.67-fold increase with all components present.[18] A separate meta-analysis reported the population-attributable fraction for MetS for diabetes as 30–52%.[19]

Cardiovascular disease

Certainly MetS increases the risk of cardiovascular disease, including coronary artery disease and stroke. The presence of MetS in children can even predict cardiovascular disease in adults 25 years later. A recent study found that children who had MetS had a nearly 15-fold risk for developing cardiovascular disease as adults, emphasizing the importance of recognizing and treating this condition among the pediatric population.[20]

Among adults with MetS, an observational study of over 1200 Finnish men found a 2.9–4.2 times increased chance of dying of coronary artery disease, after adjusting for conventional risk factors.[21] A separate meta-analysis of longitudinal studies with over 90,000 participants found a relative risk of cardiovascular events and death of 1.78, with a higher risk in women.[22] The same data also revealed a relative risk for stroke of 1.6 to 2.2.[23] In the Northern Manhattan study with over 3000 participants, the authors predicted that elimination of MetS would result in a 19% reduction in overall stroke, a 30% reduction of stroke in women, and a 35% reduction of stroke among Hispanics.[24]

All cause mortality

The above study of Finnish men found not only an increased risk of dying from coronary artery disease, but also a nearly 2-fold increase in all-cause mortality, with higher risk associated with greater number of components present.[21]

Other

Having MetS is also an independent risk factor for nonalcoholic fatty liver disease (NAFLD). A recent study found a 2.37-fold risk of NAFLD among those with MetS compared to those without.[25] MetS has also been associated with chronic kidney disease,[26,27] polycystic ovary syndrome (PCOS),[28] and obstructive sleep apnea (OSA).[29]

Causes and risk factors of the metabolic syndrome

Obesity

Perhaps the condition most closely associated with MetS is obesity, particularly central obesity. The index of central obesity, a ratio of waist circumference and height, has recently been shown to be one of the most sensitive screens for MetS.[30] The proposed mechanism by which obesity contributes to insulin resistance and the components of MetS is through an increase in non-esterified free fatty acids and inflammatory compounds[31] (see Figure 4.2). With adipose tissue producing and releasing a greater amount of free fatty acids, insulin's action is inhibited, including insulin's suppression of hepatic glucose production and glucose uptake in peripheral cells. Additionally, an inflammatory cascade is triggered, which includes the activation of NF-KappaB, which may directly influence insulin sensitivity,[31] and protein kinase C (PKC). These, in turn, decrease tyrosine phosphorylation of the insulin receptor substrate 1 or 2, which further inhibits the metabolic actions of insulin. Elevated C-reactive protein carries a 3-(nearly)6-fold increase in risk for MetS.[32,33,34]

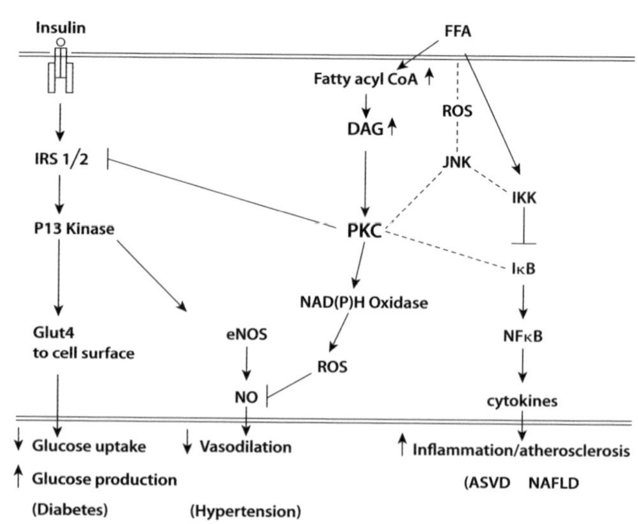

Figure 4.2 Mechanisms by which obesity contributes to diabetes and other conditions. From: Boden G. Obesity and free fatty acids. *Endocrinol Metab Clin North Am.* 2008 Sep;37(3):635-46, viii-ix. Used with permission from Elsevier.

Physical inactivity

Inactivity has a significant and direct relationship with MetS, diabetes, and cardiovascular disease. In a study that followed 800 men over 20 years, physical inactivity and obesity were both found to be independent predictors of insulin resistance, suggesting that there is not a complete overlap between these two risk factors.[35] It has been estimated that prolonged TV and computer time can more than double the risk for MetS. Lipoprotein lipase suppression may be responsible for some of the dyslipidemia, insulin resistance, and hypertension seen,[36] and low preheparin serum lipoprotein levels have been suggested as a biomarker for MetS.[37] Fortunately, a combination of diet and exercise has proven to be a very powerful modifier of metabolic abnormalities; in the Diabetes Prevention Program trial, incidence of MetS was reduced by 41% in the lifestyle group, and only 17% in the metformin group (P = 0.03), compared with placebo.[38]

Diet

Along with physical inactivity, dietary patterns have also been strongly associated with MetS. Specifically, a diet high in fruits, vegetables, fibers, polyunsaturated and omega-3 fatty acids, and low in saturated fat, refined carbohydrates, and trans fats has been found to decrease the risk for MetS.[39] Figure 4.3 summarizes some of the mechanisms by which dietary factors lead to coronary artery disease. Numerous trials have demonstrated that a higher intake of dietary fiber is a cornerstone of dietary planning for diabetics.[184,186,187] Dietary fiber intake is associated with higher adiponectin levels in men[40] and women.[41] Additionally, fiber improves glycemic control, satiety, and reduces inflammation (see Figure 4.4).[42] The viscosity of the fiber has been shown to be directly proportional to postprandial glycemia.[43,44]

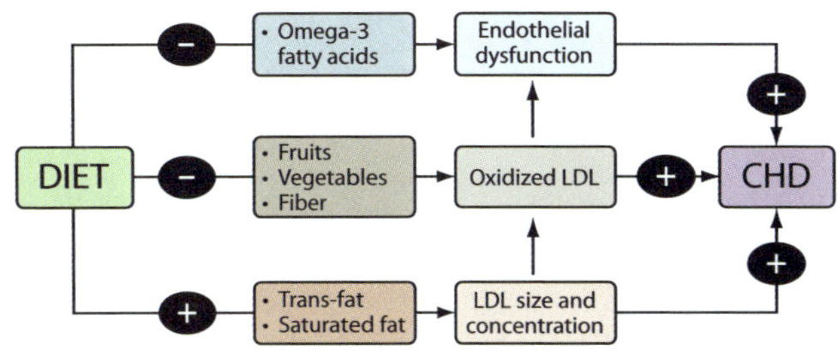

Figure 4.3 Mechanisms for dietary impact on coronary heart disease. From: Giugliano D, Ceriello A, Esposito K. The effects of diet on inflammation: emphasis on the metabolic syndrome. *J Am Coll Cardiol.* 2006 Aug 15;48(4):677-85. Used with permission from Elsevier.

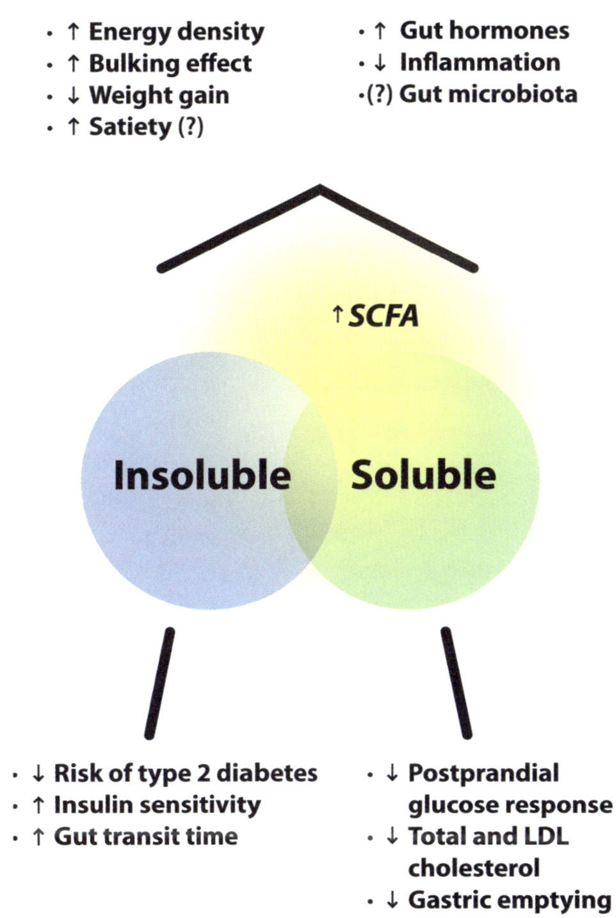

Figure 4.4 Effects of fiber types on insulin sensitivity and type 2 diabetes. From: Weickert MO, Pfeiffer AF. Metabolic effects of dietary fiber consumption and prevention of diabetes. *J Nutr.* 2008 Mar;138(3):439-42. Used with permission from the American Society for Nutrition.

Vitamin D and magnesium

Other dietary components associated with MetS include insufficient essential fatty acid intake, vitamin D, and magnesium.[45] Data from the NHANES 2003–2004 study found that the odds ratio for MetS in the highest quintile of serum 25(OH)D compared with the lowest quintile was 0.27, after adjusting for age, sex, race/ethnicity, income, lifestyle factors, total calcium, and energy intake.[46] A prospective study also found that baseline vitamin D levels also predict future insulin resistance and hyperglycemia.[47] Genetic polymorphisms appear to influence insulin sensitivity as well: the BsmI vitamin D receptor polymorphism influences body mass index, while the FokI polymorphism affects insulin sensitivity and serum HDL levels.[48] Magnesium intake has also been associated with MetS, BMI, and serum glucose, with higher intakes shown to reduce the risk. This effect may be mediated by reductions in inflammation and/or increases in serum adiponectin levels.[40,49,50]

Environmental toxins

Environmental toxins have been found to increase insulin resistance and risk for MetS. Analysis of the 1999–2003 NHANES data revealed an association between MetS and persistent organic pollutants, with the subcategory of organochlorine (OC) pesticides most consistently and strongly associated (OR of 5.3 in the highest quartile).[51] Dioxin-like PCBs were also associated with increased insulin resistance.[52]

Type 1 Diabetes Mellitus

Epidemiology and etiology

NHANES data from 1999–2004 projected that 7.8% of the United States adult population had diabetes mellitus; approximately 5–10% of those individuals were estimated to have type 1 diabetes mellitus (T1D).[53] T1D is thought to be a chronic immune-mediated disease, with a subclinical prodromal period characterized by selective loss of the insulin-secreting pancreatic beta-cells in genetically susceptible subjects. There seems to be a spectrum of glandular dysfunction (beta-cell destruction) associated with islet cell autoimmunity ranging from latency through prediabetes (impaired fasting glucose or impaired glucose tolerance) and a clinical phenotype of type 2 diabetes mellitus (T2D) (probably precipitated by insulin resistance from overweight) to ketosis-prone T1D. Although islet cell and other antibodies are used to help make a diagnosis, they are neither 100% sensitive nor absolutely specific, and a significant percentage of individuals diagnosed with either T1D or T2D may be misclassified. Additionally, latent autoimmune diabetes in adults (LADA) shares many features of T1D but has a much later onset, and beta-cell function appears to not diminish as rapidly. It is currently a matter of debate whether LADA is part of a spectrum between T1D and T2D, or whether it is T1D with a later onset.

Although the etiology of T1D is certainly autoimmune pancreatic beta-cell destruction, the triggers of this destruction appear to be multifactorial, including genetic, dietary, and other environmental factors (see Figure 4.5). Autoreactive T-cell recognition (both CD4 and CD8 cells) of islet autoantigenic epitopes is a key step in the autoimmune cascade. Various autoantigens have been identified in T1D: insulin (IAA), glutamic acid decarboxylase (GAD or GAA), the protein tyrosine phosphatase-related islet antigen 2 (IA-2 or ICA512), and most recently the zinc transporter Slc30A8 residing in the insulin secretory granule of the beta-cell.[56] It may be that the number of antibodies, rather than any individual antibody, is most predictive of progression to overt diabetes. It is thought that haplotypes of the HLA class convey the most significant genetic disease susceptibility. Specifically, DQB1*0302 is a strong susceptibility gene and the heterozygous combination of DQA1*0301-DQB1*0302 on the HLA-DR4 haplotype and DQA1*0501-DQB1*0201 on the HLA-DR3 haplotype results in a synergistically increased risk of T1D.[57]

Much evidence indicates that the function of the gut immune system is central in the pathogenesis of T1D.[58] This may explain in part the connection

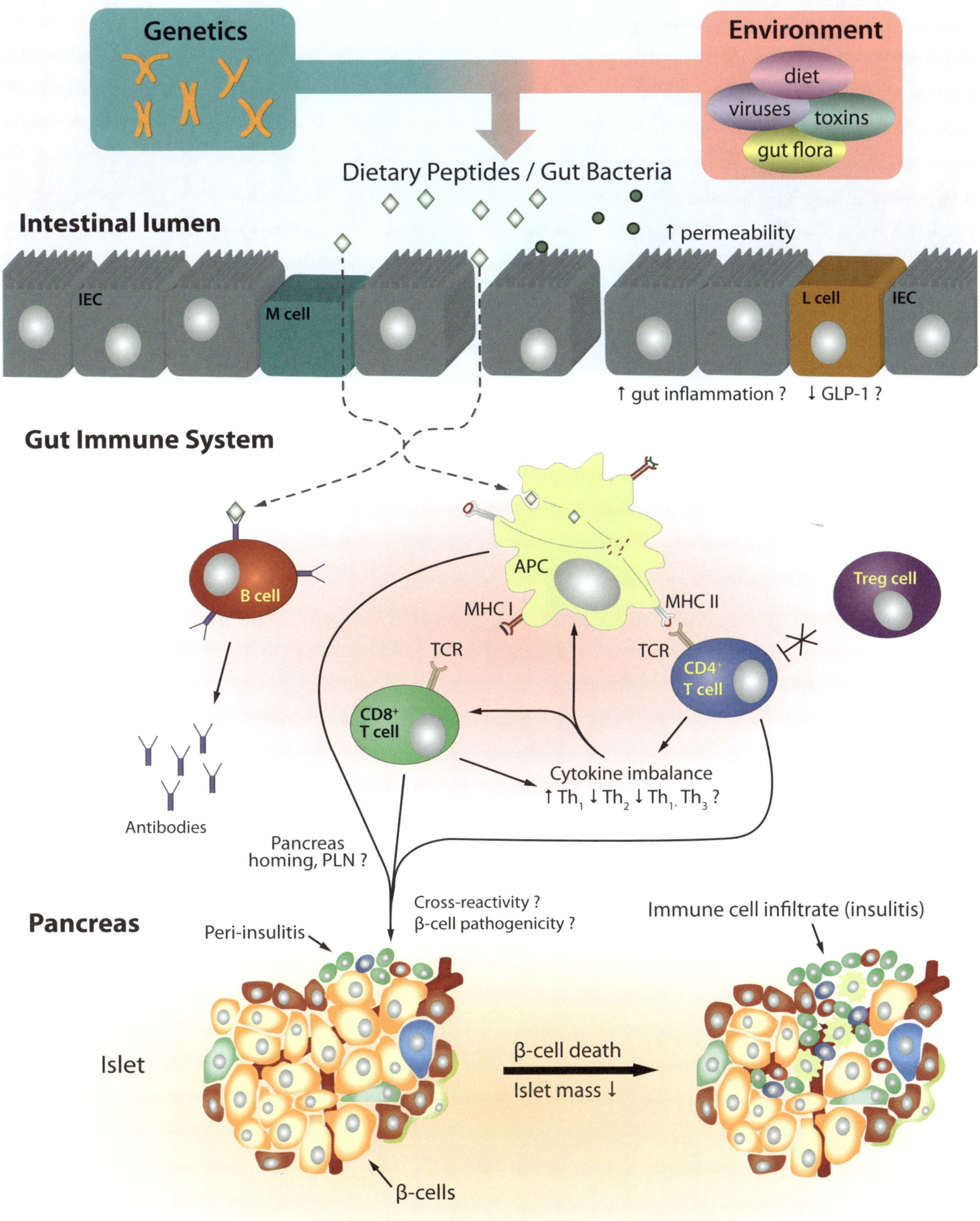

Figure 4.5 A multifactorial model for modification of type 1 diabetes with diet. From: Lefebvre DE, Powell KL, Strom A, et al. Dietary proteins as environmental modifiers of type 1 diabetes mellitus. *Annu Rev Nutr.* 2006;26:175-202. Reproduced with permission of Annual Reviews Inc.

between enterovirus infection and T1D; epidemiological data have shown an association between enterovirus infections and type 1 diabetes, and a prospective trial has confirmed this link.[59,60] One possible mechanism posits enterovirus as augmenting immune responses to dietary antigens; these viruses replicate in gut-associated lymphoid tissues. Among the dietary antigens under suspicion, cow's milk and gluten stand out, though it has been suggested that poor digestion of dietary protein is the culprit, rather than any one specific protein.[61] A dysregulated immune response to oral antigens may also be involved.[62,63]

Risk factors for the development of type 1 diabetes

Genetic

Genetic factors in the development of T1D are present, although the genetic contribution to disease lessens with age, indicating environmental factors contribute more significantly. While the average risk of T1D is 0.4% in the general population, the average prevalence risk in siblings is 7%, and in a child of a diabetic 6%.[59] Thus, if a child has T1D, siblings are at a 15-times greater risk of developing diabetes than a member of the general population.[59]

The genes involved are primarily HLA related (40–50%), suggestive of inappropriate early T-cell selection and maturation.[59] But these are not the only genes that increase risk; polymorphisms in the vitamin D receptor gene also appear to increase the risk. A recent analysis that included an assessment of seasonal UV exposure strengthened the case for this association, which may also explain the association of T1D risk with season of birth.[64] When considered in isolation, the genetic predisposition may not be sufficient to cause disease, but when combined with the right environmental circumstances, such as low vitamin D activity, the genetic susceptibility leads to illness.[65,66]

Immune abnormalities

One consistent association with T1D is early exposure to cow's milk. In a study of over 17,000 newborns, infants exposed to cow's milk formulas at <2 months of age were found to have a nearly 3-fold risk for having T1D antibodies.[67] And infants with antibodies to proteins in cow's milk are more likely to develop T1D later in childhood. This is thought to be due to an enhanced humoral immune response to various cow's milk proteins in infancy, and suggests that a dysregulated immune response to oral antigens may be an early event in the pathogenesis of T1D.[68] Additionally, increased intestinal permeability due to early introduction of cow's milk has also been demonstrated in infants,[69] as well as an increased risk for T1D antibodies (OR 2.5–3.5) as a result of shorter duration of both total and exclusive breastfeeding.[70]

Celiac disease

Individuals with celiac disease, an autoimmune intolerance to gluten, are known to have a higher incidence of T1D. Also, having family members with celiac disease is known to increase the risk (e.g., celiac disease in grandparents has an OR of 2.2). Many cases of celiac disease among those with T1D and their family members remain undiagnosed.[71]

The likely explanation for the comorbidity between these two diseases is a shared HLA genotype.[59] But a link between the gut immune system and T1D has been suggested both in animal models and in humans, suggesting a failure of oral tolerance in both conditions.[72] Gluten is also proposed as a shared causative factor between T1D and celiac, though no evidence yet exists for this.[73] However, an increased risk for islet cell autoimmunity associated with the timing of gluten introduction has been documented. In infants at higher risk for T1D, a window of lowest risk occurs with introduction between 4–6 months. Earlier and later introductions are associated with a 5.55- and a 12.53-fold increase in risk, respectively. This effect is heavily influenced by HLA status.[74]

Diet

In addition to gluten and cow's milk intake, egg and soft-drink consumption have also been associated with an increased risk of T1D.[75] Omega-3 fatty acid consumption in children at greater risk of T1D has been found to have a protective effect, with a hazard ratio for autoantibody production of 0.23-0.45 with higher intake. Higher red blood cell n-3 levels are also associated with reduced risk.[76] Given the abnormal T-cell activity found in T1D, omega-3 fatty acids may be of benefit by diminishing T-lymphocyte proliferation and IL-2 production, as well as improving oxidative cellular status.[77]

T1D, like other autoimmune diseases, has been found to be associated with low vitamin D in both mothers and their children. Observational studies suggest that supplementation of vitamin D in children reduces risk, with a dose-dependent effect that is somewhat dependent on timing.[78,79,80,81]

Infection

An additional factor long considered to play a role in the etiology of T1D is infection, particularly viral infection. Although not limited to enteroviruses, this class of virus has shown the greatest association with T1D.[82] At least 75% of adults with T1D have been shown to have persistent enterovirus infection in the gut mucosa, vs. 10% of controls.[83] And maternal enterovirus infection has also been associated with T1D risk in children.[84] Because breastfeeding has been shown to reduce enterovirus infection in children, this may at least partly explain the reduced risk of T1D in breast-fed children.[85]

Environmental toxins

Although inconsistent, the nitrate content in drinking water has been associated with increased risk in some studies.[84,86] A review of the associations between T1D and environmental contaminants found a higher intake of nitrates, nitrites, and N-nitroso compounds, as well as higher serum levels of polychlorinated biphenyls, to be associated with increased risk, though findings were inconsistent.[87]

Insulin resistance

The "accelerator hypothesis," first published in 2001, proposes that insulin resistance accelerates development of type 1 diabetes in people with islet autoimmunity and insulin deficiency. The increasing rates of obesity, which promotes insulin resistance, could help to account for the rising incidence of type 1 diabetes.[88]

Type 2 Diabetes Mellitus

Etiology and epidemiology

Returning to the NHANES data from 1999–2004, among the 7.8% of the U.S. adult population with diabetes mellitus, approximately 90–95% individuals were estimated to have T2D.[55] In 2007, the CDC reported that approximately 23.6 million people in the U.S. had diabetes, with about one-fourth unaware of it; that number is expected to double by 2050. Total health care costs for diabetes reached $174 billion in 2007.[89] Additionally, the NHANES 2005–2006 found that, in people aged ≥20 years, the crude prevalence of impaired fasting glucose was 25.7% and of impaired glucose tolerance was 13.8%, with almost 30% having one or the other. Thus, over 40% of individuals had diabetes or pre-diabetes.

T2D is a disease characterized by progressive worsening of glycemic control (see Figure 4.6), which starts with mild alterations in postprandial glucose homeostasis, followed by an increase in fasting plasma glucose. It is well-established that the hyperglycemia is the result of two major defects: the development of insulin resistance and defective beta-cell function. Hepatic insulin resistance is marked by an inappropriately high rate of hepatic glucose, despite elevated insulin concentrations. The inability of endogenous insulin to increase plasma glucose uptake by peripheral tissues indicates peripheral insulin resistance. It is estimated that beta-cell function may already be reduced by 50% by the time of diagnosis, resulting from an earlier phase of gradual decline and decompensation preceding overt diabetes and followed by a phase of rapid acceleration of impaired insulin secretion and beta-cell apoptosis, perhaps due to glucose and lipotoxicity.[90]

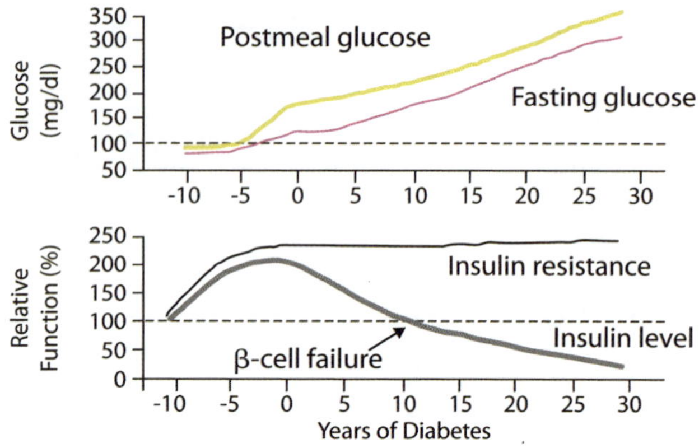

Figure 4.6 Natural history of type 2 diabetes. From: LeRoith D. Beta-cell dysfunction and insulin resistance in type 2 diabetes: role of metabolic and genetic abnormalities. *Am J Med.* 2002 Oct 28;113 Suppl 6A:3S-11S. Used with permission from Elsevier.

Complications of diabetes affect many tissues and organs, causing retinopathy, nephropathy, neuropathy, cardiovascular diseases, peripheral vascular diseases, stroke, and periodontal pathologies. Additionally, insulin resistance even without diabetes has recently been shown to damage both retinal and cerebral vasculature.[91]

Generalized endothelial dysfunction in diabetes (see Figure 4.7) can result from disparate metabolic insults that include hyperglycemia, dyslipidemia, hypertension, hyperinsulinemia, elevated levels of fatty acids, increased production of reactive oxygen species, hyperleptinemia, cytokine-mediated inflammation, activation of the sympathoadrenal

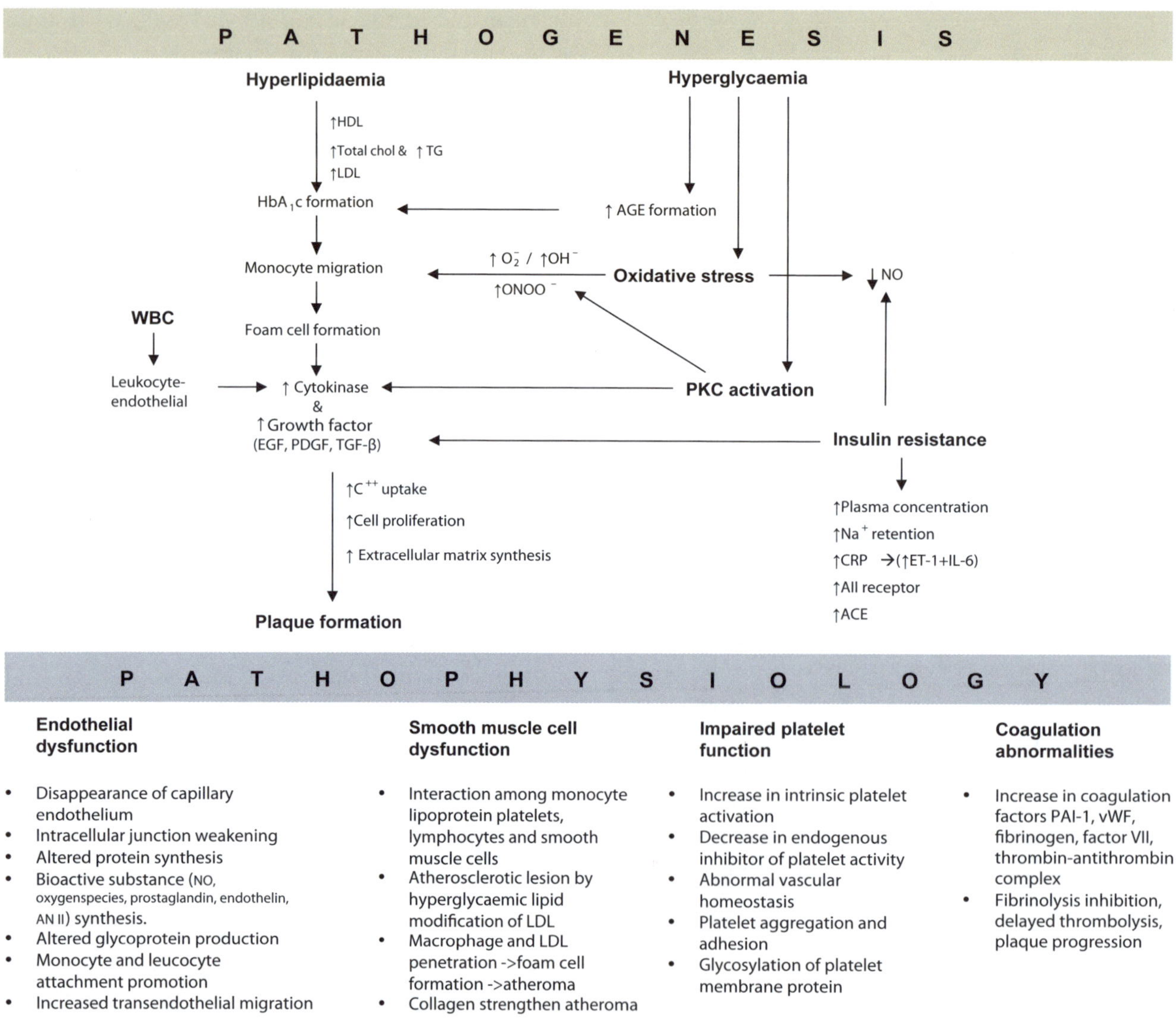

Figure 4.7 Diabetes-associated macrovasculopathy: pathophysiology and pathogenesis. From: Rahman S, Rahman T, et al. Diabetes-associated macrovasculopathy: pathophysiology and pathogenesis. *Diabetes Obes Metab.* 2007 Nov;9(6):767-80. Used with permission from John Wiley & Sons, Inc.

system, and activation of protein kinase C. While cardiovascular disease is the major cause of morbidity and mortality in people with diabetes, and coronary artery disease the most common cause of death, diabetes is also the leading cause of end-stage renal failure, visual impairment, blindness, and non-traumatic lower limb amputations.[92,93]

The causes of T2D, like those of MetS, are multifactorial, but most can be attributed largely to changes in nutrition and lifestyle, which have led to increased rates of obesity and decreased levels of physical activity. There is, however, a genetic component to T2D, and environmental exposures also influence diabetes risk.

Risk factors for type 2 diabetes mellitus

Obesity

Central obesity is strongly associated with the development of T2D, just as it is with MetS and insulin resistance. Waist circumference is positively associated with the incidence of type 2 diabetes, with an OR of 1.6–2.66. Higher BMI and waist-to-hip ratios appear to have similar risks.[94,95] Both obesity and T2D are associated with greater cancer risk and overall mortality, perhaps via insulin resistance.[96] Waist-to-height ratio may be the best discriminator predictor of cardiovascular disease.[97]

Physical inactivity

Through mechanisms that do not entirely overlap with obesity, physical activity is known to decrease the risk for T2D, as well as for diabetic complications. In a study of over 50,000 women, sedentary behaviors (especially TV watching), independent of exercise levels, were associated with significantly elevated risk of obesity and T2D, whereas even light to moderate activity was associated with substantially lower risk.[98] Similar findings were documented in a study of ~38,000 men.[99]

Unfortunately, many people with diabetes are not meeting basic recommendations for physical activity. The odds for adults with diabetes meeting physical activity recommendations were significantly lower than in adults without diabetes even after multivariate adjustment.[100]

Diet

Good nutrition certainly is a powerful predictor of diabetes development and progression. A diet high in refined carbohydrates and foods with a high glycemic index, elevating the total glycemic load, substantially increases risk, while higher fiber and cereal intake reduces risk.[101,102] A low intake of fruits, vegetables, legumes, whole grain, and fiber is the dietary pattern associated with the greatest risk.[103,104,105] Figure 4.8 shows the relationship between cereal fiber intake, glycemic index, and risk of type 2 diabetes.

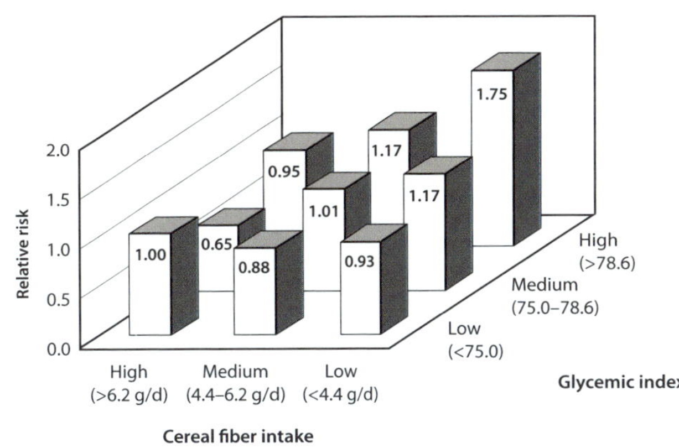

Figure 4.8 Relative risk of type 2 diabetes by different levels of cereal fiber intake and glycemic index. From: Schulze MB, Liu S, Rimm EB, et al. Glycemic index, glycemic load, and dietary fiber intake and incidence of type 2 diabetes in younger and middle-aged women. *Am J Clin Nutr.* 2004 Aug;80(2):348-56. Used with permission from the American Society for Nutrition.

The importance of food with a high glycemic index can be explained by the effect of foods on blood glucose levels after meals, i.e., postprandial hyperglycemia. Recent epidemiological studies strongly indicate that hyperglycemia, specifically postprandial hyperglycemia, is a greater risk factor for morbidity and mortality in type 2 diabetes, and for the development of cardiovascular disease, than fasting glucose.[106,107] And the foods which lead to the smallest increase in postprandial glycemia appear to be those high in fiber, particularly viscous fiber. Fiber's viscosity has been shown to be inversely proportional to postprandial glycemia.[43,44]

Consumption of legumes, soybeans in particular, was inversely associated with T2D risk in women, with a RR of 0.53 for overall legume intake.[108] Compared with low intake, high antioxidant intake has been independently associated with 59% and 46% lower risks of diabetes, after adjustment for lifestyle and metabolic factors, respectively, in a study of over 800 Swedish men.[109]

Food insecurity also increases the risk of T2D. Those with limited financial resources and food insecurity have an OR of 2.1 for developing T2D, largely because available foods are often calorically dense and nutritionally poor.[110]

Family history/ethnicity/genetics

Genes associated with T2D risk include CAPN10, PPARG, KCNJ11, and TCF7L2. The latter has the greatest effect currently known, with one allele conferring ~40% risk, whereas two copies confer 80% risk.[111] Having parents with diabetes increases the chance that the children will develop diabetes one day. The child of a diabetic parent has a 40% chance of developing diabetes, in contrast to a population risk of ~7%; if both parents are affected, the risk rises to 70%.[113] However, genetic and familial associations with T2D risk are heavily influenced by lifestyle factors, as clearly shown by the Pima Indians.

In Pima Indians, the population with the highest reported prevalence of diabetes (nearly all T2D), the incidence is 2.3 times higher in individuals with one diabetic parent and 3.9 times higher in individuals with two diabetic parents.[112] Although there is a strong genetic component, Pima Indians living in Mexico have a prevalence of T2D of 6.9%, less than one-fifth that in the U.S. Pima Indians (38%).[113] Certainly the influence of lifestyle greatly modifies genetic risk, at least in this population. Other ethnicities with greater risk for T2D include Asians, Hispanics, and African-Americans.[114]

Other genes have been shown to influence diabetes risk as well. The fat mass and obesity-associated (FTO) gene has been consistently associated with elevated BMI and obesity, and a recent analysis found that low physical activity magnifies the effect of an FTO polymorphism.[115] As mentioned earlier, polymorphisms of the adipoQ gene, apolipoprotein E gene promoter, and hepatic lipase gene promoter all influence the impact of dietary choices on insulin resistance. For example, a dietary intervention replacing white rice with whole grains and an increase in vegetable intake had a greater effect on insulin resistance and adiponectin levels in those homozygous for an adipoQ polymorphism.[116]

Hypertension and prediabetes

Elevated blood pressure is a risk factor for both T2D development and complications.[117] Roughly 40% of individuals with T2D have hypertension at diagnosis. Tight blood pressure control appears to reduce diabetic complications, but only if maintained.[118]

Impaired fasting glucose (IFG) and glucose tolerance (IGT) predict insulin resistance in children and identify future risk of T2D.[119] Dyslipidemia also contributes; higher amounts of oxidized LDL combined with IFG or IGT may increase the risk of T2D 10-fold.[120]

Environmental toxins

Bisphenol A (BPA) has recently come into the spotlight for a number of reasons, one of which is increased risk for diabetes. Higher urinary BPA concentrations were associated with T2D, with an OR of 1.39 per 1 standard deviation increase, found in NHANES data collected from nearly 1500 adults.[121] Arsenic has also been shown to increase diabetes risk. The odds ratios for T2D, comparing participants at the 80th vs. the 20th percentiles, were 3.58 for the level of total arsenic, 1.57 for dimethylarsenate, and 0.69 for arsenobetaine in a cross-sectional study of nearly 800 adults in the NHANES study.[122] A dose-dependent effect was also seen in a Mexican study with 200 cases and 200 controls.[123]

Polychlorinated biphenyls (PCBs) have also been associated with insulin sensitivity in non-diabetic pregnant women,[124] and phthalates with obesity and insulin resistance. In a national cross-section of U.S. men, concentrations of several prevalent phthalate metabolites showed statistically significant correlations with abdominal obesity and insulin resistance.[125] Data from NHANES also found associations between phthalates and body mass index and waist circumference, particularly in men.[126]

Testosterone

An analysis of 26 studies found an association in men between hypogonadism and an adverse metabolic profile. This analysis reported that as many as 20–64% of men with T2D may have low testosterone levels.[127,128]

Depression

A review of available studies found that the presence of depression had a fully adjusted relative risk estimate of 1.25 for T2D.[129,13]

Assessment

Evaluating insulin resistance is useful in the assessment and treatment of MetS and diabetes mellitus, and is performed through a variety of measures. Diagnosis of MetS is based on central obesity, dyslipidemia, insulin resistance, and hypertension, though the criteria vary to some degree from one organization to another. The diagnosis of diabetes recommended by the American Diabetes Association has more consistency, and is the same for types 1 and 2. Differentiating between the two types is not always possible, but evaluation may include an investigation of autoantibodies, insulin levels, C-peptide, and symptomatology.[94]

Insulin resistance diagnosis[133]

Currently, no perfect assessment is available for measuring insulin resistance. While direct measures, such as the glucose clamp technique, are considered to be the gold standard, they are rarely used, given the difficulty of administration. More practical measures include the oral glucose tolerance test, mathematical models such as the homeostasis model assessment (HOMA) or quantitative insulin sensitivity check index (QUICKI), and physical parameters such as BMI and waist circumference. Other laboratory markers have also recently emerged that may prove to be excellent indicators of insulin resistance, such as adiponectin and Fetuin-A.

Oral glucose tolerance test (OGTT)

One of the more widely used tests in clinical practice, the oral glucose tolerance test reflects the efficiency of the body's ability to dispose of glucose after an oral glucose load. After an overnight fast, blood samples for determinations of glucose and insulin concentrations are taken at 0, 30, 60, and 120 minutes following a standard glucose load (75 g). While often used as an indirect measure of insulin resistance, the OGTT is dependent upon both insulin secretion and sensitivity, as well as other factors such as incretin secretion.[132] An impaired glucose tolerance (IGT) is more likely to indicate insulin resistance, while impaired fasting glucose (IFG) is more indicative of basal insulin secretion deficiency.[134]

Minimal model analysis of frequently sampled intravenous glucose tolerance test

After an intravenous bolus of glucose is delivered, serum glucose is measured repeatedly over a 3-hour period. From this, information about insulin sensitivity, glucose effectiveness, and beta-cell function is derived from a single dynamic test. However, because an IV form of glucose is used, the test is not frequently employed.

Homeostasis model assessment (HOMA) and quantitative insulin sensitivity check index (QUICKI)

HOMA-IR and QUICKI are often used to determine insulin sensitivity in clinical trials; both are mathematical models based upon fasting insulin and fasting glucose levels. For an individual with "normal" insulin sensitivity, HOMA-IR equals 1.0. It is often considered to have a reasonable linear correlation with the glucose clamp and minimal model estimates of insulin sensitivity/resistance.

WHO, 1998 (15)	EGIR, 199 (12)	NCEP:ATPIII, 2001 (1)	AACE, 2003 (18)	IDF, 2006 (13)
High insulin levels, IFG or IGT, and two of the following:	Top 25% of the fasting insulin values among nondiabetic individuals and two of the following:	Three or more of the following:	IGT and two or more of the following:	Central obesity as defined by the ethnic/racial specific WC, and two of the following:
Abdominal obesity: WHR >0.9, BMI ≥30 kg/m^2, WC >37 inches	WC: ≥94 cm for men ≥80 cm for women	WC: >40 inches for men, >35 inches for women	Triglycerides ≥150 mg/dl	Triglycerides ≥150 mg/dl
Lipid panel with triglycerides > 150 mg/dl, HDL-C <35 mg/dl	Triglycerides ≥2.0 mmol/ liter and HDL-C <1.0 mg/dl	Triglycerides ≥150 mg/dl	HDL-C: <40 mg/dl for men, <50 mg/dl for women	HDL-C: <40 mg/dl for men, <50 mg/dl for women
BP >140/90 mm Hg	BP >140/90 mm Hg or antihypertensive medication	HDL-C: <40 mg/dl for men, <50 mg/dl for women	BP >130/85 mm Hg	BP >130/85 mm Hg
	Fasting glucose ≥6.1 mmol/liter	BP >130/85 mm Hg		FPG ≥100 mg/dl
		FPG ≥100 mg/dl*		

Reference numbers are shown in *parentheses*. WHR, Waist-to-hip ratio; BP, blood pressure; FPG, fasting plasma glucose.
* In 2003, the ADA changed the criteria for IFG tolerance from >110 mg/dl to <100 mg /dl (16,17).

Figure 4.9 Criteria for the MetS definitions. From: Cornier MA, Dabelea D, Hernandez RC, et al. The metabolic syndrome. *Endocr Rev.* 2008 Dec;29(7):777-822. Epub 2008 Oct 29. Legend: WHO, World Health Organization; EGIR, European Group for the Study of Insulin Resistance; NCEP:ATPIII, National Cholesterol Education Program's Adult Treatment Panel III; AACE, American Association of Clinical Endocrinologists; IDF, International Diabetes Federation. Copyright 2008 Endocrine Society Used with permission from the Endocrine Society.

(HOMA-IR) = {[fasting insulin (mU/ml)] * [fasting glucose (mmol/l)]}/22.5.

Also a mathematical model, QUICKI may be significantly better at predicting the reference standard glucose clamp than HOMA-IR, and is a reproducible and reasonably accurate index of insulin sensitivity. Including fasting free fatty acid concentrations, along with fasting glucose and insulin, was recently shown to improve the association of QUICKI, but not HOMA-IR, with insulin sensitivity in adults, but not children.[133]

QUICKI = 1/[log (fasting insulin, mU/ml) + log (fasting glucose, mg/dl)].

Log (HOMA) and QUICKI are generally the most accurate surrogate indexes for determining insulin sensitivity, but they both have similar drawbacks.[134] The downside with these models is that they are based on fasting glucose and insulin levels, so they are much more reflective of hepatic insulin resistance, which occurs later, than they are for peripheral or skeletal muscle insulin resistance.[135]

Other markers

Serum adiponectin has emerged as a potentially excellent marker for insulin sensitivity, though it has not yet been fully evaluated. Serum adiponectin levels are linked to blood glucose levels in oral glucose tolerance testing, HOMA, and QUICKI, as well as insulin sensitivity markers in frequently sampled intravenous glucose tolerance testing and clamp studies. Levels are also negatively correlated with body mass index (BMI), waist circumference, waist/hip ratio, intra-abdominal fat, and percentage body fat.[136] Recent data suggests that adiponectin isoforms, particularly the high molecular weight isoform (HMW), are more strongly associated with visceral adiposity and insulin resistance, in some populations.[137,138,139]

Fetuin-A is a hepatic secretory protein that binds the insulin receptor and inhibits insulin action. Levels have been associated with incident diabetes, independent of other markers of insulin resistance.[140,141,142]

The TyG index, the product of fasting triglycerides and glucose levels, has shown a reasonable sensitivity (84.0%), although a poor specificity (45.0%), for detecting individuals with insulin resistance.[143]

BMI and waist circumference (WC) are also used as predictors of insulin resistance. A recent trial of over 200 men and 200 women found that a WC

>88 cm alone is nearly as good at predicting insulin resistance in women as MetS criteria. A WC >96 cm in men is also predictive, but not nearly as good as WC is in women.[144] Body mass index, muscle strength, and cardiorespiratory fitness were better predictors in men.[145]

Metabolic syndrome diagnosis

Currently there are several methods for diagnosing MetS, all of which include low HDL-C, elevated blood pressure and triglycerides, and either abnormal fasting plasma glucose or impaired glucose tolerance. Some methods also include measures of central obesity, such as the International Diabetes Federation criteria, which requires it for diagnosis. Two of the definitions shown in Figure 4.9 include as one of the criteria impaired fasting plasma glucose, which detects the degree of decompensation but not insulin resistance.[134]

Diabetes diagnosis and monitoring

The diagnosis of diabetes is more standardized, and has traditionally been made in one of three ways (Figure 4.10): a fasting plasma glucose ≥126 mg/dl; symptoms of hyperglycemia with a random glucose ≥200 mg/dl; or a 2-hour plasma glucose ≥200 mg/dl during an oral glucose tolerance test (see figure Figure 4.10)

1	FPG ≥126 mg/dl (7.0 mmol/dl). Fasting is defined as no caloric intake for at least 8 h.*
	OR
2	Symptoms of hyperglycemia and a casual plasma glucose ≥200 mg/dl (11.1 mmol/l). Casual is defined as any time of day without regard to time since last meal. The classic symptoms of hyperglycemia include polyuria, polydipsia, and unexplained weight loss.
	OR
3	2-h plasma glucose ≥200 mg/dl (11.1 mmol/l) during an OGTT. The test should be performed as described by the World Health Organization, using a glucose load containing the equivalent of 75 mg anhydrous glucose dissolved on water.*

*In the absence of unequivocal hyperglycemia, these criteria should be confirmed by repeat testing on a different day (5).

Figure 4.10 Criteria for the diagnosis of diabetes. From: American Diabetes Association. Standards of medical care in diabetes—2008. *Diabetes Care*. 2008 Jan;31 Suppl 1:S12-54. Reprinted with permission from The American Diabetes Association.

Although fasting glucose alone is often used to screen for diabetes, it is thought to miss approximately 30% of cases.[146] It is an insensitive tool because it does not reflect the earlier rises in postprandial glycemia associated with poor glucose tolerance. Only after the beta-cell function has declined enough for an elevated fasting glucose will these patients be detected, after the disease has progressed. Indeed, a recent analysis found that asymptomatic individuals with early stage T2D and impaired glucose tolerance have much more pronounced beta-cell defects than previously estimated by HOMA.[147] These patients may go undetected if fasting plasma glucose alone is used as for screening. Additionally, patients with both impaired fasting glucose and impaired glucose tolerance develop diabetes twice as often as those with only one of these abnormalities, emphasizing the importance of both tests for prognosis.

In addition to fasting blood glucose, there are several ways to monitor the efficacy of diabetes therapy, as well as the need for insulin. Chief among them is hemoglobin A1C (HbA1c), which is the American Diabetes Association's (ADAs) recommended primary target for glycemic control. It has also recently been approved for the diagnosis of diabetes (levels >6.5).[148] It does reflect the average serum glucose over several months (see Figure 4.11), but does not give good data for daily fluctuations in blood sugar; it misses the sharp rises and drops in blood sugar associated with meals that closer monitoring may detect.[94]

A1C (%)	Mean plasma glucose	
	mg/dl	mmol/l
6	135	7.5
7	170	9.5
8	205	11.5
9	240	13.5
10	275	15.5
11	310	17.5
12	345	19.5

Figure 4.11 Correlation between A1C level and mean plasma glucose levels. From: American Diabetes Association. Standards of medical care in diabetes—2008. *Diabetes Care*. 2008 Jan;31 Suppl 1:S12-54. Copyright 2008 American Diabetes Association. Reprinted with permission from The American Diabetes Association.

Improved glycemic control can be achieved with self-monitoring of glucose levels, particularly continuous monitoring. Self-monitoring has been associated with better glucose control in T2D, and is considered essential in T1D.[149,150] And continuous glucose monitoring is associated not only with better glucose control in adult diabetics, it can be used as a motivational tool for dietary and lifestyle changes. Perhaps most important, it can detect postprandial glucose excursions.[151,152] Recent epidemiological studies strongly indicate that hyperglycemia, specifically postprandial hyperglycemia, is a greater risk factor for morbidity and mortality in type 2 diabetes and for the development of cardiovascular disease than fasting glucose.[153,154] Additionally, reductions in HbA1c do not necessarily indicate a reduction in postprandial hyperglycemia, which may explain why reductions in HbA1c did not significantly reduce cardiovascular disease risk in recent studies.[155]

Because HbA1c may miss postprandial glucose increases, relying strictly on those test results can be misleading. For example, the patients in Figure 4.12 have roughly the same HbA1c and mean glucose, but quite different daily fluctuations in serum glucose levels, which certainly affect prognosis.

Another method to assess disease progression is the ankle-brachial index (ABI), a ratio of the blood pressure in the brachial artery to the dorsalis pedis or posterior tibial artery, whichever has a higher pressure. A low ABI was independently associated with a high risk of all-cause and CVD mortality in Chinese patients with T2D, as well as participants in the Framingham study.[156,157,158]

C-peptide is sometimes used to assess the degree of remaining pancreatic function, and may be useful in determining the necessity of insulin treatment. Measurement of C-peptide rather than insulin shortly after OGTT (15 minutes) helps in the assessment of first-phase insulin secretion.[159,160,161]

Regular screening for other diabetic complications is essential. This includes screening for retinopathy, nephropathy, neuropathy, gastrointestinal pathology (gastroparesis, intestinal enteropathy, and nonalcoholic fatty liver disease), periodontal disease, and other comorbitities.[94,162] Additionally, for individuals with T1D, a screen for celiac disease is recommended annually after diagnosis, for a minimum of 2 years.[163]

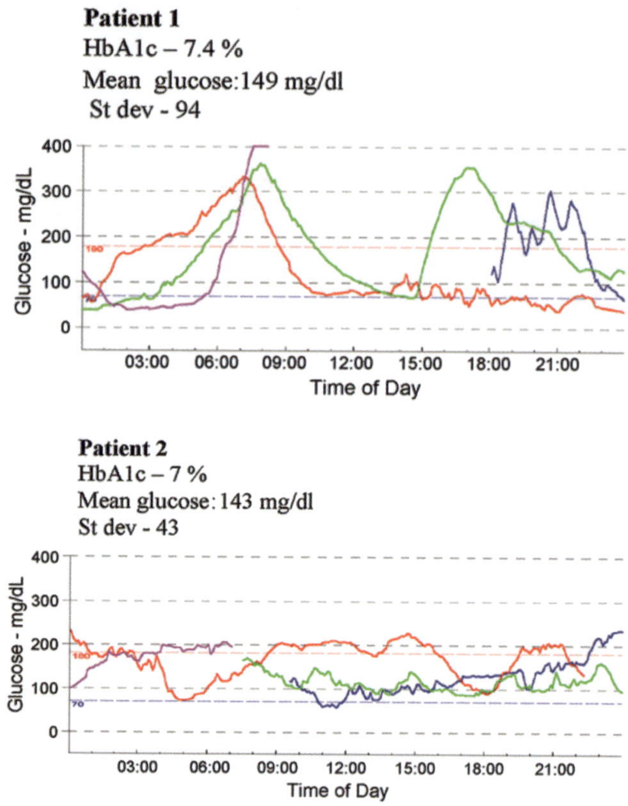

Figure 4.12 Continuous glucose monitoring of two patients at HbA1c target. From: Harman-Boehm I. Continuous glucose monitoring in type 2 diabetes. *Diabetes Res Clin Pract.* 2008 Dec 15;82 Suppl 2:S118-21. Used with permission from Elsevier.

Intervention

Treatment of insulin resistance, MetS, and diabetes and its complications can be complex, but is most successfully done with a combination of interventions, including lifestyle changes such as increasing physical activity and improving diet and nutrition, as well as targeted nutritional and botanical supplementation. Addressing underlying causes, achieving good glycemic control, preserving beta-cell function, reducing or eliminating central obesity, correcting nutritional deficiencies, and reducing inflammation are all important goals of treatment.

Diet and physical activity

Diet and activity combined

The combination of diet and physical activity is likely to have the greatest impact of any interventions for restoring insulin sensitivity and for improving glycemic control. In a trial of over 3000 non-diabetic individuals with elevated fasting and post-load plasma glucose concentrations, lifestyle interventions reduced the incidence of T2D by 58%, and metformin only by 31%, compared with placebo. The lifestyle intervention was significantly more effective than metformin. Interventions were designed to achieve a 7% weight loss, and 150 minutes aerobic exercise per week.[164]

In the Diabetes Prevention Program, a randomized trial, the same lifestyle interventions reduced the incidence of the metabolic syndrome 41% vs. only 17% in the metformin group, compared with placebo.[165] Interestingly, in a cost-based analysis of this study, they found that compared, with the placebo intervention, the lifestyle and metformin interventions were estimated to delay the development of T2D by 11 and 3 years, respectively.[166] And the cost for each program per quality-adjusted life year (QALY) was approximately $1100 for the lifestyle intervention and $31,300 for the metformin intervention.[168] Thus, not only did the lifestyle interventions delay the development of T2D almost 4 times as long as metformin, it incurred only a fraction of the cost. In a related trial of nearly 600 adults with impaired glucose tolerance, diet and lifestyle interventions over 6 years were found to prevent or delay diabetes for up to 14 years after the active intervention.[167]

In older individuals, lifestyle modification has been shown to be exceptionally effective in preventing diabetes, while metformin has very limited benefit, perhaps due to age-related differences in insulin action and secretion.[168]

Physical activity

Physical activity alone has significant benefit for individuals with poor insulin sensitivity. Muscle strengthening activity has been shown to be independently associated with higher insulin sensitivity among U.S. adults.[169] In a study of 250 adults, the absolute change in the HbA1c value was -0.51 percentage point in an aerobic training group, and -0.38 percentage point in a resistance training group. Combined exercise training resulted in an additional change in the HbA1c value of -0.46 percentage point compared with aerobic training alone and -0.59 percentage point compared with resistance training alone.[170] Mild to moderate aerobic exercise has also been found to prevent the cognitive decline seen in T2D.[171]

Diet

The Mediterranean diet can be particularly useful in the prevention of diabetes; it has been shown to improve glycemic control in normoglycemic populations, with mixed results in a diabetic population.[172] In a study of over 3000 men and women, greater adherence to the Mediterranean diet was associated with 51% lower odds of being obese and 59% lower odds of having central obesity.[173] In a study of nearly 14,000 Spanish university graduates, adherence was directly associated with a reduced incidence of diabetes, with those in the group of highest adherence having an OR of 0.17 compared to those with the least.[174]

A low glycemic index (GI) diet has also shown tremendous benefit for diabetes prevention as well as treatment (see Figures 4.13 and 4.14). The best evidence of the clinical usefulness of the GI has been reported in diabetic patients in whom low-GI foods have consistently shown beneficial effects on blood glucose control in both the short term and the long term.[175] In a review of 37 prospective cohort studies, the relative risk of T2D was 1.40 for those consuming a high vs. low glycemic index diet.[176] A high glycemic index meal has been shown to triple NF-KappaB activation in young lean subjects, activating inflammatory pathways as well as contributing to hyperglycemia.[177] An ideal approach would be to emphasize low-GI foods along with appropriate choices for

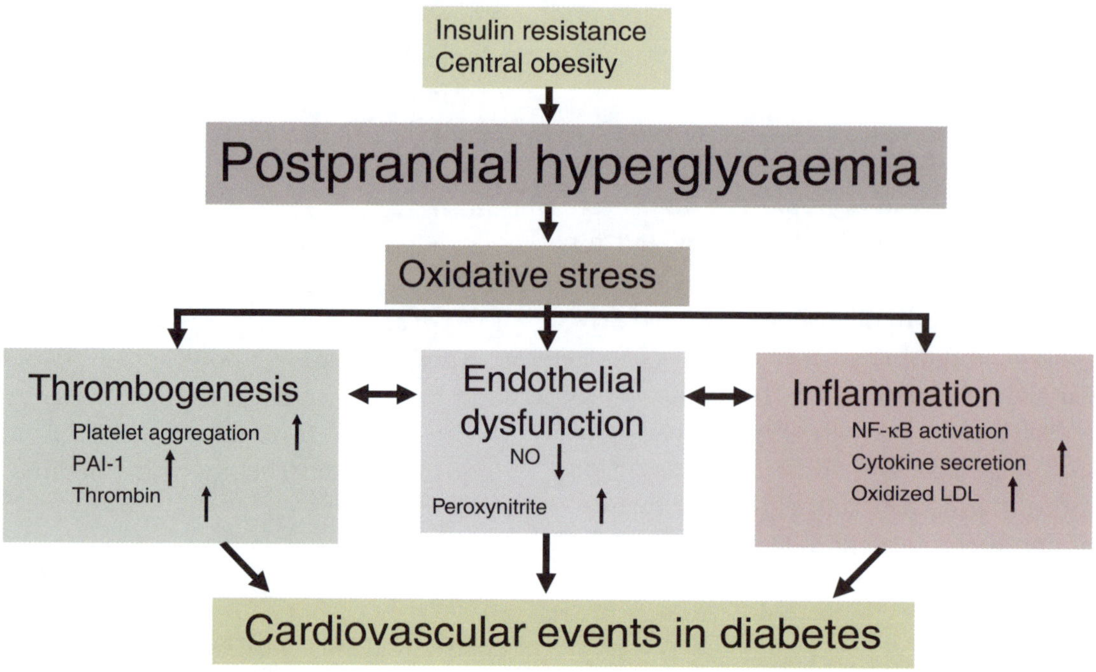

Figure 4.15 Molecular mechanisms for postprandial hyperglycemia-elicited CVD in diabetes. From: Yamagishi SI, Nakamura K, Matsui T, et al. Role of postprandial hyperglycaemia in cardiovascular disease in diabetes. *Int J Clin Pract.* 2007 Jan;61(1):83-7. Used with permission from John Wiley & Sons, Inc.

other relevant food characteristics, i.e., energy content, amount of other macronutrients, available carbohydrates, and dietary fiber.[178]

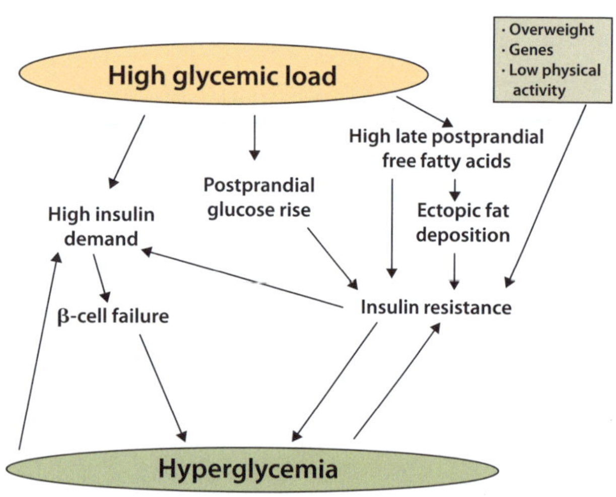

Figure 4.13 Mechanisms by which a high glycemic load leads to diabetes. From: Riccardi G, Rivellese AA, Giacco, R, et al. Role of glycemic index and glycemic load in the healthy state, in prediabetes, and in diabetes. *Am J Clin Nutr.* 2008 Jan;87(1):269S-274S. Used with permission from the American Society for Nutrition.

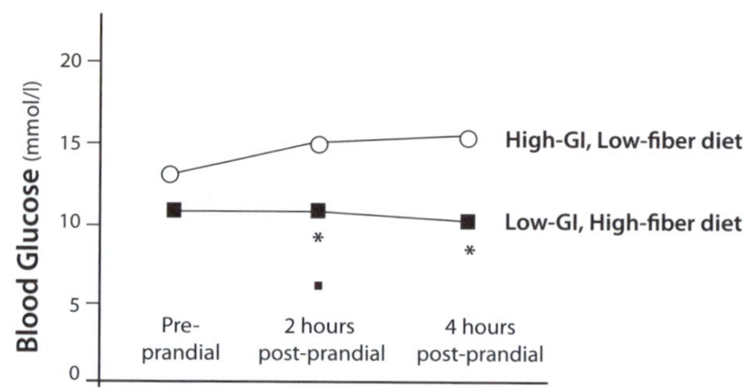

Figure 4.14 Postprandial blood glucose concentrations in patients with type 1 diabetes treated with a low glycemic index (GI), high-fiber diet or with a high-GI, low-fiber diet. From: Riccardi G, Rivellese AA, Giacco, R, et al. Role of glycemic index and glycemic load in the healthy state, in prediabetes, and in diabetes. *Am J Clin Nutr.* 2008 Jan;87(1):269S-274S. Used with permission from the American Society for Nutrition.

Dietary fiber

Both a low glycemic index diet and the Mediterranean diet tend to be high in fiber, a key ingredient for controlling postprandial glycemia. For example, a low glycemic load meal containing psyllium soluble fiber at breakfast significantly improves the postprandial glycemic, insulinemic, and free fatty acid responses in adults with T2D, and also has a beneficial effect on the next meal.[179]

Fiber intake is often assessed by cereal and/or whole grain consumption. In a prospective cohort study of 59,000 black women, intake of cereal fiber was inversely associated with risk of diabetes, with an incidence rate ratio of 0.82 from the highest compared to the lowest consumption.[180] In another study of over 2000 men and 2000 women, the relative risk for diabetes between the highest and lowest quartiles of whole-grain consumption was 0.65. In this study, cereal fiber intake was also associated with a reduced risk of T2D; the relative risk of the highest vs. the lowest quartile of cereal fiber intake was 0.39.[181]

Furthermore, dietary fiber has the potential to reduce one of the greatest consequences of poor blood glucose control—postprandial hyperglycemia. To repeat for emphasis: postprandial hyperglycemia is a greater risk factor than abnormal fasting plasma glucose for the mortality and morbidity associated with diabetes, including the risk for cardiovascular disease (see Figure 4.15).

More viscous fibers have consistently shown benefit in improving blood glucose levels, as seen by reductions in postprandial glucose, insulin, and C-peptide responses in subjects with T2D, with similar benefits in insulin resistance subjects.[182,183,184,185]

Dietary fats

Monounsaturated fats (MUFA) appear to have benefit for restoring both beta-cell function and insulin sensitivity. Both of these variables progressively improve in the postprandial state as the ratio of monounsaturated fats to saturated fats increases.[186] Using NHANES data, adults with diabetes had a lower incidence of peripheral neuropathy with a higher intake of MUFA, most likely due to alpha-linolenic acid intake.[187,188] Polymorphisms in the adiponectin gene have been associated with the effect of MUFA on insulin resistance, and may allow better targeting of this intervention, with similar findings for the apoB gene. Both saturated fats and trans fats are known to increase postprandial insulinemia in obese patients with T2D, and saturated fats have also been shown to impair endothelial function in T2D patients, an effect not seen with monounsaturated fats.[189,190]

Meal regularity and timing

Using continuous glucose monitoring, a study of 23 diabetic subjects found that evenly spaced carbohydrate consumption throughout the day did not optimize blood glucose control, although having the largest carbohydrate intake at lunch was associated with the most favorable postprandial profile.[191] In a study of over 3600 individuals, the adjusted OR for having the greatest number of components of MetS in subjects who were regular eaters was 0.27, using subjects who did not fulfill any criteria for MetS as a reference group. Eating meals regularly was also inversely related to insulin resistance, with an OR of 0.68.[192]

Nutritional and botanical supplementation

The key goals of supplementation are to impact one or all of the following:

1. Reduce after-meal elevations in blood sugar levels
2. Provide optimal nutrient status
3. Improve insulin function and sensitivity
4. Prevent nutritional and oxidative stress

Fiber supplementation

Numerous trials have demonstrated the benefit of whole foods and fiber for glucose control (with more viscous fibers having a greater benefit), particularly postprandial hyperglycemia. Fiber supplementation can also improve insulin sensitivity, reduce appetite, and increase weight loss, targeting many of the underlying dysfunctions of insulin resistance.

Multivitamin/multimineral

Given the wide variety of nutrients shown to have benefit for glucose control, a multivitamin/mineral is often part of basic therapy. Specific improvements have been shown for broad antioxidant support, B vitamins, chromium, and magnesium as part of a multiple vitamin.[193,194] Vitamin C has been found to improve endothelial function, glycemic control, arterial stiffness, hypertension, and oxidation status.[195,196] Vitamin E reduces inflammation, though there may be greater benefit with gamma or mixed tocopherols than alpha only.[197] When combined with beta-carotene, these antioxidants increased adiponectin levels and improved markers of insulin resistance.[198]

Chromium is thought to improve insulin sensitivity by increasing the activity of insulin receptor tyrosine kinase; chromium picolinate supplementation in subjects with T2D who are taking sulfonylurea agents produced significant improvements in insulin sensitivity and glucose control.[199,200] In a randomized trial of more than 400 T2D patients with poor glucose control receiving antidiabetic therapy, HbA1c decreased 0.54% in those patients given chromium and biotin. The decrease in HbA1c was most pronounced in chromium picolinate/biotin subjects whose baseline HbA1c was ≥10%.[201,202] Benefits have also been shown for weight loss, improving fasting plasma glucose, and reducing central obesity.[201]

In a review of nine randomized trials with T2D patients, magnesium was shown to have raised HDL and lowered fasting plasma glucose.[203] In a study of over 1100 adults, hypomagnesemia was found to be independently associated with the development of impaired glucose tolerance (IGT) with or without impaired fasting glucose (IFG), and type 2 diabetes, although not with isolated IFG, i.e., IFG without concurrent IGT.[204]

Omega-3 fatty acids

In addition to improving insulin sensitivity, omega-3 fatty acids have been shown to provide significant benefit for cardiovascular disease prevention, the major cause of morbidity and mortality in diabetic patients.[205,206] There may also be a preventive effect for T1D; overall consumption of omega-3s was inversely associated with risk of T1D among children at risk, with a hazard ratio of 0.45.[207]

Omega-3s have also been shown to lower triglycerides and very low density lipoproteins (VLDL), although they may raise LDL cholesterol among T2D patients.[208] However, LDL particle size increases from small, dense, atherogenic particles to larger, buoyant particles that are less likely to contribute to atherosclerotic vascular disease.[209,210] And when combined with gamma-linolenic acid (GLA), an anti-inflammatory essential fatty acid, they provide benefit for the prevention and treatment of diabetic neuropathy.[211,212]

Vitamin D

Insufficient vitamin D increases the risk of insulin resistance and inflammation, and is involved in the pathogenesis of T1D and T2D.[213] Although supplemental vitamin D has been shown to improve insulin production and release, early studies suggested that the benefit might be limited to correcting an existing deficiency, a problem we now know to be widespread.[214,215] Two recent studies suggest that vitamin D supplementation of non-diabetic individuals with central obesity improves postprandial insulin sensitivity, and that plasma 25-OH vitamin D is directly associated with insulin resistance in non-diabetic adults.[216,217]

Antioxidant support

CoQ10 has very broad spectrum benefits for diabetic and prediabetic populations. It has been shown to improve blood pressure, oxidative status, HbA1c, and glycemic control in diabetic patients.[218,219,220] It also improves mitochondrial function, which is impaired in individuals with insulin resistance and T2D, and also in their offspring.[221] Fasting mitochondrial function is 14–40% lower in the presence of insulin resistance than in controls, as seen in those with type 2 diabetes, their insulin-resistant relatives or the obese.[222] One review suggests mitochondrial function is central to insulin resistance.[223]

Alpha-lipoic acid is also an important antioxidant for blood sugar control, and for preventing complications of hyperglycemia. It has been found to reduce oxidative damage, and improve glycemic control and insulin resistance.[224,225] It also improves symptoms of polyneuropathy at a dose of 600 mg per day, with higher doses having more adverse effects.[226]

Botanical support

A number of herbs have shown benefit in the treatment of diabetes and insulin resistance, and may have synergistic effects when taken in combination. Fenugreek produced improvements in fasting plasma glucose and oral glucose tolerance in T1D patients.[227] In a randomized trial of 25 patients with T2D, it was also found to improve glycemic control and decrease insulin resistance.[228] *Gymnema sylvestre* has little clinical research, but what exists is suggestive of benefits for beta-cell activity in both T1D and T2D.[229,230] Panax ginseng has been shown to reduce fasting plasma glucose, HbA1c, and postprandial hyperglycemia in trials with non-diabetic and T2D patients.[231] *Momordica charantia* was recently studied in a randomized clinical trial of 40 adult patients, and showed a very slight decrease in HbA1c compared to placebo.[232] Although initial trials with this herb were not randomized, they found a moderate hypoglycemic effect.[233] Mulberry powder has been found to suppress elevations of postprandial glucose.[234] Green tea has had mixed clinical findings,[235] but a recent randomized trial found a reduction in HbA1c in patients taking a powdered extract.[236] It may also have thermogenic effects, providing assistance with weight loss.[237]

Other treatments

Nicotinamide may have a role in treating children with T1D. It has been shown to have beta-cell sparing effects, prolonging the need for insulin in children.[238,239,240] Acetyl-L-carnitine, particularly in patients with diabetes and neuropathy, demonstrates beneficial effects on nerve conduction slowing, neuropathic pain, axonal degenerative changes, and nerve fiber regeneration.[241]

References

1. Muniyappa R, Lee S, Chen H, et al. Current approaches for assessing insulin sensitivity and resistance *in vivo*: advantages, limitations, and appropriate usage. *Am J Physiol Endocrinol Metab.* 2008 Jan;294(1):E15-26. 17957034.
2. Fonseca VA. Early identification and treatment of insulin resistance: impact on subsequent prediabetes and type 2 diabetes. *Clin Cornerstone.* 2007;8 Suppl 7:S7-18 18159645.
3. Tabák AG, Jokela M, Akbaraly TN, et al. Trajectories of glycaemia, insulin sensitivity, and insulin secretion before diagnosis of type 2 diabetes: an analysis from the Whitehall II study. *Lancet.* 2009 Jun 27;373(9682):2215-21.
4. Ioannou GN, Bryson CL, Boyko EJ. Prevalence and trends of insulin resistance, impaired fasting glucose, and diabetes. *J Diabetes Complications.* 2007 Nov-Dec;21(6):363-70.17967708.
5. Ogden CL, Carroll MD, Curtin LR, et al. Prevalence of overweight and obesity in the United States, 1999-2004. *JAMA.* 2006 Apr 5;295(13):1549-55 16595758.
6. Gregg EW, Cheng YJ, Narayan KM, et al. The relative contributions of different levels of overweight and obesity to the increased prevalence of diabetes in the United States: 1976-2004. *Prev Med.* 2007 Nov;45(5):348-52. 17889292.
7. Stefan N, Kantartzis K, Machann J, et al. Identification and characterization of metabolically benign obesity in humans. *Arch Intern Med.* 2008 Aug 11;168(15):1609-16. 18695074.
8. Chiarelli F, Marcovecchio ML. Insulin Resistance and Obesity in Childhood. *Eur J Endocrinol.* 2008 Sep 19. Epub ahead of print. 18805916.
9. Reilly MP, Lehrke M, Wolfe ML, et al. Resistin is an inflammatory marker of atherosclerosis in humans. *Circulation.* 2005 Feb 22;111(7):932-9. 15710760.
10. Hivert MF, Sullivan LM, Fox CS, et al. Associations of adiponectin, resistin, and tumor necrosis factor-alpha with insulin resistance. *J Clin Endocrinol Metab.* 2008 Aug;93(8):3165-72. 18492747.
11. Pérez-Martínez P, López-Miranda J, Cruz-Teno C, et al. Adiponectin gene variants are associated with insulin sensitivity in response to dietary fat consumption in Caucasian men. *J Nutr.* 2008 Sep;138(9):1609-14. 18716158.
12. Moreno JA, Pérez-Jiménez F, Marín C, et al. The apolipoprotein E gene promoter (-219G/T) polymorphism determines insulin sensitivity in response to dietary fat in healthy young adults. *J Nutr.* 2005 Nov;135(11):2535-40. 16251607.
13. Gómez P, Pérez-Jiménez F, Marín C, et al. The -514 C/T polymorphism in the hepatic lipase gene promoter is associated with insulin sensitivity in a healthy young population. *J Mol Endocrinol.* 2005 Apr;34(2):331-8. 15821100.
14. Cornier MA, Dabelea D, Hernandez TL, et al. The Metabolic Syndrome. *Endocr Rev.* 2008 Oct 29. Epub ahead of print. 18971485.
15. Ford ES. Prevalence of the metabolic syndrome defined by the International Diabetes Federation among adults in the U.S. *Diabetes Care.* 2005 Nov;28(11):2745-9. 16249550.
16. Cook S, Auinger P, Li C, et al. Metabolic syndrome rates in United States adolescents, from the National Health and Nutrition Examination Survey, 1999-2002. *J Pediatr.* 2008 Feb;152(2):165-70. 18206683.
17. Ford ES, Li C. Metabolic syndrome and health-related quality of life among U.S. adults. *Ann Epidemiol.* 2008 Mar;18(3):165-71. 18280918.
18. Klein BE, Klein R, Lee KE. Components of the metabolic syndrome and risk of cardiovascular disease and diabetes in Beaver Dam. *Diabetes Care.* 2002 Oct;25(10):1790-4. 12351479.
19. Ford ES. Risks for all-cause mortality, cardiovascular disease, and diabetes associated with the metabolic syndrome: a summary of the evidence. *Diabetes Care.* 2005 Jul;28(7):1769-78. 15983333.
20. Morrison JA, Friedman LA, Gray-McGuire C. Metabolic syndrome in childhood predicts adult cardiovascular disease 25 years later: the Princeton Lipid Research Clinics Follow-up Study. *Pediatrics.* 2007 Aug;120(2):340-5. 17671060.
21. Lakka HM, Laaksonen DE, Lakka TA, et al. The metabolic syndrome and total and cardiovascular disease mortality in middle-aged men. *JAMA.* 2002 Dec 4;288(21):2709-16. 12460094.
22. Gami AS, Witt BJ, Howard DE, et al. Metabolic syndrome and risk of incident cardiovascular events and death: a systematic review and meta-analysis of longitudinal studies. *J Am Coll Cardiol.* 2007 Jan 30;49(4):403-14. 17258085.
23. Li W, Ma D, Liu M, et al. Association between metabolic syndrome and risk of stroke: a meta-analysis of cohort studies. *Cerebrovasc Dis.* 2008;25(6):539-47. 18480607.
24. Boden-Albala B, Sacco RL, Lee HS, et al. Metabolic syndrome and ischemic stroke risk: Northern Manhattan Study. *Stroke.* 2008 Jan;39(1):30-5. 18063821.
25. Tsai CH, Li TC, Lin CC. Metabolic syndrome as a risk factor for nonalcoholic fatty liver disease. *South Med J.* 2008 Sep;101(9):900-5. 18708987.
26. Lastra G, Manrique C, Sowers JR. Obesity, cardiometabolic syndrome, and chronic kidney disease: the weight of the evidence. *Adv Chronic Kidney Dis.* 2006 Oct;13(4):365-73. 17045222.
27. Kawamoto R, Kohara K, Tabara Y, et al. An association between metabolic syndrome and the estimated glomerular filtration rate. *Intern Med.* 2008;47(15):1399-406. 18670145.
28. Cheung LP, Ma RC, Lam PM, et al. Cardiovascular risks and metabolic syndrome in Hong Kong Chinese women with polycystic ovary syndrome. *Hum Reprod.* 2008 Jun;23(6):1431-8. 18359783.

29. Lam JC, Ip MS. *Curr Opin Pulm Med.* 2007 Nov;13(6):484-9. 17901753.

30. Parikh RM, Joshi SR, Pandia K. Index of Central Obesity Is Better than Waist Circumference in Defining Metabolic Syndrome. *Metab Syndr Relat Disord.* 2009 Jun 26. Epub ahead of print. 19558273.

31. Boden G. Obesity and free fatty acids. *Endocrinol Metab Clin North Am.* 2008 Sep;37(3):635-46, VIII-IX 18775356.

32. Ishikawa S, Kayaba K, Gotoh T, et al. Metabolic syndrome and C-reactive protein in the general population: JMS Cohort Study. *Circ J.* 2007 Jan;71(1):26-31. 17186974.

33. Ye X, Yu Z, Li H, et al. Distributions of C-reactive protein and its association with metabolic syndrome in middle-aged and older Chinese people. *J Am Coll Cardiol.* 2007 May 1;49(17):1798-805. 17466231.

34. Laaksonen DE, Niskanen L, Nyyssönen K, et al. C-reactive protein and the development of the metabolic syndrome and diabetes in middle-aged men. *Diabetologia.* 2004 Aug;47(8):1403-10. 15309290.

35. Ingelsson E, Arnlöv J, Sundström J, et al. Relative importance and conjoint effects of obesity and physical inactivity for the development of insulin resistance. *Eur J Cardiovasc Prev Rehabil.* 2009 Feb;16(1):28-33.

36. Hamilton MT, Hamilton DG, Zderic TW. Role of low energy expenditure and sitting in obesity, metabolic syndrome, type 2 diabetes, and cardiovascular disease. *Diabetes.* 2007 Nov;56(11):2655-67. 17827399.

37. Saiki A, Oyama T, Endo K, et al. Preheparin serum lipoprotein lipase mass might be a biomarker of metabolic syndrome. *Diabetes Res Clin Pract.* 2007 Apr;76(1):93-101. 16956692.

38. Orchard TJ, Temprosa M, Goldberg R, et al. The effect of metformin and intensive lifestyle intervention on the metabolic syndrome: the Diabetes Prevention Program randomized trial. *Ann Intern Med.* 2005 Apr 19;142(8):611-9. 15838067.

39. Giugliano D, Ceriello A, Esposito K. The effects of diet on inflammation: emphasis on the metabolic syndrome. *J Am Coll Cardiol.* 2006 Aug 15;48(4):677-85. 16904534.

40. Qi L, Rimm E, Liu S, et al. Dietary glycemic index, glycemic load, cereal fiber, and plasma adiponectin concentration in diabetic men. *Diabetes Care.* 2005 May;28(5):1022-8. 15855561.

41. Qi L, Meigs JB, Liu S, et al. Dietary fibers and glycemic load, obesity, and plasma adiponectin levels in women with type 2 diabetes. *Diabetes Care.* 2006 Jul;29(7):1501-5. 16801569.

42. Weickert MO, Pfeiffer AF. Metabolic effects of dietary fiber consumption and prevention of diabetes. *J Nutr.* 2008 Mar;138(3):439-42. 18287346.

43. Jenkins DJ, Wolever TM, Leeds AR, et al. Dietary fibres, fibre analogues, and glucose tolerance: importance of viscosity. *Br Med J.* 1978 May 27;1(6124):1392-4. 647304.

44. Brenelli SL, Campos SD, Saad MJ. Viscosity of gums *in vitro* and their ability to reduce postprandial hyperglycemia in normal subjects. *Braz J Med Biol Res.* 1997 Dec;30(12):1437-40. 9686163.

45. Kabagambe EK, Tsai MY, Hopkins PN, et al. Erythrocyte fatty acid composition and the metabolic syndrome: a National Heart, Lung, and Blood Institute GOLDN study. *Clin Chem.* 2008 Jan;54(1):154-62. 17998266.

46. Reis JP, von Mühlen D, Miller ER 3rd. Relation of 25-hydroxyvitamin D and parathyroid hormone levels with metabolic syndrome among US adults. *Eur J Endocrinol.* 2008 Jul;159(1):41-8. 18426812.

47. Forouhi NG, Luan J, Cooper A, et al. Baseline serum 25-hydroxy vitamin d is predictive of future glycemic status and insulin resistance: the Medical Research Council Ely Prospective Study 1990-2000. *Diabetes.* 2008 Oct;57(10):2619-25. 18591391.

48. Filus A, Trzmiel A, Kuliczkowska-Płaksej J, et al. Relationship between vitamin D receptor BsmI and FokI polymorphisms and anthropometric and biochemical parameters describing metabolic syndrome. *Aging Male.* 2008 Sep;11(3):134-9. 18821289.

49. McKeown NM, Jacques PF, Zhang XL, et al. Dietary magnesium intake is related to metabolic syndrome in older Americans. *Eur J Nutr.* 2008 Jun;47(4):210-6. 18560789.

50. Song Y, Ridker PM, Manson JE, et al. Magnesium intake, C-reactive protein, and the prevalence of metabolic syndrome in middle-aged and older U.S. women. *Diabetes Care.* 2005 Jun;28(6):1438-44. 15920065.

51. Lee DH, Lee IK, Porta M, et al. Relationship between serum concentrations of persistent organic pollutants and the prevalence of metabolic syndrome among non-diabetic adults: results from the National Health and Nutrition Examination Survey 1999-2002. *Diabetologia.* 2007 Sep;50(9):1841-51. 17624515.

52. Lee DH, Lee IK, Jin SH, et al. Association between serum concentrations of persistent organic pollutants and insulin resistance among nondiabetic adults: results from the National Health and Nutrition Examination Survey 1999-2002. *Diabetes Care.* 2007 Mar;30(3):622-8. 17327331.

53. Ong KL, Cheung BM, Wong LY, et al. Prevalence, treatment, and control of diagnosed diabetes in the U.S. National Health and Nutrition Examination Survey 1999-2004. *Ann Epidemiol.* 2008 Mar;18(3):222-9. 18201902.

54. Leslie RD, Kolb H, Schloot NC, et al. Diabetes classification: grey zones, sound and smoke: Action LADA 1. *Diabetes Metab Res Rev.* 2008 Oct;24(7):511-9. 18615859.

55. Knip M, Siljander H. Autoimmune mechanisms in type 1 diabetes. *Autoimmun Rev.* 2008 Jul;7(7):550-7.18625444.

56. Wenzlau JM, Juhl K, Yu L, et al. The cation efflux transporter ZnT8 (Slc30A8) is a major autoantigen in human type 1 diabetes. *Proc Natl Acad Sci U S A.* 2007 Oct 23;104(43):17040-5. 17942684.

57. Cerná M. Genetics of autoimmune diabetes mellitus. *Wien Med Wochenschr.* 2008;158(1-2):2-12. 18286244.

58. Akerblom HK, Vaarala O, Hyöty H, et al. Environmental factors in the etiology of type 1 diabetes. *Am J Med Genet.* 2002 May 30;115(1):18-29. 12116173.

59. Oikarinen M, Tauriainen S, Honkanen T, et al. Detection of enteroviruses in the intestine of type 1 diabetic patients. *Clin Exp Immunol.* 2008 Jan;151(1):71-5. 17991291.

60. Roivainen M. Enteroviruses: new findings on the role of enteroviruses in type 1 diabetes. *Int J Biochem Cell Biol.* 2006;38(5-6):721-5. 16226050.

61. Barbeau WE, Bassaganya-Riera J, Hontecillas R. Putting the pieces of the puzzle together–a series of hypotheses on the etiology and pathogenesis of type 1 diabetes. *Med Hypotheses.* 2007;68(3):607-19. 17045415.

62. Franzese A, Lombardi F, Valerio G, et al. Update on coeliac disease and type 1 diabetes mellitus in childhood. *J Pediatr Endocrinol Metab.* 2007 Dec;20(12):1257-64. 18341084.

63. Kohno T, Kobashiri Y, Sugie Y, et al. Antibodies to food antigens in Japanese patients with type 1 diabetes mellitus. *Diabetes Res Clin Pract.* 2002 Jan;55(1):1-9. 11755473.

64. Lewy H, Hampe CS, Kordonouri O, et al. Seasonality of month of birth differs between type 1 diabetes patients with pronounced beta-cell autoimmunity and individuals with lesser or no beta-cell autoimmunity. *Pediatr Diabetes.* 2008 Feb;9(1):46-52. 18036133.

65. Bener A, Alsaied A, Al-Ali M, et al. High prevalence of vitamin D deficiency in type 1 diabetes mellitus and healthy children. *Acta Diabetol.* 2008 Oct 10. Epub ahead of print. 18846317.

66. Ponsonby AL, Pezic A, Ellis J, et al. Variation in associations between allelic variants of the vitamin D receptor gene and onset of type 1 diabetes mellitus by ambient winter ultraviolet radiation levels: a meta-regression analysis. *Am J Epidemiol.* 2008 Aug 15;168(4):358-65. 18552362.

67. Wahlberg J, Fredriksson J, Nikolic E, et al. Environmental factors related to the induction of beta-cell autoantibodies in 1-yr-old healthy children. *Pediatr Diabetes.* 2005 Dec;6(4):199-205. 16390388.

68. Luopajärvi K, Savilahti E, Virtanen SM, et al. Enhanced levels of cow's milk antibodies in infancy in children who develop type 1 diabetes later in childhood. *Pediatr Diabetes.* 2008 Oct;9(5):434-41. 18503496.

69. Catassi C, Bonucci A, Coppa GV, et al. Intestinal permeability changes during the first month: effect of natural versus artificial feeding. *J Pediatr Gastroenterol Nutr.* 1995 Nov;21(4):383-6. 8583288.

70. Holmberg H, Wahlberg J, Vaarala O, et al. Short duration of breast-feeding as a risk-factor for beta-cell autoantibodies in 5-year-old children from the general population. *Br J Nutr.* 2007 Jan;97(1):111-6. 17217566.

71. Wahlberg J, Fredriksson J, Nikolic E, et al. Environmental factors related to the induction of beta-cell autoantibodies in 1-yr-old healthy children. *Pediatr Diabetes.* 2005 Dec;6(4):199-205. 16390388.

72. Franzese A, Lombardi F, Valerio G, et al. Update on coeliac disease and type 1 diabetes mellitus in childhood. *J Pediatr Endocrinol Metab.* 2007 Dec;20(12):1257-64. 18341084.

73. Frisk G, Hansson T, Dahlbom I, et al. A unifying hypothesis on the development of type 1 diabetes and celiac disease: gluten consumption may be a shared causative factor. *Med Hypotheses.* 2008;70(6):1207-9. 18249499.

74. Norris JM, Barriga K, Klingensmith G, et al. Timing of initial cereal exposure in infancy and risk of islet autoimmunity. *JAMA.* 2003 Oct 1;290(13):1713-20. 14519705.

75. Benson VS, Vanleeuwen JA, Taylor J, et al. Food consumption and the risk of type 1 diabetes in children and youth: a population-based, case-control study in Prince Edward Island, Canada. *J Am Coll Nutr.* 2008 Jun;27(3):414-20. 18838530.

76. Norris JM, Yin X, Lamb MM, et al. Omega-3 polyunsaturated fatty acid intake and islet autoimmunity in children at increased risk for type 1 diabetes. *JAMA.* 2007 Sep 26;298(12):1420-8. 17895458.

77. Merzouk SA, Saker M, Reguig KB, et al. N-3 polyunsaturated fatty acids modulate *in vitro* T cell function in type 1 diabetic patients. *Lipids.* 2008 Jun;43(6):485-97. 18392872.

78. Ponsonby AL, Pezic A, Ellis J, et al. Variation in associations between allelic variants of the vitamin D receptor gene and onset of type 1 diabetes mellitus by ambient winter ultraviolet radiation levels: a meta-regression analysis. *Am J Epidemiol.* 2008 Aug 15;168(4):358-65. 18552362.

79. Zipitis CS, Akobeng AK. Vitamin D supplementation in early childhood and risk of type 1 diabetes: a systematic review and meta-analysis. *Arch Dis Child.* 2008 Jun;93(6):512-7. 18339654.

80. Brekke HK, Ludvigsson J. Vitamin D supplementation and diabetes-related autoimmunity in the ABIS study. *Pediatr Diabetes.* 2007 Feb;8(1):11-4. 17341286.

81. Bener A, Alsaied A, Al-Ali M, et al. High prevalence of vitamin D deficiency in type 1 diabetes mellitus and healthy children. *Acta Diabetol.* 2008 Oct 10. Epub ahead of print. 18846317.

82. Akerblom HK, Vaarala O, Hyöty H, et al. Environmental factors in the etiology of type 1 diabetes. *Am J Med Genet.* 2002 May 30;115(1):18-29. 12116173.

83. Oikarinen M, Tauriainen S, Honkanen T, et al. Detection of enteroviruses in the intestine of type 1 diabetic patients. *Clin Exp Immunol.* 2008 Jan;151(1):71-5. 17991291.

84. Viskari H, Ludvigsson J, Uibo R, et al. Relationship between the incidence of type 1 diabetes and maternal enterovirus antibodies: time trends and geographical variation. *Diabetologia.* 2005 Jul;48(7):1280-7. 15902401.

85. Sadeharju K, Knip M, Virtanen SM, et al. Maternal antibodies in breast milk protect the child from enterovirus infections. *Pediatrics*. 2007 May;119(5):941-6. 17473095.

86. Moltchanova E, Rytkönen M, Kousa A, et al. Zinc and nitrate in the ground water and the incidence of type 1 diabetes in Finland. 2004 Mar;21(3):256-61. 15008836.

87. Longnecker MP, Daniels JL. Environmental contaminants as etiologic factors for diabetes. *Environ Health Perspect*. 2001 Dec;109 Suppl 6:871-6. 11744505.

88. Fourlanos S, Harrison LC, Colman PG. The accelerator hypothesis and increasing incidence of type 1 diabetes. *Curr Opin Endocrinol Diabetes Obes*. 2008 Aug;15(4):321-5. 18594271.

89. Centers for Disease Control and Prevention (CDC). State-specific incidence of diabetes among adults—participating states, 1995-1997 and 2005-2007. *MMWR Morb Mortal Wkly Rep*. 2008 Oct 31;57(43):1169-73. 18971918.

90. Lupi R, Del Prato S. Beta-cell apoptosis in type 2 diabetes: quantitative and functional consequences. *Diabetes Metab*. 2008 Feb;34 Suppl 2:S56-64. 18640587.

91. Tirsi A, Bruehl H, Sweat V, et al. Retinal vessel abnormalities are associated with elevated fasting insulin levels and cerebral atrophy in nondiabetic individuals. *Ophthalmology*. 2009 Jun;116(6):1175-81.

92. American Diabetes Association. Standards of medical care in diabetes—2008. *Diabetes Care*. 2008 Jan;31 Suppl 1:S12-54. 18165335.

93. Rahman S, Rahman T, Ismail AA, et al. Diabetes-associated macrovasculopathy: pathophysiology and pathogenesis. *Diabetes Obes Metab*. 2007 Nov;9(6):767-80. 17924861.

94. Vazquez G, Duval S, Jacobs DR Jr, et al. Comparison of body mass index, waist circumference, and waist/hip ratio in predicting incident diabetes: a meta-analysis. *Epidemiol Rev*. 2007;29:115-28. 17494056.

95. Snijder MB, Dekker JM, Visser M, et al. Associations of hip and thigh circumferences independent of waist circumference with the incidence of type 2 diabetes: the Hoorn Study. *Am J Clin Nutr*. 2003 May;77(5):1192-7. 12716671.

96. LeRoith D, Novosyadlyy R, Gallagher EJ, et al. Obesity and type 2 diabetes are associated with an increased risk of developing cancer and a worse prognosis; epidemiological and mechanistic evidence. *Exp Clin Endocrinol Diabetes*. 2008 Sep;116 Suppl 1:S4-6. 18777452.

97. Lee CM, Huxley RR, Wildman RP, et al. Indices of abdominal obesity are better discriminators of cardiovascular risk factors than BMI: a meta-analysis. *J Clin Epidemiol*. 2008 Jul;61(7):646-53. 18359190.

98. Hu FB, Li TY, Colditz GA, et al. Television watching and other sedentary behaviors in relation to risk of obesity and type 2 diabetes mellitus in women. *JAMA*. 2003 Apr 9;289(14):1785-91. 12684356.

99. Hu FB, Leitzmann MF, Stampfer MJ, et al. Physical activity and television watching in relation to risk for type 2 diabetes mellitus in men. *Arch Intern Med*. 2001 Jun 25;161(12):1542-8. 11427103.

100. Zhao G, Ford ES, Li C, et al. Compliance with physical activity recommendations in US adults with diabetes. *Diabet Med*. 2008 Feb;25(2):221-7. 18201213.

101. Schulze MB, Liu S, Rimm EB, et al. Glycemic index, glycemic load, and dietary fiber intake and incidence of type 2 diabetes in younger and middle-aged women. *Am J Clin Nutr*. 2004 Aug;80(2):348-56. 15277155.

102. Barclay AW, Petocz P, McMillan-Price J, et al. Glycemic index, glycemic load, and chronic disease risk—a meta-analysis of observational studies. *Am J Clin Nutr*. 2008 Mar;87(3):627-37. 18326601.

103. Sargeant LA, Khaw KT, Bingham S, et al. Fruit and vegetable intake and population glycosylated haemoglobin levels: the EPIC-Norfolk Study. *Eur J Clin Nutr*. 2001 May;55(5):342-8. 11378807.

104. Harding AH, Wareham NJ, Bingham SA, et al. Plasma vitamin C level, fruit and vegetable consumption, and the risk of new-onset type 2 diabetes mellitus: the European prospective investigation of cancer—Norfolk prospective study. *Arch Intern Med*. 2008 Jul 28;168(14):1493-9. 18663161.

105. Bazzano LA, Li TY, Joshipura KJ, et al. Intake of fruit, vegetables, and fruit juices and risk of diabetes in women. *Diabetes Care*. 2008 Jul;31(7):1311-7. 18390796.

106. Qiao Q, Tuomilehto J, Borch-Johnsen K. Post-challenge hyperglycaemia is associated with premature death and macrovascular complications. *Diabetologia*. 2003 Mar;46 Suppl 1:M17-21.

107. Gao W, Qiao Q, Tuomilehto J. Post-challenge hyperglycaemia rather than fasting hyperglycaemia is an independent risk factor of cardiovascular disease events. *Clin Lab*. 2004;50(9-10):609-15.

108. Villegas R, Gao YT, Yang G, et al. Legume and soy food intake and the incidence of type 2 diabetes in the Shanghai Women's Health Study. *Am J Clin Nutr*. 2008 Jan;87(1):162-7. 18175751.

109. Arnlöv J, Zethelius B, Risérus U, et al. Serum and dietary beta-carotene and alpha-tocopherol and incidence of type 2 diabetes mellitus in a community-based study of Swedish men: report from the Uppsala Longitudinal Study of Adult Men (ULSAM) study. *Diabetologia*. 2008 Nov 5. Epub ahead of print. 18985315.

110. Seligman HK, Bindman AB, Vittinghoff E, et al. Food insecurity is associated with diabetes mellitus: results from the National Health Examination and Nutrition Examination Survey (NHANES) 1999-2002. *J Gen Intern Med*. 2007 Jul;22(7):1018-23. 17436030.

111. Moore AF, Florez JC. Genetic susceptibility to type 2 diabetes and implications for antidiabetic therapy. *Annu Rev Med*. 2008;59:95-111. 17937592.

112. Knowler WC, Pettitt DJ, Savage PJ, et al. Diabetes incidence in Pima indians: contributions of obesity and parental diabetes. *Am J Epidemiol.* 1981 Feb;113(2):144-56. 7468572.

113. Schulz LO, Bennett PH, Ravussin E, et al. Effects of traditional and western environments on prevalence of type 2 diabetes in Pima Indians in Mexico and the U.S. *Diabetes Care.* 2006 Aug;29(8):1866-71. 16873794.

114. Shai I, Jiang R, Manson JE, et al. Ethnicity, obesity, and risk of type 2 diabetes in women: a 20-year follow-up study. *Diabetes Care.* 2006 Jul;29(7):1585-90. 16801583

115. Andreasen CH, Stender-Petersen KL, Mogensen MS, et al. Low physical activity accentuates the effect of the FTO rs9939609 polymorphism on body fat accumulation. *Diabetes.* 2008 Jan;57(1):95-101.

116. Chung HK, Chae JS, Hyun YJ, et al. Influence of adiponectin gene polymorphisms on adiponectin level and insulin resistance index in response to dietary intervention in overweight-obese patients with impaired fasting glucose or newly diagnosed type 2 diabetes. *Diabetes Care.* 2009 Apr;32(4):552-8.

117. Hypertension in Diabetes Study (HDS): I. Prevalence of hypertension in newly presenting type 2 diabetic patients and the association with risk factors for cardiovascular and diabetic complications. *J Hypertens.* 1993 Mar;11(3):309-17. 8387089.

118. Holman RR, Paul SK, Bethel MA, et al. Long-term follow-up after tight control of blood pressure in type 2 diabetes. *N Engl J Med.* 2008 Oct 9;359(15):1565-76. 18784091.

119. Morrison JA, Glueck CJ, Horn PS, et al. Pre-teen insulin resistance predicts weight gain, impaired fasting glucose, and type 2 diabetes at age 18-19 y: a 10-y prospective study of black and white girls. *Am J Clin Nutr.* 2008 Sep;88(3):778-88. 18779296.

120. Garrido-Sánchez L, Cardona F, García-Fuentes E, et al. Anti-oxidized low-density lipoprotein antibody levels are associated with the development of type 2 diabetes mellitus. *Eur J Clin Invest.* 2008 Sep;38(9):615-21. 18837736.

121. Lang IA, Galloway TS, Scarlett A, et al. Association of urinary bisphenol A concentration with medical disorders and laboratory abnormalities in adults. *JAMA.* 2008 Sep 17;300(11):1303-10. 18799442.

122. Navas-Acien A, Silbergeld EK, Pastor-Barriuso R, et al. Arsenic exposure and prevalence of type 2 diabetes in US adults. *JAMA.* 2008 Aug 20;300(7):814-22. 18714061.

123. Coronado-González JA, Del Razo LM, García-Vargas G, et al. Inorganic arsenic exposure and type 2 diabetes mellitus in Mexico. *Environ Res.* 2007 Jul;104(3):383-9. 17475235.

124. Chen JW, Wang SL, Liao PC, et al. Relationship between insulin sensitivity and exposure to dioxins and polychlorinated biphenyls in pregnant women. *Environ Res.* 2008 Jun;107(2):245-53. 18313660.

125. Stahlhut RW, van Wijngaarden E, Dye TD, et al. Concentrations of urinary phthalate metabolites are associated with increased waist circumference and insulin resistance in adult U.S. males. *Environ Health Perspect.* 2007 Jun;115(6):876-82. 17589594.

126. Hatch EE, Nelson JW, Qureshi MM, et al. Association of urinary phthalate metabolite concentrations with body mass index and waist circumference: a cross-sectional study of NHANES data, 1999-2002. *Environ Health.* 2008 Jun 3;7:27. 18522739.

127. Farrell JB, Deshmukh A, Baghaie AA. Low testosterone and the association with type 2 diabetes. *Diabetes Educ.* 2008 Sep-Oct;34(5):799-806. 18832284.

128. Kalyani RR, Dobs AS. Androgen deficiency, diabetes, and the metabolic syndrome in men. *Curr Opin Endocrinol Diabetes Obes.* 2007 Jun;14(3):226-34. 17940444.

129. Cosgrove MP, Sargeant LA, Griffin SJ. Does depression increase the risk of developing type 2 diabetes? *Occup Med* (Lond). 2008 Jan;58(1):7-14. 17965449.

130. Li C, Ford ES, Strine TW, et al. Prevalence of depression among U.S. adults with diabetes: findings from the 2006 behavioral risk factor surveillance system. *Diabetes Care.* 2008 Jan;31(1):105-7. 17934145.

131. Muniyappa R, Lee S, Chen H, et al. Current approaches for assessing insulin sensitivity and resistance *in vivo*: advantages, limitations, and appropriate usage. *Am J Physiol Endocrinol Metab.* 2008 Jan;294(1):E15-26. 17957034.

132. Faerch K, Vaag A, Holst JJ, et al. Impaired fasting glycaemia vs. impaired glucose tolerance: similar impairment of pancreatic alpha and beta cell function but differential roles of incretin hormones and insulin action. *Diabetologia.* 2008 May;51(5):853-61. 18317726.

133. Ijzerman RG, Stehouwer CD, Serné EH, et al. Incorporation of the fasting free fatty acid concentration into quantitative insulin sensitivity check index improves its association with insulin sensitivity in adults, but not in children. *Eur J Endocrinol.* 2009 Jan;160(1):59-64.

134. Chen H, Sullivan G, Quon MJ. Assessing the predictive accuracy of QUICKI as a surrogate index for insulin sensitivity using a calibration model. *Diabetes.* 2005 Jul;54(7):1914-25. 15983190.

135. Hoffman RP. Indices of insulin action calculated from fasting glucose and insulin reflect hepatic, not peripheral, insulin sensitivity in African-American and Caucasian adolescents. *Pediatr Diabetes.* 2008 Jun;9(3 Pt 2):57-61.

136. Szmitko PE, Teoh H, Stewart DJ, et al. Adiponectin and cardiovascular disease: state of the art? *Am J Physiol Heart Circ Physiol.* 2007 Apr;292(4):H1655-63.

137. Kaser S, Tatarczyk T, Stadlmayr A, et al. Effect of obesity and insulin sensitivity on adiponectin isoform distribution. *Eur J Clin Invest.* 2008 Nov;38(11):827-34.

138. Leung KC, Xu A, Craig ME, et al. Adiponectin isoform distribution in women—relationship to female sex steroids and insulin sensitivity. *Metabolism.* 2009 Feb;58(2):239-45.

139. Jürimäe J, Jürimäe T, Ring-Dimitriou S, et al. Plasma adiponectin and insulin sensitivity in overweight and normal-weight middle-aged premenopausal women. *Metabolism.* 2009 May;58(5):638-43.

140. Ix JH, Wassel CL, Kanaya AM, et al. Fetuin-A and incident diabetes mellitus in older persons. *JAMA.* 2008 Jul 9;300(2):182-8. 18612115.

141. Stefan N, Fritsche A, Weikert C, et al. Plasma fetuin-A levels and the risk of type 2 diabetes. *Diabetes.* 2008 Oct;57(10):2762-7. 18633113.

142. Reinehr T, Roth CL. Fetuin-a and its relation to metabolic syndrome and fatty liver disease in obese children before and after weight loss. *J Clin Endocrinol Metab.* 2008 Nov;93(11):4479-85. 18728159.

143. Simental-Mendía LE, Rodríguez-Morán M, et al. The product of fasting glucose and triglycerides as surrogate for identifying insulin resistance in apparently healthy subjects. *Metab Syndr Relat Disord.* 2008 Winter;6(4):299-304.

144. Nilsson G, Hedberg P, Jonason T, et al. Waist circumference alone predicts insulin resistance as good as the metabolic syndrome in elderly women. *Eur J Intern Med.* 2008 Nov;19(7):520-6.

145. Chen CN, Chuang LM, Wu YT. Clinical measures of physical fitness predict insulin resistance in people at risk for diabetes. *Phys Ther.* 2008 Nov;88(11):1355-64. 18801854.

146. Aroda VR, Ratner R. Approach to the patient with prediabetes. *J Clin Endocrinol Metab.* 2008 Sep;93(9):3259-65.

147. Festa A, Williams K, Hanley AJ, et al. Beta-cell dysfunction in subjects with impaired glucose tolerance and early type 2 diabetes: comparison of surrogate markers with first-phase insulin secretion from an intravenous glucose tolerance test. *Diabetes.* 2008 Jun;57(6):1638-44.

148. Executive summary: standards of medical care in diabetes—2011. *Diabetes Care.* 2011 Jan;34 Suppl 1:S4-10.

149. Hoeks LB, Greven WL, de Valk HW, et al. Real-time continuous glucose monitoring system for treatment of diabetes: a systematic review. *Diabet Med.* 2011 Apr;28(4):386-94.

150. Murata GH, Duckworth WC, Shah JH, et al. Blood Glucose Monitoring is Associated with Better Glycemic Control in Type 2 Diabetes: A database study. *J Gen Intern Med.* 2008 Oct 31. Epub ahead of print. 18975035.

151. Lecomte P, Romon I, Fosse S, et al. Self-monitoring of blood glucose in people with type 1 and type 2 diabetes living in France: the Entred study 2001. *Diabetes Metab.* 2008 Jun;34(3):219-26. 18343703.

152. Juvenile Diabetes Research Foundation Continuous Glucose Monitoring Study Group, et al. Continuous glucose monitoring and intensive treatment of type 1 diabetes. *N Engl J Med.* 2008 Oct 2;359(14):1464-76. 18779236.

153. Yoo HJ, An HG, Park SY, et al. Use of a real time continuous glucose monitoring system as a motivational device for poorly controlled type 2 diabetes. *Diabetes Res Clin Pract.* 2008 Oct;82(1):73-9. 18701183.

154. Qiao Q, Tuomilehto J, Borch-Johnsen K. Post-challenge hyperglycaemia is associated with premature death and macrovascular complications. *Diabetologia.* 2003 Mar;46 Suppl 1:M17-21.

155. Gao W, Qiao Q, Tuomilehto J. Post-challenge hyperglycaemia rather than fasting hyperglycaemia is an independent risk factor of cardiovascular disease events. *Clin Lab.* 2004;50(9-10):609-15.

156. Yamagishi SI, Nakamura K, Matsui T, et al. Role of postprandial hyperglycaemia in cardiovascular disease in diabetes. *Int J Clin Pract.* 2007 Jan;61(1):83-7.

157. Li J, Luo Y, Xu Y, et al. Risk factors of peripheral arterial disease and relationship between low ankle–brachial index and mortality from all-cause and cardiovascular disease in Chinese patients with type 2 diabetes. *Circ J.* 2007 Mar;71(3):377-81. 17322639.

158. Ankle Brachial Index Collaboration, Fowkes FG, Murray GD, Butcher I, et al. Ankle brachial index combined with Framingham Risk Score to predict cardiovascular events and mortality: a meta-analysis. *JAMA.* 2008 Jul 9;300(2):197-208. 18612117.

159. Mostaza JM, Suarez C, Manzano L, et al. Sub-clinical vascular disease in type 2 diabetic subjects: relationship with chronic complications of diabetes and the presence of cardiovascular disease risk factors. *Eur J Intern Med.* 2008 Jun;19(4):255-60. 18471673.

160. Brandenburg D. History and diagnostic significance of C-peptide. *Exp Diabetes Res.* 2008;2008:576862. 18509495.

161. Murao S, Kondo S, Ohashi J, et al. Anti-thyroid peroxidase antibody, IA-2 antibody, and fasting C-peptide levels predict beta cell failure in patients with latent autoimmune diabetes in adults (LADA)—a 5-year follow-up of the Ehime study. *Diabetes Res Clin Pract.* 2008 Apr;80(1):114-21. 18342387.

162. Bacha F, Gungor N, Arslanian SA. Measures of beta-cell function during the oral glucose tolerance test, liquid mixed-meal test, and hyperglycemic clamp test. *J Pediatr.* 2008 May;152(5):618-21. 18410762.

163. Shakil A, Church RJ, Rao SS. Gastrointestinal complications of diabetes. *Am Fam Physician.* 2008 Jun 15;77(12):1697-702. 18619079.

164. Larsson K, Carlsson A, Cederwall E, et al. Annual screening detects celiac disease in children with type 1 diabetes. *Pediatr Diabetes.* 2008 Aug;9(4 Pt 2):354-9. 18774995.

165. Knowler WC, Barrett-Connor E, Fowler SE, et al. Reduction in the incidence of type 2 diabetes with lifestyle intervention or metformin. *N Engl J Med.* 2002 Feb 7;346(6):393-403.11832527.

166. Orchard TJ, Temprosa M, Goldberg R, et al. The effect of metformin and intensive lifestyle intervention on the metabolic syndrome: the Diabetes Prevention Program randomized trial. *Ann Intern Med.* 2005 Apr 19;142(8):611-9. 15838067.

167. Herman WH, Hoerger TJ, Brandle M, et al. The cost-effectiveness of lifestyle modification or metformin in preventing type 2 diabetes in adults with impaired glucose tolerance. *Ann Intern Med.* 2005 Mar 1;142(5):323-32. 15738451.

168. Li G, Zhang P, Wang J, et al. The long-term effect of lifestyle interventions to prevent diabetes in the China Da Qing Diabetes Prevention Study: a 20-year follow-up study. *Lancet.* 2008 May 24;371(9626):1783-9. 18502303.

169. Diabetes Prevention Program Research Group, et al. The influence of age on the effects of lifestyle modification and metformin in prevention of diabetes. *J Gerontol A Biol Sci Med Sci.* 2006 Oct;61(10):1075-81. 17077202.

170. Cheng YJ, Gregg EW, De Rekeneire N, et al. Muscle-strengthening activity and its association with insulin sensitivity. *Diabetes Care.* 2007 Sep;30(9):2264-70. 17586746.

171. Sigal RJ, Kenny GP, Boulé NG, et al. Effects of aerobic training, resistance training, or both on glycemic control in type 2 diabetes: a randomized trial. *Ann Intern Med.* 2007 Sep 18;147(6):357-69. 17876019.

172. Colberg SR, Somma CT, Sechrist SR. Physical activity participation may offset some of the negative impact of diabetes on cognitive function. *J Am Med Dir Assoc.* 2008 Jul;9(6):434-8. 18585646.

173. Panagiotakos DB, Tzima N, Pitsavos C, et al. The association between adherence to the Mediterranean diet and fasting indices of glucose homoeostasis: the ATTICA Study. *J Am Coll Nutr.* 2007 Feb;26(1):32-8. 17353581.

174. Panagiotakos DB, Chrysohoou C, Pitsavos C, et al. Association between the prevalence of obesity and adherence to the Mediterranean diet: the ATTICA study. *Nutrition.* 2006 May;22(5):449-56. 16457990.

175. Martínez-González MA, de la Fuente-Arrillaga C, Nunez-Cordoba JM, et al. Adherence to Mediterranean diet and risk of developing diabetes: prospective cohort study. *BMJ.* 2008 Jun 14;336(7657):1348-51. 18511765.

176. Riccardi G, Rivellese AA, Giacco R. Role of glycemic index and glycemic load in the healthy state, in prediabetes, and in diabetes. *Am J Clin Nutr.* 2008 Jan;87(1):269S-274S. 18175767.

177. Barclay AW, Petocz P, McMillan-Price J, et al. Glycemic index, glycemic load, and chronic disease risk—a meta-analysis of observational studies. *Am J Clin Nutr.* 2008 Mar;87(3):627-37. 18326601.

178. Dickinson S, Hancock DP, Petocz P, et al. High-glycemic index carbohydrate increases nuclear factor-kappaB activation in mononuclear cells of young, lean healthy subjects. *Am J Clin Nutr.* 2008 May;87(5):1188-93. 18469238.

179. Riccardi G, Rivellese AA, Giacco R. Role of glycemic index and glycemic load in the healthy state, in prediabetes, and in diabetes. *Am J Clin Nutr.* 2008 Jan;87(1):269S-274S. 18175767.

180. Clark CA, Gardiner J, McBurney MI, et al. Effects of breakfast meal composition on second meal metabolic responses in adults with Type 2 diabetes mellitus. *Eur J Clin Nutr.* 2006 Sep;60(9):1122-9. 16670695.

181. Krishnan S, Rosenberg L, Singer M, et al. Glycemic index, glycemic load, and cereal fiber intake and risk of type 2 diabetes in US black women. *Arch Intern Med.* 2007 Nov 26;167(21):2304-9. 18039988.

182. Montonen J, Knekt P, Järvinen R, et al. Whole-grain and fiber intake and the incidence of type 2 diabetes. *Am J Clin Nutr.* 2003 Mar;77(3):622-9. 12600852.

183. Flammang AM, Kendall DM, Baumgartner CJ, et al. Effect of a viscous fiber bar on postprandial glycemia in subjects with type 2 diabetes. *J Am Coll Nutr.* 2006 Oct;25(5):409-14. 17031010.

184. Chow J, Choe YS, Noss MJ, et al. Effect of a viscous fiber-containing nutrition bar on satiety of patients with type 2 diabetes. *Diabetes Res Clin Pract.* 2007 Jun; 76(3):335-40. 17023088.

185. Vuksan V, Sievenpiper JL, Owen R, et al. Beneficial effects of viscous dietary fiber from Konjac-mannan in subjects with the insulin resistance syndrome: results of a controlled metabolic trial. *Diabetes Care.* 2000 Jan; 23(1):9-14. 10857960.

186. Vuksan V, Jenkins DJ, Spadafora P, et al. Konjac-mannan (glucomannan) improves glycemia and other associated risk factors for coronary heart disease in type 2 diabetes. A randomized controlled metabolic trial. *Diabetes Care.* 1999 Jun;22(6):913-9. 10372241.

187. López S, Bermúdez B, Pacheco YM, et al. Distinctive postprandial modulation of beta cell function and insulin sensitivity by dietary fats: monounsaturated compared with saturated fatty acids. *Am J Clin Nutr.* 2008 Sep; 88(3):638-44. 18779278.

188. Tao M, McDowell MA, Saydah SH, et al. Relationship of polyunsaturated fatty acid intake to peripheral neuropathy among adults with diabetes in the National Health and Nutrition Examination Survey (NHANES) 1999–2004. *Diabetes Care.* 2008 Jan; 31(1):93-5. 17914029.

189. Ziegler D, Ametov A, Barinov A, et al. Oral treatment with alpha-lipoic acid improves symptomatic diabetic polyneuropathy: the SYDNEY 2 trial. *Diabetes Care.* 2006 Nov;29(11):2365-70. 17065669.

190. Christiansen E, Schnider S, Palmvig B, et al. Intake of a diet high in trans monounsaturated fatty acids or saturated fatty acids. Effects on postprandial insulinemia and glycemia in obese patients with NIDDM. *Diabetes Care.* 1997 May;20(5):881-7. 9135961.

191. Tentolouris N, Arapostathi C, Perrea D, et al. Differential effects of two different isoenergetic meals one rich in saturated and one rich in monounsaturated fat on endothelial function in subjects with type 2 diabetes mellitus. *Diabetes Care.* 2008 Oct 3. Epub ahead of print. 18835957.

192. Pearce KL, Noakes M, Keogh J, et al. Effect of carbohydrate distribution on postprandial glucose peaks with the use of continuous glucose monitoring in type 2 diabetes. *Am J Clin Nutr.* 2008 Mar;87(3):638-44. 18326602.

193. Sierra-Johnson J, Undén AL, Linestrand M, et al. Eating meals irregularly: a novel environmental risk factor for the metabolic syndrome. *Obesity* (Silver Spring). 2008 Jun;16(6):1302-7. 18388902.

194. Jakus V. The role of free radicals, oxidative stress and antioxidant systems in diabetic vascular disease. *Bratisl Lek Listy.* 2000;101(10):541-51.

195. Vega-López S, Devaraj S, Jialal I, et al. Oxidative stress and antioxidant supplementation in the management of diabetic cardiovascular disease. *J Investig Med.* 2004 Jan;52(1):24-32.

196. Antoniades C, Tousoulis D, Tountas C, et al. Vascular endothelium and inflammatory process, in patients with combined Type 2 diabetes mellitus and coronary atherosclerosis: the effects of vitamin C. *Diabet Med.* 2004 Jun;21(6):552-8. 15154938.

197. Mullan BA, Young IS, Fee H, et al. Ascorbic acid reduces blood pressure and arterial stiffness in type 2 diabetes. *Hypertension.* 2002 Dec;40(6):804-9. 12468561.

198. Jiang Q, Ames BN. Gamma-tocopherol, but not alpha-tocopherol, decreases proinflammatory eicosanoids and inflammation damage in rats. *FASEB J.* 2003 May;17(8):816-22. 12724340.

199. Vincent HK, Bourguignon CM, Weltman AL, et al. Effects of antioxidant supplementation on insulin sensitivity, endothelial adhesion molecules, and oxidative stress in normal-weight and overweight young adults. *Metabolism.* 2009 Feb;58(2):254-62.

200. Wang H, Kruszewski A, Brautigan DL. Cellular chromium enhances activation of insulin receptor kinase. *Biochemistry.* 2005 Jun 7;44(22):8167-75. 15924436.

201. Martin J, Wang ZQ, Zhang XH, et al. Chromium picolinate supplementation attenuates body weight gain and increases insulin sensitivity in subjects with type 2 diabetes. *Diabetes Care.* 2006 Aug;29(8):1826-32. 16873787.

202. Albarracin CA, Fuqua BC, Evans JL, et al. Chromium picolinate and biotin combination improves glucose metabolism in treated, uncontrolled overweight to obese patients with type 2 diabetes. *Diabetes Metab Res Rev.* 2008 Jan-Feb;24(1):41-51. 17506119.

203. Singer GM, Geohas J. The effect of chromium picolinate and biotin supplementation on glycemic control in poorly controlled patients with type 2 diabetes mellitus: a placebo-controlled, double-blinded, randomized trial. *Diabetes Technol Ther.* 2006 Dec;8(6):636-43. 17109595.

204. Song Y, He K, Levitan EB, et al. Effects of oral magnesium supplementation on glycaemic control in Type 2 diabetes: a meta-analysis of randomized double-blind controlled trials. *Diabet Med.* 2006 Oct;23(10):1050-6. 16978367.

205. Guerrero-Romero F, Rascón-Pacheco RA, Rodríguez-Morán M, et al. Hypomagnesaemia and risk for metabolic glucose disorders: a 10-year follow-up study. *Eur J Clin Invest.* 2008 Jun;38(6):389-96. 18489400.

206. Abete I, Parra D, Crujeiras AB, et al. Specific insulin sensitivity and leptin responses to a nutritional treatment of obesity via a combination of energy restriction and fatty fish intake. *J Hum Nutr Diet.* 2008 Dec;21(6):591-600.

207. Wang C, Harris WS, Chung M, et al. n-3 fatty acids from fish or fish-oil supplements, but not alpha-linolenic acid, benefit cardiovascular disease outcomes in primary- and secondary-prevention studies: a systematic review. *Am J Clin Nutr.* 2006 Jul;84(1):5-17. 16825676.

208. Norris JM, Yin X, Lamb MM, et al. Omega-3 polyunsaturated fatty acid intake and islet autoimmunity in children at increased risk for type 1 diabetes. *JAMA.* 2007 Sep 26;298(12):1420-8. 17895458.

209. Hartweg J, Perera R, Montori V, et al. Omega-3 polyunsaturated fatty acids (PUFA) for type 2 diabetes mellitus. *Cochrane Database Syst Rev.* 2008 Jan 23;(1):CD003205. 18254017.

210. Suzukawa M, Abbey M, Howe PR, et al. Effects of fish oil fatty acids on low density lipoprotein size, oxidizability, and uptake by macrophages. *J Lipid Res.* 1995 Mar;36(3):473-84. 7775859.

211. Montori VM, Farmer A, Wollan PC, et al. Fish oil supplementation in type 2 diabetes: a quantitative systematic review. *Diabetes Care.* 2000 Sep;23(9):1407-15. 10977042.

212. Kapoor R, Huang YS. Gamma-linolenic acid: an anti-inflammatory omega-6 fatty acid. *Curr Pharm Biotechnol.* 2006 Dec;7(6):531-4. 17168669.

213. Horrobin DF. The use of gamma-linolenic acid in diabetic neuropathy. *Agents Actions Suppl.* 1992;37:120-44. 1321553.

214. Palomer X, González-Clemente JM, Blanco-Vaca F, et al. Role of vitamin D in the pathogenesis of type 2 diabetes mellitus. *Diabetes Obes Metab.* 2008 Mar;10(3):185-97. 18269634.

215. Borissova AM, Tankova T, Kirilov G, et al. The effect of vitamin D3 on insulin secretion and peripheral insulin sensitivity in type 2 diabetic patients. *Int J Clin Pract.* 2003 May;57(4):258-61. 12800453.

216. Mathieu C, Gysemans C, Giulietti A, et al. Vitamin D and diabetes. *Diabetologia.* 2005 Jul;48(7):1247-57. 15971062.

217. Liu E, Meigs JB, Pittas AG, et al. Plasma 25-hydroxyvitamin d is associated with markers of the insulin resistant phenotype in nondiabetic adults. *J Nutr.* 2009 Feb;139(2):329-34.

218. Nagpal J, Pande JN, Bhartia A. A double-blind, randomized, placebo-controlled trial of the short-term effect of vitamin D3 supplementation on insulin sensitivity in apparently healthy, middle-aged, centrally obese men. *Diabet Med.* 2009 Jan;26(1):19-27.

219. Tsuneki H, Sekizaki N, Suzuki T, et al. Coenzyme Q10 prevents high glucose-induced oxidative stress in human umbilical vein endothelial cells. *Eur J Pharmacol.* 2007 Jul 2;566(1-3):1-10. 17434478.

220. Hodgson JM, Watts GF, Playford DA, et al. Coenzyme Q10 improves blood pressure and glycaemic control: a controlled trial in subjects with type 2 diabetes. *Eur J Clin Nutr.* 2002 Nov;56(11):1137-42. 12428181.

221. Watts GF, Playford DA, Croft KD, et al. Coenzyme Q(10) improves endothelial dysfunction of the brachial artery in Type II diabetes mellitus. *Diabetologia.* 2002 Mar;45(3):420-6. 11914748.

222. Petersen KF, Dufour S, Befroy D, et al. Impaired mitochondrial activity in the insulin-resistant offspring of patients with type 2 diabetes. *N Engl J Med.* 2004 Feb 12;350(7):664-71. 14960743.

223. Szendroedi J, Roden M. Mitochondrial fitness and insulin sensitivity in humans. *Diabetologia.* 2008 Dec;51(12):2155-67. 18802678.

224. Kim JA, Wei Y, Sowers JR. Role of mitochondrial dysfunction in insulin resistance. *Circ Res.* 2008 Feb 29;102(4):401-14. 18309108.

225. Bradley R, Oberg EB, Calabrese C, et al. Algorithm for complementary and alternative medicine practice and research in type 2 diabetes. *J Altern Complement Med.* 2007 Jan-Feb;13(1):159-75. 17309390

226. Kamenova P. Improvement of insulin sensitivity in patients with type 2 diabetes mellitus after oral administration of alpha-lipoic acid. *Hormones* (Athens). 2006 Oct-Dec;5(4):251-8. 17178700.

227. Tang J, Wingerchuk DM, Crum BA, et al. Alpha-lipoic acid may improve symptomatic diabetic polyneuropathy. *Neurologist.* 2007 May;13(3):164-7. 17495764.

228. Sharma RD, Raghuram TC, Rao NS. Effect of fenugreek seeds on blood glucose and serum lipids in type I diabetes. *Eur J Clin Nutr.* 1990 Apr;44(4):301-6. 2194788.

229. Gupta A, Gupta R, Lal B. Effect of *Trigonella foenum-graecum* (fenugreek) seeds on glycaemic control and insulin resistance in type 2 diabetes mellitus: a double blind placebo controlled study. *J Assoc Physicians India.* 2001 Nov;49:1057-61. 11868855.

230. Shanmugasundaram ER, Rajeswari G, Baskaran K, et al. Use of *Gymnema sylvestre* leaf extract in the control of blood glucose in insulin-dependent diabetes mellitus. *J Ethnopharmacol.* 1990 Oct;30(3):281-94. 2259216.

231. Baskaran K, Kizar Ahamath B, Radha Shanmugasundaram K, et al. Antidiabetic effect of a leaf extract from *Gymnema sylvestre* in non-insulin-dependent diabetes mellitus patients. *J Ethnopharmacol.* 1990 Oct;30(3):295-300. 2259217.

232. Vuksan V, Sung MK, Sievenpiper JL, et al. Korean red ginseng (*Panax ginseng*) improves glucose and insulin regulation in well-controlled, type 2 diabetes: results of a randomized, double-blind, placebo-controlled study of efficacy and safety. *Nutr Metab Cardiovasc Dis.* 2008 Jan;18(1):46-56. 16860976.

233. Dans AM, Villarruz MV, Jimeno CA, et al. The effect of *Momordica charantia* capsule preparation on glycemic control in type 2 diabetes mellitus needs further studies. *J Clin Epidemiol.* 2007 Jun;60(6):554-9. 17493509.

234. Basch E, Gabardi S, Ulbricht C. Bitter melon (*Momordica charantia*): a review of efficacy and safety. *Am J Health Syst Pharm.* 2003 Feb 15;60(4):356-9. 12625217.

235. Kimura T, Nakagawa K, Kubota H, et al. Food-grade mulberry powder enriched with 1-deoxynojirimycin suppresses the elevation of postprandial blood glucose in humans. *J Agric Food Chem.* 2007 Jul 11;55(14):5869-74. 17555327.

236. Mackenzie T, Leary L, Brooks WB. The effect of an extract of green and black tea on glucose control in adults with type 2 diabetes mellitus: double-blind randomized study. *Metabolism.* 2007 Oct;56(10):1340-4. 17884442.

237. Fukino Y, Ikeda A, Maruyama K, et al. Randomized controlled trial for an effect of green tea-extract powder supplementation on glucose abnormalities. *Eur J Clin Nutr.* 2008 Aug;62(8):953-60. 17554248.

238. Boschmann M, Thielecke F. The effects of epigallocatechin-3-gallate on thermogenesis and fat oxidation in obese men: a pilot study. *J Am Coll Nutr.* 2007 Aug;26(4):389S-395S. 17906192.

239. Chianelli M, Parisella MG, Visalli N, et al. Pancreatic scintigraphy with 99mTc-interleukin-2 at diagnosis of type 1 diabetes and after 1 year of nicotinamide therapy. *Diabetes Metab Res Rev.* 2008 Feb;24(2):115-22. 17918277.

240. Kamal M, Abbasy AJ, Muslemani AA, et al. Effect of nicotinamide on newly diagnosed type 1 diabetic children. *Acta Pharmacol Sin.* 2006 Jun;27(6):724-7. 16723091.

241. Crinó A, Schiaffini R, Ciampalini P, et al. A two year observational study of nicotinamide and intensive insulin therapy in patients with recent onset type 1 diabetes mellitus. *J Pediatr Endocrinol Metab.* 2005 Aug;18(8):749-54. 16200840.

242. De Grandis D, Minardi C. Acetyl-L-carnitine (levacecarnine) in the treatment of diabetic neuropathy. A long-term, randomised, double-blind, placebo-controlled study. *Drugs R D.* 2002;3(4):223-31. 12455197.

A Comprehensive Approach to Inflammation

Overview

Inflammation is an adaptive, coordinated, and protective response, primarily triggered by injury or infection, which is generally thought to be of benefit when it is well-controlled and self-limited. It has been described as a "system of information flow in response to injury and infection."[1] The inflammatory response probably evolved as a means to restore homeostasis and functionality to tissues, because it plays a key role in warding off infectious agents, clearing killed pathogens, cell debris, and damaged or injured tissue, and assisting in necessary tissue proliferation and remodeling. Controlled inflammation appears to be necessary to keep tissues functioning at a high level; for example, the recruitment of resident macrophages and additional leukocytes to a tissue with a large number of dead or malfunctioning cells allows that tissue to recover from an injury it could not adapt to on its own.[2] Perhaps best termed "physiological" or adaptive inflammation, this reparative process is often contrasted with the "pathological" or maladaptive chronic expression of inflammation, which seems to be increasing in prevalence and is linked to a number of chronic diseases, including cardiovascular disease, allergies, type 2 diabetes, cancer, and arthritis.

A great deal of progress has been made in understanding the cellular and molecular events that occur during acute local inflammation, particularly in response to infection. While the adaptive value of acute local inflammation is now well recognized, much less is understood about chronic or pathological inflammation, particularly systemic inflammation. This area is currently being intensely researched, with an emphasis on understanding the underlying physiological differences between acute and chronic inflammation, and how inflammation becomes pathological. Rather than attempting a simplistic approach of "turning off" inflammation, more appropriate goals seem to be supporting healthy inflammation and the resolution of acute inflammatory processes, and reducing the factors that lead to a more chronic state. Lifestyle patterns, particularly dietary choices and physical activity, as well as targeted nutritional supplementation can have a significant impact on reducing cellular stress and optimizing cellular function, thereby limiting the induction of inflammatory processes. An understanding of the physiology behind inflammation offers insight into effective therapeutic strategies (Figure 5.1).

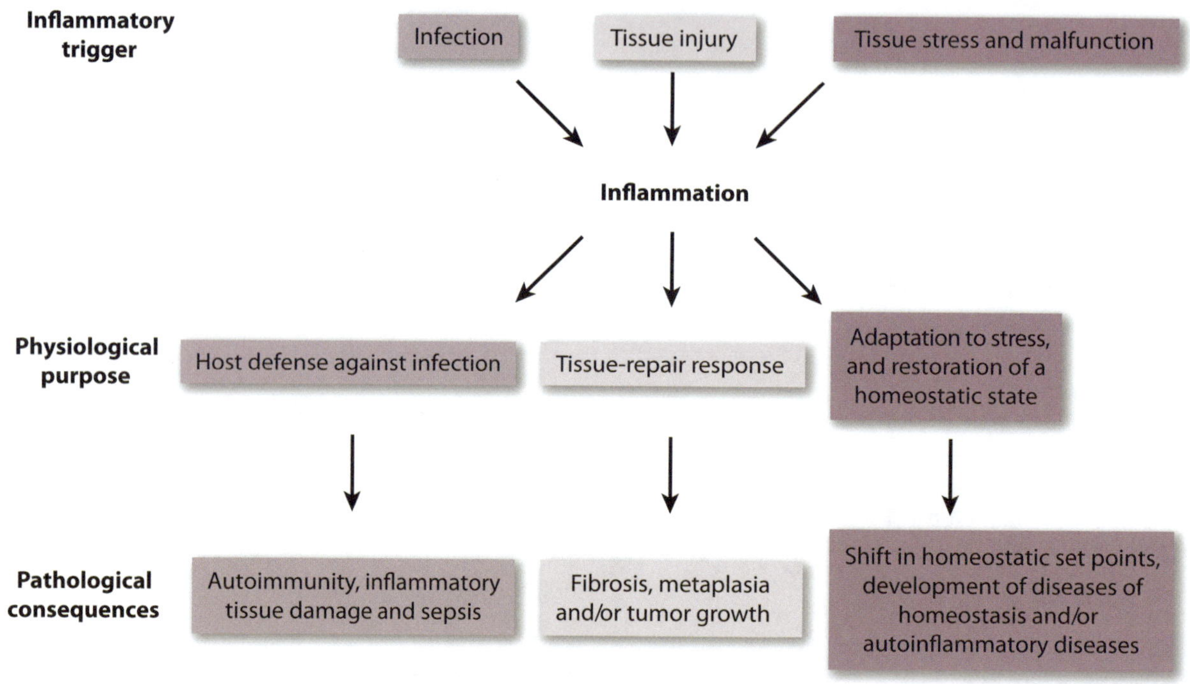

Figure 5.1 Causes and outcomes of inflammation. From: Medzhitov R. Origin and physiological roles of inflammation. *Nature.* 2008 Jul 24;454(7203):428-35. Reproduced with permission from Macmillan Publishers Ltd.

Physiology of Acute Inflammation

Infection or tissue damage

Acute inflammation is characterized by four phases: the recognition of either infection or tissue damage; a recruitment of cells to the site of inflammation; an elimination of the microbial threat; and, finally, the resolution of inflammation. While we usually think of the first phase of inflammation as being triggered by an infection, it may be brought on by both exogenous sources, microbial and non-microbial, and endogenous sources.[2] Endogenous sources include cellular stress and malfunctioning tissues, advanced glycation end-products (AGEs), and oxidized lipoproteins. In fact, some evidence suggests that, in environments laden with oxidative stress or elevated glucose levels, the effect of endogenous inducers of inflammation may be to transform what would normally be repair processes to those that drive more chronic inflammation.[4] AGEs—which accumulate under pro-oxidative and hyperglycemic conditions via their chief signaling receptor, the AGE-specific receptor (RAGE)—are known to generate reactive oxygen species and activate inflammatory signaling cascades.[3,4] One mechanism by which a Western diet initiates inflammation is by the activation of RAGE due to a high level of AGEs, an event demonstrated in animal-based research.[5]

The initial events of the inflammatory process are mediated by the innate immune system.[6] Innate receptors on macrophages and mast cells target highly conserved features of microbes, allowing for the detection of a wide range of microbial diversity (examples include LPS and peptidoglycan from the cell walls of gram-negative and gram-positive bacteria, respectively.) This strategy has been termed "pattern recognition" and the innate receptors employing it are called "pattern-recognition receptors" (PRRs).[6] The most well characterized of the PRRs are toll-like receptors (TLRs), with others including nucleotide-binding oligomerization domain-like (NOD-like) receptors (NLRs), and retinoic acid-inducible gene I-like (RIG-I) receptors (RLRs).

Recruitment of cells to the site of infection

The activation of a PRR triggers an inflammatory cascade, which recruits plasma proteins and leukocytes (mostly neutrophils [PMNs]) to the site of infection or tissue damage. This occurs through the activation of endothelium, allowing for selective extravasation of neutrophils.[2] The initiation of an inflammatory cascade has the dual purposes of containing infection and activating the adaptive immune response.

Varied inflammatory mediators are released, including chemokines, cytokines, vasoactive amines, vasoactive peptides, lipid mediators, fragments of complement components, and proteolytic enzymes (Figure 5.2). Lipid mediators are derived from phospholipids present in the inner leaflet of cellular membranes, such as phosphatidylcholine. Intracellular calcium ions activate the enzyme phospholipase A_2, which generates arachidonic acid (AA) and lysophosphatidic acid. As will be discussed in detail below, arachidonic acid is converted either by cyclooxygenases (COX-1 and COX-2) to generate prostaglandins and thromboxanes, or by lipoxygenases to form leukotrienes and lipoxins, while lysophosphatidic acid is acetylated to generate platelet-activating factors.[2]

The entire process culminates in the activation of NF-kB and IFN-regulatory factor (IRF) transcription factors, which drive the expression of

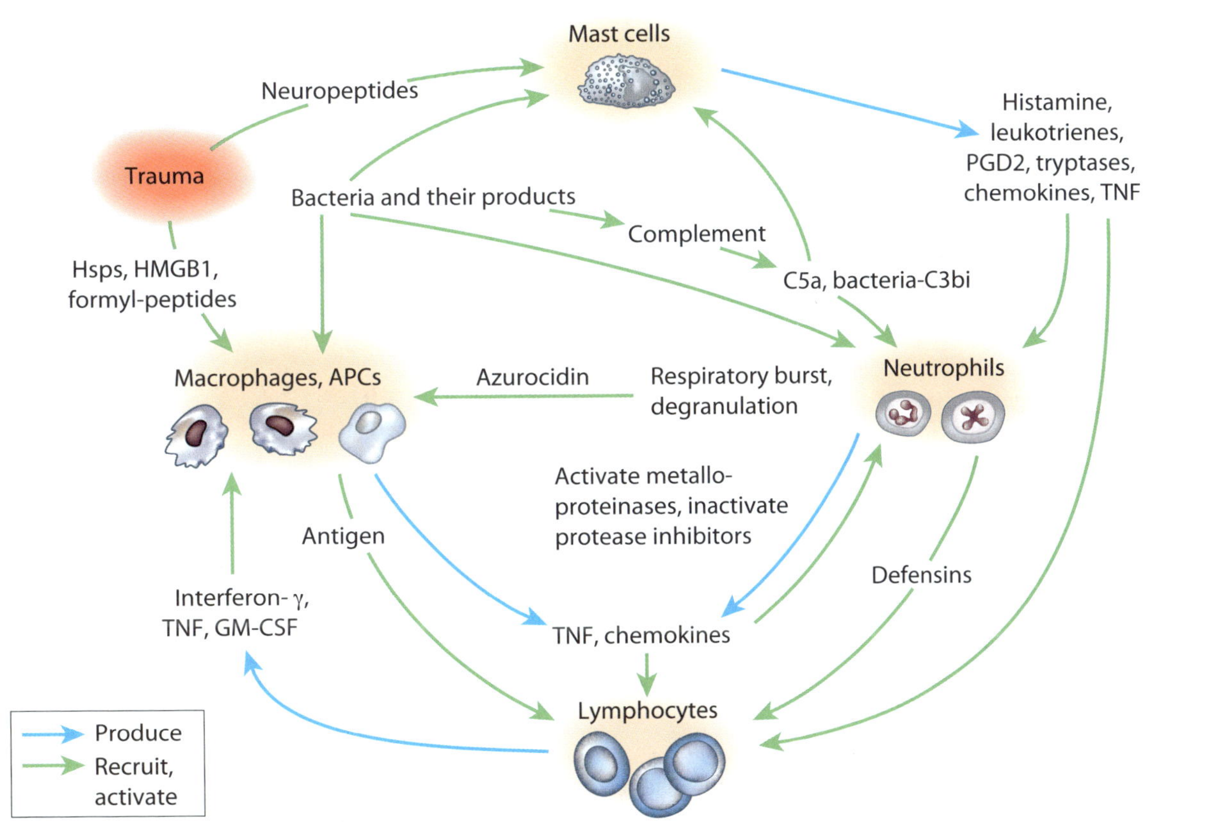

Figure 5.2 Information flow of inflammatory response following mild trauma with infection. From: Nathan C. Points of control in inflammation. *Nature.* 2002 Dec 19-26;420(6917):846-52. Reproduced with permission from Macmillan Publishers Ltd.

pro-inflammatory genes (such as TNF-alpha and IL-1), and increase the production of signals that initiate adaptive immunity.[6]

Elimination of the microbe

Once recruited to the site, neutrophils and macrophages are largely responsible for clearing the infection. Neutrophils possess granules loaded with proteases capable of degrading phagocytosed material, and they also produce reactive oxygen and nitrogen species that denature proteins, disrupt lipids, and damage DNA. After entering the site of inflammation, neutrophils phagocytose any available microbes and direct the contents of their granules toward these phagosomes.[6] Macrophages engulf and degrade microbes and apoptotic neutrophils.

Resolution (return to homeostasis)

If the inflammatory response effectively contains the microbial infection, then the overall response is shifted toward anti-inflammatory signals and resolution of inflammation. It has only recently been determined that resolution is an active process, one that is preprogrammed and tightly controlled.[7] It is mediated by a number of signals, primarily lipoxins, protectins, and resolvins, that are derived from polyunsaturated essential fatty acids. Although most of the classic prostaglandins and leukotrienes are pro-inflammatory, various counterregulatory substances are generated during the resolution of acute inflammation. Lipoxins, for example, are eicosanoids derived from arachidonic acid that bind cellular receptors, block the influx of neutrophils, promote the uptake of apoptotic neutrophils by macrophages, and recruit additional monocytes to help clear away dead cells and tissue debris. As shown in Figure 5.3, the initiation of acute inflammation is mediated by arachidonate-derived prostaglandins which regulate early events such as changes in blood flow. Lipoxins appear to mediate complete resolution to inflammation, a process which occurs over time.

The last phase (resolution of inflammation) is particularly important, both because poor resolution of inflammation is what drives chronic and pathological inflammation, and also because it can be greatly enhanced with natural therapies. For example, resolvins and protectins, derived from omega-3 fatty acids, have a crucial role in the resolution of inflammation, including the initiation of tissue repair.[8] Resolvins are derived

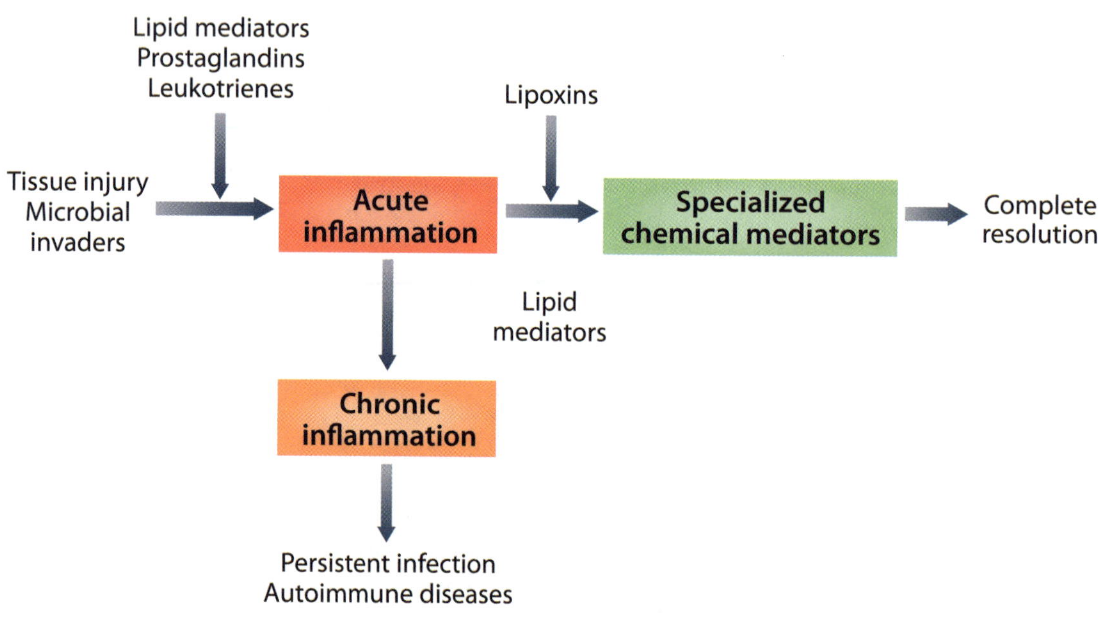

Figure 5.3 Lipid mediators and outcomes of acute inflammation. From: Mittal A., et al. Omega fatty acids and resolution of inflammation: A new twist in an old tale. *J Indian Soc Periodontol.* 2010 Jan;14(1):3-7. Reproduced from Open Access article distributed under the terms of the Creative Commons Attribution License.

either from the essential fatty acids EPA and DHA; they limit neutrophil infiltration and protect the GI tract from damage. Protectins are derived from DHA and have anti-inflammatory and neuroprotective actions.[7] Low levels of one specific protectin (neuroprotectin D1) have been documented in Alzheimer's disease, and *in vitro* evidence has shown that it may promote brain cell survival via the induction of anti-apoptotic and neuroprotective gene-expression programs, and by limiting amyloid-beta toxicity.[9] Protectins are also found to have wound healing and repair functions, protecting retinal, lung, and liver tissue from damage.[7,10,11]

Very recently, a new class of DHA-derived compounds was discovered, coined Maresins (macrophage mediators in resolving inflammation), which may also be linked to homeostasis, inflammation resolution, wound healing, and cancer.[12] Given the importance of these compounds as well as the poor supply of omega-3 fatty acids in most diets, it helps to explain why the resolution phase of inflammation is so frequently dysfunctional.

Para-inflammation/Meta-inflammation and Cellular Stress

Para-inflammation and macrophage differentiation

While acute inflammation is well understood, the mechanisms behind chronic inflammation are not as well delineated and may be quite different. The terms "para-inflammation" and "meta-inflammation" have been used recently to describe the low-grade inflammation seen in many chronic metabolic diseases, such as diabetes, atherosclerosis, asthma, and neurodegenerative diseases.[2] "Para" refers to a middle-ground between acute inflammation and the basal or homeostatic state of a cell. Essentially, it can be switched on without the presence of infection or injury, but turns on if tissue malfunction is present (Figure 5.4). If the malfunction lasts for a sustained period, para-inflammation can become chronic.

Sustained malfunctions can result from genetic mutations or environmental factors, such as a high-calorie and nutrient-poor diet, a low level of physical

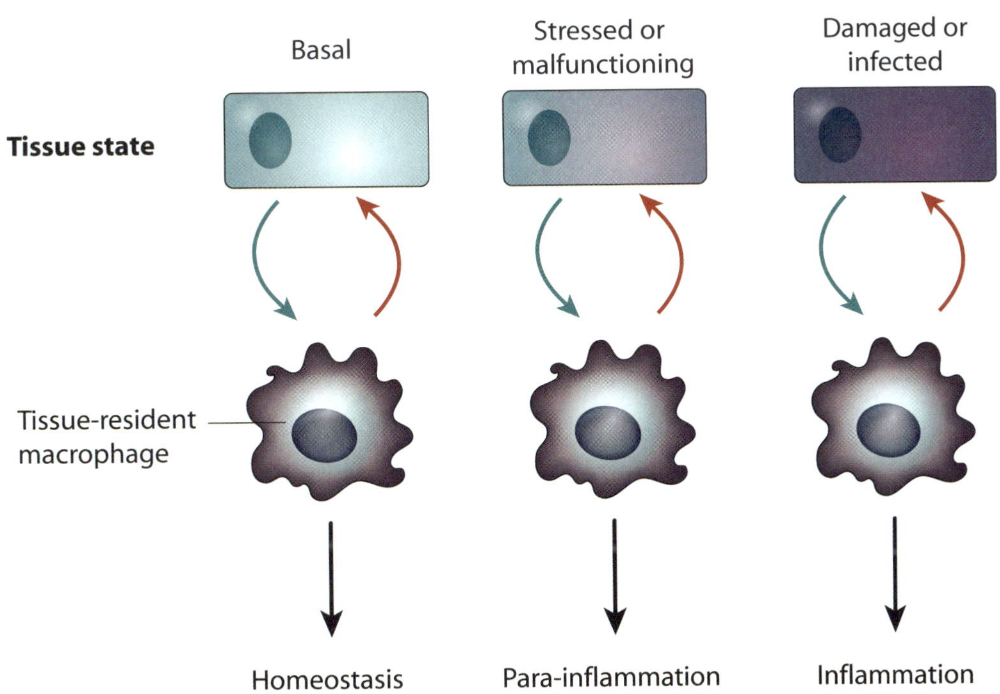

Figure 5.4 Three modes of adaptation and maintenance of tissue homeostasis. LEGEND: Blue arrows indicate signals reporting tissue states to macrophages, and red report macrophage-derived signals that control tissue adaptation. From: Medzhitov R. Origin and physiological roles of inflammation. *Nature*. 2008 Jul 24;454(7203):428-35. Reproduced with permission from Macmillan Publishers Ltd.

activity, exposure to toxic compounds, or advanced age. It can also be caused by maladaptive traits that are responsible for modern human diseases, such as allergy and obesity, characteristics that may have had evolutionary advantages at one time, but do not provide benefit in the modern environment.[2]

One consequence of a chronic low-level of inflammation may be a change in the set-point for physiological homeostasis, such as a change in insulin sensitivity or blood pressure. For example, secretion of MCP-1 (aka CC-chemokine ligand 2) from malfunctioning adipocytes directly triggers the recruitment of macrophages to adipose tissue. The infiltrated macrophages may in turn secrete a variety of chemokines and other cytokines that further promote a local inflammatory response and affect gene expression in adipocytes, resulting in systemic insulin resistance.[13]

It has been suggested that a cell's underlying metabolic state is vital for efficient cellular function, and that nuclear receptors are responsible for coordinating metabolic and inflammatory signals. Indeed, it is the cross-talk between lipid metabolism and inflammation that seems to be fundamental to the pathogenesis of human diseases such as type 2 diabetes and atherosclerosis. For example, PPAR and LXR nuclear receptors appear to function as transducers and reinforcers of particular metabolic programs required to support particular inflammatory programs. In addition, these nuclear receptors may modulate inflammatory signals that alter or disrupt a cell's "preferred" metabolic state, consistent with the concept of low-level inflammation altering a cell's homeostatic set-point.[14] This concept is illustrated by the differentiation of macrophages, leading to

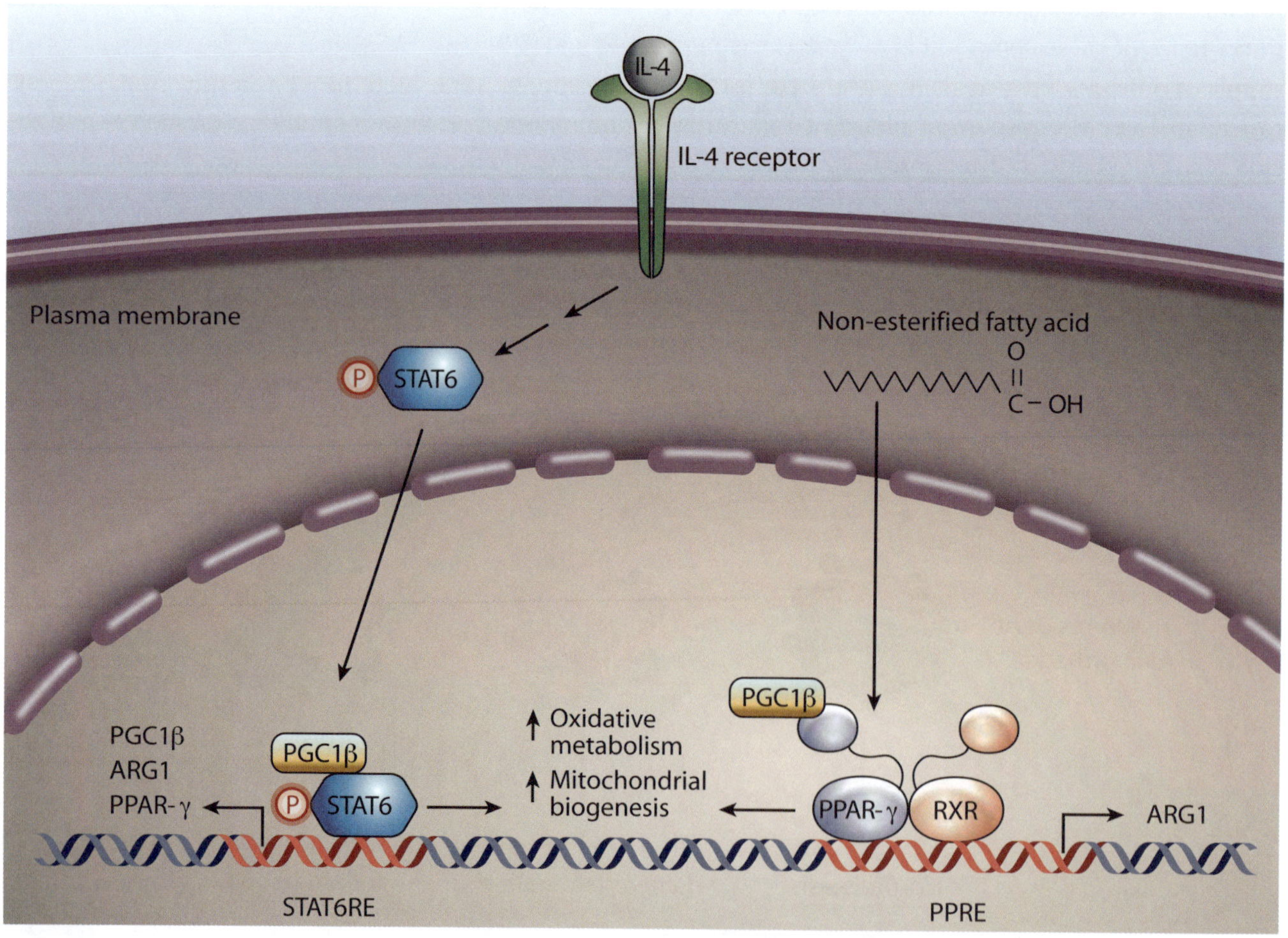

Figure 5.5 Integration of lipid and cytokine signals by PPAR-g and PGC1b. From: Bensinger SJ, Tontonoz P. Integration of metabolism and inflammation by lipid-activated nuclear receptors. *Nature*. 2008 Jul 24;454(7203):470-7. Reproduced with permission from Macmillan Publishers Ltd.

either an M1 or M2 subset, akin to the Th1 and Th2 differentiation of T cells. Activation of PPAR-gamma encourages production of the M2 subset (macrophages that generate anti-inflammatory products, mediate tissue repair, and have anti-parasite activity), rather than M1 macrophages, which generate pro-inflammatory cytokines. In Figure 5.5, IL-4 signaling as well as endogenous lipid ligands (i.e., non-esterified fatty acids) induce transcription of genes involved in the M2 subset, as well as those for mitochondrial biogenesis and oxidative metabolism.

From a clinical standpoint, the importance of the interaction between PPAR genotype and metabolism was recently analyzed in research exploring the relationship between dietary intake, PPAR genotype, and body composition. In a study of nearly 2000 elderly participants, researchers identified 6 dietary patterns and found in comparing groups that men and women with a specific genotype for PPAR (Pro/Pro) did not differ in body composition. However, men who carried an Ala allele (instead of a Pro) and consumed greater amounts of foods such as low-fat dairy products, fruit, whole grains, poultry, fish, and vegetables had significantly lower levels of all measures of adiposity, while women with an Ala allele consuming these foods had reduced thigh adiposity.[15] Essentially, dietary intake modulated the genetic influence on adiposity.

Meta-inflammation

Also introduced recently is the concept of "meta-inflammation" (metabolically triggered inflammation), a condition principally caused by nutrient excess and metabolic surplus, which engages a similar set of molecules and signaling pathways to those involved in classical inflammation (Figure 5.6).[16] This concept recognizes the many links between immune and metabolic responses, including the overlapping pathways that regulate both functions through common key regulatory molecules and signaling systems. The co-localization of metabolic and immune cells (e.g., the close proximity of adipocytes or hepatocytes and Kupffer cells or

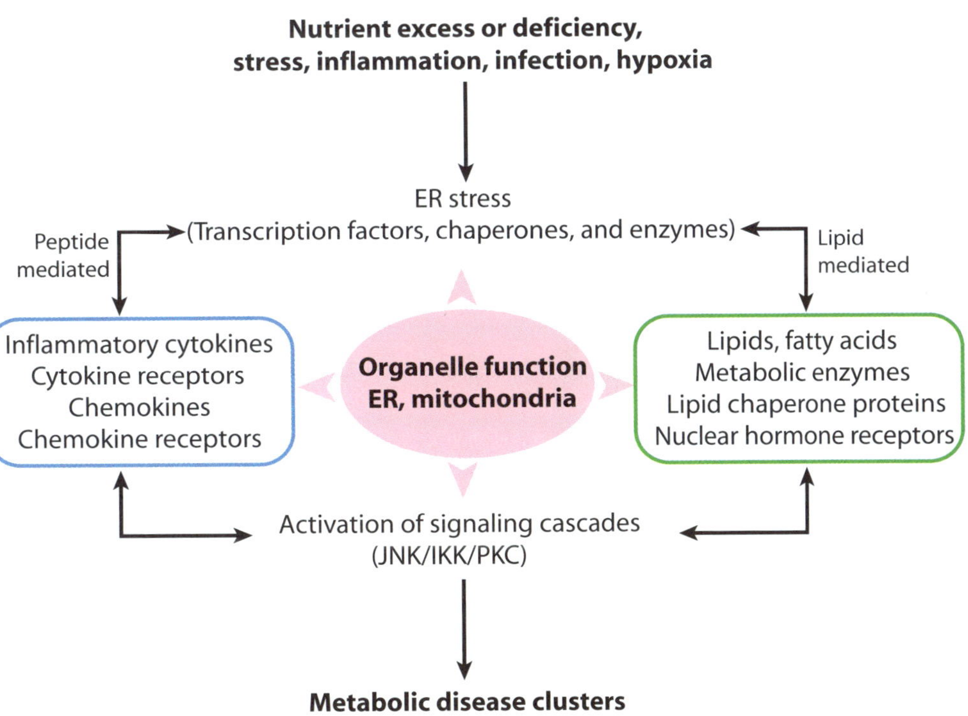

Figure 5.6 Therapeutic targets at the interface between metabolic and inflammatory pathways. From: Hotamisligil GS. Inflammation and metabolic disorders. *Nature*. 2006 Dec 14;444(7121):860-7. Reproduced with permission from Macmillan Publishers Ltd.

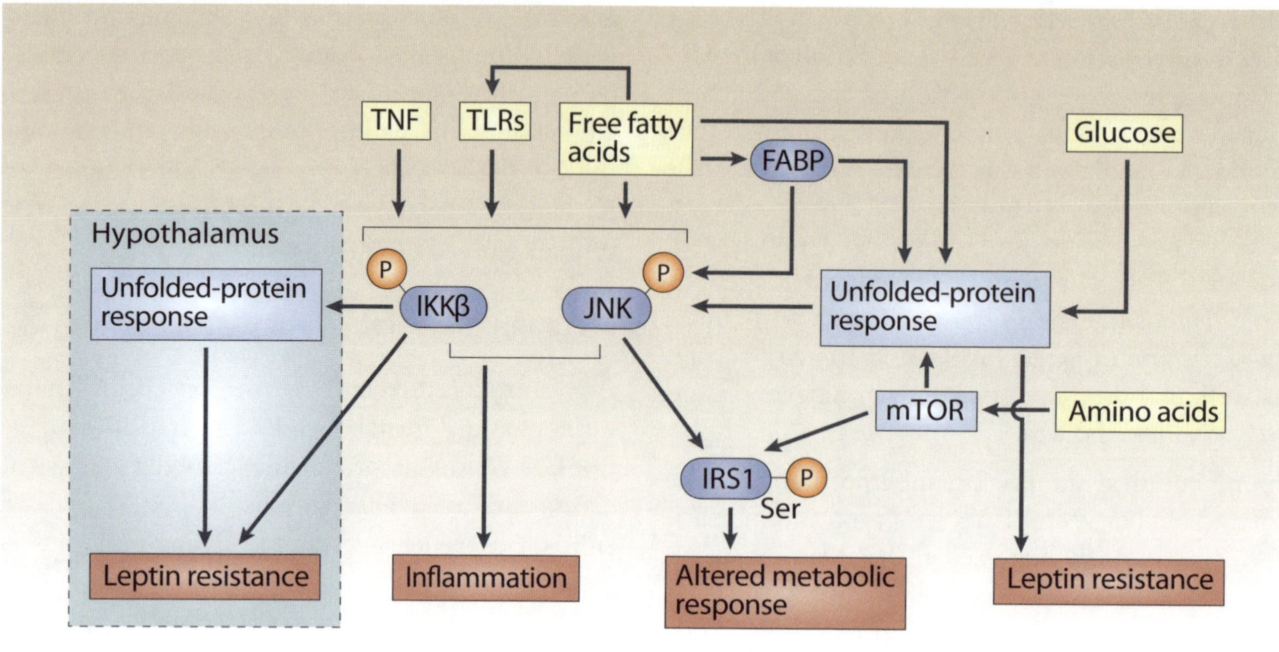

Figure 5.7 Nutrient sensing and inflammation. Notes: Many pathways that monitor nutrient availability interact with each other, such as the UPR (unfolded-protein response) in the ER (endoplasmic reticulum). Nutrients as well as dysregulation of crosstalk between pathways may culminate in altered metabolic responses, inflammation, and leptin resistance. From: Hotamisligil GS, Erbay E. Nutrient sensing and inflammation in metabolic diseases. *Nat Rev Immunol.* 2008 Dec;8(12):923-34. Reproduced with permission from Macmillan Publishers Ltd.

macrophages, as well as the embedding of lymph nodes in adipose tissue) and even the genetic and functional overlap between fully differentiated adipocytes and macrophages are examples of such links.[16,17]

Cellular/organelle stress and inflammation

One of the established ways that metabolic stress may lead to inflammation is also demonstrated by the nutrient-sensing capacity of the endoplasmic reticulum (ER), which activates the "unfolded-protein response" (UPR) in response to stress, one of several pathways which links nutrient intake and metabolic function (Figure 5.7). The ER is known mainly as a protein-folding factory, responsible for the biosynthesis, folding, assembly, and modification of numerous soluble proteins and membrane proteins. Approximately one-third of all cellular proteins are translocated into the lumen of the ER, where post-translational modification, folding, and oligomerization occur, before being targeted to various cellular organelles or transported to the surface of the cell. In addition, the ER is the major signal-transducing organelle within the cell that continuously responds to environmental cues, including growth factors, hormones, and stimuli that perturb cellular energy levels, nutrient availability, or redox status. The ER is exquisitely sensitive to alterations in homeostasis, where, upon a variety of different stimuli, signals are transduced from the ER to the cytoplasm and the nucleus to eventually result in adaptation for survival or induction of apoptosis.[18]

Physiological states that increase the demand for protein folding, or stimuli that disrupt the reactions by which proteins fold, create an imbalance between the protein-folding load and the capacity of the ER, causing unfolded or misfolded proteins to accumulate in the ER lumen—a condition referred to as ER stress. In addition to ER stress, hypoxia, infections, toxins, nutrient overload, and energy deprivation are all known to activate the UPR, which has both protective and inflammatory functions.[19] UPR activation increases cytokines which have a role in insulin resistance,[20] NF-κB which upregulates a series of inflammatory genes, including COX-2, and a number of acute-phase proteins, including C-reactive protein (CRP) and serum amyloid P-component (saP).[17]

Thus, in response to stressful cellular states, at least at the level of the organelle, a cascade of signals is induced, one effect of which is to increase inflammatory signals. While the ER's response is well understood, it is probable that dysfunction or stress in other organelles also contributes to inflammation. Inter-organelle communication makes it likely that stress in another organelle, such as the mitochondria, affects stress in the ER, or vice versa, through a specialized sub-domain of the ER called the mitochondrial-associated membrane (MAM).[21] For example, mitochondrial structural defects have been documented in nonalcoholic steatohepatitis (NASH), which leads to increased fatty acid beta oxidation, which may cause abnormal cytokine production and insulin resistance, crucial pathophysiologic factors of NASH.[22,23] This metabolic induction of inflammation may play a role in many chronic diseases, and appears to initiate a vicious cycle, as many metabolic diseases (e.g., obesity) are known to cause inflammation. It should be noted that many of the physiological signals are nutrient related, including excess free fatty acids, glucose, and amino acids.

Cross-talk between the UPR and inflammatory molecules is exemplified in cell types that have metabolic or immune functions, including hepatocytes, β-cells, adipocytes, macrophages, and oligodendrocytes. Many *in vitro* studies suggest that pathological conditions that interfere with ER homeostasis

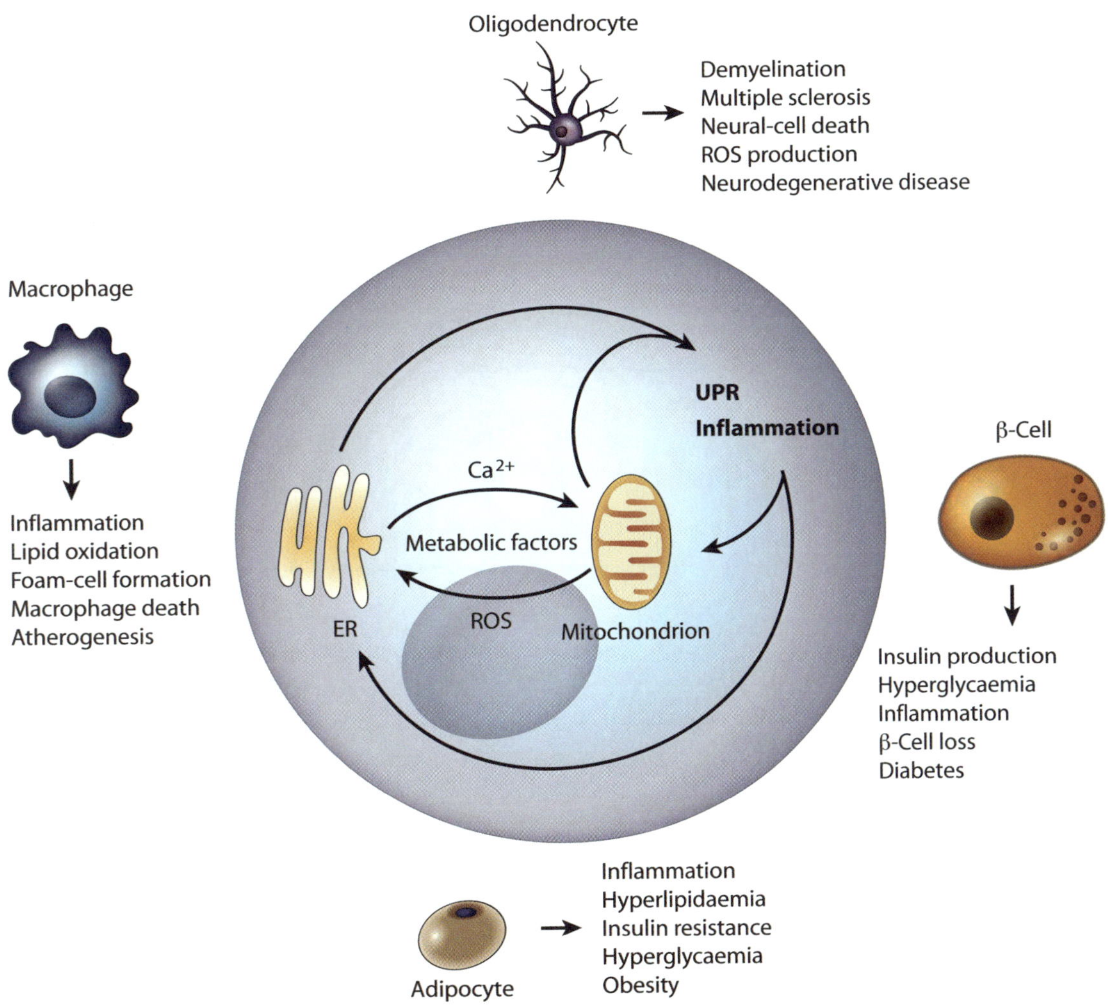

Figure 5.8 The ER-stress-inflammation loop in specialized cells. From: Zhang K, Kaufman RJ. From endoplasmic-reticulum stress to the inflammatory response. *Nature.* 2008 Jul 24;454(7203):455-62. Reproduced with permission from Macmillan Publishers Ltd.

and/or mitochondrial metabolism result in chronic activation of the UPR, and thus inflammation. The coupling of the UPR and inflammation in specialized cells and tissues might be fundamental to the pathogenesis of metabolic, neurodegenerative and infectious diseases (Figure 5.8).[19]

Contributors to Inflammation

Diet

The pro-inflammatory Western diet is a significant contributor to chronic inflammation, mostly due to its excess of sugars and arachidonic acid, and the insufficiency of omega-3 fatty acids and phytonutrients. The typical Western diet is also high in corn and corn oil, containing high amounts of the omega-6 fatty acid linoleic acid, which upregulates inflammatory gene transcription, increases low-density lipoprotein oxidation and the severity of coronary atherosclerosis, increases platelet aggregation, and interferes with the incorporation of EPA and DHA in cell membrane phospholipids.[24] What has also emerged as a critical factor in driving inflammation is the ratio of omega-3 to omega-6 fatty acids. The last 150 years has seen a dramatic increase in vegetable seed oil, rich in omega-6 fatty acids, and a parallel decrease of foods rich in omega-3 fatty acids. As a result, the omega-6/omega-3 ratio in Western diet ranges

Table 5.1 Omega-3 and omega-6 fatty acid-derived messengers and physiological effects

	Arachidonic acid (n-6) derived messengers	Physiological effects	Physiological effects	EPA and DHA (n-3) derived messengers
Prostaglandins	PGD_2			PGD_3
	PGE_2	Pro-arrhythmic	Anti-arrhythmic	PGE_3
	PGF_2			PGF_3
	PGI_2	Pro-arrhythmic	Anti-arrhythmic	PGI_3
Thromboxanes	TXA_2	Platelat activator	Platelat inhibitor	TXA_3
	TXB_2	Vasoconstriction	Vasodilation	TXB_3
Leukotrienes	LTA_4			LTA_5
	LTB_4	Pro-inflammatory	Anti-inflammatory	LTB_5
	LTC_4			LTC_5
	LTD_4			LTD_5
	LTE_4			LTE_5
Epoxyeicosatrienoic derivatives	5,6-EET			
	8,9-EET			
	11,12-EET	Inflammatory		
	14,15-EET			
Hydroxyleicosatetraenoic derivatives	5-HETE			
	12-HETE			
	15-HETE			
Lipoxins	LXA_4			
Resolvins			Anti-inflammatory	RVE1
			Anti-inflammatory	RVD
Neuroprotectin			Anti-inflammatory	NPD1

The opposing effects of omega-3 and omega-6 fatty acids. From: Schmitz G, Ecker J. *Prog Lipid Res.* 2008 Mar;47(2):147-55. Reproduced with permission from Elsevier Science & Technology Journals.

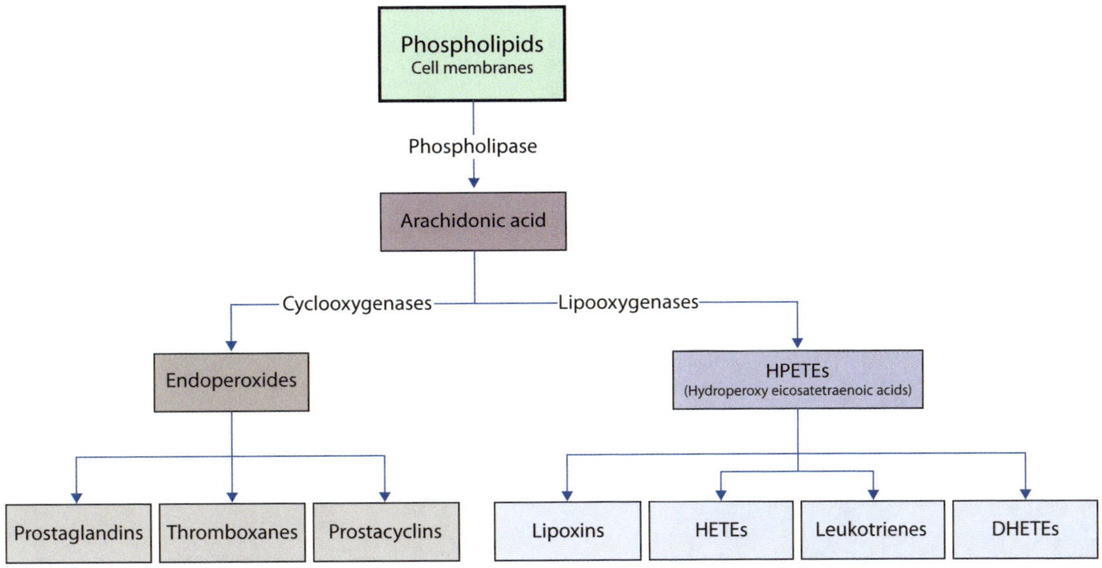

Figure 5.9 Pro-inflammatory derivatives of arachidonic acid.

between 15:1 and 20:1—far different from the nearly 1:1 ratio humans evolved on as a species.

Omega-3 to omega-6 ratio

As shown in Table 5.1 and Figures 5.9 and 5.10, most mediators formed from omega-3 precursors are anti-inflammatory, while those derived from omega-6 (ultimately arachidonic acid) are pro-inflammatory.[25] Arachidonic acid increases the production of the prostaglandin and thromboxane 2-series and leukotriene 4-series, as well as lipoxins, while omega-3 derivatives increase the prostaglandin and thromboxane 3-series and leukotriene 5-series, as well as the resolvins and protectins.[25]

However, some prostaglandin effects are more complex. For example, PGE2 is generally thought to be pro-inflammatory. Although it initially does have a pro-inflammatory effect (by inducing COX-2), it later becomes an inducer of subsequent anti-inflammatory pathways, in part via its roles in amplifying lipoxin expression,[26] and also by inhibiting 5-lipoxygenase and the leukotriene 4-series expression.[25] This may help to explain why, although omega-3 and omega-6 fatty acids are both necessary, it is the ratio between them that may be most important. For example, in a study of over 400 healthy men and 450 healthy women, only at high omega-6 intakes were omega-3 intakes inversely associated with markers of inflammation, and a combination of both was associated with the lowest inflammation.[27]

EPA, DHA, and AA are competitive substrates for enzymes involved in autacoid biosynthesis. Increased dietary consumption of EPA and DHA results in higher concentrations of these fatty acids compared to arachidonic acid in cellular phospholipids and glycerides, as well as in cellular and organelle lipid membranes.[25] Also, omega-3 fatty acids favorably affect gene expression of nuclear receptors and nuclear transcription factors related to inflammation, such as peroxisome proliferator-activated receptor alpha (PPAR alpha) expression in adipose tissue.[28,29]

For some individuals, conversion of plant-based omega-3 fatty acids to DHA and EPA is more difficult. Delta-6-desaturase is the rate-limiting enzyme in long-chain fatty acid synthesis, and polymorphisms in this gene (FADS2) may impair conversion from plant-based omega-3 fatty acids containing alpha-linolenic acid.[30] Additionally, trans fats have been shown to inhibit desaturase activity in animals.[31]

Unfortunately, the typical Western diet of fast foods and packaged dinners tends to be rich in

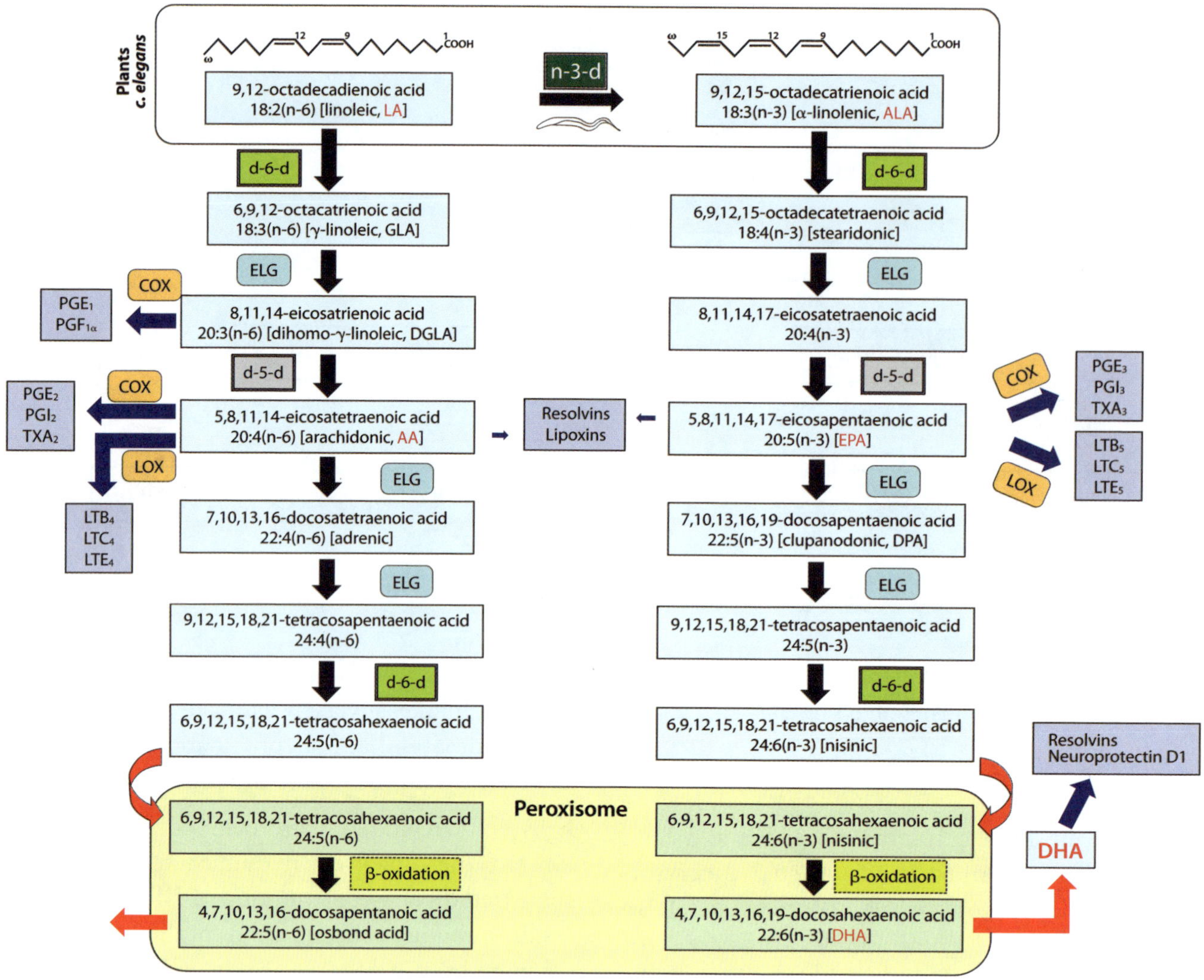

Figure 5.10 Detailed diagram of fatty acid and prostaglandin biosynthesis. From: Russo GL. *Biochem Pharmacol.* 2009;77(6):937-46. Note: Omega-3-d is not present in mammals, which is why humans can't convert omega-6 to omega-3. Reproduced with permission from Elsevier Science & Technology Journals.

saturated fats and hydrogenated oils (trans fats) and lacking in essential fatty acids (EFAs). A diet rich in beef and dairy products from corn-fed land animals and low in nuts, seeds, and fish has a much higher ratio of 6/3 fatty acids. This results in a substantial increase in the risk of chronic inflammation, which is associated with many common chronic diseases such as heart disease and cancer. For example, breast cancer directly correlates with the dietary omega-6/omega-3 ratio.[32] Studies of patients with many diseases have found a higher omega-6/omega-3 ratio than in those without the disease. For example, children with ADHD have a 36% higher ratio than children without.[33]

Unfortunately, years of press reports about the associations between dietary fat, calories, and cholesterol with cancer and heart disease have resulted in a misunderstanding that fats are unhealthy. This is simply not true. The problem is not fat per se, but rather the ratio of fatty acids in the fats. Just as a diet too high in omega-6 fatty acids can increase the risk of disease, a diet too low in fat can result in many health problems as well. A large amount of research now shows that replacing high omega-6 oils with oils lower in omega-6 and higher in omega-3 has many health benefits. For example, replacing corn oil (high in LA) with olive and canola oil (low in LA) to reach a 4:1 ratio of LA/ALA results in a remarkable 70% decrease in total mortality![85]

Other dietary factors

In general, a low glycemic load and low calorie Mediterranean-style diet rich in fruits and vegetables has the greatest benefit for reducing inflammation. Meals with a high glycemic load increase C-reactive protein and other markers of inflammation. For example, in a study of over 200 apparently healthy women, glycemic load was found to be significantly and positively associated with plasma hsCRP, independently of conventional risk factors for ischemic heart disease.[34] In another study of nearly 1000 Dutch men and women, researchers also found an inverse association between glycemic index and C-reactive protein levels.[35] Data from the Women's Health Initiative found high dietary fiber (typically a sign of a low glycemic load diet) to be associated with lower levels of the inflammatory markers IL-6 and TNF-alpha-R2, although it was not associated with CRP levels.[36]

The Mediterranean diet specifically has been found to be of great benefit. In a study following over 1500 men and 1500 women, the greatest adherence to a Mediterranean diet resulted in, on average, 20% lower CRP levels, 17% lower IL-6 levels, 15% lower homocysteine levels, 14% lower white blood cell counts, and 6% lower fibrinogen levels, as compared with those in the lowest tertile.[37] In another study, 120 obese women given information about the Mediterranean diet and increasing physical activity had a reduction in weight, insulin resistance, CRP, and other inflammatory cytokines.[38] In a study of nearly 350 twins, adherence to a Mediterranean diet was associated with reduced levels of interleukin-6 but not C-reactive protein, after adjustment for total energy intake, other nutritional factors, known cardiovascular risk factors, and use of supplements and medications.[39]

Weight loss is also an effective strategy for reducing inflammation, because obesity is closely tied to inflammation, as well as to the metabolic syndrome. Adiponectin appears to reduce CRP levels, and the hypoadiponectin levels observed with excessive adipose tissue may be a causal mechanism.[40] In a study of 7540 individuals, central adiposity was the strongest independent predictor of inflammation, with an OR of 3.45.[41] Interestingly, data from this study also indicated that inflammatory markers partly explained the association between psychosocial stress and obesity, suggesting that inflammation may be a link between stress and obesity.[42] Finally, calorie-restricted diets have been associated with a reduction in a number of inflammatory markers in animal-based studies.[43]

In a study of over 7000 Japanese men and women, high intakes of vegetables, fruit, soy products, and fish were significantly and inversely related to hsCRP concentrations, even after adjustment for age, body mass index, smoking, alcohol consumption, and physical activity in both men and women.[44] High flavonoid content also appears to be protective. When data from NHANES 1999–2002 were analyzed, researchers found that among over 8000 US adults, total flavonoid intake was associated with a reduced CRP, as were individual flavonol, anthocyanidin, and isoflavone intakes.[45]

Sufficient intake of several nutrients has also been shown to be important in reducing inflammation—specifically, magnesium, betaine, and choline. Data from the Nurses' Health Study cohort found that the highest quintile of Mg intake was associated with a 24% lower CRP.[46] And the Attica Study, which enrolled over 1500 men and 1500 women, found that those consuming >360 mg/d of betaine had, on average, 10% lower concentrations of homocysteine, 19% lower concentrations of C-reactive protein, and 12% lower concentrations of TNF-alpha than did those who consumed <260 mg/d. Compared with the lowest tertile of choline intake (<250 mg/d), participants who consumed >310 mg/d had, on average, 22% lower concentrations of C-reactive protein, 26% lower concentrations of interleukin-6, and 6% lower concentrations of TNF-alpha.[47]

Finally, a number of food additives may contribute to an increasing degree of inflammation. Carrageenan, for example, was found to increase NF-κB production by activating toll-like receptor 4, an innate immune receptor.[48] This may explain its ability to induce inflammation in animal models of colitis. Other additives implicated include sulfites, MSG, tartrazine, benzoates, and aspartame.[49,50,51]

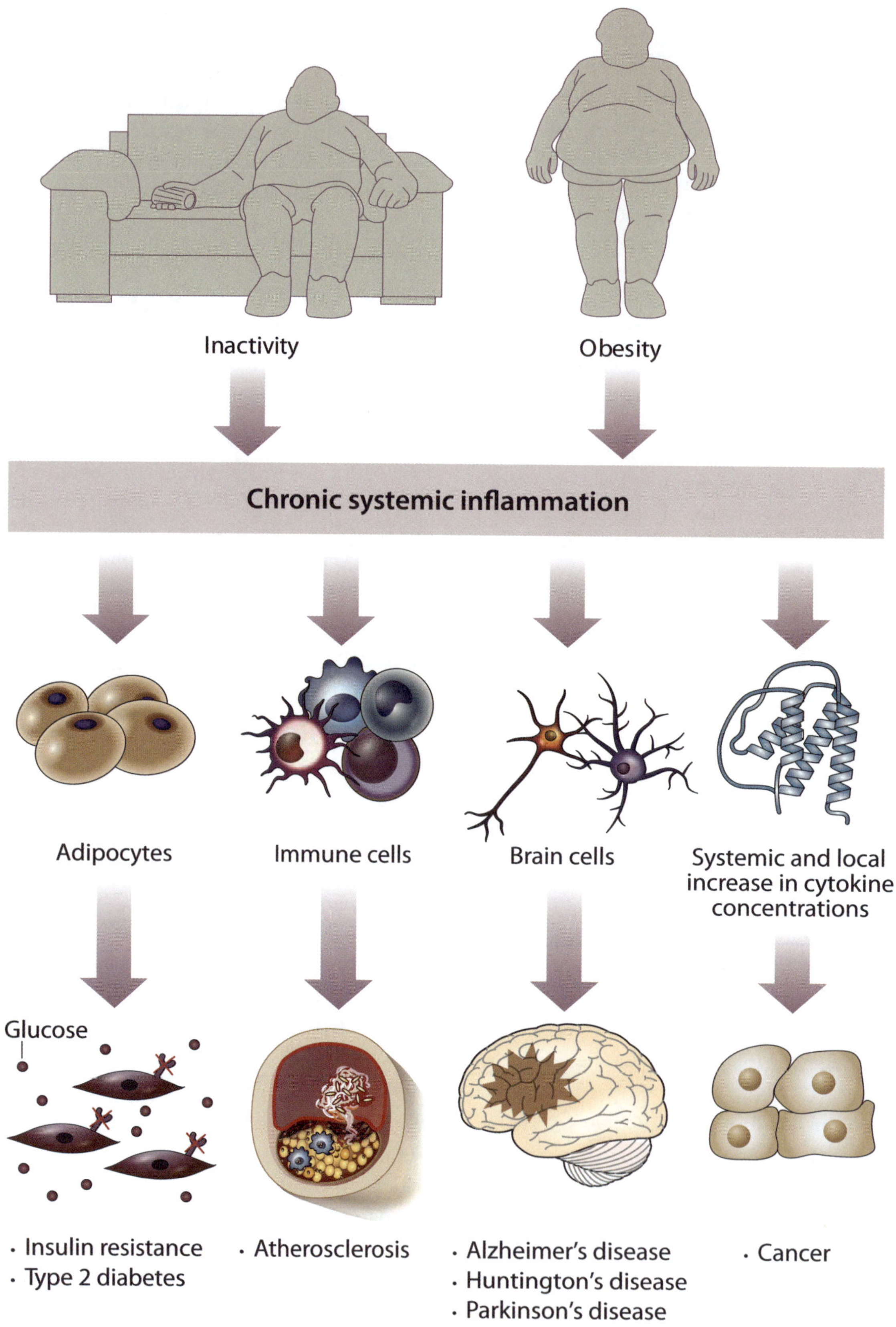

Figure 5.11 Contributions of inactivity and obesity to inflammation and chronic disease. From: Handschin C, Spiegelman BM. The role of exercise and PGC1alpha in inflammation and chronic disease. *Nature.* 2008 Jul 24;454(7203):463-9. Reproduced with permission from Macmillan Publishers Ltd.

Physical activity

Physical activity is tightly linked to inflammation in a complex manner. Regular, moderate exercise reduces the level of systemic inflammation, while high intensity training for a prolonged period increases systemic inflammation.[52] Figure 5.11 depicts how obesity and inactivity affect specific cellular functions, contributing to a number of chronic diseases.

A new view of muscle tissue as an endocrine organ has emerged; the inflammatory mediators tied to physical activity have only recently been discovered. A number of "myokines" (cytokines produced and secreted by muscle) are now known to be released; the best understood of these may be IL-6, IL-8, and IL-15.[53]

IL-6 levels undergo somewhat paradoxical changes with exercise. While exercise may increase IL-6 production from muscles nearly 100-fold, basal levels of IL-6 are lower in those who exercise regularly. It is generally thought that transient fluctuations in local and systemic myokine concentrations after physical activity might contribute to the beneficial effects of exercise on non-muscle tissues in a hormone-like manner, whereas a chronic increase in the concentration of many of these molecules is likely to be pro-inflammatory and detrimental. Thus, the cytokines secreted by muscle during exercise, and the subsequent return of these cytokine concentrations to basal levels, should be tightly regulated.[52]

Clinical studies have generally found that regular moderate exercise may not only reduce inflammation, but also that inflammation is associated with disability and muscle atrophy. In a study of 424 elderly men and women who underwent a 12-month moderate-intensity physical activity program, lower systemic concentrations of IL-6 were found, especially in those at the greatest risk for disability and subsequent loss of independence.[54] Higher levels of basal IL-6 and CRP have also been found to increase the risk of muscle strength loss (sarcopenia) in older men and women.[55] It should be noted that CRP levels are probably not a good marker for physical activity, and usually do not change with exercise.[56] CRP is probably a better marker for the effects of physical activity on BMI.[57]

Gastrointestinal permeability

Compromised barrier integrity represents the first step in the pathway to macrophage activation and establishment of chronic inflammation, and its sequelae in underlying tissues (Figure 5.12). This may be due to microbial toxins, environmental insults (such as toxins or food allergies), or the genetic predisposition of the host.[58] Epithelial barriers, such as those found in the skin, kidneys, lungs, or GI tract, define the interface between separate body compartments and between the body and the external world. The challenge in the GI tract is significantly greater than other barrier functions, because it must balance the need for a barrier against a hostile environment with the necessity of active and passive transport of desirable substances. An intact intestinal barrier is, therefore, critical to normal physiological function and prevention of disease.[59] Disruption of the epithelial barrier may allow commensal microorganisms access to the TLRs on macrophages that reside in the lamina propria, resulting in TLR-mediated induction of tissue repair responses in the intestine.[2]

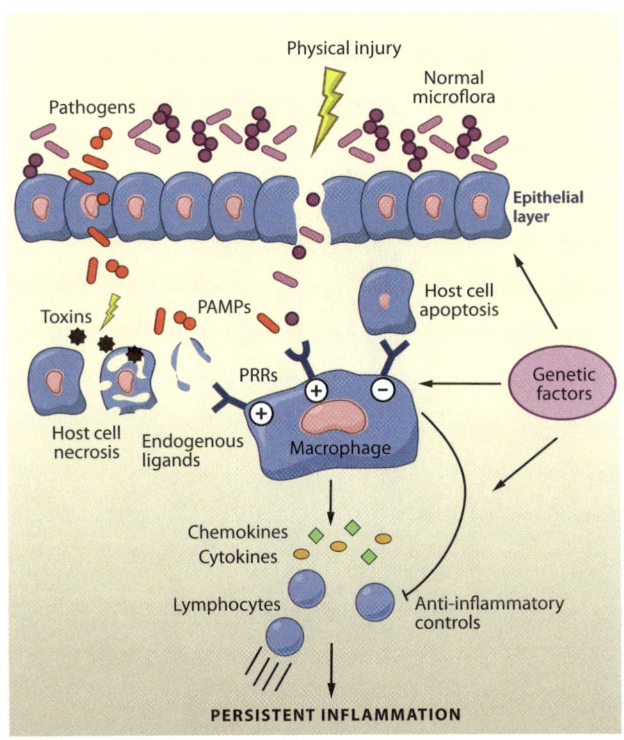

Figure 5.12 Compromised epithelial function leads to persistent inflammation. From: Karin M, Lawrence T, Nizet V. Innate immunity gone awry: linking microbial infections to chronic inflammation and cancer. *Cell.* 2006 Feb 24;124(4):823-35. Reproduced with permission from Elsevier Science & Technology Journals.

Celiac disease has been used as a model of how impaired intestinal permeability initiates a chronic inflammatory process (Figure 5.13). Recent research has proposed the exciting hypothesis that repairing damaged intestinal permeability may halt this inflammatory process and the resultant autoimmune damage.[60] In addition to therapeutics that restore GI integrity, probiotics appear to be crucial to maintaining GI integrity, and for reducing inflammation mediators.[61]

Vitamin D deficiency

Substantial evidence is now available documenting that the deficiency of vitamin D is pandemic, and that lower levels are associated with a number of chronic diseases, including cardiovascular and autoimmune diseases. Vitamin D is also a significant factor in a number of physiological functions, specifically as a biological inhibitor of inflammatory hyperactivity, perhaps explaining why a deficiency (or even an insufficiency) can be so detrimental.[62,63,64] Clinically, vitamin D produces dose-dependent reductions in IL-6 and CRP, with either an associated deficiency or a supplemental benefit demonstrated for osteoarthritis, multiple sclerosis, type 1 diabetes, Graves' disease, ankylosing spondylitis, SLE, and rheumatoid arthritis.[65,66,67]

Sleep

Sleep deprivation causes both somnolence and fatigue, and it has also been shown to increase daytime IL-6 levels. Post-deprivation was associated with decreases in nighttime IL-6 which may explain why it leads to a deeper sleep.[68] Thus, poor sleep increases total exposure to the inflammatory effects of IL-6. Both acute total and short-term partial sleep deprivation have resulted in elevated hsCRP concentrations. It has been suggested that sleep loss may be one of the ways in which inflammatory processes are activated and contribute to the association of sleep complaints, short sleep duration, and cardiovascular morbidity observed in epidemiologic surveys.[69] For example, obstructive sleep apnea has been associated with elevated plasma CRP concentrations, as well as an

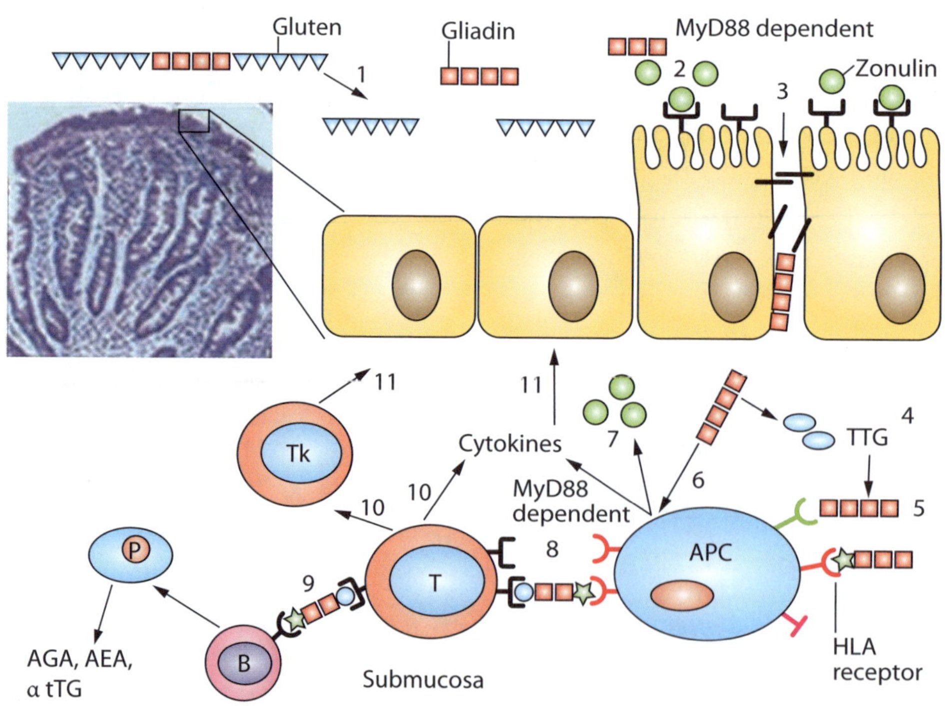

Figure 5.13 Proposed role of abnormal intestinal permeability in the pathogenesis of celiac disease. From: Fasano A, Shea-Donohue T. Mechanisms of disease: the role of intestinal barrier function in the pathogenesis of gastrointestinal autoimmune diseases. *Nat Clin Pract Gastroenterol Hepatol.* 2005 Sep;2(9):416-22. Reproduced with permission from Macmillan Publishers Ltd.

increased risk for many cormorbidities.[70] For more information on strategies to improve sleep quality, please see Clinical Focus 6—Stress, Anxiety, Depression and Insomnia.

Inhibition of Inflammation Resolution/ Inadequate Quenching

Because we now understand that resolution of inflammation is an active process, we can begin to change how we treat inflammation. For example, direct inhibition of many of the mediators involved in the process may actually stall or prevent successful resolution. One example of this is the inhibition of cyclooxygenases by NSAIDs (Figure 5.14), especially selective enzyme inhibition of these enzymes.[8] While NSAIDs prevent prostaglandin biosynthesis and are effective anti-inflammatories because they reduce the levels of prostaglandin as well as the cardinal signs of inflammation, they are actually now considered "resolution-toxic" because they prolong the time to resolve inflammation, and may even extend its spread.[7] Although the COX enzymes have been demonized by many pharmaceutical advertisements, we now recognize that COX-2 is not the cause of inflammation, and actually has an active role in its resolution.

Selectively inhibiting COX-2 suppresses its beneficial roles, resulting in adverse drug reactions. For example, prostacyclin (an eicosanoid whose production is lowered when COX is targeted) normally reduces both blood pressure and platelet aggregation. Additionally the same prostaglandins that are inhibited by NSAIDs have protective roles in the body, such as gastric mucosal defense. The consequences of such selective inhibition

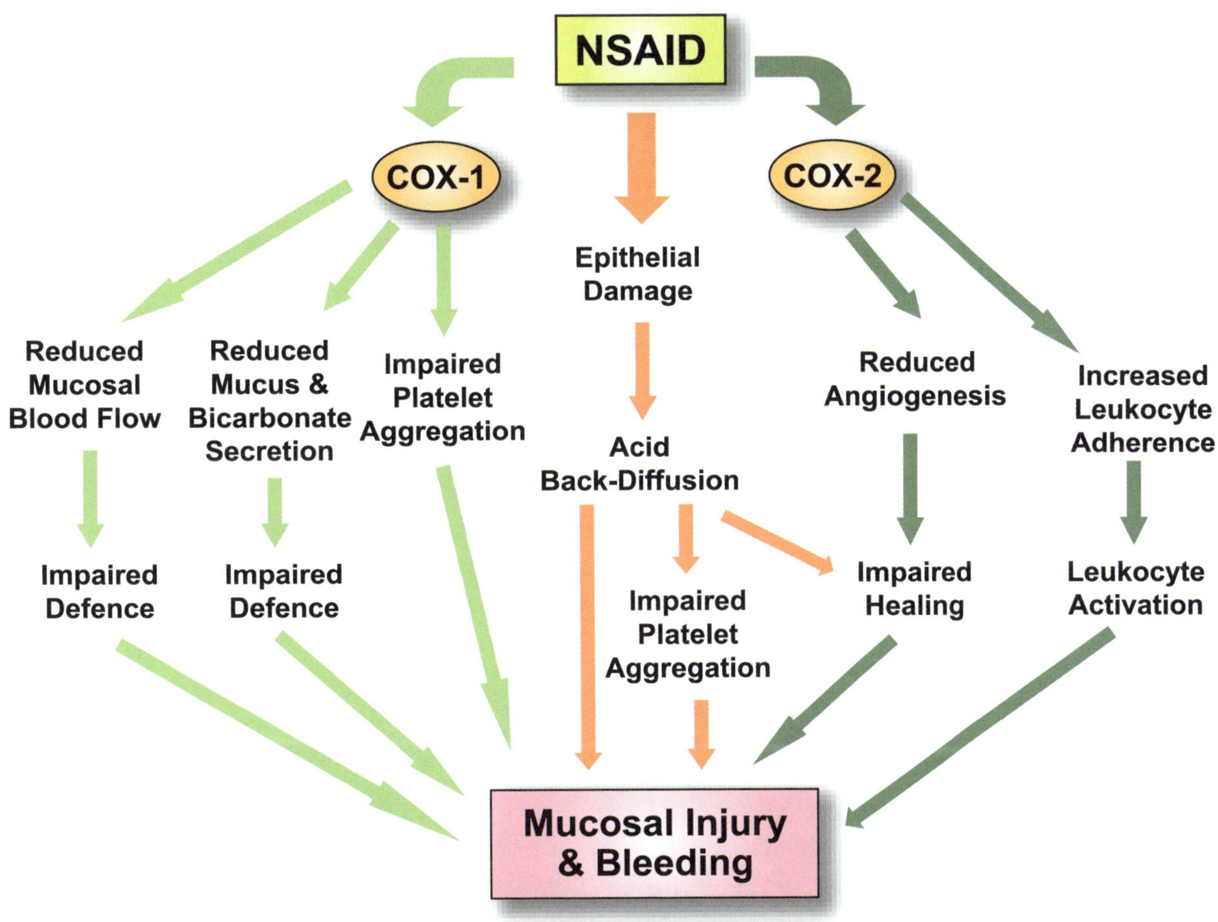

Figure 5.14 Pathogenesis of NSAID-induced gastric injury and bleeding. From: Wallace JL. Prostaglandins, NSAIDs, and gastric mucosal protection: why doesn't the stomach digest itself? *Physiol Rev.* 2008 Oct;88(4):1547-65. Reproduced with permission from the American Physiological Society.

have been quite severe. Chronic use of COX-2 inhibitors injured at least 160,000 and killed an estimated 26,000–55,000.[71,72,73] Other problems associated with selective inhibition of eicosanoid pathways are presented in Figure 5.15.

- Bioactive lipids mediating the same phenomena might be synthesized by more than one pathway (e.g., COX-2 and 5-LOX), so blocking one pathway might divert AA metabolism along an alternative route which might exacerbate the pathological condition.
- Bioactive eicosanoids with inhibitory and stimulating properties are produced by the same pathway (e.g., PGE2/PGD2 versus PGI2/TXA2) and selective inhibition might adversely destabilize the delicate balance between the physiological actions of these products.
- The same eicosanoids can be pathogenic at the beginning of the inflammatory response, but might exert pro-resolving effects at a later stage (e.g., PGE2> lipoxins or PGD2> 15dPGJ2). Therefore, blocking production also suppresses their anti-inflammatory activities.
- The same eicosanoids initiate a pathological condition in one tissue/organ (e.g., PGE2 in IBD) but might ameliorate it in another organ/tissue (e.g., PGE2 in asthma). Moreover, some eicosanoids have essential physiological functions (e.g., PGE2 in labour/neuro- and gastro-protection). Therefore, complete elimination by a systemic drug might treat inflammation at one site but might have adverse effects in other sites/organs.

Figure 5.15 Problems associated with selective inhibition of eicosanoid pathways. From: Yedgar S, Krimsky M, Cohen Y, et al. Treatment of inflammatory diseases by selective eicosanoid inhibition: a double-edged sword? *Trends Pharmacol Sci.* 2007 Sep;28(9):459-64. Epub 2007 Aug 10. Reproduced with permission from Elsevier Science & Technology Journals.

Selective inhibition of enzymatic activity is characteristic of pharmaceutical approaches, but not of natural medicine therapeutics. The main advantages of a multi-faceted natural medicine approach are that they allow the body's regulatory systems to continue to function while encouraging the resolution of inflammation through the use of lipoxins, resolvins, and protectins. A natural approach reduces inflammation by quenching the mediators of inflammation, by supporting antioxidant status, quenching many of the reactive oxygen and reactive nitrogen species that initiate and propagate inflammatory pathways and damage cellular organelles and lipid membranes. For example, vitamin C decreases oxidant stress related to macrophage activation, decreases uptake and degradation of oxidized LDL, and enhances several aspects of macrophage function.[74]

Assessment

A number of conditions are associated with increased inflammation. For example, ulcerative colitis and asthma are both good predictors of excess inflammation. In addition to a clinical evaluation, a number of laboratory assessments are available. C-reactive protein is considered a sensitive marker for inflammation and a predictive risk factor for cardiovascular disease.[75,76] Indeed, of the current inflammatory markers, hsCRP provides the most conclusive information in clinical practice with regard to cardiovascular risk. Results are typically divided into three different risk categories: low risk (<1 mg/l), average risk (1–3 mg/l), and high risk (>3 mg/l).[77]

The ESR (erythrocyte sedimentation rate) is also often used because of its availability and low cost, but other factors (including non-inflammatory conditions) such as anemia, hyperlipoproteinemia, abnormal immunoglobulin, diabetes, estrogen, and progesterone can all increase the ESR. Other conventional markers of acute inflammation include procalcitonin, serum amyloid A, ferritin, and apolipoprotein A-I. For example apoA-I levels decrease by at least 25% during inflammation, as IL-6, IL-1, and TNF inhibit its synthesis by hepatocytes. ApoA-I is the principal protein constituent of HDL, which has antioxidant, anti-inflammatory, and anti-thrombotic properties. Thus a decreased production of apoA-I lessens the protection provided by HDL.[77]

In addition to standard markers of inflammation, nutritional markers should also be evaluated. Low omega-3 blood levels indicate the need for a greater intake of DHA and EPA. For example, data from nearly 33,000 women in the Nurses' Health Study found that higher plasma concentrations of EPA and DPA (and DHA nonsignificantly) were associated with lower risk of nonfatal myocardial infarction. RBC levels were more weakly associated and nonsignificant.[78] Similarly, because of the prevalence of insufficient vitamin D levels, this should be routinely ordered to evaluate inflammatory risk.

Given the contribution of reactive oxygen species to cellular dysfunction and inflammation, two markers are recommended to assess antioxidant status, 8-oxo-7,8-dihydro-2'-deoxyguanosine (8-oxodG, an oxidized nucleoside of DNA) and gamma-glutamyltransferase (GGT). 8-oxodG indicates damaged nuclear or mitochondrial DNA. Along with GGT, 8-oxodG will provide a good estimate of overall mortality risk, as well as cardiovascular and cancer risk.

Finally, assessment of gastrointestinal integrity, food allergies, and gut microbiota will help the clinician better understand the patient's risk of inflammation. In addition to a food allergy panel and/or elimination diet, the lactulose/mannitol test along with either DNA analysis or culture of GI flora should be a part of a comprehensive assessment for inflammation.

Interventions

Diet

As discussed above, a Mediterranean-type diet with a high omega-3 to omega-6 ratio is the most effective dietary pattern for reducing inflammation. Additionally, given the effects of hyperglycemia and AGEs on inflammation, an anti-inflammatory diet should contain a low glycemic load, with emphasis on whole, natural foods such as fruits, vegetables, nuts, seeds, and berries (high in flavonoids). These foods are generally rich sources of phytonutrients that have antioxidant and anti-inflammatory properties that can help to quench inflammatory triggers.

Although a general anti-inflammatory dietary approach is likely sufficient for most patients, more aggressive changes may be necessary for those with more severe inflammation. A gluten-free vegan diet has been used successfully by patients with rheumatoid arthritis, inducing changes that are potentially atheroprotective and anti-inflammatory, including decreased LDL and oxLDL levels and raised anti-PC IgM and IgA levels.[79] This benefit may be due to decreased immunoreactivity to food antigens, as demonstrated in a previous trial, which also showed clinical benefit. In the earlier study, 40.5% of the vegan group fulfilled the American College of Rheumatology improvement criteria, compared with 4% in the non-vegan group.[80] A vegetarian diet was also found to have clinical benefit for rheumatoid arthritis, and was thought to augment the effect of fish oil supplementation because it is lower in arachidonic acid.[81] Also, as discussed previously, a diet rich in magnesium, betaine, and choline may also offer specific benefit in reducing inflammation.

Physical activity and stress reduction

The anti-inflammatory benefits of moderate-intensity regular physical activity appear to exceed those of high-intensity prolonged exercise.[52] The ability of such exercise to reduce inflammation also helps to prevent age-associated decline in muscle strength. Again, CRP is not a good marker for the effects of physical activity on inflammation.

Reducing stress also plays an important role in minimizing inflammation. Several therapies may offer benefit by helping to reduce stress. For example, music therapy has been shown to decrease plasma cortisol, decrease bronchial asthma symptoms, and reduce latex-induced wheals in patients with latex sensitization.[82] Stress reduction has also been shown to reduce experimental neurogenic inflammation.[83] For more information on strategies to lower stress, please see Clinical Focus 6—Stress, Anxiety, Depression, and Insomnia.

Nutritional and botanical therapies

As part of a comprehensive treatment plan, a combination of botanicals, foods, and nutrients is integrated into a multiphase approach to treating inflammation. Antioxidants, quenchers of inflammatory mediators, enzyme inhibitors, and therapies that directly enhance the resolution phase of inflammation are all essential to successful treatment.

Natural enhancers of resolution

Supplemental fish oil (DHA and EPA) is another very important supplement consideration in inflammatory conditions. Many of the natural substances that bring about resolution of inflammation (e.g., lipoxins, resolvins, and protectins) are derived from omega-3 fatty acids. A combination of both fatty acids is preferred; while EPA may have more immediate anti-inflammatory properties,[84] DHA is the precursor for the resolvins and protectins.

Of course, improving the omega-6/omega-3 ratio is pretty straightforward, but it takes time to convert the cell membranes, and eventually the fat stores, to the healthy ratio. Thus, along with omega-3 supplementation, a diet that reduces consumption of omega-6 oils and that is also rich in alpha-linolenic acid, monounsaturated fat, and low-mercury fish should be adopted. See Table 5.2 for dietary sources of omega-3 and omega-6 fatty acids.

Table 5.2 Dietary sources of omega-6 (LA + AA) and omega-3 (ALA + EPA/DHA)[85]

Product	LA	ALA	AA	EPA+DHA
η-6 FA rich foods				
Corn oil	50000	900		
Cotton seed oil	47800	1000		
Peanut oil	23900			
Soybean oil	53400	7600		
Sunflower oil	60200	500		
Safflower oil	74000	470		
Margarine	17600	1900		
Lard	8600	1000	1070	
Chicken egg	3800	220		
Bacon	6080	250	250	
Ham	2480	160	130	
Soya bean	8650	1000		
Maize	1630	40		
Almond	9860	260		
Brazil nut	24900			
Peanut	13900	530		
Walnut	34100	6800	590	
η-3 FA rich foods				
Canola oil	19100	8600		
Linseed oil	13400	55300		
Herring	150	61.66	36.66	1700
Salmon	440	550	300	1200
Trout	74		30	500
Tuna	260	270	280	400
Cod	4	2	3	300

Data reported as mg/100 g.

Content of η-6, η-3 FAs may slightly vary according to species, sources and analytical methods.

From: Russo GL. *Biochem Pharmacol.* 2009;77(6):937-46. Reproduced with permission from Elsevier Science & Technology Journals.

Natural antioxidants

Antioxidant use is indicated for patients with excess inflammation, particularly those with increased oxidative stress. As mentioned previously, those with elevated levels of gamma-glutamyltransferase (GGT) and/or 8-oxodG have an increased need for antioxidant compounds.

In addition to a diet rich in antioxidants, a number of foods contain compounds that exert some specific benefit for reducing inflammation. Among these are blueberry/bilberry (*Vaccinium myrtillus*), chocolate (*Theobroma cacao*), cranberry (*Vaccinium macrocarpon*), garlic (*Allium sativum*), ginger (*Zingiber officinalis*), grape (*Vitis vinifera*), green tea (*Camellia sinensis*), and turmeric (*Curcuma longa*).

In particular, the yellow pigment of turmeric, curcumin, has been shown to be a potent antioxidant[86] and it also inhibits NF-κB production, likely through the toll-like receptor TLR-4.[87]

Curcumin has had potent benefits in clinical trials for inflammatory conditions.[88] For example, in one double-blind crossover clinical trial in patients with rheumatoid arthritis, curcumin (1200 mg/day) was compared with phenylbutazone (300 mg/day). The improvements in the duration of morning stiffness, walking time, and joint swelling were comparable in both groups.[89] In another study, which used the postoperative inflammation model for evaluating nonsteroidal anti-inflammatory drugs (NSAIDs), curcumin was again shown to exert comparable anti-inflammatory action to phenylbutazone, but without significant side effects.[90] The results of these studies indicate that turmeric or curcumin may provide benefit in the treatment of inflammation.

Withania is a potent antioxidant, and extracts of withania have been shown to be a novel class of NF-κB activation inhibitors, as well as blocking NF-κB gene expression.[91,92] Cranberry juice has been shown to inhibit IL-6, IL-8, and PGE2 responses of gingival fibroblasts, demonstrating clinical benefit in the treatment of periodontitis.[93] Finally, garlic has been shown to attenuate reactive oxygen species from neutrophils,[94] as well as to inhibit leukocyte migration through endothelial cells.[95]

Anti-inflammatory botanicals

Many botanicals have also shown the ability to inhibit enzymes involved in inflammation, without associated adverse effects found in similar medications, and have been used clinically for pain relief. For example, *Allium cepa* (onion) is a potent inhibitor of the COX and lipoxygenase enzymes.[96,97,98] *Boswellia serrata* (Boswellia) has emerged as a potent inhibitor of 5-lipoxygenase, and has been shown to suppress NF-κB production.[99,100,101] In a clinical trial of osteoarthritis patients, an extract from Boswellia was shown to confer prompt and significant pain relief and improvement in physical ability in as few as 7 days.[102]

Camellia sinensis (green tea) has been shown to inhibit COX-2 and IL-1β-induced MUC5AC gene expression and secretion, an important contributor to inflammation.[103,104,105] *Ginkgo biloba* inhibits PAF, NF-κB, TNF-α, and IL-6.[106,107]

Table 5.3 Percentage of pain-free patients and relative change in the modified Arthus Index and its pain component

Study	Willow bark High dose	Willow bark Low dose	Conventional therapy or placebo	p
NRCT, all patients taking willow bark				
Pain-free at week 4 (end), % of patients	40	19	18	<0.001
Arhus Index, % relative change over 4 weeks	22	11	17	<0.001
Arhus pain component, % relative change	35	18	25	0.0062
NRCT, all patients taking willow bark extract only				
Pain-free at week 4 (end), % of patients	41	8	18	–
RCDT				
Pain-free at week 4 (5 days), % of patients	39	21	6	<0.001
Arhus Index, % relative change over 4 weeks	54	44	0	0.022
Arhus pain component, % relative change over 4 wks	67	40	0	<0.001

Legend: * Relative change in the modified Arhus Index (AI) = (AI, begin – AI, end)/AI, begin × 100. NRCT = non-randomized controlled trial; RCDT = randomized, controlled, double-blind trial. From: Chrubasik S, Pollak S, Black A, et al. Willow bark extract, a useful alternative for the treatment of osteoarthritis. *Arthritis Rheum.* 2003;48:278-80.Reproduced with permission from John Wiley & Sons, Inc.

Glycyrrhiza glabra (licorice) acts via a number of mechanisms, including the inhibition of phospholipase A2 and IL-18 production.[108,109,110] *Salix spp.* (willow bark), a herb with a long history of use as an anti-inflammatory, inhibits both cyclooxygenase and lipoxygenase enzymes. A head-to-head study of 228 patients comparing willow bark with Vioxx found them equally effective, but willow bark was less expensive (see Table 5.3).[111,112]

Uncaria spp. (cat's claw) also acts via multiple mechanisms, and has been shown to reduce NF-κB, TNF-α, COX-2, and PGE2. In a clinical trial of 30 patients with osteoarthritis of the knees, cat's claw was shown to reduce pain by 36% at 4 weeks.[113] Modest benefit was also reported in a one-year study of patients with rheumatoid arthritis.[114] Also, *Zingiber officinale* (ginger) inhibits 5-lipoxygenase and cyclooxygenase.[115,116,117]

Resveratrol has many biological effects as demonstrated by *in vitro* studies, including anti-inflammatory and chondroprotective effects. It exerts synergistic effects with curcumin. In a study in human chondrocytes, the synergistic effect of curcumin and resveratrol used together was greater than either alone, because they act on multiple and complementary steps of inflammation.[118] In chondrocytes, resveratrol modulates the NF-κB pathway by inhibiting the proteasome, while curcumin modulates the activation of NF-κB by inhibiting upstream kinases (Akt).[119] This is a clear example of the benefit of natural therapies working on multiple sites without the consequences of selective single enzyme inhibition (Figure 5.16).

Anti-inflammatory hormones

Two hormones have powerful anti-inflammatory benefits: DHEA and vitamin D. DHEA inhibits NF-κB and secretion of IL-6 and IL-12.[120] In a clinical trial for patients with type 2 diabetes, DHEA was shown to downregulate the TNF-α/TNF-α receptor system, and thereby prevent advanced glycation end product formation.[121] Levels of DHEA are low in systemic lupus erythematosus and inflammatory bowel disease

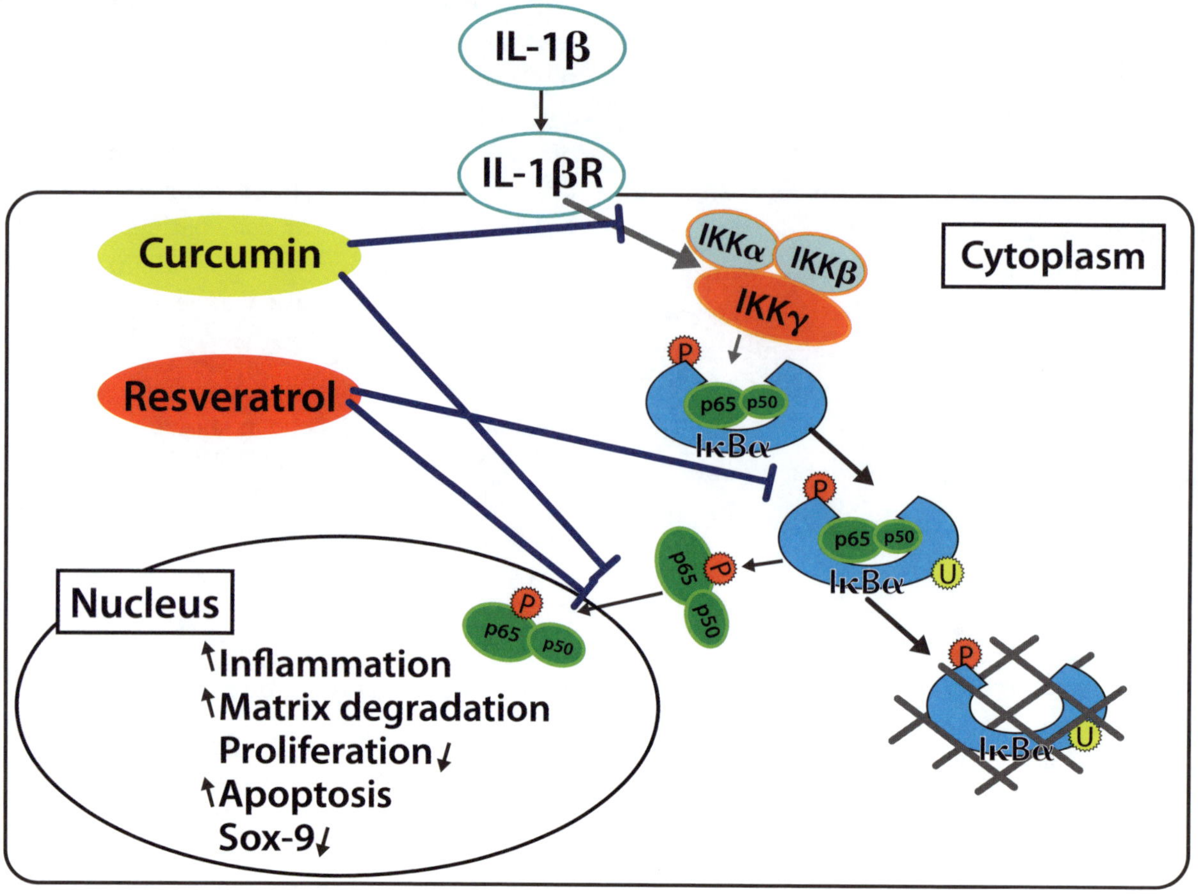

Figure 5.16 Inhibitory effects of resveratrol and curcumin on IL-1b-induced NF-κB activation in human chrondocytes. From: Csaki C, Mobasheri A, Shakibaei M. Synergistic chondroprotective effects of curcumin and resveratrol in human articular chondrocytes: inhibition of IL-1beta-induced NF-kappaB-mediated inflammation and apoptosis. *Arthritis Res Ther*. 2009;11(6):R165. Epub 2009 Nov 4. Reproduced from Open Access article distributed under the terms of the Creative Commons Attribution License.

(both Crohn's disease and ulcerative colitis), with DHEA administration often leading to clinical improvement.[122,123]

As mentioned earlier, vitamin D deficiency is pandemic, which is particularly relevant to inflammation because it has been shown to modulate both the immune and inflammatory response. Determination of S-DHEA and 25-OH vitamin D levels may help to guide therapy with these hormones.

References

1. Nathan C. Points of control in inflammation. *Nature.* 2002 Dec;19-26;420(6917):846-52.
2. Medzhitov R. Origin and physiological roles of inflammation. *Nature.* 2008 Jul 24;454(7203):428-35.
3. Herold K, Moser B, Chen Y, et al. Receptor for advanced glycation end products (RAGE) in a dash to the rescue: inflammatory signals gone awry in the primal response to stress. *J Leukoc Biol.* 2007 Aug;82(2):204-12.
4. Yan SF, Ramasamy R, Schmidt AM. Mechanisms of disease: advanced glycation end-products and their receptor in inflammation and diabetes complications. *Nat Clin Pract Endocrinol Metab.* 2008 May;4(5):285-93.
5. Tikellis C, Thomas MC, Harcourt BE, et al. Cardiac inflammation associated with a Western diet is mediated via activation of RAGE by AGEs. *Am J Physiol Endocrinol Metab.* 2008 Aug;295(2):E323-30.
6. Barton GM. A calculated response: control of inflammation by the innate immune system. *J Clin Invest.* 2008 Feb;118(2):413-20.
7. Serhan CN. Resolution phase of inflammation: novel endogenous anti-inflammatory and proresolving lipid mediators and pathways. *Annu Rev Immunol.* 2007;25:101-37.
8. Yedgar S, Krimsky M, Cohen Y, et al. Treatment of inflammatory diseases by selective eicosanoid inhibition: a double-edged sword? *Trends Pharmacol Sci.* 2007 Sep;28(9):459-64.
9. Lukiw WJ, Cui JG, Marcheselli VL. A role for docosahexaenoic acid-derived neuroprotectin D1 in neural cell survival and Alzheimer disease. *J Clin Invest.* 2005 Oct;115(10):2774-83.
10. González-Périz A, Planagumà A, Gronert K, Docosahexaenoic acid (DHA) blunts liver injury by conversion to protective lipid mediators: protectin D1 and 17S-hydroxy-DHA. *FASEB J.* 2006 Dec;20(14):2537-9.
11. Levy BD, Kohli P, Gotlinger K, et al. Protectin D1 is generated in asthma and dampens airway inflammation and hyperresponsiveness. *J Immunol.* 2007 Jan 1;178(1):496-502.
12. Serhan CN, Yang R, Martinod K, et al. Maresins: novel macrophage mediators with potent anti-inflammatory and proresolving actions. *J Exp Med.* 2008 Dec 22. Epub ahead of print.
13. Kanda H, Tateya S, Tamori Y, et al. MCP-1 contributes to macrophage infiltration into adipose tissue, insulin resistance, and hepatic steatosis in obesity. *J Clin Invest.* 2006 Jun;116(6):1494-505.
14. Bensinger SJ, Tontonoz P. Integration of metabolism and inflammation by lipid-activated nuclear receptors. *Nature.* 2008 Jul 24;454(7203):470-7.
15. Anderson AL, Harris TB, Houston DK, et al. Relationships of dietary patterns with body composition in older adults differ by gender and PPAR-gamma Pro12Ala genotype. *Eur J Nutr.* 2010 Feb 21. Epub ahead of print.
16. Hotamisligil GS. Inflammation and metabolic disorders. *Nature.* 2006 Dec 14;444(7121):860-7.
17. Hotamisligil GS, Erbay E. Nutrient sensing and inflammation in metabolic diseases. *Nat Rev Immunol.* 2008 Dec;8(12):923-34.
18. Kaufman RJ. Stress signaling from the lumen of the endoplasmic reticulum: coordination of gene transcriptional and translational controls. *Genes Dev.* 1999 May 15;13(10):1211-33.
19. Zhang K, Kaufman RJ. From endoplasmic-reticulum stress to the inflammatory response. *Nature.* 2008 Jul 24;454(7203):455-62.
20. Ozcan U, Cao Q, Yilmaz E, et al. Endoplasmic reticulum stress links obesity, insulin action, and type 2 diabetes. *Science.* 2004 Oct 15;306(5695):457-61.
21. Levine T, Loewen C. Inter-organelle membrane contact sites: through a glass, darkly. *Curr Opin Cell Biol.* 2006 Aug;18(4):371-8.
22. Sanyal AJ, Campbell-Sargent C, Mirshahi F, et al. Nonalcoholic steatohepatitis: association of insulin resistance and mitochondrial abnormalities. *Gastroenterology.* 2001 Apr;120(5):1183-92.
23. Tilg H, Hotamisligil GS. Nonalcoholic fatty liver disease: Cytokine-adipokine interplay and regulation of insulin resistance. *Gastroenterology.* 2006 Sep;131(3):934-45.
24. Simopoulos AP. The importance of the omega-6/omega-3 fatty acid ratio in cardiovascular disease and other chronic diseases. *Exp Biol Med* (Maywood). 2008 Jun;233(6):674-88.
25. Schmitz G, Ecker J. The opposing effects of omega-3 and omega-6 fatty acids. *Prog Lipid Res.* 2008 Mar;47(2):147-55.
26. Levy BD, Clish CB, Schmidt B, et al. Lipid mediator class switching during acute inflammation: signals in resolution. *Nat Immunol.* 2001 Jul;2(7):612-9.
27. Pischon T, Hankinson SE, Hotamisligil GS, et al. Habitual dietary intake of omega-3 and omega-6 fatty acids in relation to inflammatory markers among US men and women. *Circulation.* 2003 Jul 15;108(2):155-60.
28. Lee JY, Hwang DH. Docosahexaenoic acid suppresses the activity of peroxisome proliferator-activated receptors in a colon tumor cell line. *Biochem Biophys Res Commun.* 2002 Nov 15;298(5):667-74.
29. Deckelbaum RJ, Worgall TS, Seo T. Omega-3 fatty acids and gene expression. *Am J Clin Nutr.* 2006 Jun;83 (6 Suppl):1520S-1525S.
30. Baylin A, Ruiz-Narvaez E, Kraft P, et al. Alpha-linolenic acid, Delta6-desaturase gene polymorphism, and the risk of nonfatal myocardial infarction. *Am J Clin Nutr.* 2007 Feb;85(2):554-60.
31. Kummerow FA, Zhou Q, Mahfouz MM, et al. Trans fatty acids in hydrogenated fat inhibited the synthesis of the polyunsaturated fatty acids in the phospholipid of arterial cells. *Life Sci.* 2004 Apr 16;74(22):2707-23.

32. Thiébaut AC, Chajès V, Gerber M, et al. Dietary intakes of omega-6 and omega-3 polyunsaturated fatty acids and the risk of breast cancer . *Int J Cancer.* 2008 Sep 9. Epub ahead of print.

33. Antalis CJ, Stevens LJ, Campbell M, et al. Omega-3 fatty acid status in attention-deficit/hyperactivity disorder. *Prostaglandins, Leukotrienes and Essential Fatty Acids* 2006;75:299-308.

34. Liu S, Manson JE, Buring JE, et al. Relation between a diet with a high glycemic load and plasma concentrations of high-sensitivity C-reactive protein in middle-aged women. *Am J Clin Nutr.* 2002 Mar;75(3):492-8.

35. Du H, van der A DL, van Bakel MM, et al. Glycemic index and glycemic load in relation to food and nutrient intake and metabolic risk factors in a Dutch population. *Am J Clin Nutr.* 2008 Mar;87(3):655-61.

36. Ma Y, Hébert JR, Li W, et al. Association between dietary fiber and markers of systemic inflammation in the Women's Health Initiative Observational Study. *Nutrition.* 2008 Oct;24(10):941-9.

37. Chrysohoou C, Panagiotakos DB, Pitsavos C, et al. Adherence to the Mediterranean diet attenuates inflammation and coagulation process in healthy adults: The ATTICA Study. *J Am Coll Cardiol.* 2004 Jul 7;44(1):152-8.

38. Esposito K, Pontillo A, Di Palo C. Effect of weight loss and lifestyle changes on vascular inflammatory markers in obese women: a randomized trial. *JAMA.* 2003 Apr 9; 289(14):1799-804.

39. Dai J, Miller AH, Bremner JD, et al. Adherence to the Mediterranean diet is inversely associated with circulating interleukin-6 among middle-aged men: a twin study. *Circulation.* 2008 Jan 15;117(2):169-75.

40. Devaraj S, Torok N, Dasu MR, et al. Adiponectin decreases C-reactive protein synthesis and secretion from endothelial cells: evidence for an adipose tissue-vascular loop. *Arterioscler Thromb Vasc Biol.* 2008 Jul;28(7):1368-74.

41. Hamer M, Stamatakis E. The accumulative effects of modifiable risk factors on inflammation and haemostasis. *Brain Behav Immun.* 2008 Oct;22(7):1041-3.

42. Hamer M, Stamatakis E. Inflammation as an intermediate pathway in the association between psychosocial stress and obesity. *Physiol Behav.* 2008 Jul 5;94(4):536-9.

43. Fontana L. Neuroendocrine factors in the regulation of inflammation: excessive adiposity and calorie restriction. *Exp Gerontol.* 2009 Jan-Feb;44(1-2):41-5.

44. Nanri A, Yoshida D, Yamaji T, et al. Dietary patterns and C-reactive protein in Japanese men and women. *Am J Clin Nutr.* 2008 May;87(5):1488-96.

45. Chun OK, Chung SJ, Claycombe KJ. Serum C-reactive protein concentrations are inversely associated with dietary flavonoid intake in U.S. adults. *J Nutr.* 2008 Apr;138(4):753-60.

46. Song Y, Li TY, van Dam RM. Magnesium intake and plasma concentrations of markers of systemic inflammation and endothelial dysfunction in women. *Am J Clin Nutr.* 2007 Apr;85(4):1068-74.

47. Detopoulou P, Panagiotakos DB, Antonopoulou S, et al. Dietary choline and betaine intakes in relation to concentrations of inflammatory markers in healthy adults: the ATTICA study. *Am J Clin Nutr.* 2008 Feb;87(2):424-30.

48. Bhattacharyya S, Gill R, Chen ML, et al. Toll-like receptor 4 mediates induction of the Bcl10-NFkappaB-interleukin-8 inflammatory pathway by carrageenan in human intestinal epithelial cells. *J Biol Chem.* 2008 Apr 18;283(16):10550-8.

49. Wilson BG, Bahna SL. Adverse reactions to food additives. *Ann Allergy Asthma Immunol.* 2005 Dec;95(6): 499-507.

50. Asero R. Food additives intolerance: does it present as perennial rhinitis? *Curr Opin Allergy Clin Immunol.* 2004 Feb;4(1):25-9.

51. Spergel JM, Fiedler J. Food allergy and additives: triggers in asthma. *Immunol Allergy Clin North Am.* 2005 Feb;25(1):149-67.

52. Handschin C, Spiegelman BM. The role of exercise and PGC1alpha in inflammation and chronic disease. *Nature.* 2008 Jul 24;454(7203):463-9.

53. Pedersen BK, Febbraio MA. Muscle as an endocrine organ: focus on muscle-derived interleukin-6. *Physiol Rev.* 2008 Oct;88(4):1379-406.

54. Nicklas BJ, Hsu FC, Brinkley TJ, et al. Exercise training and plasma C-reactive protein and interleukin-6 in elderly people. *J Am Geriatr Soc.* 2008 Nov;56(11):2045-52.

55. Schaap LA, Pluijm SM, Deeg DJ, et al. Inflammatory markers and loss of muscle mass (sarcopenia) and strength. *Am J Med.* 2006 Jun;119(6):526.e9-17.

56. Campbell KL, Campbell PT, Ulrich CM, et al. No reduction in C-reactive protein following a 12-month randomized controlled trial of exercise in men and women. *Cancer Epidemiol Biomarkers Prev.* 2008 Jul;17(7):1714-8.

57. Merrill RM, Massey MT, Aldana SG, et al. C-reactive protein levels according to physical activity and body weight for participants in the coronary health improvement project. *Prev Med.* 2008 May;46(5):425-30. Epub 2007 Dec 8.

58. Karin M, Lawrence T, Nizet V. Innate immunity gone awry: linking microbial infections to chronic inflammation and cancer. *Cell.* 2006 Feb 24;124(4):823-35.

59. Turner JR. Molecular basis of epithelial barrier regulation: from basic mechanisms to clinical application. *Am J Pathol.* 2006 Dec;169(6):1901-9.

60. Fasano A, Shea-Donohue T. Mechanisms of disease: the role of intestinal barrier function in the pathogenesis of gastrointestinal autoimmune diseases. *Nat Clin Pract Gastroenterol Hepatol.* 2005 Sep;2(9):416-22.

61. Isolauri E, Salminen S. Probiotics: use in allergic disorders: a Nutrition, Allergy, Mucosal Immunology, and

Intestinal Microbiota (NAMI) Research Group Report. *J Clin Gastroenterol.* 2008 Jul;42 Suppl 2:S91-6.

62. Holick MF. The vitamin D deficiency pandemic and consequences for nonskeletal health: Mechanisms of action. *Mol Aspects Med.* 2008 Dec;29(6):361-8.
63. Holick MF. Vitamin D deficiency. *N Engl J Med.* 2007 Jul 19;357(3):266-81.
64. Arnson Y, Amital H, Shoenfeld Y. Vitamin D and autoimmunity: new aetiological and therapeutic considerations. *Ann Rheum Dis.* 2007 Sep;66(9):1137-42.
65. Holick MF. Vitamin D: importance in the prevention of cancers, type 1 diabetes, heart disease, and osteoporosis. *Am J Clin Nutr.* 2004;79:362-71.
66. Huisman AM, White KP, Algra A, et al. Vitamin D levels in women with systemic lupus erythematosus and fibromyalgia. *J Rheumatol.* 2001;28:2535-9.
67. Goldberg P, Fleming MC, Picard EH, et al. Multiple sclerosis: decreased relapse rate through dietary supplementation with calcium, magnesium and vitamin D. *Med Hypotheses.* 1986;21:193-200.
68. Vgontzas AN, Papanicolaou DA, Bixler EO, et al. Circadian interleukin-6 secretion and quantity and depth of sleep. *J Clin Endocrinol Metab.* 1999 Aug;84(8):2603-7.
69. Meier-Ewert HK, Ridker PM, Regan MM, et al. Effect of sleep loss on C-reactive protein, an inflammatory marker of cardiovascular risk. *J Am Coll Cardiol.* 2004 Feb 18;43(4):678-83.
70. Simpson N, Dinges DF. Sleep and inflammation. *Nutr Rev.* 2007 Dec;65(12 Pt 2):S244-52.
71. Topol EJ. Failing the public health—rofecoxib, Merck, and the FDA. *NEJM* 2004;351:1707-9.
72. Topol EJ. Arthritis medicines and cardiovascular events-"house of coxibs." *JAMA* 2005;293:366-8.
73. Ray WA, Griffin MR, Stein CM, et al. Cardiovascular toxicity of valdecoxib. *NEJM* 2004;351:2767.
74. Aguirre R, May JM. Inflammation in the vascular bed: importance of vitamin C. *Pharmacol Ther.* 2008 Jul;119(1):96-103.
75. Devaraj S, Singh U, Jialal I. The Evolving Role of C-Reactive Protein in Atherothrombosis. *Clin Chem.* 2008 Dec 18. Epub ahead of print.
76. Cushman M, Arnold AM, Psaty BM, et al. C-reactive protein and the 10-year incidence of coronary heart disease in older men and women: the cardiovascular health study. *Circulation.* 2005 Jul 5;112(1):25-31.
77. Dayer E, Dayer JM, Roux-Lombard P. Primer: the practical use of biological markers of rheumatic and systemic inflammatory diseases. *Nat Clin Pract Rheumatol.* 2007 Sep;3(9):512-20.
78. Sun Q, Ma J, Campos H, et al. Blood concentrations of individual long-chain omega-3 fatty acids and risk of nonfatal myocardial infarction. *Am J Clin Nutr.* 2008 Jul;88(1):216-23.
79. Elkan AC, Sjöberg B, Kolsrud B, et al. Gluten-free vegan diet induces decreased LDL and oxidized LDL levels and raised atheroprotective natural antibodies against phosphorylcholine in patients with rheumatoid arthritis: a randomized study. *Arthritis Res Ther.* 2008;10(2):R34. Epub 2008 Mar 18.
80. Hafström I, Ringertz B, Spångberg A, et al. A vegan diet free of gluten improves the signs and symptoms of rheumatoid arthritis: the effects on arthritis correlate with a reduction in antibodies to food antigens. *Rheumatology* (Oxford). 2001 Oct;40(10):1175-9.
81. Adam O, Beringer C, Kless T, et al. Anti-inflammatory effects of a low arachidonic acid diet and fish oil in patients with rheumatoid arthritis. *Rheumatol Int.* 2003 Jan;23(1):27-36.
82. Kimata H. Listening to Mozart reduces allergic skin wheal responses and *in vitro* allergen-specific IgE production in atopic dermatitis patients with latex allergy. *Behav Med.* 2003;29:15-9.
83. Lutgendorf S, Logan H, Kirchner HL, et al. Effects of relaxation and stress on the capsaicin-induced local inflammatory response. *Psychosom Med.* 2000;62:524-34.
84. Sierra S, Lara-Villoslada F, Comalada M, et al. Dietary eicosapentaenoic acid and docosahexaenoic acid equally incorporate as docosahexaenoic acid but differ in inflammatory effects. *Nutrition.* 2008 Mar;24(3):245-54.
85. Russo GL. Dietary n-6 and n-3 polyunsaturated fatty acids: From biochemistry to clinical implications in cardiovascular prevention. *Biochem Pharmacol.* 2009 Mar 15;77(6):937-46. Epub 2008 Oct 28.
86. Mandal MN, Patlolla JM, Zheng L, et al. Curcumin protects retinal cells from light-and oxidant stress-induced cell death. *Free Radic Biol Med.* 2008 Dec 24. Epub ahead of print.
87. Lubbad A, Oriowo MA, Khan I. Curcumin attenuates inflammation through inhibition of TLR-4 receptor in experimental colitis. *Mol Cell Biochem.* 2008 Nov 11. Epub ahead of print.
88. Jurenka JS. Anti-inflammatory properties of curcumin, a major constituent of *Curcuma longa*: a review of preclinical and clinical research. *Altern Med Rev.* 2009 Jun;14(2):141-53.
89. Deodhar SD, Sethi R, Srimal RC. Preliminary studies on anti-rheumatic activity of curcumin (diferuloyl methane). *Ind J Med Res.* 1980;71:632-634.
90. Satoskar RR, Shah SJ, Shenoy SG. Evaluation of anti-inflammatory property of curcumin (diferuloyl methane) in patients with postoperative inflammation. *Int J Clin Pharmacol Ther Toxicol.* 1986;24:651-654.
91. Kaileh M, Vanden Berghe W, Heyerick A, et al. Withaferin a strongly elicits IkappaB kinase beta hyperphosphorylation concomitant with potent inhibition of its kinase activity. *J Biol Chem.* 2007 Feb 16;282(7):4253-64.

92. Ichikawa H, Takada Y, Shishodia S, et al. Withanolides potentiate apoptosis, inhibit invasion, and abolish osteoclastogenesis through suppression of nuclear factor-kappaB (NF-kappaB) activation and NF-kappaB-regulated gene expression. *Mol Cancer Ther.* 2006 Jun;5(6):1434-45.

93. Bodet C, Chandad F, Grenier D. Cranberry components inhibit interleukin-6, interleukin-8, and prostaglandin E production by lipopolysaccharide-activated gingival fibroblasts. *Eur J Oral Sci.* 2007 Feb;115(1):64-70.

94. Sankaranarayanan A, Narender T, Kumar S, et al. *Allium sativum* constituents: effect on free radical generation from rat neutrophils. *Cell Mol Biol.* (Noisy-le-grand). 2007 May 30;53(5):63-7.

95. Hofbauer R, Frass M, Gmeiner B, et al. Effects of garlic extract (*Allium sativum*) on neutrophil migration at the cellular level. *Heart Dis.* 2001 Jan-Feb;3(1):14-7.

96. Dorsch W, Ring J: Suppression of immediate and late anti-IgE-induced skin reactions by topically applied alcohol/onion extract. *Allergy.* 1984;39:43-9.

97. Dorsch W, Schneider E, Bayer T, et al. Anti-inflammatory effects of onions: Inhibition of chemotaxis of human PMNs by thiosulfinates and cepanes. *Int Arch Allergy Apply Immunol.* 1990;92:39-42.

98. Norwell DY, Tarr RS. Garlic, vampires and CHD. *Osteopathy Ann.* 1983;11:546-9.

99. Kimmatkar N, Thawani V, Hingorani L, et al. Efficacy and tolerability of *Boswellia serrata* extract in treatment of osteoarthritis of knee—a randomized double blind placebo controlled trial. *Phytomedicine.* 2003;10:3-7.

100. Ammon HP. Boswellic acids (components of frankincense) as the active principle in treatment of chronic inflammatory diseases (German) *Wien Med Wochenschr.* 2002;152:373-8.

101. Takada Y, Ichikawa H, Badmaev V, et al. Acetyl-11-keto-beta-boswellic acid potentiates apoptosis, inhibits invasion, and abolishes osteoclastogenesis by suppressing NF-kappa B and NF-kappa B-regulated gene expression. *J Immunol.* 2006 Mar 1;176(5):3127-40.

102. Sengupta K, Alluri KV, Satish AR, et al. A double blind, randomized, placebo controlled study of the efficacy and safety of 5-Loxin for treatment of osteoarthritis of the knee. *Arthritis Res Ther.* 2008;10(4):R85.

103. Asboe-Hansen G. Treatment of generalized scleroderma with inhibitors of collagen synthesis. *Int J Dermatol.* 1982;21:159-161.

104. Krahwinkel T, Willershausen B. The effect of sugar-free green tea chew candies on the degree of inflammation of the gingiva. *Eur J Med Res.* 2000;5:463-467.

105. Kim HJ, Park SH, Park SY, et al. Epigallocatechin-3-gallate inhibits interleukin-1beta-induced MUC5AC gene expression and MUC5AC secretion in normal human nasal epithelial cells. *J Nutr Biochem.* 2008.

106. Koltai M, Hosford D, Guinot P, et al. Platelet activating factor (PAF). A review of its effects, antagonists and possible future clinical implications (Part I). *Drugs.* 1991;42:9-29.

107. Zhou YH, Yu JP, Liu YF, et al. Effects of *Ginkgo biloba* extract on inflammatory mediators (SOD, MDA, TNF-alpha, NF-kappaBp65, IL-6) in TNBS-induced colitis in rats. *Mediators Inflamm.* 2006;2006(5):92642.

108. Chandler RF. Licorice, more than just a flavour. *Can Pharm J.* 1985;118:421-424.

109. Yoshida T, Abe K, Ikeda T, et al. Inhibitory effect of glycyrrhizin on lipopolysaccharide and d-galactosamine-induced mouse liver injury. *Eur J Pharmacol.* 2007;576:136-42.

110. Okimasa E, Moromizato Y, Watanabe S, et al. Inhibition of phospholipase A2 by glycyrrhizin, an anti-inflammatory drug. *Acta Med Okayama.* 1983;37:385-391.

111. Chrubasik S, Künzel O, Model A, et al. Treatment of low-back pain with a herbal or synthetic anti-rheumatic: a randomized controlled study. Willow bark extract for low-back pain. *Rheumatology.* (Oxford). 2001;40:1388-93.

112. Chrubasik S, Pollak S, Black A. Willow bark extract, a useful alternative for the treatment of osteoarthritis. *Arthritis Rheum.* 2003;48:278-80.

113. Piscoya J, Rodriguez Z, Bustamante SA, et al. Efficacy and safety of freeze-dried cat's claw in osteoarthritis of the knee: mechanisms of action of the species *Uncaria guianensis. Inflamm Res.* 2001;50:442-8.

114. Mur E, Hartig F, Eibl G, et al. Randomized double blind trial of an extract from the pentacyclic alkaloid-chemotype of *Uncaria tomentosa* for the treatment of rheumatoid arthritis. *J Rheumatol.* 2002;29:678-81.

115. Nurtjahja-Tjendraputra E, Ammit AJ, Roufogalis BD, et al. Effective anti-platelet and COX-1 enzyme inhibitors from pungent constituents of ginger. *Thromb Res.* 2003;111:259-265.

116. Tripathi S, Bruch D, Kittur DS. Ginger extract inhibits LPS induced macrophage activation and function. *BMC Comp Alt Med.* 2008;8:1.

117. Tjendraputra E, Tran VH, Liu-Brennan D, et al. Effect of ginger constituents and synthetic analogues on cyclooxygenase-2 enzyme in intact cells. *Bioorg Chem.* 2001;29:156-163.

118. Csaki C, Mobasheri A, Shakibaei M. Synergistic chondroprotective effects of curcumin and resveratrol in human articular chondrocytes: inhibition of IL-1beta-induced NF-kappaB-mediated inflammation and apoptosis. *Arthritis Res Ther.* 2009;11(6):R165. Epub 2009 Nov 4.

119. Koeberle A, Northoff H, Werz O. Curcumin blocks prostaglandin E2 biosynthesis through direct inhibition of the microsomal prostaglandin E2 synthase-1. *Mol Cancer Ther.* 2009 Aug;8(8):2348-55. Epub 2009 Aug 11.

120. Straub RH, Konecna L, Hrach S, et al. Serum dehydroepiandrosterone (DHEA) and DHEA sulfate are negatively correlated with serum interleukin-6 (IL-6), and DHEA inhibits IL-6 secretion from mononuclear cells in

man *in vitro*: possible link between endocrinosenescence and immunosenescence. *J Clin Endocrinol Metab.* 1998; 83:2012-7.

121. Brignardello E, Runzo C, Aragno M. Dehydroepiandrosterone administration counteracts oxidative imbalance and advanced glycation end product formation in type 2 diabetic patients. *Diabetes Care.* 2007 Nov;30(11):2922-7.

122. de la Torre B, Hedman M, Befrits R. Blood and tissue dehydroepiandrosterone sulphate levels and their relationship to chronic inflammatory bowel disease. *Clin Exp Rheumatol.* 1998;16:579-82.

123. Andus T, Klebl F, Rogler G, et al. Patients with refractory Crohn's disease or ulcerative colitis respond to dehydroepiandrosterone: a pilot study. *Aliment Pharmacol Ther.* 2003;17:409-14.

Stress, Anxiety, Depression, and Insomnia

Overview

Stress is defined in many ways, most commonly as any type of real or perceived disturbance, physical or emotional, which alters homeostasis and leads to a stress response that is mediated by both the central nervous system and peripheral organs. Although the homeostatic response to an acute stressor can be lifesaving, persistent and uncontrollable stress is pathogenic, mediated in part by the stress response itself, via the hypothalamic-pituitary-adrenocortical (HPA) axis. Stress and the stress response are known to contribute to both psychosocial and physiological pathology. Many conditions are affected by and/or associated with chronic stress—e.g., age-related cognitive decline, neurodegenerative diseases, cardiovascular disorders, diabetes, and abdominal obesity. Those discussed in this chapter include depression, anxiety, and insomnia. Fortunately, a number of lifestyle, nutritional, and botanical interventions help to minimize the impact of stress, and restore healthy endocrine and neurological function.

HPA Axis and the General Theory of Adaptation

The stress response was originally described by Hans Selye[1,2] as the "general adaptation syndrome"; today, the physiology is more clearly detailed. Real or perceived stress involves a large number of neuronal circuits, including the prefrontal cortex, hippocampus, amygdala, septum, and hypothalamus, resulting in an activation of the hypothalamic-pituitary-adrenocortical (HPA) axis via production of corticotrophin-releasing hormone (CRH) and arginine vasopressin (AVP) in the hypothalamus. From there, both neuropeptides reach the pituitary gland through small blood vessels (CRH) or neural projections (AVP), resulting in secretion and release of corticotrophin (adrenocorticotrophic hormone, ACTH) into the circulation, which in turn stimulates the cortex of the adrenal glands to synthesize and release glucocorticoids, in particular cortisol.[3] (Figure 6.1)

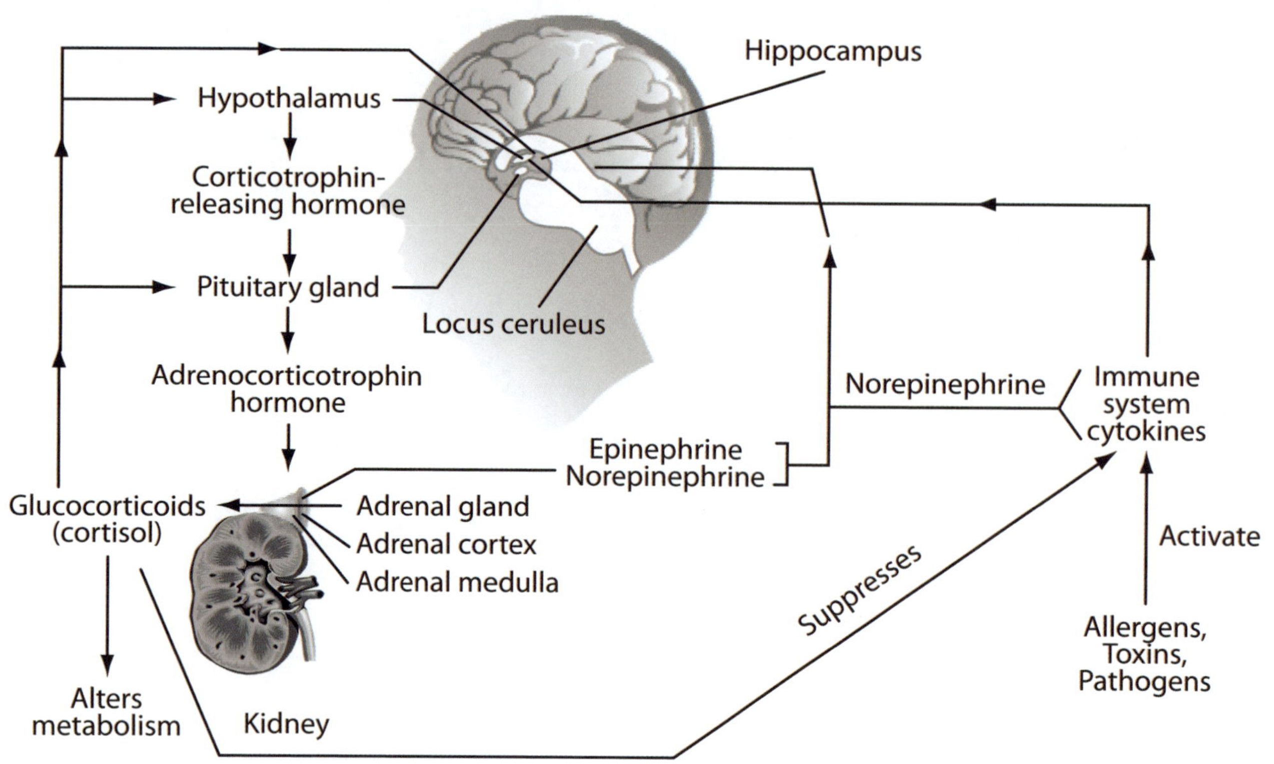

Figure 6.1 Interaction between the nervous and immune systems. © 2005 The Institute for Functional Medicine. Used with permission granted by The Institute for Functional Medicine, www.functionalmedicine.org. No part of this content may be reproduced or transmitted in any form or by any means without the express written consent of The Institute for Functional Medicine, except as permitted by applicable law.

The sympathetic nervous system is also activated, because CRH- and AVP-containing fibers are intertwined with monoaminergic fibers. This enhanced production of the catecholamines epinephrine and norepinephrine leads to the immediate "fight-or-flight" stage Selye referred to. He also characterized the subsequent "resistance" phase, primarily mediated by corticosteroids, which adapts to stress-induced demands—for example, to provide increased glucose and to maintain electrolyte balance, mainly achieved by the mineralocorticosteroid aldosterone, which is also released from the adrenal cortex. This is followed by the final phase, which he termed exhaustion, and today may be termed cacostasis, defined as suboptimal adaptation or dyshomeostasis.[4] It is this last phase that is considered pathological; for example, as a reaction to acute stress, hypercortisolemia may actually improve memory consolidation, offering significant benefit. However, prolonged elevation of cortisol is known to cause memory impairment through detrimental influences on hippocampal functions.[5] Today we understand that the damage done is largely due to chronic hormonal effects and disturbances in the HPA axis, which are influenced not only by real or perceived stress, but also by past experiences, nutritional status, and genetic influences.

HPA Dysregulation

The stress system has a basal circadian activity and also responds to stressors on demand. Continuous activity, however, and prolonged secretion of CRH, norepinephrine, cortisol, and other hormones can produce anxiety, anorexia or hyperphagia, and depression. For example, up to 20% of patients on high doses of glucocorticoids develop psychiatric disorders such as depression, mania, psychosis, or a mixed affective state; up to 75% report psychiatric symptoms that can be reversed with cessation of glucocorticoid therapy.[6] These mediators also suppress the sleep system, which causes insomnia, loss of sleep, and daytime somnolence.[4]

HPA axis dysfunction reported in patients with depression is thought to be related, at least in part, to impaired feedback inhibition by endogenous glucocorticoids. This has been attributed to glucocorticoid resistance and/or to hypersecretion of hypothalamic CRH. In a healthy system, cortisol binding to glucocorticoid receptors helps to bring the HPA axis back to baseline by providing negative feedback, not only for ACTH synthesis and release, but also for many other activities of the central nervous system, including production of CRH and AVP. Over a period of prolonged stress, some of this negative feedback is diminished, and AVP levels increase despite a decline in CRH levels. This has the net effect of increasing cortisol levels (frequency of corticosterone pulses in animals nearly doubles) while flattening or losing circadian rhythm entirely.[7]

Other Mediators of Stress

Although most chronic stress physiology is related to glucocorticoid action, a number of other mediators are also involved. For example, excitatory amino acids such as glutamate are thought to play a key role in the remodeling of the hippocampus seen after chronic stress.[8] Stress also is related to systemic inflammation. In an analysis of nearly 7000 individuals from the NHANES study, a strong association between stress and CRP levels was found, particularly among men. A history of major depression was associated with an odds ratio of 1.64 for an elevated CRP level, after adjusting for a number of other variables.[9]

An association between depression and the peptide brain-derived neurotrophic factor (BDNF) has also been recently established. Some authors have postulated that perturbations in cerebral endothelium (such as the loss of the neuroprotection afforded by BDNF) mediate neuronal dysfunction. BDNF levels have also been reported to be reduced in patients with depression, and antidepressants upregulate BDNF levels. Additionally, depression has been associated with elevated levels of coagulation factors, such as fibrinogen. Recently, BDNF was shown to increase cerebral artery levels of prostacyclin, one mechanism by which it may offer benefit.[10]

Consequences

Stress impacts nearly every system in the body, and altered HPA function contributes to a wide variety of conditions (Table 6.1). Stress inhibits the growth, reproductive, and thyroid axes, and the GI system via the vagus nerve. Thus, in adults, stress-induced hypogonadism can manifest as loss of libido and/or hypofertility, and hyperactivity of the sympathetic system can lead to essential hypertension.

Table 6.1 Conditions with altered HPA axis activity

Conditions
Increased activity of the HPA axis
• Cushing syndrome
• Chronic stress
• Melancholic depression
• Anorexia nervosa
• Obsessive–compulsive disorder
• Panic disorder
• Excessive exercise (obligate athleticism)
• Chronic, active alcoholism
• Alcohol and narcotic withdrawal
• Diabetes mellitus
• Central obesity (metabolic syndrome)
• Post-traumatic stress disorder in children
• Hyperthyroidism
• Pregnancy
Decreased activity of HPA axis
• Adrenal insufficiency
• Atypical/seasonal depression
• Chronic fatigue syndrome
• Fibromyalgia
• Premenstrual tension syndrome
• Climacteric depression
• Nicotine withdrawal
• Following cessation of glucocorticoid therapy
• Following Cushing syndrome cure
• Following chronic stress
• Post-partum period
• Adult post-traumatic stress disorder
• Hypothyroidism
• Rheumatoid arthritis
• Asthma, eczema

Abbreviation: HPA, hypothalamic–pituitary–adrenal.

Stress and disorders of the stress system. From: Chrousos GP. *Nat Rev Endocrinol.* 2009 Jul;5(7):374-81. Epub 2009 Jun 2. Reproduced with permission from Macmillan Publishers Ltd.

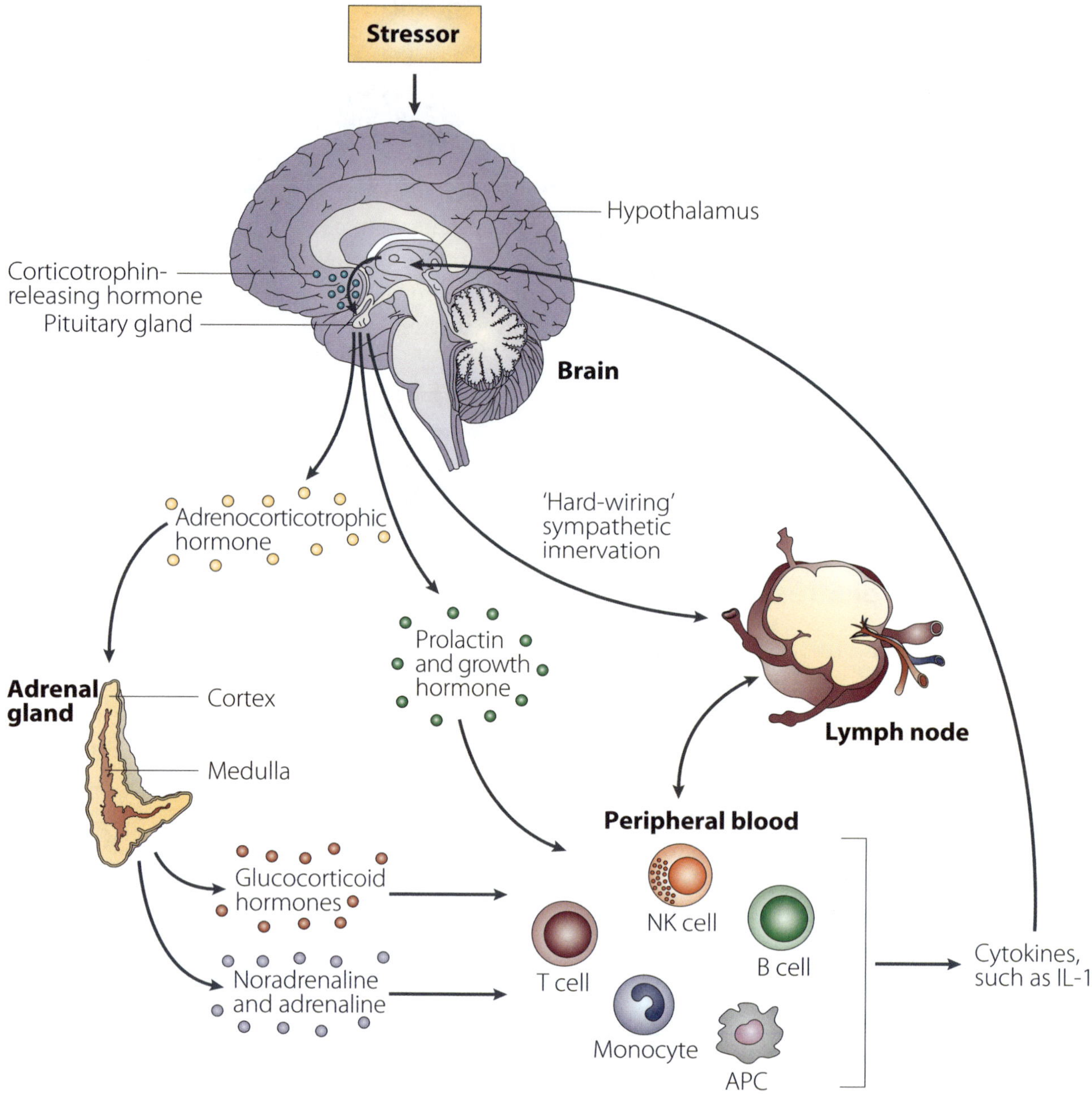

Figure 6.2 Stress associated modulation of the hormone response by the central nervous system. From: Glaser R. Stress-induced immune dysfunction: implications for health. *Nat Rev Immunol.* 2005 Mar;5(3):243-51. Reproduced with permission from Macmillan Publishers Ltd.

The immune system is also affected by chronic stress, with a switch from TH1 to TH2 increasing the vulnerability to certain infections, such as *Helicobacter pylori*, and autoimmune disorders such as Graves' disease and systemic lupus erythematosus.[11,12] Additionally, mast cell degranulation is also brought on by CRH; thus, chronic stress may increase the risk of allergy and asthma, as well as migraine headaches (via histamine release in meningeal blood vessels that causes local vasodilation and increased permeability of the blood-brain barrier). Figure 6.2 depicts some of the mechanisms by which stress modulates hormonal influences on immune function. Stress has also been found to reduce NK cell activity, lower total lymphocyte count, decrease antibody production, and to modulate cytokine production.[13]

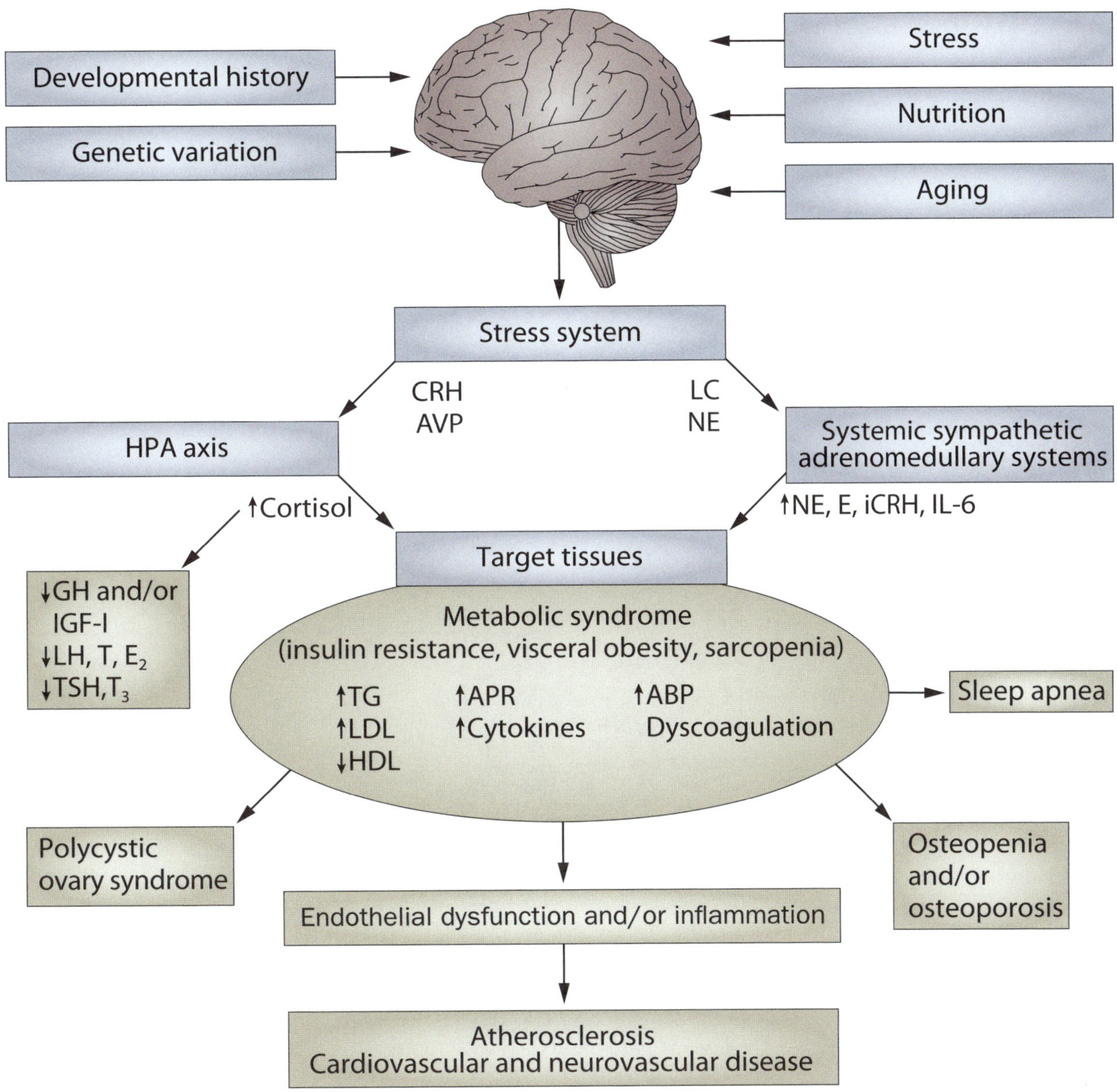

Figure 6.3 Chronic stress can contribute to the metabolic syndrome. From: Chrousos GP. Stress and disorders of the stress system. *Nat Rev Endocrinol.* 2009 Jul;5(7):374-81. Epub 2009 Jun 2. Reproduced with permission from Macmillan Publishers Ltd.

Stress also appears to be a major contributor to cardiovascular disease and diabetes, with a bidirectional association.[14] For example, severity of heart disease is a significant predictor of depression, while depressed mood, anhedonia, and feelings of hopelessness are recognized risk factors for heart disease-related morbidity and mortality.[15,16] Compared to a prevalence of approximately 2–3% (men) and 5–9% (women) of depression in the general population, its prevalence in patients following a myocardial infarction may be as high as 45%; approximately 20–50% of patients who die from myocardial infarction may have experienced an episode of depression prior to the infarction.[14]

Stress and Diabetes/Metabolic Syndrome

Stress also plays a role in the metabolic syndrome (Figure 6.3). Prolonged activation of the HPA axis (chronic hypercortisolism) has been shown to contribute to visceral fat accumulation, and insulin hypersecretion. In a recent study of women in the Mediterranean area, a pathological HPA axis response was associated with greater abdominal fat distribution and with a higher dietary saturated and total fat intake. They measured both morning and evening cortisol levels, as well as cortisol secretion following a dexamethasone suppression test. Pathological HPA response was characterized by a lack of effective suppression by dexamethasone, as well as a flattened cortisol diurnal curve (i.e., lacking the normal high in the morning and low in the evening).[17]

Type 2 diabetes is associated with reduced hippocampal volume as well as poor glucose control.[18] Hyperglycemia may directly contribute to the reduction in hippocampal volume, which in turn leads to HPA axis hyperactivation and cognitive impairment.[19] Interestingly, in an animal study, supplementation with omega-3 fatty acids was shown to increase hippocampal volume and BDNF production, as well as having antidepressant-like effects.[20]

In the British Whitehall II study, over 4000 adults were screened for depression and were given oral glucose tolerance tests. A U-shaped association between fasting glucose and CES-D (scale for depression symptoms) was reported, with elevated depression scores seen at both ends of the glucose distribution and hemoglobin A1c levels, suggesting that normoglycemic individuals have the lowest depression risk (Figure 6.4).[21]

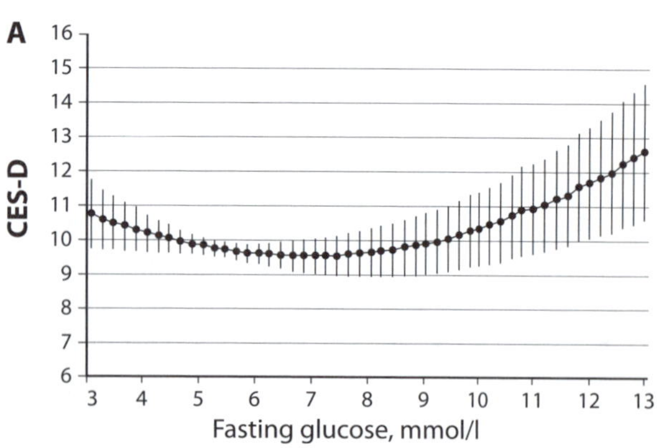

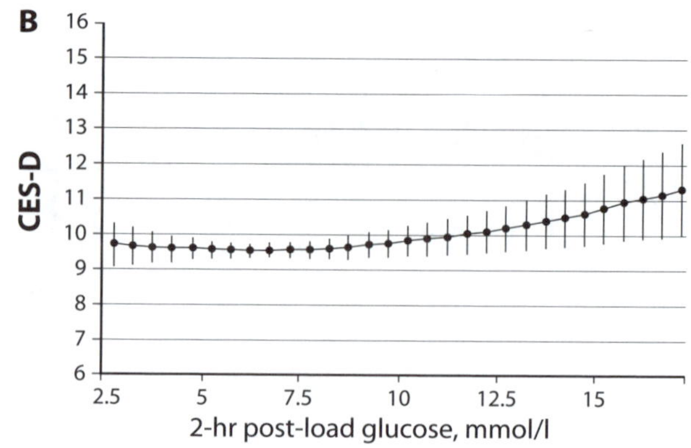

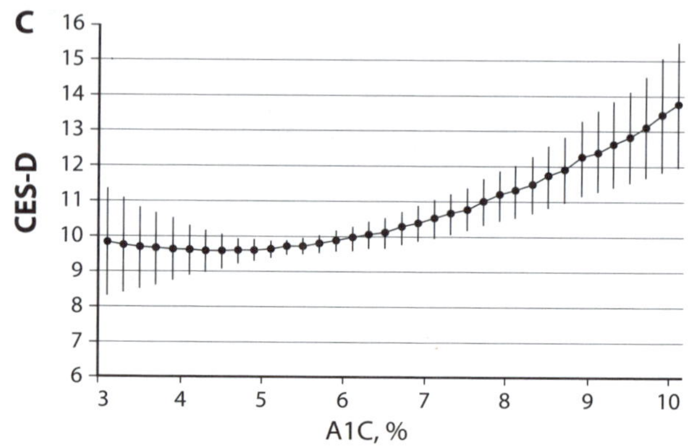

Figure 6.4 Association of glucose control and HbA1c with CES-D (Center for Epidemiologic Studies Depression scale). From: Kivimaki M, Tabak AG, Batty GD, et al. Hyperglycemia, type 2 diabetes, and depressive symptoms: the British Whitehall II study. *Diabetes Care.* 2009 Oct;32(10):1867-9. © 2009 American Diabetes Association. Reproduced with permission from the American Diabetes Association.

Genetic Predisposition and Early Life Experiences

Genetic factors and early life experiences are of great importance in determining the impact of stress. A growing body of evidence suggests that resilience to the effects of stress is influenced by both elements. Several gene candidates have been studied which partly explain this. For example, normally, activation of the glucocorticoid and mineralocorticoid receptors (GR and MR) by cortisol should be an effective negative feedback mechanism, with each receptor having a complementary role in stopping activation of the HPA axis. For this same reason, dysfunctional alterations in GR and/or MR genes are associated with a greater susceptibility to stress and risk for stress-related conditions, such as depression. In a recent study comparing nearly 500 control subjects with almost as many depressive patients, researchers found that two polymorphisms in the GR gene (BclI and ER22/23EK) were associated with susceptibility to developing major depression, with the ER22/23EK polymorphism also associated with a faster clinical response to antidepressant treatment.[22] The BDNF gene also appears to be important. Researchers recently found that those with the BDNF Val66Met polymorphism had not only a smaller hippocampus, but a smaller parahippocampal gyrus and amygdala, structural changes associated with several disorders, including schizophrenia and depression.[23]

Family and twin studies have demonstrated the importance of genetic factors in vulnerability to major depressive disorder (MDD). Being a first-degree family member of an MDD patient increases the risk of developing the disorder by a factor of almost three. And in a large meta-analysis of available twin study data, it was observed that about 40% of the risk of developing major depression is accounted for by additive genetic factors. The authors also reported that there do not appear to be genetic factors that uniquely increase the risk of depression, but rather that clusters of genes increase the risk of depression and anxiety disorders.[24,25,26]

Interactions between genetic predisposition and life experiences have also been documented. In a study of 100 healthy men, the combined effects of a past history of severe stressful life events (SLEs) and the genotype for the serotonin transporter polymorphism (5-HTTLPR) on cortisol levels before and after a stressful event (public speaking) were examined. In subjects homozygous for the s-allele of this gene, and with a previous history of stressful life events, the cortisol peak after public speaking was significantly higher than for all other groups, despite a similar baseline cortisol (Figure 6.5).[27] This suggests hyperreactivity of the HPA axis in response to stressful events, possibly accounting for the higher incidence of depression, early alcohol use, alcohol consumption, drug use, and violent behavior in those who carry an s-allele and also have a history of stressful experiences.

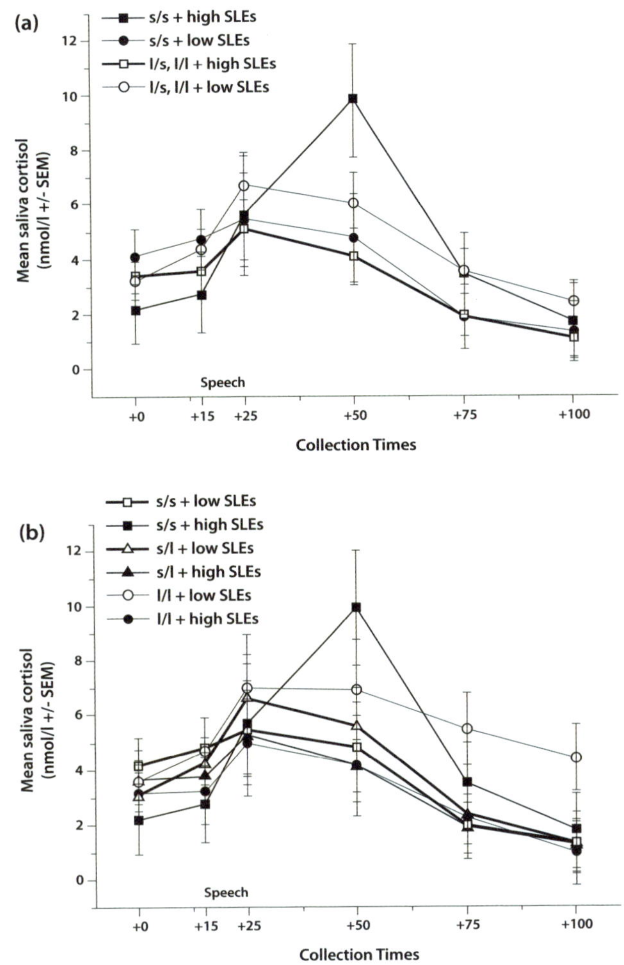

Figure 6.5 Salivary cortisol response to public speaking as a function of 5-HTTLPR genotype and stressful life events. From: Alexander N, Kuepper Y. Gene-environment interactions predict cortisol responses after acute stress: implications for the etiology of depression. *Psychoneuroendocrinology.* 2009; 34(9):1294-303. Reproduced with permission from Elsevier.

In addition to genetic factors, epigenetics and early life experiences are also emerging as important factors in HPA axis regulation. For example, in animal studies, maternal behavior toward offspring induces long-term changes in gene expression (including the GR gene) that are associated with alterations in histone acetylation, DNA methylation, and NGFI-A transcription factor binding. These changes may be reversed in adult rats through dietary changes, as well as by administration of L-methionine, suggesting that the methyl donor content in an adult's diet may modify epigenetically influenced gene expression.[28]

Depression and Anxiety

Depression and anxiety are remarkably common. In a survey of nearly 10,000 U.S. residents aged 18 and older, the lifetime prevalence of major depressive disorder (the odds of ever having depression during a lifetime) was found to be 16.2%, with a 12-month prevalence of 6.6%.[29] Data from the same survey found the 12-month prevalence of an anxiety disorder to be 18.1%.[30] Depression and anxiety have such a high degree of comorbidity that some researchers advocate that they be grouped together as "distress" that varies along a continuum from less severe to more severe, rather than discrete, categorical disorders.[31,32] In the above survey, the lifetime comorbidity rate of major depressive disorder with other DSM-IV disorders was over 70%, with nearly 60% for comorbid anxiety.[29] Surprisingly, the authors found that "no more than 21.6% of all respondents with 12-month MDD received adequate treatment in the year of the interview."

Recent data also suggest that the overlap between depression and anxiety is quite significant, including the genetic risk for each. For example, in a study of over 37,000 twins (the Swedish Twin Registry), they found a very high genetic correlation between major depression and generalized anxiety disorder, particularly among women.[33] However, environmental risk factors for the two disorders were less strongly correlated, leading the authors to suggest that environmental risk factors may influence how the underlying psychopathology is manifested.

In addition to HPA dysregulation, genetic influences, and early life experiences, a number of other factors are known to contribute to both depression and anxiety, among them nutritional and environmental factors. For example, using NHANES data for adults aged 20–39, high blood lead levels were found to significantly increase the risk of depression and panic disorder.[34] Researchers found that individuals with blood lead levels in the highest quintile had 2.3 times the odds of major depressive disorder and 4.9 times the odds of panic disorder as those in the lowest quintile. Mercury exposure also appears to increase the risks, although the data are influenced by genetic predisposition. In several published papers by the *Battelle Centers for Public Health Research and Evaluation* in Seattle, WA, many symptoms, including anxiety and depression (as well as memory loss, confusion, etc.), were associated with mercury exposure, even at very low levels, and particularly among dental assistants (women) vs. dentists (men). These associations also seemed to be generally influenced by genotype, including polymorphisms for the BDNF, catechol-O-methyltransferase (COMT), coproporphyrinogen oxidase (CPOX4), and the serotonin transporter (5-HTTLPR) genes.[35,36,37] Lifestyle and nutritional factors also contribute to anxiety and depression. In an analysis of over 10,000 initially healthy participants from the Spanish SUN study, adherence to a Mediterranean diet was found to be inversely associated with risk of depression, with adjusted hazard ratios of (for the four upper successive categories of adherence) 0.74, 0.66, 0.49, and 0.58.[39] As discussed earlier, depression is associated with endothelial dysfunction and reduced BDNF levels. It is suggested that one of the potential mechanisms by which adherence to a Mediterranean diet lowers depression risk is by improving BDNF production through restoration of endothelial function. Additionally, a Mediterranean diet may assist in maintaining a healthy weight, itself associated with decreased risk. Using NHANES data, a relationship was found between body weight and risk of depression and anxiety, with obesity conferring an approximately 25% increase in odds of mood and anxiety disorders.[40]

Intake of omega-3 fatty acids is also closely linked to affective disorders. Data from the Coronary Artery Risk Development in Young Adults study found that intake of EPA, DHA, and fish oil was associated with the risk of depression, particularly in women. "For the total number of occasions with depressive symptoms, the multivariable adjusted odds ratios (95% confidence level) in women were 0.75 for fish intake, 0.66 for EPA, 0.66 for DHA, and 0.71 for EPA + DHA when comparing the highest with the lowest quintiles."[41] This association is certainly seen in pregnant women.[42]

A number of mechanisms may explain the relationship between omega-3 fatty acids and depression risk. The content of omega-3s is known to affect membrane fluidity and the functioning of enzymes, ion channels, and receptor binding affinity and expression; omega-3 levels have been found to be low in RBC membranes of depressed patients.[43] Omega-3s also affect neuroplasticity and cell survival through their impact on neurotrophins such as BDNF, levels of which are known to be associated with depression risk. Omega-3 fatty acids affect gene expression and the production of pro-inflammatory cytokines such as interleukin-1beta and tumor necrosis factor-alpha, which have been shown to be elevated in depressed patients and inhibited by some antidepressant medications.[44]

Vitamin D levels are associated with risk of depression. In a trial of over 400 overweight men and women, serum levels of 25(OH)D were associated with scores on the Beck Depression Inventory. Additionally, supplementation of either 20,000 or 40,000 IU per week was associated with improved scores compared to placebo.[45] Additionally, in a small study of patients with fibromyalgia, a vitamin D deficiency was not only common, but was also more commonly associated with both depression and anxiety.[46]

A number of other nutrients have been linked to risk of depression and/or anxiety, particularly B vitamins. For example, low folate levels have been found in many studies of depressive patients, possibly because it is necessary for production of the methyl donor S-adenosyl methionine (SAM). In a trial of nearly 3000 participants, low RBC and/or serum folate was found in patients who met the criteria for major depression.[47] Polymorphisms in the MTHFR gene, which is involved in folate metabolism, have been reported to influence depression risk in some, but not all, studies.[48,49] Similarly, low levels of B6 and B12 have also been associated with greater risk.[50,51]

Insomnia

Insomnia is the most common sleep disorder, with a prevalence that varies considerably based on the definition used. While one-fourth to one-half of the general population reports difficulty falling and/or staying asleep, about 10% present chronic complaints and seek medical help for insomnia.[52,53] Insomnia is an underappreciated problem, as only ~40% of patients suffering insomnia seek help. The most often used definition is the DSM-IV, which defines insomnia as a complaint of difficulty initiating or maintaining sleep, early awakening, and interrupted or non-restorative sleep; nighttime symptoms are accompanied by clinically significant impairment in daytime function, for which no identifiable cause is found. Other known causes are medical disorders, such as chronic pain, cardiovascular disease, thyroid dysfunction, and a number of medications.

A number of factors contribute to insomnia, including emotional/personality factors. "Insomniacs, compared to controls, tend to be more discontent, both as children and as adults, have less satisfying interpersonal relations, and relatively poor self concepts, leading to inadequate coping mechanisms for dealing with stress."[52] Models such as the "internalization hypothesis" model describes a vicious cycle in which the poor coping with stress and the internalization of emotions leads to hyperarousal at night, preventing both sleep initiation and a return to sleep. This is compounded and intensified by a "fear of sleeplessness," which exacerbates the hyperarousal. Certainly depression, anxiety, inhibition of emotions, and an inability to express anger are more common in insomniacs. In many cases, it may be difficult to ascertain if depression/anxiety is causing insomnia, or vice versa.

Insomnia: Hyperarousal and inflammation

Similarly to depression and anxiety, stress is often a significant contributor to insomnia. Stress has been associated with activation of the HPA axis, while CRH and cortisol are known to cause arousal and sleeplessness; sleep and particularly deep sleep have an inhibitory effect on the stress system, including its two major components, the HPA axis and the sympathetic system. Indeed, more recent data suggest that insomnia is only one manifestation of a 24-hour hyperarousal, which includes activation

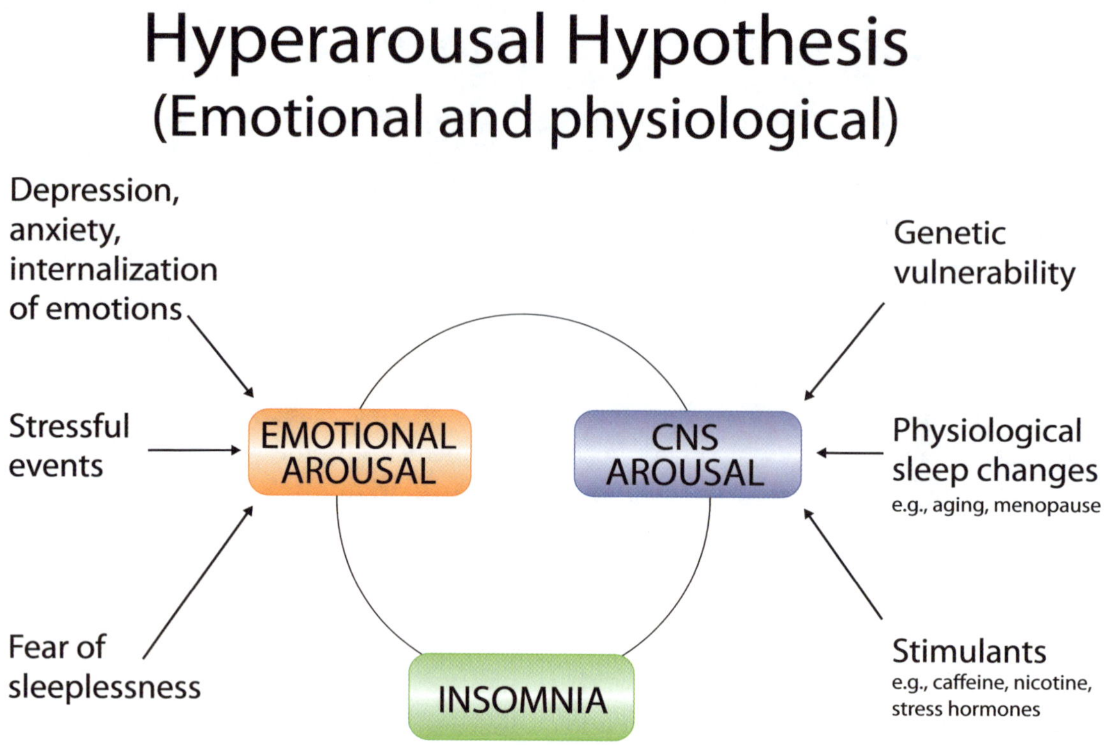

Figure 6.6 Hyperarousal model of insomnia. From: Basta M, Chrousos GP, Vela-Bueno A, et al. Chronic insomnia and stress system. *Sleep Med Clin.* 2007 Jun;2(2):279-291. Reproduced with kind permission from Dr. Alexandros N Vgontzas.

of the sympathetic nervous system as well as the HPA axis.[54,55] In a trial comparing insomniacs with healthy adults, the authors found an overall increase of ACTH and cortisol secretion in insomniacs who sustained a normal circadian pattern, a finding consistent with a disorder of central nervous system hyperarousal rather than one of sleep loss.[56] Current understanding points to HPA activation as at least partly causal for insomnia (Figure 6.6), as compared to the HPA activation found in obstructive sleep apnea which is considered to be a consequence rather than a cause of that condition.[57]

In addition to hyperactivity of the HPA axis, insomnia has also been associated with an increase in inflammatory markers, particularly IL-6. Although the overall amount secreted within a 24-hour period appears to be unchanged, sleep-deprived subjects had daytime oversecretion and nighttime undersecretion of IL-6, with the former potentially responsible for daytime somnolence and fatigue, the latter for the better quality (depth) of sleep.[58] Interestingly, daytime napping following a night of sleep loss has been shown to reverse the effects on IL-6.[59]

Insomnia and insulin resistance

Another consequence of poor sleep is an increase in insulin resistance. Sleep deprivation increases sympathetic nervous activity, evening cortisol, and daytime growth hormone levels, all of which may increase insulin resistance and impair glucose tolerance. Additionally, the reduced leptin and increased ghrelin levels found with sleep loss correlate with increases in subjective hunger and may have an additive effect to increase the risk of metabolic disease, diabetes, and obesity (Figure 6.7).[60]

Assessment

Evaluating depression, anxiety, and insomnia requires a multidimensional approach that encompasses a medical history, physical exam,

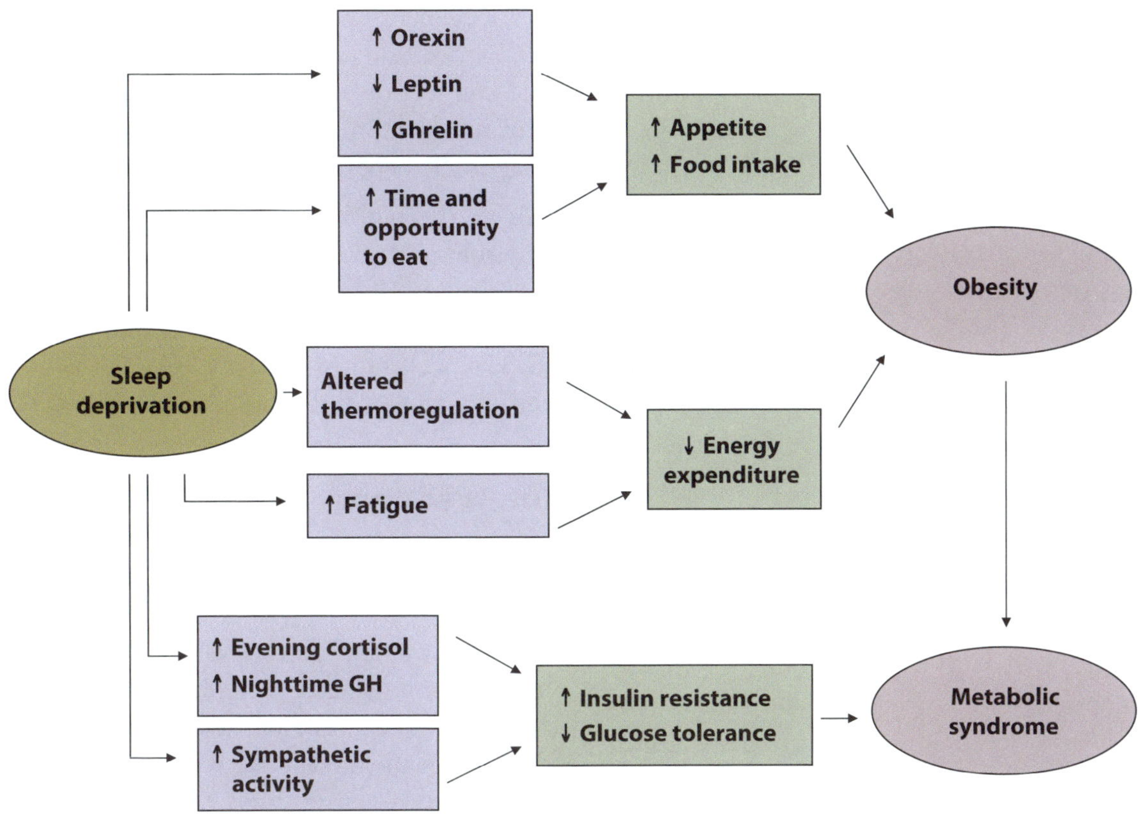

Figure 6.7 Schematic of possible pathways leading from sleep loss to metabolic syndrome and obesity risk. From: Garaulet M. The chronobiology, etiology and pathophysiology of obesity. *Int J Obes* (Lond). 2010 Jun 22. Reproduced with permission from Macmillan Publishers Ltd.

record of dietary intake and environmental exposures, sleep history, record of legal and illegal drugs and other substances used, and often a psychiatric assessment. As discussed earlier, stressful events and/or poor coping patterns often contribute to these conditions, and may require retraining through cognitive or insight-oriented psychotherapy.

Given the role that overactivation of the HPA axis plays in all of these conditions, evaluation of its functioning is recommended, traditionally done by combining dexamethasone-induced HPA axis suppression with HPA stimulation by an intravenous bolus of CRH. As discussed earlier, the negative feedback from cortisol provides an important check to prevent HPA axis hyperactivity. Dexamethasone, a glucocorticoid agonist, should effectively prevent cortisol release, and elevation in cortisol therefore demonstrates impaired negative feedback. The addition of CRH promotes the escape of cortisol from dexamethasone suppression, offering a more sensitive gauge of HPA axis regulation. In healthy individuals, pretreatment with dexamethasone prevents substantial release of ACTH and cortisol after additional administration of CRH. In depressed patients, however, increased secretion of ACTH and cortisol is observed, due to poor negative feedback by dexamethasone (and ultimately cortisol).[61] The cortisol release following this combined dexamethasone(dex)/CRH test is considered to sensitively gauge HPA regulation and has been used as a biomarker to monitor the clinical course of depression.

Alternative assessment tools are based on salivary cortisol levels. Salivary hormone levels are reproducible, comparable to plasma levels, and easy to assess. Salivary cortisol determination is a sensitive, specific, and pain-free procedure.[62] Additionally, salivary levels reflect the circulating level of free steroid rather than total circulating levels, which are confounded by the presence of circulating binding proteins. Salivary cortisol levels parallel those in plasma following ACTH and CRH stimulation, and following exercise-induced stress.[63]

One test which uses salivary hormone levels is the cortisol-awakening response (CAR), a reasonably good predictor of HPA dysregulation. The CAR is a measure of cortisol production as a response to the stress of awakening, a separate function than the HPA circadian rhythm. Salivary levels generally show a sharp rise upon awakening and during the first hour after wake-up. Generally, an initially hyperactive HPA response results in elevated cortisol levels, while more chronic stress may blunt this effect. For example, a blunted cortisol response to awakening has been found in a non-clinical sample of women from the community with mild to moderate depressive symptomatology.[64] Lower cortisol levels immediately after awakening were further found to be related to poor sleep quality in patients with primary insomnia.[65]

Given that cortisol levels fluctuate throughout the day and are important measures of HPA axis function (i.e., a total 24-hour cortisol level is not a sensitive test), salivary cortisol measured throughout the day is a useful evaluation. Often combined with a salivary DHEA level, this test allows for interpretation of the DHEA-to-cortisol ratio and altered circadian rhythm of cortisol. One pattern associated with chronic stress is elevated cortisol combined with reduced DHEA, indicating a shift toward glucocorticoid production and away from sex hormone steroid production. For example, caregivers of Alzheimer's patients, who have a high degree of chronic stress, were compared to non-caregivers; caregivers had reduced DHEA-S levels and an increased cortisol/DHEA-S ratio, despite having similar cortisol levels to the controls. They also had an impaired HPA axis response to Dex.[66]

Lastly, excess visceral adipose tissue may be an indicator of disturbed HPA axis function. In a recent study, researchers found that higher fat mass index, waist circumference, and waist-to-hip ratio were related to HPA axis dysfunction.[67] This has been a consistent finding in other studies, as has an association with hyperinsulinemia.[68] Again, the connection between HPA axis dysregulation and the metabolic syndrome may also offer some diagnostic benefit.

Given their close associations with the pathophysiology of depression, anxiety, and insomnia, assessment of glucose regulation (oral glucose tolerance, hemoglobin A1C, etc.) and serum levels of 25-OH vitamin D and C-reactive protein may indicate the need for more specific therapy.

Interventions

General

Healthy dietary and physical activity patterns have been associated with healthy sleep patterns and a reduced risk of depression and anxiety. Although most studies were of small sample size, physical activity has been shown to reduce depression in a number of randomized trials, including endurance, mindful, and non-mindful exercise.[69,70] Several mechanisms are probably involved, including an increase in BDNF due to physical activity, and a blunting of the adrenal response to ACTH.[71,72]

Among dietary patterns, the Mediterranean diet (or one closely approximating that) appears to offer the best protection, and may have specific benefit for restoring normal HPA axis activity. In a trial of women living in the Mediterranean area, researchers found that HPA dysregulation was associated with increased abdominal fat, as well as a higher total and saturated fat intake. Women most closely following a Mediterranean diet had the least HPA dysregulation.[73] Additionally, the relationship between HPA activation and insulin resistance suggests another mechanism for benefit from the Mediterranean diet. Animal studies, and to a lesser degree human studies, are beginning to outline a mechanism by which chronic stress facilitates the need to consume high-calorie foods, which in turn leads to abdominal obesity and insulin resistance.[74] Figure 6.8 represents a hypothetical schema for this process.

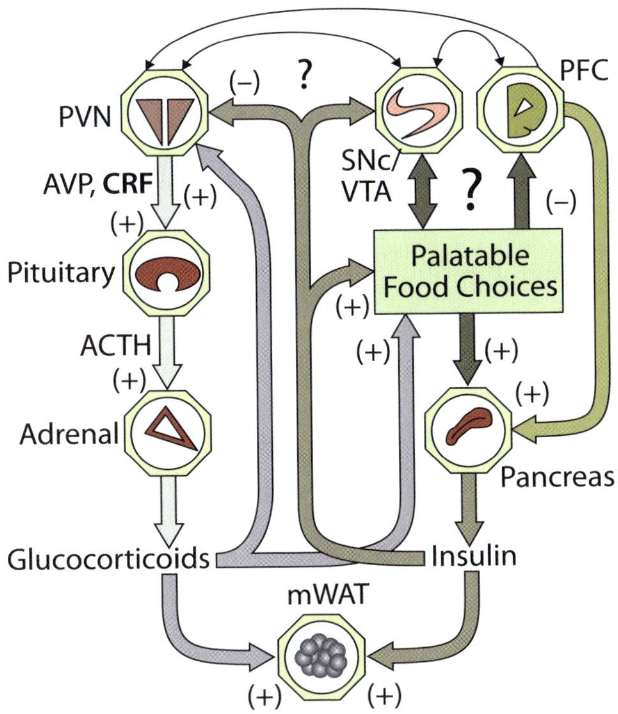

Figure 6.8 Hypothetical schema for the mechanisms by which palatable food intake, glucocorticoids and insulin interact to regulate metabolic and neurological pathways. From: Warne JP. Shaping the stress response: interplay of palatable food choices, glucocorticoids, insulin and abdominal obesity. *Mol Cell Endocrinol.* 2009 Mar 5;300(1-2):137-46. Epub 2008 Oct 15. Reproduced with permission from Elsevier Science & Technology Journals.

In addition to diet and physical activity, stress-reduction activities, possibly in conjunction with individual psychotherapy, may be indicated. While cognitive-behavioral stress reduction (CBSR) techniques have been shown to reduce symptoms of stress and depression, and help to develop a positive affect, a recent comparison between CBSR and mindfulness-based stress reduction (MBSR) found a greater benefit from MBSR, particularly in regard to mindfulness, energy, pain, and a trend for binge eating. MBSR included a combination of meditation, body scans, gentle Hatha yoga, and group discussion.[75] A number of mechanisms have been suggested for this outcome; electroencephalographic (EEG) studies have revealed a significant increase in alpha and theta activity during meditation, and neuroimaging has shown increased activity in areas of the brain related to activity.[76]

Nutritional and botanical supplementation

Broad spectrum multivitamin/mineral and vitamin D

A high potency, broad-spectrum multiple vitamin and mineral formula is indicated for several reasons, including the fact that a number of vitamins have been shown to be associated with symptoms of depression, anxiety, and insomnia, and are necessary for adrenal function, including folate, B6, B12, and vitamin C (see above). In addition, ensuring optimal vitamin D levels is important, given the relationship between stress symptoms, depression, and serum levels of 25(OH) vitamin D. Supplementation with vitamin D has been shown to reduce symptoms of depression compared to placebo.[77] A second placebo-controlled trial also found that daily supplementation increased positive affect when given to healthy subjects during the winter.[78]

Omega-3 fatty acids

As discussed earlier, omega-3 fatty acid intake has been directly correlated to symptoms of depression and to reduced anger and anxiety levels in substance users.[79] Fish oil has been shown to blunt the increase in cortisol and epinephrine following a stressful exposure.[80] Given the anti-inflammatory function of fish oil, it is likely to reduce the inflammatory component of insomnia, although no clinical trials have been done.[81]

Adaptogens

Adaptogens have been defined as "medicinal plants that enhance the 'state of non-specific resistance' of an organism to stress, augmenting resistance to physical, biological, chemical and psychological stresses, and increasing concentration, performance and endurance during fatigue".[82] Several herbal adaptogens have been shown to be of significant clinical benefit in the treatment of depression, anxiety, and/or insomnia, likely through modulation of the HPA axis. A recent study suggests that another mechanism by which adaptogens work is by increasing production of molecular chaperones, proteins that promote correct folding of other proteins, prevent their aggregation, and assist in re-folding of misfolded or unfolded proteins, which would otherwise interfere with cellular function and increase apoptotic signals in response to stress.[82,83]

Among adaptogens, the Indian herb ashwagandha has been shown to prevent a number of adverse reactions to stress in animals, including changes in blood sugar, adrenal weight, and cortisol levels.[84] In one human double-blinded study, chronically stressed subjects taking a standardized extract of ashwagandha had significant reductions in a modified Hamilton anxiety (mHAM-A) scale, serum cortisol, C-reactive protein, pulse rate, and blood pressure, and significant increases of serum DHEA-S and hemoglobin, compared to the placebo group. In addition, there were dose-dependent responses in lowering fasting blood glucose and improving the serum lipid levels.[85]

Other adaptogens with significant clinical benefit include *Rhodiola rosea*, and *Lavandula angustifolia*. In a randomized, placebo-controlled trial of 60 patients with stress-related fatigue, rhodiola was found to have an anti-fatigue effect that increased mental performance, particularly the ability to concentrate, as well as decreased the cortisol response to awakening stress.[86] In another placebo-controlled 6-week trial of patients with depression, rhodiola was found to reduce depressive symptoms and insomnia and improve emotional stability compared to placebo.[87] And in a small preliminary trial, rhodiola was also found to improve symptoms of anxiety.[88] *Lavandula angustifolia* is another herb which has shown significant benefit in clinical trials. In a randomized trial, it was found to increase the effect of the antidepressant imipramine, compared to imipramine alone, when given to depressed patients.[89] When essential oil of lavender was humidified, it was shown to have a positive, yet small, change in blood pressure and pulse, pain, anxiety, depression, and sense of well-being in cancer hospice patients.

GABA

Gamma-aminobutyric acid (GABA) is a major neurotransmitter that is abundantly and widely distributed throughout the central nervous system (CNS), known to influence levels of the neurotransmitters dopamine, serotonin, norepinephrine, and glutamate, generally increasing alpha brain wave activity. Within the brain, GABA is formed in neuronal cells by the α-decarboxylation of glutamic acid and further metabolized by GABA-α-keto-glutarate transaminase and then returned to the tricarboxylic acid cycle (TCA) cycle. Plasma membrane depolarization induces the release of GABA from the nerve terminals and GABA binds to GABA receptors, such as the $GABA_A$ receptor and the $GABA_B$ receptor, which are distributed on the post-synaptic cell membranes. Among other effects, GABA is known to mediate pre-synaptic inhibition of primary afferent fibers in the motor system and may also be involved in post-synaptic forms of motor neuron inhibition.

The neurotransmitter actions of GABA in the synaptic cleft are terminated by its reuptake by either pre-synaptic neurons or nearby glial cells via specific and high-affinity transporters that are believed to be the major mechanism for reducing its concentration in the extracellular fluid within the brain.

Low levels or decreased GABA function in the brain is associated with several psychiatric and neurological disorders, but most primarily anxiety, depression, insomnia, and epilepsy.[91,92] Some antidepressant medications, such as benzodiazepines, work by increasing brain levels of GABA, leading to a state of relaxation and sleep. In one small study, participants with a fear of heights were asked to cross a suspension bridge, and were then given either GABA or placebo. Those given GABA had an increase in salivary IgA levels, compared to a drop in those given placebo, indicating a stressful response.[93]

L-theanine

L-theanine is an amino acid found in tea leaves; it appears to increase production of alpha brain waves and reduce beta brain waves, effects likely to induce calmness, reduce hyperactivity and nervousness, and focus attention.[94,95] In one small trial, it was found to improve cognitive performance and improve mood.[96]

5-HTP

5-HTP is the metabolic precursor of both serotonin and melatonin. 5-HTP bypasses the rate-limiting enzyme tryptophan hydroxylase, which normally limits the conversion of tryptophan to serotonin. Combined with GABA in a randomized, placebo-controlled trial, 5-HTP was shown to reduce time to fall asleep, decrease sleep latency, increase the duration of sleep, and improve the quality of sleep.[97] In a trial of children with nightmares (sleep terrors), 5-HTP was shown to bring about a positive response in over 90% of patients after 1 month of treatment, compared to a group without drug therapy, of which 71.4% showed persistence of episodes with the same frequency as before.[98]

Melatonin

Melatonin has a long history of use for sleep disorders, and significant clinical support for its use. It has a circadian rhythm with considerable daily variation as well as a sensitivity to light, which suppresses its activity. It also has seasonable variability.[99] When used as a supplement, melatonin appears to have the greatest benefit for sleep disorders when it is used to restore a rhythm disorder, such as jet lag or a phase-shift, but it also has benefit for primary insomnia. For example, when given to 170 patients with primary insomnia, it was shown to significantly improve quality of sleep and morning alertness, with no withdrawal effects.[100]

Chamomile

Chamomile has a long history of use for its calming properties. In a recent randomized trial with 61 patients diagnosed with generalized anxiety disorder, chamomile was shown to improve Hamilton Anxiety Rating (HAM-A) scores compared to placebo.[101]

Saffron

A number of clinical trials have recently been done indicating a benefit of the herb saffron for mild to moderate depression. In two trials which enrolled adult outpatients diagnosed with depression, saffron was found to have similar efficacy to the conventional antidepressant fluoxetine.[102,103] In a second trial, saffron was found to have similar benefit to imipramine, with a lower rate of adverse effects.[104]

Other

Sleep habits should always be a part of a comprehensive treatment plan to address insomnia. This includes avoidance of alcohol and caffeine, total darkness and a quiet environment, using the bedroom specifically for sleeping, and maintaining a slightly warmer environment. Elderly subjects showed such a pronounced sensitivity to a 0.4°C increase in skin temperature that it was sufficient to almost double the proportion of nocturnal slow wave sleep and to decrease the probability of early morning awakening from 0.58 to 0.04.[105]

Phototherapy has also been used successfully for a number of conditions, including circadian rhythm disorders, mood disorders, dementia, and primary insomnia. Although early trials suggested a 20-minute application was sufficient, more recent work suggests that 45 minutes has a greater effect and a longer lasting benefit.[106] Bright morning light has also been used with success in the treatment of sleep-onset insomnia, while early morning awakening insomnia has been treated with bright light in the evening.[107,108]

References

1. Le Moal M. Historical approach and evolution of the stress concept: a personal account. *Psychoneuroendocrinology.* 2007 Aug;32 Suppl 1:S3-9.
2. Selye H. A syndrome produced by diverse nocuous agents, *Nature 38* (1936), p. 32.
3. Holsboer F, Ising M. Stress hormone regulation: biological role and translation into therapy. *Annu Rev Psychol.* 2010;61:81-109, C1-11.
4. Chrousos GP. Stress and disorders of the stress system. *Nat Rev Endocrinol.* 2009 Jul;5(7):374-81. Epub 2009 Jun 2.
5. León-Carrión J, Atutxa AM, et al. A clinical profile of memory impairment in humans due to endogenous glucocorticoid excess. *Clin Endocrinol* (Oxf). 2009 Feb;70(2):192-200.
6. Marques AH, Silverman MN, et al. Glucocorticoid dysregulations and their clinical correlates. From receptors to therapeutics. *Ann N Y Acad Sci.* 2009 Oct;1179:1-18.
7. Lightman SL. The neuroendocrinology of stress: a never ending story. *J Neuroendocrinol.* 2008 Jun;20(6):880-4.
8. McEwen BS. Central effects of stress hormones in health and disease: Understanding the protective and damaging effects of stress and stress mediators. *Eur J Pharmacol.* 2008 Apr 7;583(2-3):174-85.
9. Ford DE, Erlinger TP. Depression and C-reactive protein in US adults: data from the Third National Health and Nutrition Examination Survey. *Arch Intern Med.* 2004 May 10;164(9):1010-4.
10. Santhanam AV, Smith LA, Katusic ZS, et al. Brain-derived neurotrophic factor stimulates production of prostacyclin in cerebral arteries. *Stroke.* 2010 Feb;41(2):350-6. Epub 2009 Dec 17.
11. Elenkov IJ, Chrousos GP. Stress system—organization, physiology and immunoregulation. *Neuroimmunomodulation.* 2006;13(5-6):257-67.
12. Calcagni E, Elenkov I. Stress system activity, innate and T helper cytokines, and susceptibility to immune-related diseases. *Ann N Y Acad Sci.* 2006 Jun;1069:62-76.
13. Webster Marketon JI, Glasser R. Stress hormones and immune function. *Cell Immunol.* 2008 Mar-Apr;252(1-2):16-26.
14. Grippo AJ, Johnson AK. Stress, depression and cardiovascular dysregulation: a review of neurobiological mechanisms and the integration of research from preclinical disease models. *Stress.* 2009;12(1):1-21.
15. Freedland KE, Rich MW, Skala JA, et al. Prevalence of depression in hospitalized patients with congestive heart failure. *Psychosom Med.* 2003 Jan-Feb;65(1):119-28.
16. Van der Kooy K, van Hout H, Marwijk H, et al. Depression and the risk for cardiovascular diseases: systematic review and meta analysis. *Int J Geriatr Psychiatry.* 2007 Jul;22(7):613-26.
17. García-Prieto MD, Tébar FJ. Cortisol secretary pattern and glucocorticoid feedback sensitivity in women from a Mediterranean area: relationship with anthropometric characteristics, dietary intake and plasma fatty acid profile. *Clin Endocrinol* (Oxf). 2007 Feb;66(2):185-91.
18. Gold SM, Dziobek I, Sweat V, et al. Hippocampal damage and memory impairments as possible early brain complications of type 2 diabetes. *Diabetologia.* 2007 Apr; 50(4):711-9.
19. Bruehl H, Rueger M, Dziobek I, et al. Hypothalamic-pituitary-adrenal axis dysregulation and memory impairments in type 2 diabetes. *J Clin Endocrinol Metab.* 2007 Jul;92(7):2439-45.
20. Venna VR, Deplanque D, Allet C, et al. PUFA induce antidepressant-like effects in parallel to structural and molecular changes in the hippocampus. *Psychoneuroendocrinology.* 2009 Feb;34(2):199-211.
21. Kivimaki M, Tabak AG, Batty GD, et al. Hyperglycemia, type 2 diabetes, and depressive symptoms: the British Whitehall II study. *Diabetes Care.* 2009 Oct;32(10):1867-9.
22. van Rossum EF, Binder EB, Majer M, et al. Polymorphisms of the glucocorticoid receptor gene and major depression. *Biol Psychiatry.* 2006 Apr 15;59(8):681-8.
23. Montag C, Weber B, Fliessbach K, et al. The BDNF Val66Met polymorphism impacts parahippocampal and amygdala volume in healthy humans: incremental support for a genetic risk factor for depression. *Psychol Med.* 2009 Nov;39(11):1831-9.
24. Kendler KS, Gatz M, Gardner C, et al. A Swedish national twin study of lifetime major depression. *Am J Psychiatry.* 2006 Jan;163(1):109-14.
25. Claes S. Glucocorticoid receptor polymorphisms in major depression. *Ann N Y Acad Sci.* 2009 Oct;1179:216-28.
26. Hettema JM, Neale MC, Myers JM, et al. A population-based twin study of the relationship between neuroticism and internalizing disorders. *Am J Psychiatry.* 2006 May; 163(5):857-64
27. Alexander N, Kuepper Y. Gene-environment interactions predict cortisol responses after acute stress: implications for the etiology of depression. *Psychoneuroendocrinology.* 2009 Oct;34(9):1294-303.
28. McGowan PO, Meaney MJ, Szyf M, et al. Diet and the epigenetic (re)programming of phenotypic differences in behavior. *Brain Res.* 2008 Oct 27;1237:12-24.
29. Kessler RC, Berglund P, Demler O, et al. The epidemiology of major depressive disorder: results from the National Comorbidity Survey Replication (NCS-R). *JAMA.* 2003 Jun 18;289(23):3095-105.
30. Kessler RC, Chiu WT, Demler O, et al. Prevalence, severity, and comorbidity of 12-month DSM-IV disorders in the National Comorbidity Survey Replication. *Arch Gen Psychiatry.* 2005 Jun;62(6):617-27.
31. Watson D. Rethinking the mood and anxiety disorders: a quantitative hierarchical model for DSM-V. *J Abnorm Psychol.* 2005 Nov;114(4):522-36.

32. King-Kallimanis B, Gum AM, Kohn R. Comorbidity of depressive and anxiety disorders for older Americans in the national comorbidity survey-replication. *Am J Geriatr Psychiatry*. 2009 Sep;17(9):782-92.

33. Kendler KS, Gardner CO, Gatz M, et al. The sources of co-morbidity between major depression and generalized anxiety disorder in a Swedish national twin sample. *Psychol Med*. 2007 Mar;37(3):453-62. Epub 2006 Nov 23.

34. Bouchard MF, Bellinger DC. Blood lead levels and major depressive disorder, panic disorder, and generalized anxiety disorder in US young adults. *Arch Gen Psychiatry*. 2009 Dec;66(12):1313-9.

35. Heyer NJ, Echeverria D, Wood JS, et al. Chronic low-level mercury exposure, BDNF polymorphism, and associations with self-reported symptoms and mood. *Toxicol Sci*. 2004 Oct;81(2):354-63. Epub 2004 Jul 14.

36. Heyer NJ, Echeverria D, Farin FM, et al. The association between serotonin transporter gene promoter polymorphism (5-HTTLPR), self-reported symptoms, and dental mercury exposure. *J Toxicol Environ Health A*. 2008;71(19):1318-26.

37. Heyer NJ, Echeverria D, Martin MD, et al. Catechol O-methyltransferase (COMT) VAL158MET functional polymorphism, dental mercury exposure, and self-reported symptoms and mood. *J Toxicol Environ Health A*. 2009;72(9):599-609.

38. Echeverria D, Woods JS, Heyer NJ, et al. The association between a genetic polymorphism of coproporphyrinogen oxidase, dental mercury exposure and neurobehavioral response in humans. *Neurotoxicol Teratol*. 2006 Jan-Feb;28(1):39-48. Epub 2005 Dec 15.

39. Sánchez-Villegas A, Delgado-Rodríguez M, Alonso A, et al. Association of the Mediterranean dietary pattern with the incidence of depression: the Seguimiento Universidad de Navarra/University of Navarra follow-up (SUN) cohort. *Arch Gen Psychiatry*. 2009 Oct;66(10):1090-8.

40. Simon GE, Von Korff M, Sanders K, et al. Association between obesity and psychiatric disorders in the US adult population. *Arch Gen Psychiatry*. 2006 Jul;63(7):824-30.

41. Colangelo LA, He K, Whooley MA, et al. Higher dietary intake of long-chain omega-3 polyunsaturated fatty acids is inversely associated with depressive symptoms in women. *Nutrition*. 2009 Oct;25(10):1011-9. Epub 2009 Feb 4.

42. Leung BM, Kaplan BJ. Perinatal depression: prevalence, risks, and the nutrition link—a review of the literature. *J Am Diet Assoc*. 2009 Sep;109(9):1566-75.

43. Edwards R, Peet M, Shay J, et al. Omega-3 polyunsaturated fatty acid levels in the diet and in red blood cell membranes of depressed patients. *J Affect Disord*. 1998 Mar;48(2-3):149-55.

44. Owen C, Rees AM, Parker G. The role of fatty acids in the development and treatment of mood disorders. *Curr Opin Psychiatry*. 2008 Jan;21(1):19-24.

45. Jorde R, Sneve M, Figenschau Y, et al. Effects of vitamin D supplementation on symptoms of depression in overweight and obese subjects: randomized double blind trial. *J Intern Med*. 2008 Dec;264(6):599-609. Epub 2008 Sep 10.

46. Armstrong DJ, Meenagh GK, Bickle I, et al. Vitamin D deficiency is associated with anxiety and depression in fibromyalgia. *Clin Rheumatol*. 2007 Apr;26(4):551-4. Epub 2006 Jul 19.

47. Morris MS, Fava M, Jacques PF, et al. Depression and folate status in the US Population. *Psychother Psychosom*. 2003 Mar-Apr;72(2):80-7.

48. Arinami T, Yamada N. Methylenetetrahydrofolate reductase variant and schizophrenia/depression. *Am J Med Genet*. 1997 Sep 19;74(5):526-8.

49. Gilbody S, Lewis S, Lightfoot T. Methylenetetrahydrofolate reductase (MTHFR) genetic polymorphisms and psychiatric disorders: a HuGE review. *Am J Epidemiol*. 2007 Jan 1;165(1):1-13. Epub 2006 Oct 30.

50. Ng TP, Feng L, Niti M, et al. Folate, vitamin B12, homocysteine, and depressive symptoms in a population sample of older Chinese adults. *J Am Geriatr Soc*. 2009 May;57(5):871-6.

51. Merete C, Falcon LM, Tucker KL. Vitamin B6 is associated with depressive symptomatology in Massachusetts elders. *J Am Coll Nutr*. 2008 Jun;27(3):421-7.

52. Riemann D, Spiegelhalder K, Feige B, et al. The hyperarousal model of insomnia: a review of the concept and its evidence. *Sleep Med Rev*. 2010 Feb;14(1):19-31. Epub 2009 May 28.

53. Basta M, Chrousos GP, Vela-Bueno A, et al. Chronic insomnia and stress system. *Sleep Med Clin*. 2007 Jun;2(2):279-291.

54. Vgontzas AN, Mastorakos G, Bixler EO, et al. Sleep deprivation effects on the activity of the hypothalamic-pituitary-adrenal and growth axes: potential clinical implications. *Clin Endocrinol* (Oxf). 1999 Aug;51(2):205-15.

55. Irwin M, Clark C, Kennedy B, et al. Nocturnal catecholamines and immune function in insomniacs, depressed patients, and control subjects. *Brain Behav Immun*. 2003 Oct;17(5):365-72.

56. Vgontzas AN, Bixler EO, Alexandros N, et al. Chronic insomnia is associated with nyctohemeral activation of the hypothalamic-pituitary-adrenal axis: clinical implications. *J Clin Endocrinol Metab*. 2001 Aug;86(8):3787-94.

57. Buckley TM, Schatzberg AF. On the interactions of the hypothalamic-pituitary-adrenal (HPA) axis and sleep: normal HPA axis activity and circadian rhythm, exemplary sleep disorders. *J Clin Endocrinol Metab*. 2005 May;90(5):3106-14. Epub 2005 Feb 22.

58. Vgontzas AN, Papanicolaou DA, Bixler EO, et al. Circadian interleukin-6 secretion and quantity and depth of sleep. *J Clin Endocrinol Metab*. 1999 Aug;84(8):2603-7.

59. Vgontzas AN, Pejovic S, Zoumakis E, et al. Daytime napping after a night of sleep loss decreases sleepiness, improves performance, and causes beneficial changes in cortisol and interleukin-6 secretion. *Am J Physiol Endocrinol Metab*. 2007 Jan;292(1):E253-61.

60. Van Cauter E, Spiegel K, Tasali E, et al. Metabolic consequences of sleep and sleep loss. *Sleep Med.* 2008 Sep;9 Suppl 1:S23-8.

61. Heuser A, Yassouridis A, Holsboer F, et al. The combined dexamethasone/CRH test: a refined laboratory test for psychiatric disorders, *Journal of Psychiatric Research.* 28 (1994), pp. 341–356.

62. Törnhage CJ. Salivary cortisol for assessment of hypothalamic-pituitary-adrenal axis function. *Neuroimmunomodulation.* 2009;16(5):284-9. Epub 2009 Jun 29.

63. Lewis JG. Steroid Analysis in Saliva: An overview. *Clin Biochem Rev.* 2006 Aug;27(3):139-46.

64. Stetler C, Miller GE. Blunted cortisol response to awakening in mild to moderate depression: regulatory influences of sleep patterns and social contacts. *J Abnorm Psychol.* 2005 Nov;114(4):697-705.

65. Backhaus J, Junghanns K, Hohagen F. Sleep disturbances are correlated with decreased morning awakening salivary cortisol. *Psychoneuroendocrinology.* 2004 Oct;29(9):1184-91.

66. Jeckel CM, Lopes RP, Berleze MC. Neuroendocrine and immunological correlates of chronic stress in 'strictly healthy' populations. *Neuroimmunomodulation.* 2010;17(1):9-18. Epub 2009 Oct 5.

67. Rutters F, Nieuwenhuizen AG, Lemmens SG, Hypothalamus/Pituitary/Adrenal (HPA) axis functioning in relation to body fat distribution. *Clin Endocrinol* (Oxf). 2009 Sep 21. Epub ahead of print.

68. Pasquali R, Gagliardi L, Vicennati V, et al. ACTH and cortisol response to combined corticotropin releasing hormone-arginine vasopressin stimulation in obese males and its relationship to body weight, fat distribution and parameters of the metabolic syndrome. *Int J Obes Relat Metab Disord.* 1999 Apr;23(4):419-24.

69. Sjösten N, Kivelä SL. The effects of physical exercise on depressive symptoms among the aged: a systematic review. *Int J Geriatr Psychiatry.* 2006 May;21(5):410-8.

70. Tsang HW, Chan EP, Cheung WM. Effects of mindful and non-mindful exercises on people with depression: a systematic review. *Br J Clin Psychol.* 2008 Sep;47(Pt 3):303-22. Epub 2008 Jan 31.

71. Seifert T, Brassard P, Wissenberg M, et al. Endurance training enhances BDNF release from the human brain. *Am J Physiol Regul Integr Comp Physiol.* 2010 Feb;298(2):R372-7. Epub 2009 Nov 18.

72. Wittert GA, Livesey JH, Espiner EA, et al. Adaptation of the hypothalamopituitary adrenal axis to chronic exercise stress in humans. *Med Sci Sports Exerc.* 1996 Aug;28(8):1015-9.

73. García-Prieto MD, Tébar FJ, Nicolás F. Cortisol secretary pattern and glucocorticoid feedback sensitivity in women from a Mediterranean area: relationship with anthropometric characteristics, dietary intake and plasma fatty acid profile. *Clin Endocrinol* (Oxf). 2007 Feb;66(2):185-91.

74. Warne JP. Shaping the stress response: interplay of palatable food choices, glucocorticoids, insulin and abdominal obesity. *Mol Cell Endocrinol.* 2009 Mar 5;300(1-2):137-46. Epub 2008 Oct 15.

75. Smith BW, Shelley BM, Dalen J. A pilot study comparing the effects of mindfulness-based and cognitive-behavioral stress reduction. *J Altern Complement Med.* 2008 Apr;14(3):251-8.

76. Chiesa A, Serretti A. A systematic review of neurobiological and clinical features of mindfulness meditations. *Psychol Med.* 2009 Nov 27:1-14. Epub ahead of print.

77. Jorde R, Sneve M, Figenschau Y, et al. Effects of vitamin D supplementation on symptoms of depression in overweight and obese subjects: randomized double blind trial. *J Intern Med.* 2008 Dec;264(6):599-609. Epub 2008 Sep 10.

78. Smith BW, Shelley BM, Dalen J. A pilot study comparing the effects of mindfulness-based and cognitive-behavioral stress reduction. *J Altern Complement Med.* 2008 Apr;14(3):251-8.

79. Buydens-Branchey L, Branchey M, Hibbeln JR. Associations between increases in plasma n-3 polyunsaturated fatty acids following supplementation and decreases in anger and anxiety in substance abusers. *Prog Neuropsychopharmacol Biol Psychiatry.* 2008 Feb 15;32(2): 568-75. Epub 2007 Nov 1.

80. Delarue J, Marzinger O, Binnert C, et al. Fish oil prevents the adrenal activation elicited by mental stress in healthy men. *Diabetes Metab.* 2003;29:289-295.

81. Delarue J, Marzinger O, Binnert C, et al. Fish oil prevents the adrenal activation elicited by mental stress in healthy men. *Diabetes Metab.* 2003;29:289-295.

82. Panossian A, Wikman G, Kaur P, et al. Adaptogens exert a stress-protective effect by modulation of expression of molecular chaperones. *Phytomedicine.* 2009 Jun;16(6-7): 617-22. Epub 2009 Feb 1.

83. Panossian A, Wikman G. Evidence-based efficacy of adaptogens in fatigue, and molecular mechanisms related to their stress-protective activity. *Curr Clin Pharmacol.* 2009 Sep;4(3):198-219. Epub 2009 Sep 1.

84. Archana R, Namasivayam A. Antistressor effect of *Withania somnifera*. *J Ethnopharmacol.* 1999 Jan;64(1):91-3.

85. Auddy B, Hazra J, Mitra A, et al. A standardized *Withania somnifera* extract significantly reduces stress-related parameters in chronically stressed humans: A double-blind, randomized, placebo-controlled study. *JANA* 2008;11:50-6.

86. Olsson EM, von Schéele B, Panossian AG. A randomised, double-blind, placebo-controlled, parallel-group study of the standardised extract shr-5 of the roots of *Rhodiola rosea* in the treatment of subjects with stress-related fatigue. *Planta Med.* 2009 Feb;75(2):105-12. Epub 2008 Nov 18.

87. Darbinyan V, Aslanyan G, Amroyan E, et al. Clinical trial of *Rhodiola rosea L.* extract SHR-5 in the treatment of mild to moderate depression. *Nord J Psychiatry.* 2007;61(5):343-8.

88. Bystritsky A, Kerwin L, Feusner JD. A pilot study of *Rhodiola rosea* (Rhodax) for generalized anxiety disorder (GAD). *J Altern Complement Med.* 2008 Mar;14(2):175-80.

89. Akhondzadeh S, Kashani L. Comparison of *Lavandula angustifolia* Mill. tincture and imipramine in the treatment of mild to moderate depression: a double-blind, randomized trial. *Prog Neuropsychopharmacol Biol Psychiatry.* 2003 Feb;27(1):123-7.

90. Louis M, Kowalski SD. Use of aromatherapy with hospice patients to decrease pain, anxiety, and depression and to promote an increased sense of well-being. *Am J Hosp Palliat Care.* 2002 Nov-Dec;19(6):381-6.

91. Kendell SF, Krystal JH, Sanacora G. GABA and glutamate systems as therapeutic targets in depression and mood disorders. *Expert Opin Ther Targets.* 2005:9:153-168.

92. Nemeroff CB. The role of GABA in the pathophysiology and treatment of anxiety disorders. *Psychopharmacol Bull.* 2003:37:133-146.

93. Abdou AM, Higashiguchi S, Horie K, et al. Relaxation and immunity enhancement effects of gamma aminobutyric acid (GABA) administration in humans. *Biofactors* 2006;26:201-208.

94. Nobre AC, Rao A, Owen GN. L-theanine, a natural constituent in tea, and its effect on mental state. *Asia Pac J Clin Nutr.* 2008;17 Suppl 1:167-8.

95. Gomez-Ramirez M, Kelly SP, Montesi JL, et al. The effects of L-theanine on alpha-band oscillatory brain activity during a visuo-spatial attention task. *Brain Topogr.* 2009 Jun;22(1):44-51. Epub 2008 Oct 9.

96. Owen GN, Parnell H, De Bruin EA, et al. The combined effects of L-theanine and caffeine on cognitive performance and mood. *Nutr Neurosci.* 2008 Aug;11(4):193-198.

97. Shell W, Bullias D, Charuvastra E, et al. A randomized, placebo-controlled trial of an amino acid preparation on timing and quality of sleep. *Am J Ther.* 2009 May 15. Epub ahead of print.

98. Bruni O, Ferri R, Miano S, et al. L -5-Hydroxytryptophan treatment of sleep terrors in children. *Eur J Pediatr.* 2004 Jul;163(7):402-7. Epub 2004 May 14.

99. Zawilska JB, Skene DJ, Arendt J. Physiology and pharmacology of melatonin in relation to biological rhythms. *Pharmacol Rep.* 2009 May-Jun;61(3):383-410.

100. Lemoine P, Nir T, Laudon M, et al. Prolonged-release melatonin improves sleep quality and morning alertness in insomnia patients aged 55 years and older and has no withdrawal effects. *J Sleep Res.* 2007 Dec;16(4):372-80.

101. Amsterdam JD, Li Y, Soeller I, et al. A randomized, double-blind, placebo-controlled trial of oral *Matricaria recutita* (chamomile) extract therapy for generalized anxiety disorder. *J Clin Psychopharmacol.* 2009 Aug;29(4):378-82.

102. Akhondzadeh Basti A, Moshiri E, Noorbala AA. Comparison of petal of *Crocus sativus L.* and fluoxetine in the treatment of depressed outpatients: a pilot double-blind randomized trial. *Prog Neuropsychopharmacol Biol Psychiatry.* 2007 Mar 30;31(2):439-42.

103. Noorbala AA, Akhondzadeh S. Hydro-alcoholic extract of *Crocus sativus L.* versus fluoxetine in the treatment of mild to moderate depression: a double-blind, randomized pilot trial. *J Ethnopharmacol.* 2005 Feb 28;97(2):281-4. Epub 2005 Jan 6.

104. Akhondzadeh S, Fallah-Pour H. Comparison of *Crocus sativus L.* and imipramine in the treatment of mild to moderate depression: a pilot double-blind randomized trial [ISRCTN45683816]. *BMC Complement Altern Med.* 2004 Sep 2;4:12.

105. Raymann RJ, Swaab DF, Van Someren EJ, et al. Skin deep: enhanced sleep depth by cutaneous temperature manipulation. *Brain* 2008;131(Pt 2):500-13.

106. Kirisoglu C, Guilleminault C. Twenty minutes versus forty-five minutes morning bright light treatment on sleep onset insomnia in elderly subjects. *J Psychosom Res.* 2004 May;56(5):537-42.

107. Lack L, Wright H, Paynter D. The treatment of sleep onset insomnia with bright morning light. *Sleep Biol Rhythms.* 2007;5:173-9.

108. Lack L, Wright H, Kemp K, et al. The treatment of early-morning awakening insomnia with 2 evenings of bright light. *Sleep.* 2005 May 1;28(5):616-23.

Immune Function

Overview

A healthy immune system is critical for optimal wellness, as the average person is exposed to a vast number of microbes on skin and mucous membranes (e.g., the respiratory and gastrointestinal tracts), as well as to the continuous formation of malignant cells. The immune system has two fundamental and complementary systems for responding to the numerous daily threats: the innate and adaptive immune systems (Figure 7.1), with the division largely defined by the speed and specificity of the response. The innate branch of the immune system is generally defined by a consistent response, no matter how often an antigen is encountered; it includes phagocytic cells such as neutrophils, monocytes, and macrophages, although physical and chemical barriers are sometimes considered a part of innate immunity. The adaptive immune system, however, improves upon repeated exposure to a given infection, because these cells develop a memory of past encounters. Thought to have developed more recently in evolutionary history, the adaptive immune system is comprised of B and T cells, which work together to create antibodies specific to an invading organism. As we will see below, the immune system is damaged by a number of factors, including environmental toxins, stress, lifestyle, nutrition, age, and inflammation; it may also be enhanced for more optimal function.

Innate Immunity

The innate immune system, considered the first line of defense against microbial pathogens, is characterized by its ability to recognize a wide range of such pathogens (e.g., viruses, bacteria, and fungi), as well as by its rapid response. Comprised of physical, chemical, and cellular elements, the underlying basis for innate immunity is recognition of microbial molecular patterns (known as pathogen-associated molecular patterns, or PAMPs) by a limited number of receptors, called pattern-recognition receptors (PRRs). Upon recognition, a rapid killing and elimination of the pathogen occurs through the activation of the acute inflammatory

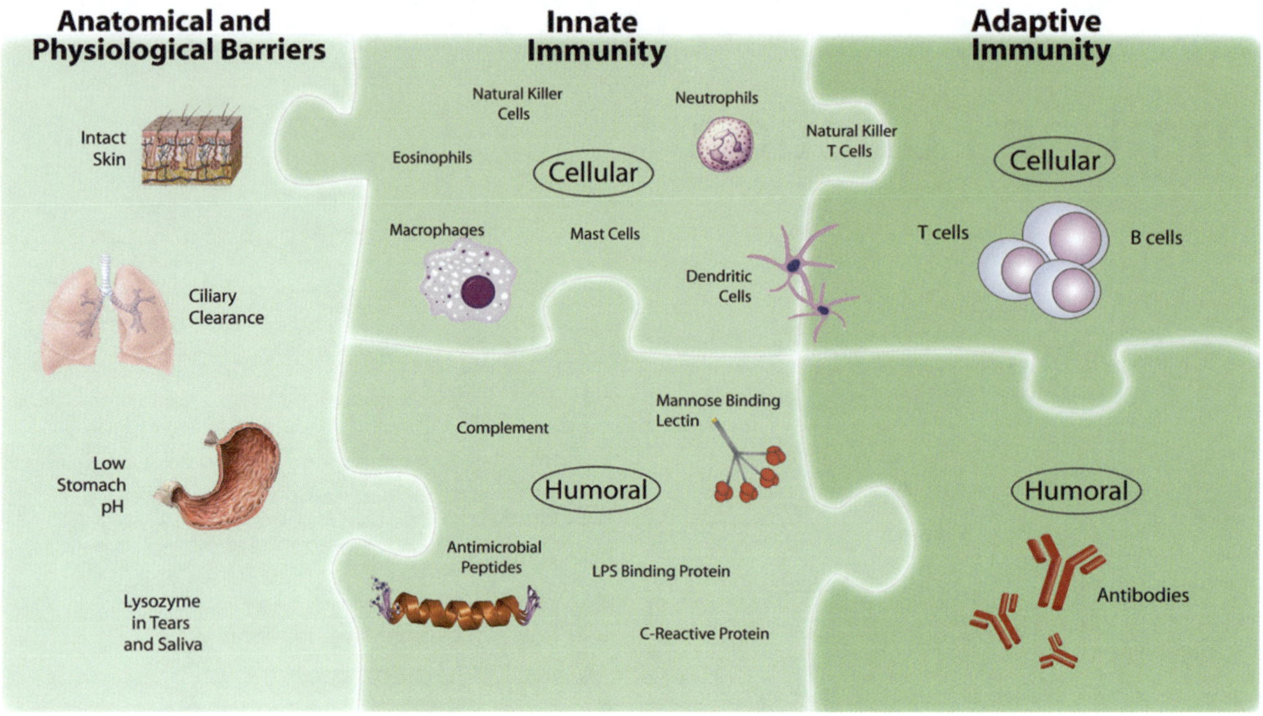

Figure 7.1 Representation of the integrated human immune system. From: Turvey SE, Broide DH. Innate immunity. *J Allergy Clin Immunol.* 2010 Feb;125(2 Suppl 2):S24-32. Reproduced with permission from Elsevier.

response, as well as the presentation of antigens to cells of the adaptive immune system.[1] PRRs are expressed by many cell types, including macrophages, monocytes, dendritic cells (DCs), neutrophils, and epithelial cells, allowing the early detection of pathogens directly at the site of infection.[2] In addition to recognizing PAMPs, the innate immune system also appears to recognize the presence of molecular patterns released by injured cells, known as danger-associated molecular patterns (DAMPs). For example, uric acid crystals are recognized by immune cells (inflammasomes), which then increase production of interleukin (IL)-1beta and IL-18, triggering an inflammatory process.[3,4]

The PRRs most well-studied are the toll-like receptors (TLRs), found on many cell types including mononuclear, endothelial, and epithelial cells. They recognize various components of the bacterial cell wall, such as LPS from gram-negative bacteria, as well as viral, fungal, and protozoan PAMPs.[5] The function of TLRs depends on a number of factors, among them vitamin D status. Indeed, vitamin D may be an important regulator of innate immunity. Using cultures from patients deficient in vitamin D, researchers found that the normal production of cathelicidin antimicrobial protein (hCAP), which kills invading bacteria, was inhibited without supplemental vitamin D. They found a direct correlation between the serum concentration of 25-hydroxyvitamin D3 and monocyte expression of hCAP, following treatment with ligands to pathogen-responsive TLRs. They also found that supplementation of patients with vitamin D insufficiency significantly enhanced innate immune responses by rescuing TLR-mediated suppression of hCAP expression.[6] The authors of that study suggested that "a key function of vitamin D... is to prevent pathogen-induced evasion of innate immunity," and they highlighted the consequences of impaired immunity in over 1 billion people worldwide whose vitamin D insufficiency would clearly benefit from supplementation.

A number of other natural therapies have been shown to enhance the function of the innate immune system by engaging TLRs. For example, *Cordyceps sinensis* (a Chinese herb) was recently shown to reduce lung metastasis occurrence in a surgical excision model of metastatic mammary

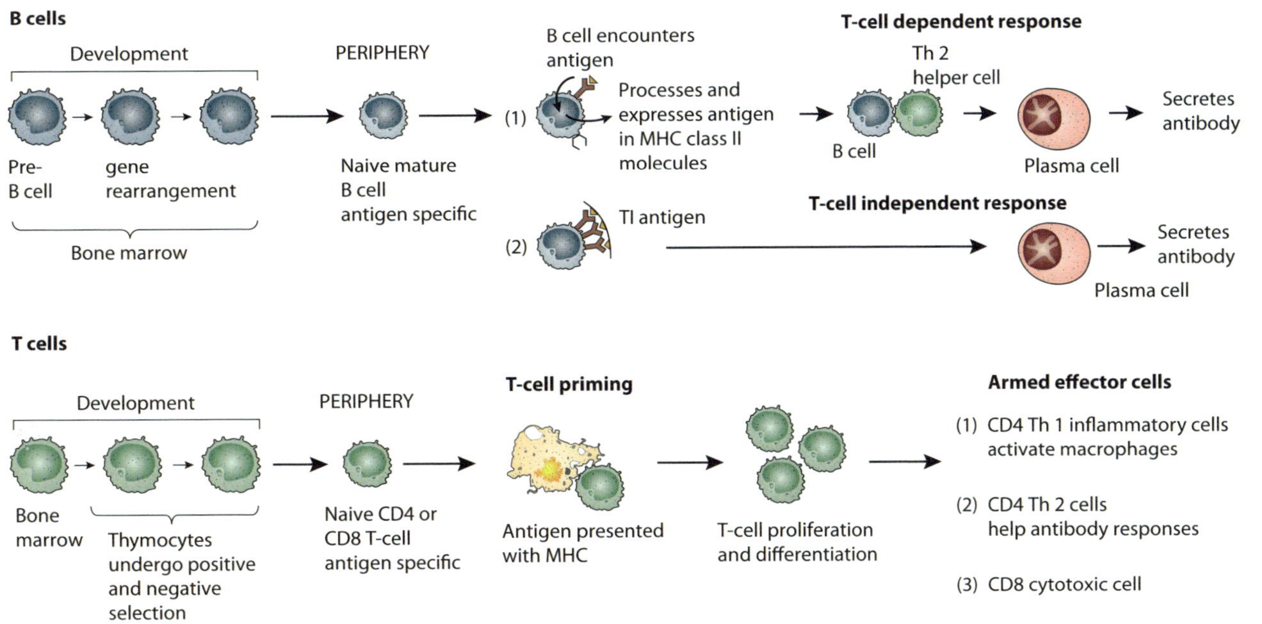

Figure 7.2 The role of T and B lymphocytes in specific immunity. From: Parkin J, Cohen B. An overview of the immune system. *The Lancet*. 2001 Jun 2;357(9270):1777-89. Reproduced with permission from Elsevier.

carcinoma,[7] an effect attributed to its activation of macrophage activity through a TLR pathway.[8]

Adaptive Immunity

In contrast to innate immunity, the adaptive immune system is characterized by a relatively slow initial response, which is activated only if the innate immune system cannot clear the infection in a relatively short period of time. However, the second time a microbe tries to invade the body, B and T memory cells help the immune system to activate much faster, because these cells have antigen-specific receptors that allow for targeted responses. B and T cell receptors are generated through somatic gene rearrangement and hypermutation, enabling the generation of a virtually infinite repertoire of antigen receptors, allowing the adaptive immune cells to recognize any specific type of microorganism (Figure 7.2). This occurs when an antigen is presented to and recognized by the antigen specific T or B cell, leading to cell priming, activation, and differentiation. Next, a response takes place, due either to the activated T cells leaving the lymphoid tissue and homing to the disease site, or to the release of antibodies from activated B cells (plasma cells) into blood and tissue fluids, and thence to the infective focus.[9] Antibodies neutralize toxins, prevent organisms from adhering to mucosal surfaces, activate complement, opsonize bacteria for phagocytosis, and sensitize tumor and infected cells for antibody-dependent cytotoxic attack by natural killer cells.[9]

The adaptive immune system is considered a more recent development in evolutionary history than the innate immune system. It has the advantage of high specificity when targeting an infection, thus sparing surrounding uninfected tissue from damage (unlike effectors of innate immunity). However, although randomly generated antigen receptors allow for recognition of a seemingly endless number of antigens, it also increases the potential of targeting self-antigens or innocuous non-self-antigens, leading to the development of autoimmunity and allergy, respectively.[10]

It now appears that the adaptive immune system is also dependent on PRRs to provide a number of checkpoints before the full immune response is generated. For example, cells of the innate immune system are thought to detect PAMPs from microbes that activate an adaptive response, although the precise signals involved are not well-understood.

Natural killer (NK) cells—involved in immune regulation, tumor surveillance, and host defense against pathogens—are now thought to be an evolutionary bridge between innate and adaptive immunity. They respond quickly and nonspecifically to an infection, but also have almost all the features of adaptive immune system cells, including memory.[11,12] NK cell activity is known to be enhanced by a number of interventions, such as lipoic acid, and is also associated with the status of zinc, vitamins A and D.[13,14,15,16] In patients with both Graves' and Hashimoto's diseases, a dysfunction recently found in a subset of NK cells normalized in a dose-dependent manner when given DHEA.[17]

Enhancing NK cell function may help to prevent some of the decline in both immune and nonimmune parameters associated with aging. For example, centenarians with the highest NK function and number of NK cells have much greater preservation of endocrine function and muscle mass.[18] Supplementation with lactobacilli and bifidobacteria have been shown to increase both NK cell activity and tumoricidal activity by up to 100%, with a greater benefit seen among the elderly than those younger than age 70.[19]

Causes of Immune Dysfunction

Immunosenescence

Broadly defined as age-related changes in the immune system, immunosenescence is thought to be partly or directly responsible for an increased susceptibility to infectious diseases, autoimmunity, and cancer, as well as to some age-related diseases, such as cardiovascular and neurodegenerative diseases, diabetes, and osteoporosis, and a decreased responsiveness to vaccination.[20] This decline in immune function has been attributed to several factors, including an involution of the thymus and thus a decreased production of newly developed T cells (Table 7.1). It has been shown that the portion of the thymus where thymopoiesis takes place shrinks to less than 10% of the total thymus volume by age 70, corresponding to a 1000-fold drop in activity. This involution results in a diminished number of circulating naive T cells and impaired adaptive immunity.

Table 7.1 Characteristics of immunosenescence

- Thymus involution with alteration in T cell subsets
- Lower levels of TREC-containing naïve T cells
- Decrease of naïve (necessary for clonal expansion) T cell subsets
- Compensatory increase of memory T cell subsets
- Oligoclonal expansion of CD8+ T cells (megaclones) caused by chronic viral infections (CMV and EBV)
- Increased number of CD8 T cells producing IFNg
- Increased resistance to apoptosis/activation-induced cell death (AICD) in T cells
- Loss of costimulatory signal CD28 (necessary for clonal expansion)
- Altered T cell proliferation (impairment of transduction signaling)
- Decreased T cell IL-2 production and IL-2 receptor expression (necessary for clonal expansion)
- Shift from Th1 to Th2 cytokine profile (in CD4 T cells)
- Changes in the cytokine profiles to a proinflammatory status (inflamm-aging)
- Decline in B cell function
- Increased nonorgan-specific autoantibodies
- Increased oxidative stress, increased DNA damage, alteration of DNA repair, increased protein glycation, telomere shortening and decreased proteasome function

Complexity of anti-immunosenescence strategies in humans. From: Capri M, Monti D, Salvioli S, et al. *Artif Organs.* 2006 Oct;30(10):730-42. Reproduced with permission from John Wiley & Sons, Inc.

Chronic low-grade inflammation, sometimes termed inflamm-aging, is also thought to play a role in the aging process, along with a decline in B cell function and an increase in reactive oxygen species.[20] Continuous inflammation leads to a paradoxical "hyperactive" yet inefficient immune response, which becomes a self-perpetuating cycle (Figure 7.3).

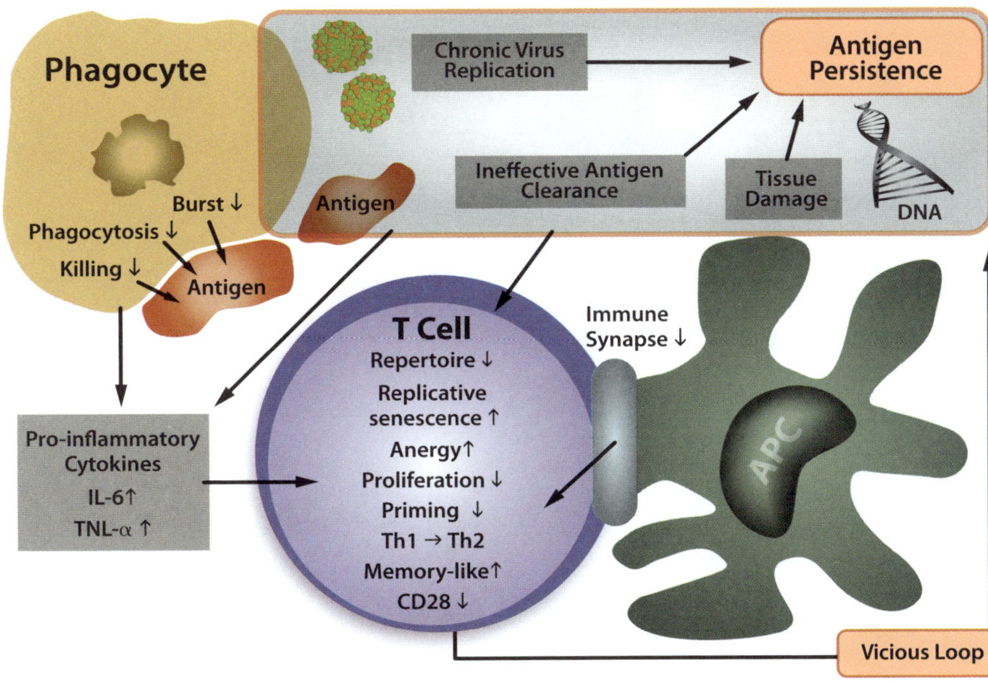

Figure 7.3 Low-grade chronic inflammation and senescence-associated immunodeficiency. From: Peters T, Weiss JM, Sindrilaru A, et al. Reactive oxygen intermediate-induced pathomechanisms contribute to immunosenescence, chronic inflammation and autoimmunity. *Mech Ageing Dev.* 2009 Sep;130(9):564-87. Reproduced with permission from Elsevier Science & Technology Journals.

Cells of the innate immune system are also affected by aging, including NK cells, neutrophils, macrophages, and eosinophils. For example, most aspects of neutrophil function are decreased in aged humans, including chemotaxis, phagocytosis of microbes, and generation of superoxide in response to stimulation by soluble host and bacterial factors (Figure 7.4). Interestingly, many of the defects in neutrophil function are thought to arise from changes to the cell membrane, possibly because of changes in membrane fluidity.[21]

Strategies to prevent and reverse immunosenescence

A number of strategies offer potential benefit for restoring the deficits seen in immunosenescence. Exercise, for example, is likely to have a broad number of immune-enhancing benefits, particularly when done long term. Physical activity has been associated with a reduced incidence of pneumonia, hospitalizations due to infection, and several markers of immune function, including lymphocyte proliferative response and NK cell cytotoxicity.[22] As mentioned above, probiotic supplementation has been shown to enhance NK cell function significantly, particularly in the elderly. Dysbiosis, i.e., the derangement of intestinal microbiota, is often present in the frail elderly, and is thought to represent an important source of continuous antigenic stimulation.[23] This heavy antigenic load of pathogens is suspected to be a significant contributor to immunosenescence, and may explain why restoration of intestinal flora offers such significant benefit.

In addition to exercise and restoring healthy intestinal microbiota, treatment of any sources of chronic inflammation, such as infections in the oral cavity or urogenital tract, should be identified and eliminated to help reduce or avert immunosenescence due to inflamm-aging. Omega-3 fatty acids have well-established anti-inflammatory effects and also improve cellular membrane function, a specific age-related deficit found in neutrophils.[21,24] A blunting of immunosenescence in aging mice given omega-3 fatty acids has been shown, probably due to an increase in Th1-stimulating cytokines, as well as a lowering of Th2-associated cytokines. In humans, fish oil supplementation

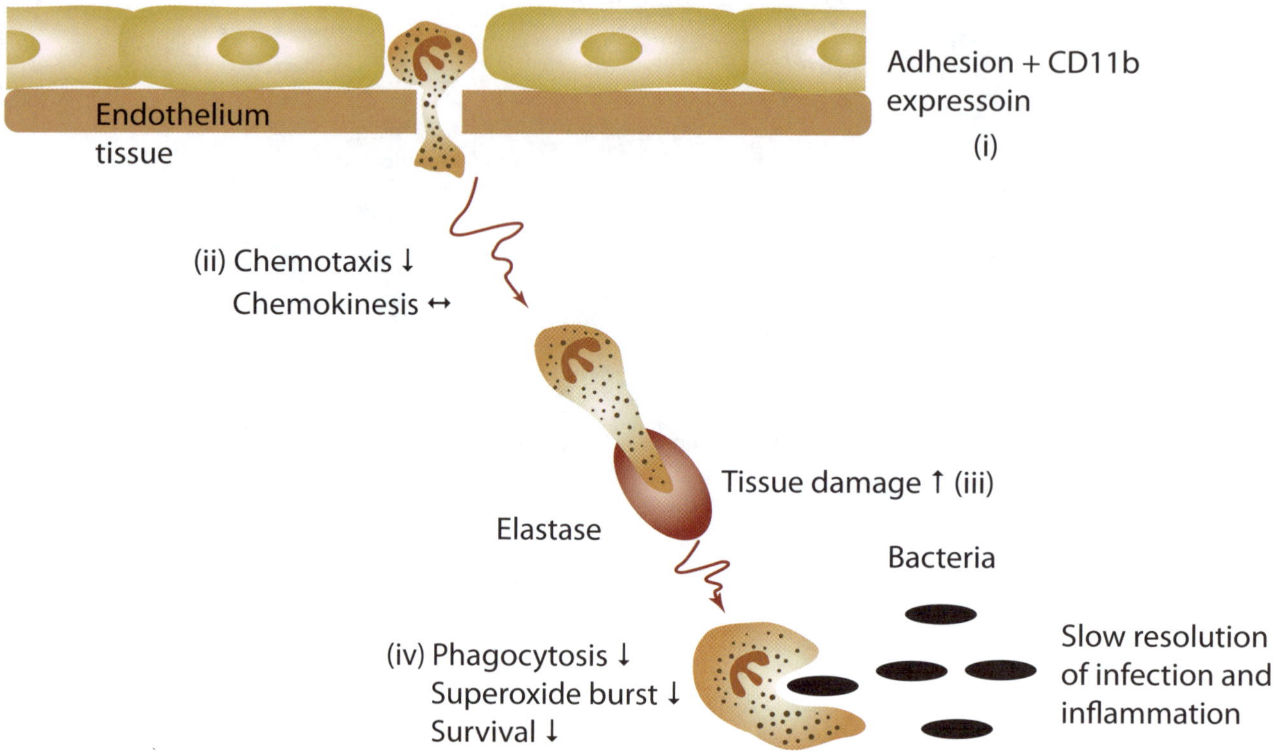

Figure 7.4 Proposed consequences of the age-related loss of human neutrophil function. From: Panda A, Arjona A, Sapey E, et al. Human innate immunosenescence: causes and consequences for immunity in old age. *Trends Immunol.* 2009 Jul;30(7):325-33. Reproduced with permission from Elsevier Science & Technology Journals.

also increased interferon-gamma production and lymphocyte proliferation.[25] A number of other nutrients may improve age-related immune function decline, among them vitamin B12, vitamin D, and zinc.[20] Vitamin D, for example, has been shown to improve a variety of immune functions, and may have a specific role in preventing thymic involution. The cytokine IL-7 has been shown to increase thymic activity; however, IL-6 may suppress this effect.[20] In a recent study of centenarians, low vitamin D (present in 99/104 individuals) was associated with an elevation of IL-6.[26] Thus, restoring optimal vitamin D status may prevent the suppression of thymic activity.

Autoimmunity/Allergy

The adaptive immune system, while offering greater specificity of response to pathogens, also brings the potential to inappropriately target human tissues and benign non-self tissues, including food antigens. Much has been learned in recent years about the etiology and triggers of autoimmune disease, both genetic and environmental. Among the more well-established mechanisms are insufficient vitamin D status and altered intestinal permeability and flora.[28,27,32]

Vitamin D has been shown to increase innate immunity while modulating adaptive immunity.[28] Insufficiency is associated with an increased prevalence of many autoimmune diseases, including multiple sclerosis, rheumatoid arthritis, SLE and inflammatory bowel disease.[28] In a study following children from birth for over 30 years, those who regularly took supplemental vitamin D at a dose of 2000 IU daily had a nearly 80% lower risk of developing type 1 diabetes compared with those who received less.[29] There also appears to be a role for inflammation in type 1 diabetes development, as an increase in specific TLRs associated with inflammatory markers on monocytes was recently found.[30] Supplemental vitamin D modulated some of the monocyte abnormalities in patients with type 1 diabetes in a recent trial.[31]

Intestinal permeability and microbiota have also emerged as key factors in the development of autoimmune disease and food allergy. Altered intestinal barrier function permits increased dietary antigen transport across the intestinal barrier and subsequent exposure of these antigens to the mucosal immune system, leading to the development of antigen-specific responses. Healthy intestinal flora contributes to the development of oral tolerance, while exposure to pathogens disrupts immune homeostasis.[32] For example, infants with higher amounts of *E. coli* or *C. difficile* had increased incidence of eczema, recurrent wheeze, or allergic sensitization, while administration of either *Lactobacillus rhamnosus* or *L. reuteri* to pregnant and/or breast-feeding mothers significantly reduced the risk of atopic eczema in their infants compared to mothers receiving placebo.[33,34,35,36]

Our understanding of celiac disease, an autoimmune process triggered by the gluten (gliadin) found in many grains, has also greatly contributed to our knowledge of the mechanisms behind autoimmunity. In a recent article published in *Nature Clinical Practice: Hepatology & Gastroenterology*, the authors outline three conditions required for autoimmune disease development:

- First, a genetic susceptibility exists, allowing the host immune system to recognize, and potentially misinterpret, an environmental antigen presented within the gastrointestinal tract. The role of NOD-like receptors (similar to TLRs) in this process is currently an area of intense research.[37] For example, mutations in NOD-like receptor genes confer an increased risk for Crohn's disease.
- The second condition for autoimmune development is that the host must be exposed to the antigen.
- Finally, the antigen must be presented to the gastrointestinal mucosal immune system, following its paracellular passage from the intestinal lumen to the gut submucosa.

The authors conclude that avoiding triggers and/or restoring intestinal integrity both have the potential to stop an autoimmune process, a very promising conclusion![39] This has been shown conclusively with celiac disease, where the trigger is known; recent research indicates that gliadin may increase susceptibility to type 1 diabetes.[40,41] This suggests that not only patients with celiac, but also those with type 1 diabetes and possibly other autoimmune conditions may benefit from gluten avoidance and a program of intestinal permeability restoration.

Dietary and environmental causes of immune dysfunction

The toxic environmental compounds we are exposed to (in increasing numbers) also impair immune function. For example, polychlorinated biphenyls (PCBs) and other organochlorine compounds have been shown to cause immune dysfunction that leads to development of diseases such as childhood leukemia, non-Hodgkin's lymphoma (NHL), asthma, and *otitis media*.[42] In a recent case-control study based in California, household dust was analyzed for PCB content. In houses where any PCBs were detected, a 2-fold risk was found for acute lymphocytic leukemia, while for those with the highest compared to the lowest exposure, a 3-fold risk was found.[43] Similarly, an increase in organochlorine exposure was also found to increase the risk for NHL, although this effect was modified by polymorphisms in immune-related genes.[44] In addition to organochlorines, many other environmental toxins, especially heavy metals, are thought to contribute to immune dysfunction. For example, mercury is known to elicit both profound immune system activation and loss of self-tolerance.[45] Clearly able to induce and exacerbate autoimmunity in animal models, it is very likely to do likewise in humans (Figure 7.5).[46] Interestingly, garlic extract was shown to prevent some of the immune dysfunction caused by mercury *in vitro*.[47]

Certainly many lifestyle factors affect immune health, including dietary intake and stress. For example, in obese patients, subsets of T-cell

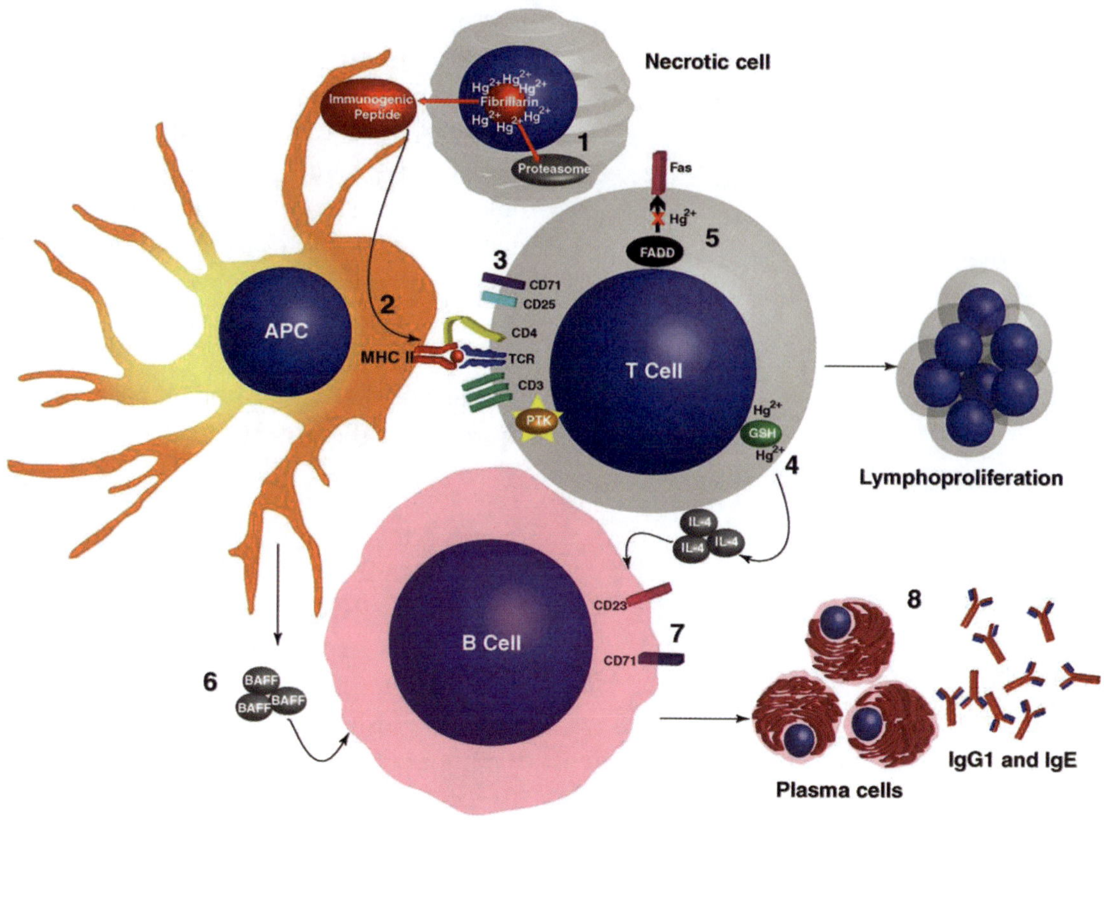

Figure 7.5 Putative mechanisms of mercury-induced autoimmunity. From: Schiraldi M, Monestier M. How can a chemical element elicit complex immunopathology? Lessons from mercury-induced autoimmunity. *Trends Immunol.* 2009 Oct;30(10):502-9. Epub 2009 Aug 24. Reproduced with permission from Elsevier Science & Technology Journals.

populations and their function appear to be reduced, particularly memory T cells. Fortunately, a reduction in BMI among obese individuals restores normal T-cell activity.[48] Other nutritional factors that impact immune function include deficits of vitamin A, vitamin C, and selenium, while an excess of sugar intake has been shown to affect innate immunity.[49] For example, in regions of China where soils are selenium depleted, a cardiomyopathy known as Keshan disease has been attributed to an endemic coxsackievirus. Supplemental selenium not only elevates antiviral immunity, but it also prevents genetic adaptations in the viral genomic RNA that lead to increased virulence and cardiac pathology. Selenium supplementation also appears to reduce cancer rates, induce better host response to viral infections, improve the effects of aging on immunity, and enhance lymphocyte counts and mitogenic responses (Th1).[50] Glucose consumption has been shown to impair monocyte function. In a trial of healthy adults given 75 g of glucose orally, NF-κB binding was shown to increase, as was TNF-alpha expression, both indicators of inflammation and increased viral susceptibility.[51] A review of nearly 40 years of research also found that "acute short-term hyperglycemia affects all major components of innate immunity and impairs the ability of the host to combat infection..." They found that chemotaxis, phagocytosis, and the formation of reactive oxygen species, hallmarks of neutrophil function, were all shown to be depressed in acute hyperglycemia.[52]

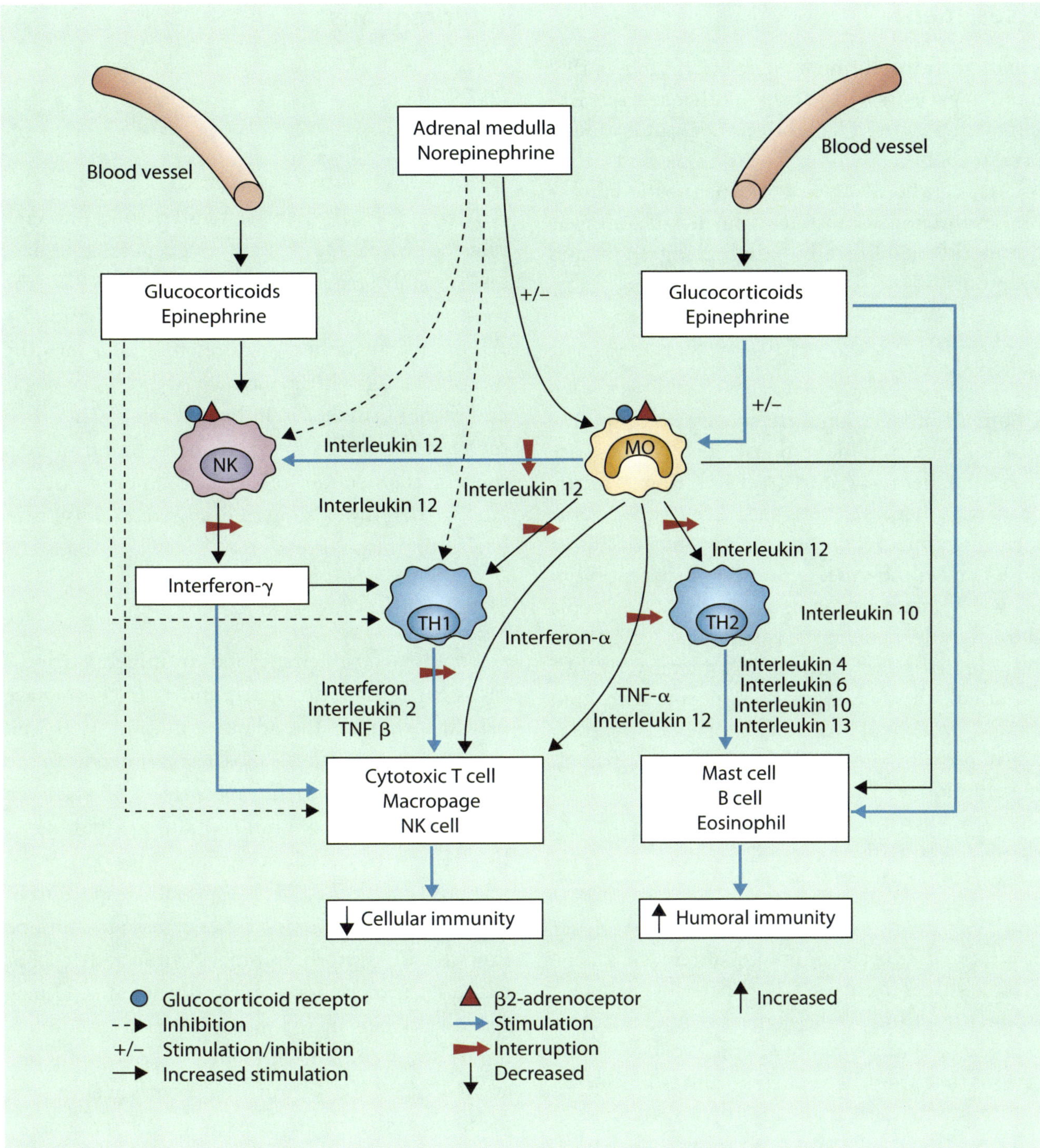

Figure 7.6 Systemic effects of the stress hormones (glucocorticoids and catecholamines) on the immune system. From: Reiche EM, Nunes SO, Morimoto HK, et al. Stress, depression, the immune system, and cancer. *Lancet Oncol.* 2004 Oct;5(10):617-25. Reproduced with permission from Elsevier.

Psychological stress has also been shown to impair immune function, in part via activation of the HPA axis, with a resultant increase in the cortisol/DHEA ratio. As discussed earlier, DHEA is tied to NK cell function.[53] A number of additional cytokines are also released which affect both innate and adaptive immunity (See Figure 7.6). For more information on the role of stress and possible interventions, please consult Clinical Focus 6—Stress, Anxiety, Depression, and Insomnia.

Assessment

Although frank immune deficiency, such as that found in patients with AIDS or other severely immunocompromised conditions, or autoimmune disease such as rheumatoid arthritis and celiac disease, can be detected with diagnostic laboratory evaluations, most assessment of immune dysfunction is clinically based, using signs and symptoms.

Weak innate response or increased susceptibility

A number of symptoms are suggestive of an impaired innate immune response. Among these are frequent upper respiratory tract infections,[54] recurrent warts, herpes,[55] boils or abscesses,[56] chronic tinea infections,[57] and respiratory syncytial virus (RSV) and rhinoviruses.[58] Increased susceptibility to a weak innate response may be found in people whose family members have had cancer[59]; those with chronic stress[53]; those with mercury,[46] DDT and organochlorine exposures[44]; people with high sugar[51,52] or alcohol[60,61] intake; people with regular aspirin use; and individuals with excessive fish oil consumption.[62]

Weak/imbalanced adaptive response or increased susceptibility

Similarly, many symptoms also suggest either an impaired adaptive immune system, or an increased susceptibility to dysfunction. Persistent and recurrent infections suggest that an adaptive response cannot be mounted efficiently, as do infections that progress to more serious conditions.[63] Autoimmune disease is certainly an example of a dysfunctional adaptive process, with B and T cells unable to distinguish self from non-self. Fatigue may be due to impaired adaptive immunity, as a chronic antigenic burden such as CMV depletes reserves.[64,65] Individuals who do not get adequate sleep,[66] have chronic stress, consume excessive alcohol,[61] have a limited and repetitive diet, and those exposed to pesticides, solvents and heavy metals are likely to have an increased susceptibility to dysfunction.[67]

Interventions

General

Diet and physical activity

A Mediterranean diet, particularly one that emphasizes whole foods, fruit and vegetable intake, and possibly fermented foods, appears to have the most significant benefit for immune function.[68,69] As discussed earlier, maintenance of a healthy weight, along with avoidance of excessive sugar and alcohol intake, is indicated for optimal immune function. Exercise has been found to help prevent the decline in immune function associated with aging, although excessive exercise is in itself immunosuppressive.

Supplementation

A broad spectrum multivitamin/mineral is indicated for most individuals, and is likely to have benefit for innate and adaptive immunity, as well as for integrity of physical barriers. A review in the *British Journal of Nutrition* recently highlighted the benefits of a multivitamin containing vitamins A, B6, B12, C, D, E, folic acid, zinc, iron, copper, and selenium (Table 7.2).[70] It is especially important in preventing the age-associated decrease in immune function and restoring proper thymic activity. For example, as mentioned previously, vitamin D may specifically benefit thymus restoration by inhibiting IL-6, a cytokine known to suppress thymic activity. Zinc and arginine have both been shown to induce thymic regrowth and activation in animal studies.[71] Supplementation of zinc significantly improves immune function in those with even a marginal zinc deficiency; in recent years, it has been established that the activity of virtually all immune cells of both the adaptive and innate systems are modulated by zinc.[72] Additionally, the decline in zinc status with aging is likely a significant contributor to immunosenescence (Figure 7.7).[73]

Table 7.2 Sites of action of micronutrients on the immune system

Epithelial barriers	Cellular immunity	Antibody protection
Vitamin A	Vitamin A	Vitamin A
Vitamin C	Vitamin B_6	Vitamin B_6
Vitamin E	Vitamin B_{12}	Vitamin B_{12}
Zinc	Vitamin C	Vitamin D
	Vitamin D	Vitamin E
	Vitamin E	Folic acid
	Folic acid	Zinc
	Iron	Copper
	Zinc	Selenium
	Copper	
	Selenium	

Selected vitamins and trace elements support immune function by strengthening epithelial barriers and cellular and humoral immune responses. From: Maggini S, Wintergerst ES, Beveridge S, et al. *British Journal of Nutrition*, Volume 98, Supplement S1, October 2007, pp S29-S35. © 2007 The Authors. Reprinted with permission from Cambridge University Press.

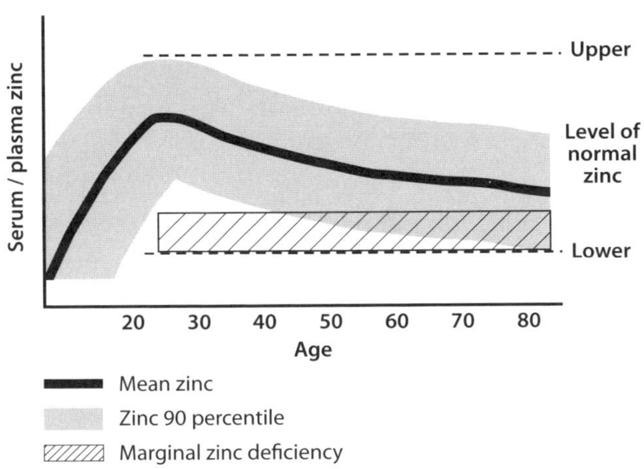

Figure 7.7 Correlation between zinc status and age. From: Haase H, Mocchegiani E, Rink L. Correlation between zinc status and immune function in the elderly. *Biogerontology*. 2006 Oct-Dec;7(5-6):421-8. Reproduced with permission from Springer Science+Business Media.

While it is unclear whether melatonin has a direct effect on thymus tissue, this hormone does appear to offer significant benefit to an aging immune system. It stimulates the production of both innate and adaptive immune cells, including progenitor cells for granulocytes and macrophages, as well as natural killer cells and CD4+ cells. Additionally, the production and release of various cytokines from natural killer cells and T-helper lymphocytes are enhanced by melatonin.[74,75]

NAC supplementation resulted in a significant decrease in the frequency of influenza-like episodes, severity, and length of time confined to bed.[76] A recent *in vitro* trial found NAC to significantly inhibit viral replication of a highly pathogenic influenza strain (H5N1).[77]

Vitamin C is certainly a vital nutrient for immune function. While a Cochrane review found that supplemental vitamin C does not reduce the incidence of the common cold, it was found to reduce the duration. Additionally, populations engaging in significant physical exercise or living in cold environments did show a 50% reduction in incidence.[78] In another study, a dose of 1000 mg per hour for 6 hours, followed by 1000 mg three times per day, at the onset of cold and flu symptoms resulted in a decrease of 85% in symptoms compared with the control group.[79]

Omega-3 fatty acids

Omega-3 supplementation is also an important consideration as long-chain omega-3 fatty acids have a role in preventing excess inflammation associated with immune activity. Clinical benefit has been shown when fish oil was given along with other supportive treatments for the prevention of *otitis media*, upper respiratory tract infection, and mortality and hospital length of stay in critically ill patients.[80,81,82]

Restoration of protective membranes

The first points of contact for many infections are the membranes that separate us from the external environment, such as the linings of the respiratory, urogenital, and gastrointestinal tracts. Damage from frequent infections, NSAID use, smoke exposure, or poor air quality may all increase the risk of future and persistent infections. Interventions that restore membrane integrity and/or prevent pathogen adhesion help to address this pathology.

To improve intestinal integrity it is important to eliminate aggravating factors, such as NSAID use and food allergies, and provide nutrients that support digestive health, including L-glutamine, quercetin, zinc, and probiotics.[83] Additionally, retinol has been shown to be important for intestinal integrity, indicating a need for sufficient vitamin A.[84] Banana powder protects gastric mucosa, an effect which may prevent NSAID erosion.[85,86]

To block the adhesion of pathogens, there are herbal remedies with established efficacy. Cranberry juice is the best-studied intervention for the prevention of urinary tract infections (UTIs).[87] A Cochrane review found that cranberry products significantly reduced the incidence of UTIs at 12 months (35%) compared with placebo/control,[88] an effect attributed to its prevention of bacterial adherence.[89] Similarly, green and black teas have been shown to prevent adhesion of *Bordetella pertussis in vitro*,[90] and berberine prevents adherence of *Streptococcus pyogenes* to epithelial cells and uropathogenic *Escherichia coli* to erythrocytes and epithelial cells.[91,92] For more information see Clinical Focus 2—Digestive Health.

Stimulate production of immune mediators

The most popular botanical approach to enhancing immune function is the use of *Echinacea* spp. While a recent review of 14 trials published in *The Lancet Infectious Disease* reported that echinacea decreased the odds of developing the common cold by 58% and the duration of a cold by 1.4 days, the review noted that results from trial with echinacea have been inconsistent.[93] Mixed results are most likely due to lack of or insufficient quantity of active compounds. The axiom for effectiveness of any herbal product is its ability to deliver an effective dosage of active compounds. If the product, by chance, had sufficient levels of active compounds, it would be effective. If not, it would likely be no more effective than a placebo. For example, in one double-blind study 160 subjects were given either echinacea or placebo and then exposed to a common cold virus. Infection occurred in 44 and 57% and illness occurred in 36 and 43% of the echinacea- and placebo-treated subjects, respectively. However, the preparation contained no echinacosides or alkamides and contained only 0.16% cichoric acid.[94]

In contrast, in a clinical trial using a well-defined echinacea extract containing alkamides, cichoric acid, and polysaccharides at concentrations of 0.25, 2.5, and 25 mg/ml, respectively, prepared from freshly harvested *Echinacea purpurea* plants, showed excellent results.[95] In this randomized, double-blind, placebo-controlled trial, 282 subjects 18–65 years old with a history of two or more colds in the previous year, but otherwise in good health, were randomized to receive either echinacea extract or placebo. They were instructed to start the echinacea or placebo at the onset of the first symptom related to a cold, consuming 10 doses the first day and four doses per day on subsequent days for 7 days. Severity of symptoms (10-point scale: 0, minimum; 9, maximum) and dosing were recorded daily. A nurse examined the subjects on the mornings of days 3 and 8 of their cold. A total of 128 subjects contracted a common cold (59 echinacea, 69 placebo).

The total daily symptom scores were found to be 23.1% lower in the echinacea group than in the placebo group. Throughout the treatment period, the response rate to treatments was greater in the echinacea group. This study indicated that early intervention with a standardized formulation of echinacea resulted in reduced symptom severity in subjects with naturally acquired upper respiratory tract infection.

Other herbs and nutrients have also shown the ability to stimulate immune function. Licorice root (*Glycyrrhiza glabra*) reduced hepatocellular damage in chronic hepatitis B and C in humans, and, in animal studies, demonstrated a reduction of mortality and viral activity in herpes simplex virus, encephalitis, and influenza A virus pneumonia.[96] These antiviral effects have been attributed to its induction of interferon-gamma in T cells, among other mechanisms. Garlic has been found to increase IL-2 production, tumor necrosis factor-alpha, and interferon-gamma, and to enhance natural killer cell, killer cell and lymphokine-activated killer cell activity.[97,98] Astragalus enhances T-cell deficits found among cancer patients, as well as NK cell activity, and, in animal studies, has demonstrated immunorestorative effects attributed to an increase in IL-2.[99,100] Other herbs with immune-stimulating properties include Shiitake mushroom (*Lentinus edodes*),[101] and Korean ginseng (*Panax ginseng*).[102]

Extracts of the herb elderberry have also recently been shown to be very clinically effective. By increasing a number of immune-related cytokines,[103] it relieved symptoms caused by influenza infection an average of 4 days earlier compared to placebo.[104] A very recent study also found that it binds to and inhibits H1N1 virus with similar efficacy to the known anti-influenza activities of Oseltamivir (Tamiflu) and Amantadine, *in vitro*.[105]

The steroid DHEA has been shown to improve immune function in patients of advanced age, perhaps due to an increase in IGF-1.[106] As mentioned above, it may restore specific deficits in NK cells as well.

Increase white cell phagocytosis

The immune-enhancing property of many herbs has also been attributed to an increase in white blood cell phagocytosis. This includes *Echinacea spp*,[107] Shiitake mushroom (*Lentinus edodes*),[108] goldenseal (*Hydrastis canadensis*), garlic (*Allium sativum*),[109] and North American ginseng (*Panax quinquefolius*). For example, North American ginseng has been shown to increase phagocytosis, as well as a number of cytokines that stimulate NK cell and adaptive immune function. In a placebo-controlled trial of over 300 individuals, an extract of this herb was found to lower the mean number of colds per person, the percentage of patients with two or more colds during the trial, overall cold symptoms, and total number of days with a cold.[110]

Similarly, garlic supplementation resulted in significantly fewer colds and quicker recovery compared to placebo.[111]

References

1. Basset C, Holton J, O'Mahony R, et al. Innate immunity and pathogen-host interaction. *Vaccine.* 2003 Jun 1;21 Suppl 2:S12-23.
2. Martinon F, Mayor A, Tschopp J. The inflammasomes: guardians of the body. *Annu Rev Immunol.* 2009;27:229-65.
3. Martinon F, Pétrilli V, Mayor A, et al. Gout-associated uric acid crystals activate the NALP3 inflammasome. *Nature.* 2006 Mar 9;440(7081):237-41.
4. Pétrilli V, Martinon F. The inflammasome, autoinflammatory diseases, and gout. *Joint Bone Spine.* 2007 Dec;74(6):571-6.
5. Kumar H, Kawai T, Akira S. Toll-like receptors and innate immunity. *Biochem Biophys Res Commun.* 2009 Oct 30;388(4):621-5.
6. Adams JS, Ren S, Liu PT. Vitamin D-directed rheostatic regulation of monocyte antibacterial responses. *J Immunol.* 2009 Apr 1;182(7):4289-95.
7. Jordan JL, Nowak A, Lee TD. Activation of innate immunity to reduce lung metastases in breast cancer. *Cancer Immunol Immunother.* 2009 Dec 3.
8. Jordan JL, Sullivan AM, Lee TD. Immune activation by a sterile aqueous extract of *Cordyceps sinensis*: mechanism of action. *Immunopharmacol Immunotoxicol.* 2008;30(1):53-70.
9. Parkin J, Cohen B. An overview of the immune system. *Lancet.* 2001 Jun 2;357(9270):1777-89.
10. Palm NW, Medzhitov R. Pattern recognition receptors and control of adaptive immunity. *Immunol Rev.* 2009 Jan;227(1):221-33.
11. Sun JC, Lanier LL. Natural killer cells remember: an evolutionary bridge between innate and adaptive immunity? *Eur J Immunol.* 2009 Aug;39(8):2059-64.
12. Sun JC, Beilke JN, Lanier LL. Adaptive immune features of natural killer cells. *Nature.* 2009 Jan 29;457(7229): 557-61.
13. Ahmad SM, Haskell MJ, Raqib R, et al. Markers of innate immune function are associated with vitamin A stores in men. *J Nutr.* 2009 Feb;139(2):377-85.
14. Yu S, Cantorna MT. The vitamin D receptor is required for iNKT cell development. *Proc Natl Acad Sci U S A.* 2008 Apr 1;105(13):5207-12.
15. Schillace RV, Pisenti N, Pattamanuch N. Lipoic acid stimulates cAMP production in T lymphocytes and NK cells. *Biochem Biophys Res Commun.* 2007 Mar 2;354(1):259-64.
16. Mocchegiani E, Giacconi R, Cipriano C, et al. NK and NKT cells in aging and longevity: role of zinc and metallothioneins. *J Clin Immunol.* 2009 Jul;29(4):416-25.
17. Solerte SB, Precerutti S, Gazzaruso C, et al. Defect of a subpopulation of natural killer immune cells in Graves' disease and Hashimoto's thyroiditis: normalizing effect of dehydroepiandrosterone sulfate. *Eur J Endocrinol.* 2005 May;152(5):703-12.
18. Candore G, Balistreri CR, Colonna-Romano G. Immunosenescence and anti-immunosenescence therapies: the case of probiotics. *Rejuvenation Res.* 2008 Apr; 11(2):425-32.
19. Gill HS, Rutherfurd KJ, Cross ML. Dietary probiotic supplementation enhances natural killer cell activity in the elderly: an investigation of age-related immunological changes. *J Clin Immunol.* 2001 Jul;21(4):264-71.
20. Capri M, Monti D, Salvioli S, et al. Complexity of anti-immunosenescence strategies in humans. *Artif Organs.* 2006 Oct;30(10):730-42.
21. Panda A, Arjona A, Sapey E, et al. Human innate immunosenescence: causes and consequences for immunity in old age. *Trends Immunol.* 2009 Jul;30(7):325-33.
22. Senchina DS, Kohut ML. Immunological outcomes of exercise in older adults. *Clin Interv Aging.* 2007;2(1):3-16.
23. van Tongeren SP, Slaets JP, Harmsen HJ, et al. Fecal microbiota composition and frailty. *Appl Environ Microbiol* 2005;71:6438-42.
24. Gorjão R, Azevedo-Martins AK, Rodrigues HG, et al. Comparative effects of DHA and EPA on cell function. *Pharmacol Ther.* 2009 Apr;122(1):56-64.
25. Watson RR, Zibadi S, Vazquez R, et al. Nutritional regulation of immunosenescence for heart health. *J Nutr Biochem.* 2005 Feb;16(2):85-7.
26. Passeri G, Pini G, Troiano L, et al. Low vitamin D status, high bone turnover, and bone fractures in centenarians. *J Clin Endocrinol Metab.* 2003 Nov;88(11):5109-15.
27. Bikle DD. Vitamin D and the immune system: role in protection against bacterial infection. *Curr Opin Nephrol Hypertens.* 2008 Jul;17(4):348-52.
28. Adorini L, Penna G. Control of autoimmune diseases by the vitamin D endocrine system. *Nat Clin Pract Rheumatol.* 2008 Aug;4(8):404-12.
29. Hyppönen E, Läärä E, Reunanen A, et al. Intake of vitamin D and risk of type 1 diabetes: a birth-cohort study. *Lancet.* 2001 Nov 3;358(9292):1500-3.
30. Devaraj S, Dasu MR, Rockwood J, et al. Increased toll-like receptor (TLR) 2 and (TLR)4 expression in monocytes from patients with type 1 diabetes: further evidence of a proinflammatory state. *J Clin Endocrinol Metab.* 2008 Feb;93(2):578-83.
31. Du T, Zhou ZG, You S, et al. Regulation by 1, 25-dihydroxy-vitamin D3 on altered TLRs expression and response to ligands of monocyte from autoimmune diabetes. *Clin Chim Acta.* 2009 Apr;402(1-2):133-8.
32. Edelman SM, Kasper DL. Symbiotic commensal bacteria direct maturation of the host immune system. *Curr Opin Gastroenterol.* 2008 Nov;24(6):720-4.
33. Penders J, Thijs C, van den Brandt PA, et al. Gut microbiota composition and development of atopic manifestations in infancy: the KOALA Birth Cohort Study. *Gut.* 2007 May;56(5):661-7. Epub 2006 Oct 17.

34. Rautava S, Kalliomäki M, Isolauri E. Probiotics during pregnancy and breast-feeding might confer immunomodulatory protection against atopic disease in the infant. *J Allergy Clin Immunol.* 2002 Jan;109(1):119-21.

35. Böttcher MF, Abrahamsson TR, Fredriksson M, et al. Low breast milk TGF-beta2 is induced by *Lactobacillus reuteri* supplementation and associates with reduced risk of sensitization during infancy. *Pediatr Allergy Immunol.* 2008 Sep;19(6):497-504.

36. Wickens K, Black PN, Stanley TV, et al. A differential effect of 2 probiotics in the prevention of eczema and atopy: a double-blind, randomized, placebo-controlled trial. *J Allergy Clin Immunol.* 2008 Oct;122(4):788-94.

37. Rosenstiel P, Schreiber S. NOD-like receptors—pivotal guardians of the immunological integrity of barrier organs. *Adv Exp Med Biol.* 2009;653:35-47.

38. Strober W, Kitani A, Fuss I, et al. The molecular basis of NOD2 susceptibility mutations in Crohn's disease. *Mucosal Immunol.* 2008 Nov;1 Suppl 1:S5-9.

39. Fasano A, Shea-Donohue T. Mechanisms of disease: the role of intestinal barrier function in the pathogenesis of gastrointestinal autoimmune diseases. *Nat Clin Pract Gastroenterol Hepatol.* 2005 Sep;2(9):416-22.

40. Krause I, Anaya JM, Fraser A, et al. Anti-infectious antibodies and autoimmune-associated autoantibodies in patients with type I diabetes mellitus and their close family members. *Ann N Y Acad Sci.* 2009 Sep;1173:633-9.

41. Visser J, Rozing J, Sapone A, et al. Tight junctions, intestinal permeability, and autoimmunity: celiac disease and type 1 diabetes paradigms. *Ann N Y Acad Sci.* 2009 May;1165:195-205.

42. Glynn A, Thuvander A, Aune M. Immune cell counts and risks of respiratory infections among infants exposed pre- and postnatally to organochlorine compounds: a prospective study. *Environ Health.* 2008 Dec 4;7:62.

43. Ward MH, Colt JS, Metayer C, et al. Residential exposure to polychlorinated biphenyls and organochlorine pesticides and risk of childhood leukemia. *Environ Health Perspect.* 2009 Jun;117(6):1007-13.

44. Colt JS, Rothman N, Severson RK, et al. Organochlorine exposure, immune gene variation, and risk of non-Hodgkin lymphoma. *Blood.* 2009 Feb 26;113(9):1899-905. Epub 2008 Dec 9.

45. Schiraldi M, Monestier M. How can a chemical element elicit complex immunopathology? Lessons from mercury-induced autoimmunity. *Trends Immunol.* 2009 Oct;30(10):502-9. Epub 2009 Aug 24.

46. Vas J, Monestier M. Immunology of mercury. *Ann N Y Acad Sci.* 2008 Nov;1143:240-67.

47. Abdalla FH, Bellé LP, De Bona KS, et al. *Allium sativum L.* extract prevents methyl mercury-induced cytotoxicity in peripheral blood leukocytes (LS). *Food Chem Toxicol.* 2009 Oct 29. Epub ahead of print.

48. Tanaka S, Isoda F, Ishihara Y, et al. T lymphopaenia in relation to body mass index and TNF-alpha in human obesity: adequate weight reduction can be corrective. *Clin Endocrinol* (Oxf). 2001 Mar;54(3):347-54.

49. Wang C, Wang H, Luo J, et al. Selenium deficiency impairs host innate immune response and induces susceptibility to *Listeria monocytogenes* infection. *BMC Immunol.* 2009 Oct 24;10:55.

50. Hoffmann PR, Berry MJ. The influence of selenium on immune responses. *Mol Nutr Food Res.* 2008 Nov;52(11):1273-80.

51. Aljada A, Friedman J, Ghanim H, et al. Glucose ingestion induces an increase in intranuclear nuclear factor kappaB, a fall in cellular inhibitor kappaB, and an increase in tumor necrosis factor alpha messenger RNA by mononuclear cells in healthy human subjects. *Metabolism.* 2006 Sep;55(9):1177-85.

52. Turina M, Fry DE, Polk HC Jr. Acute hyperglycemia and the innate immune system: clinical, cellular, and molecular aspects. *Crit Care Med.* 2005 Jul;33(7):1624-33.

53. Bauer ME, Jeckel CM, Luz C. The role of stress factors during aging of the immune system. *Ann N Y Acad Sci.* 2009 Feb;1153:139-52.

54. Don M, Fasoli L, Gregorutti V, et al. Recurrent respiratory infections and phagocytosis in childhood. *Pediatr Int.* 2007 Feb;49(1):40-7.

55. Peng T, Zhu J, Klock A, et al. Evasion of the mucosal innate immune system by herpes simplex virus type 2. *J Virol.* 2009 Dec;83(23):12559-68.

56. Levy R, Shriker O, Porath A, et al. Vitamin C for the treatment of recurrent furunculosis in patients with imparied neutrophil functions. *J Infect Dis.* 1996 Jun;173(6):1502-5.

57. Di Silverio A, Zeccara C, Serra F. Specific and non-specific parameters of the host defence system in patients with superficial fungal infections. *Mycoses.* 1995 Nov-Dec;38(11-12):453-8.

58. Halfhide C, Smyth RL. Innate immune response and bronchiolitis and preschool recurrent wheeze. *Paediatr Respir Rev.* 2008 Dec;9(4):251-62. Epub 2008 Oct 23.

59. Stein QP, Flanagan JD. Genetic and familial factors influencing breast, colon, prostate and lung cancers. *S D Med.* 2010;Spec No:16-22.

60. Happel KI, Nelson S. Alcohol, immunosuppression, and the lung. *Proc Am Thorac Soc.* 2005;2(5):428-32.

61. Szabo G, Mandrekar P. A recent perspective on alcohol, immunity, and host defense. *Alcohol Clin Exp Res.* 2009 Feb;33(2):220-32.

62. Kelley DS. Modulation of human immune and inflammatory responses by dietary fatty acids. *Nutrition.* 2001 Jul-Aug;17(7-8):669-73.

63. Wingate PJ, McAulay KA, Anthony IC. Regulatory T cell activity in primary and persistent Epstein-Barr virus infection. *J Med Virol.* 2009 May;81(5):870-7.

64. Mihaylova I, DeRuyter M, Rummens JL, et al. Decreased expression of CD69 in chronic fatigue syndrome in relation to inflammatory markers: evidence for a severe disorder in the early activation of T lymphocytes and natural killer cells. *Neuro Endocrinol Lett.* 2007 Aug;28(4):477-83.
65. Lorusso L, Mikhaylova SV, Capelli E. Immunological aspects of chronic fatigue syndrome. *Autoimmun Rev.* 2009 Feb;8(4):287-91.
66. Lange T, Dimitrov S, Fehm HL, et al. Shift of monocyte function toward cellular immunity during sleep. *Arch Intern Med.* 2006 Sep 18;166(16):1695-700.
67. Duramad P, Tager IB, Holland NT. Cytokines and other immunological biomarkers in children's environmental health studies. *Toxicol Lett.* 2007 Jul 30;172(1-2):48-59.
68. Schoen C, Schulz A, Schweikart J, et al. Regulatory effects of a fermented food concentrate on immune function parameters in healthy volunteers. *Nutrition.* 2009 May;25(5):499-505. Epub 2009 Jan 3.
69. Li L, Werler MM. Fruit and vegetable intake and risk of upper respiratory tract infection in pregnant women. *Public Health Nutr.* 2009 Jun 25:1-7.
70. Maggini S, Wintergerst ES, Beveridge S, et al. Selected vitamins and trace elements support immune function by strengthening epithelial barriers and cellular and humoral immune responses. *Br J Nutr.* 2007 Oct;98 Suppl 1:S29-35.
71. Mocchegiani E, Santarelli L, Costarelli L, et al. Plasticity of neuroendocrine-thymus interactions during ontogeny and ageing: role of zinc and arginine. *Ageing Res Rev.* 2006 Aug;5(3):281-309. Epub 2006 Aug 14.
72. Haase H, Rink L. Functional significance of zinc-related signaling pathways in immune cells. *Annu Rev Nutr.* 2009;29:133-52.
73. Haase H, Mocchegiani E, Rink L. Correlation between zinc status and immune function in the elderly. *Biogerontology.* 2006 Oct-Dec;7(5-6):421-8.
74. Cardinali DP, Esquifino AI, Srinivasan V, et al. Melatonin and the immune system in aging. *Neuroimmunomodulation.* 2008;15(4-6):272-8. Epub 2008 Nov 26.
75. Srinivasan V, Spence DW, Trakht I, et al. Immunomodulation by melatonin: its significance for seasonally occurring diseases. *Neuroimmunomodulation.* 2008; 15(2):93-101. Epub 2008 Aug 5.
76. De Flora S, Grassi C, Carati L. Attenuation of influenza-like symptomatology and improvement of cell-mediated immunity with long-term N-acetylcysteine treatment. *Eur Respir J.* 1997 Jul;10(7):1535-41.
77. Geiler J, Michaelis M, Naczk P, et al. N-acetyl-L-cysteine (NAC) inhibits virus replication and expression of pro-inflammatory molecules in A549 cells infected with highly pathogenic H5N1 influenza A virus. *Biochem Pharmacol.* 2010 Feb 1;79(3):413-20. Epub 2009 Sep 2.
78. Douglas RM, Hemilä H, Chalker E, et al. Vitamin C for preventing and treating the common cold. *Cochrane Database Syst Rev.* 2007 Jul 18;(3):CD000980.
79. Gorton HC, Jarvis K. The effectiveness of vitamin C in preventing and relieving the symptoms of virus-induced respiratory infections. *J Manipulative Physiol Ther.* 1999 Oct;22(8):530-3.
80. Linday LA, Shindledecker RD, Tapia-Mendoza J, et al. Effect of daily cod liver oil and a multivitamin-mineral supplement with selenium on upper respiratory tract pediatric visits by young, inner-city, Latino children: randomized pediatric sites. *Ann Otol Rhinol Laryngol.* 2004 Nov;113(11):891-901.
81. Linday LA, Dolitsky JN, Shindledecker RD, et al. Lemon-flavored cod liver oil and a multivitamin-mineral supplement for the secondary prevention of *Otitis media* in young children: pilot research. *Ann Otol Rhinol Laryngol.* 2002 Jul;111(7 Pt 1):642-52.
82. Marik PE, Zaloga GP. Immunonutrition in critically ill patients: a systematic review and analysis of the literature. *Intensive Care Med.* 2008 Nov;34(11):1980-90. Epub 2008 Jul 15.
83. Chen P, Soares AM, Lima AA. Association of vitamin A and zinc status with altered intestinal permeability: analyses of cohort data from northeastern Brazil. *J Health Popul Nutr.* 2003 Dec;21(4):309-15.
84. Quadro L, Gamble MV, Vogel S, et al. Retinol and retinol-binding protein: gut integrity and circulating immunoglobulins. *J Infect Dis.* 2000 Sep;182 Suppl 1:S97-S102.
85. Mukhopadhyaya K, Bhattacharya D, Chakraborty A, et al. Effect of banana powder (*Musa sapientum var. paradisiaca*) on gastric mucosal shedding. *J Ethnopharmacol.* 1987 Sep-Oct;21(1):11-9.
86. Lewis DA, Fields WN, Shaw GP. A natural flavonoid present in unripe plantain banana pulp (*Musa sapientum L. var. paradisiaca*) protects the gastric mucosa from aspirin-induced erosions. *J Ethnopharmacol.* 1999 Jun; 65(3):283-8.
87. Pérez-López FR, Haya J, Chedraui P. *Vaccinium macrocarpon*: an interesting option for women with recurrent urinary tract infections and other health benefits. *J Obstet Gynaecol Res.* 2009 Aug;35(4):630-9.
88. Jepson RG, Craig JC. Cranberries for preventing urinary tract infections. *Cochrane Database Syst Rev.* 2008 Jan 23;(1):CD001321.
89. Pinzón-Arango PA, Liu Y, Camesano TA. Role of cranberry on bacterial adhesion forces and implications for *Escherichia coli*-uroepithelial cell attachment. *J Med Food.* 2009 Apr;12(2):259-70.
90. Horiuchi Y, Toda M, Okubo S, et al. Protective activity of tea and catechins against *Bordetella pertussis*. *Kansenshogaku Zasshi.* 1992 May;66(5):599-605.
91. Sun D, Abraham SN, Beachey EH. Berberine sulphate blocks adherence of *Streptococcus pyogenes* to epithelial cells, fibronectin and hexadecane. *Agents Chemother.* 32:1370-4, 1988.

92. Sun D, Abraham SN, Beachey EH. Influence of berberine sulfate on synthesis and expression of Pap fimbrial adhesin in uropathogenic *Escherichia coli. Antimicrob Agents Chemother.* 1988 Aug;32(8):1274-7.

93. Shah SA, Sander S, White CM. Evaluation of echinacea for the prevention and treatment of the common cold: a meta-analysis. *Lancet Infect Dis.* 2007 Jul;7(7):473-80.

94. Turner RB, Riker DK, Gangemi JD. Ineffectiveness of echinacea for prevention of experimental rhinovirus colds. *Antimicrob Agents Chemother* 2000;44:1708-1709.

95. Goel V, Lovlin R, Barton R, et al. Efficacy of a standardized echinacea preparation (Echinilin) for the treatment of the common cold: a randomized, double-blind, placebo-controlled trial. *J Clin Pharm Ther.* 2004;29:75-83.

96. Fiore C, Eisenhut M, Krausse R, et al. Antiviral effects of Glycyrrhiza species. *Phytother Res.* 2008 Feb;22(2):141-8.

97. Morioka N, Sze LL, Morton DL, et al. A protein fraction from aged garlic extract enhances cytotoxicity and proliferation of human lymphocytes mediated by interleukin-2 and conconavalin *Cancer Immunol Immunother.* 1993 Oct;37(5):316-22.

98. Lamm DL, Riggs DR. Enhanced immunocompetence by garlic: role in bladder cancer and other malignancies. *J Nutr.* 2001 Mar;131(3s):1067S-70S.

99. Cho WC, Leung KN. *In vitro* and *in vivo* anti-tumor effects of *Astragalus membranaceus. Cancer Lett.* 2007 Jul 8;252(1):43-54. Epub 2007 Jan 16.

100. Cho WC, Leung KN. *In vitro* and *in vivo* immunomodulating and immunorestorative effects of *Astragalus membranaceus. J Ethnopharmacol.* 2007 Aug 15;113(1): 132-41.

101. Lee HH, Lee JS, Cho JY, et al. Study on immunostimulating activity of macrophage treated with purified polysaccharides from liquid culture and fruiting body of *Lentinus edodes. J Microbiol Biotechnol.* 2009 Jun;19(6): 566-72.

102. Kim MH, Byon YY, Ko EJ, et al. Immunomodulatory activity of ginsan, a polysaccharide of *panax ginseng*, on dendritic cells. *Korean J Physiol Pharmacol.* 2009 Jun;13(3): 169-73.

103. Barak V, Birkenfeld S, Halperin T, et al. The effect of herbal remedies on the production of human inflammatory and anti-inflammatory cytokines. *Isr Med Assoc J.* 2002 Nov;4(11 Suppl):919-22.

104. Zakay-Rones Z, Thom E, Wollan T, et al. Randomized study of the efficacy and safety of oral elderberry extract in the treatment of influenza A and B virus infections. *J Int Med Res.* 2004 Mar-Apr;32(2):132-40.

105. Roschek B Jr, Fink RC, McMichael MD, et al. Elderberry flavonoids bind to and prevent H1N1 infection *in vitro. Phytochemistry.* 2009 Jul;70(10):1255-61.

106. Khorram O, Vu L, Yen SS. Activation of immune function by dehydroepiandrosterone (DHEA) in age-advanced men. *J Gerontol A Biol Sci Med Sci.* 1997 Jan;52(1):M1-7.

107. Groom SN, Johns T, Oldfield PR. The potency of immunomodulatory herbs may be primarily dependent upon macrophage activation. *J Med Food.* 2007 Mar;10(1):73-9.

108. Lee HH, Lee JS, Cho JY, et al. Structural characteristics of immunostimulating polysaccharides from *Lentinus edodes. J Microbiol Biotechnol.* 2009 May;19(5):455-61.

109. Ghazanfari T, Hassan ZM, Khamesipour A. Enhancement of peritoneal macrophage phagocytic activity against Leishmania major by garlic (*Allium sativum*) treatment. *J Ethnopharmacol.* 2006 Feb 20;103(3):333-7. Epub 2005 Oct 5.

110. Predy GN, Goel V, Lovlin R, et al. Efficacy of an extract of North American ginseng containing poly-furanosyl-pyranosyl-saccharides for preventing upper respiratory tract infections: a randomized controlled trial. *CMAJ.* 2005 Oct 25;173(9):1043-8.

111. Josling P. Preventing the common cold with a garlic supplement: a double-blind, placebo-controlled survey. *Adv Ther.* 2001 Jul-Aug;18(4):189-93.

Endocrine Balance

Overview

Most metabolic processes are regulated by the endocrine system, ranging from the thyroid's control of the metabolic rate to the regulation of glucose metabolism by the pancreas. Given the potency of even small amounts of the hormones secreted by all endocrine organs and the tight control required for optimal function, endocrine imbalances are fairly common, affecting 25–50% of adults.[1,2] This susceptibility to dysfunction is often due to nutritional deficiencies and excesses, reduced physical activity, lifestyle factors, and increasingly to environmental toxins. This chapter reviews the epidemiology, etiology, and assessment of some common endocrine dysfunctions, as well as clinically effective treatments to restore optimal endocrine function.

Thyroid

Hypothyroidism

Hypothyroidism is characterized by reduced thyroid hormone production and/or effect, which effectively lowers cellular metabolism throughout the body. Thyroid hormones regulate the rate of metabolic function of most tissues, in part by increasing the number and size of mitochondria, and by inducing transcription of enzymes of the respiratory chain and membrane Na+-K+ ATPase. Most actions of thyroid hormones result from the interaction of nuclear thyroid hormone receptors that have a preferential affinity for T3 and their specific target gene promoters.[3]

Epidemiology and etiology

Thyroid disorders are the second most common endocrine disorder after diabetes.[2] The prevalence of hypothyroidism is typically cited as ranging from 1–10% of adults, but this range depends on the criteria used. Data analysis from the National Health and Nutrition Examination Survey (NHANES 1999–2002) found the prevalence of TSH >4.5 mIU/l to be 3.7%, although individuals aged 80 years or more had 5 times greater odds for hypothyroidism than those aged 12–49.[1]

Primary hypothyroidism occurs when thyroid failure results from disease of the thyroid gland itself, and it accounts for more than 99% of all cases of hypothyroidism. The most common cause of primary hypothyroidism is chronic autoimmune thyroiditis (Hashimoto's disease)[3]; most other causes are iatrogenic, including surgical removal of the thyroid gland, thyroid gland ablation or irradiation, or drugs such as lithium, amiodarone, or α-interferon. Secondary causes of hypothyroidism include pituitary and hypothalamic disease.[3]

Thyroid hormone regulation

The regulation of the thyroid gland is dependent on the negative feedback loop between the hypothalamus, anterior pituitary, and the thyroid gland (Figure 8.1), and in some cases this regulatory system fails.[4] This can be explained in part by the different rates at which T4 is converted intracellularly to T3 in different locations.[5]

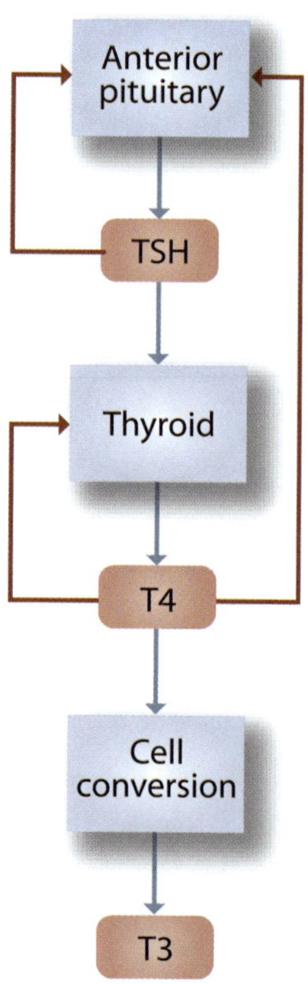

Figure 8.1 Negative feedback loop between the hypothalamus, anterior pituitary, and the thyroid.

The negative feedback of thyroid hormones primarily reduces the response of pituitary thyrotrophs to TRH, and to a lesser degree reduces the secretion rate of TRH. The sensitivity of the thyrotrophs to TRH depends not only on circulating levels of T4, but more so on the intracellular level of T3 in the pituitary, 80% of which is from the intrapituitary conversion of the prohormone T4.[3] Additionally, T4 is also taken up by hypothalamic glial cells, converted to T3, and then transported to the TRH-producing neurons in the paraventricular nucleus (PVN).[6] Thus, in both the pituitary and the hypothalamus, the local conversion of T4 to T3 is what determines the set-point for TRH and TSH secretion, and the local conversion may not reflect more systemic levels.[7] In both of these tissues, T3 content is largely determined by local deiodinase type 2 (D2) activity,[8] while in many other tissues throughout the body, including the liver (the main site of T3 production), kidney, and intestines, deiodinase type 1 is responsible for the conversion (see Figure 8.2 for role of D2 in TSH feedback). Thus if the pituitary conversion of T4 to T3 by D2 is more efficient than the conversion in other tissues, those cells may experience a local hypothyroidism, regardless of the TSH and free T4 levels.[9]

Sources of thyroid disruption

Thyroid activity can be affected by a number of mechanisms, including decreased TSH and/or T4 production, poor or inconsistent (between different tissues) conversion of T4 to T3, and reduced cellular response to T3. For example, stress of various types appears to inhibit TSH production, possibly due to the inhibition of the pituitary's response to TRH.[10,11,12]

Toxins

Environmental factors play a significant role in thyroid disruption. Cadmium has been shown to reduce TSH levels,[13] although this effect is completely blunted in animals given zinc and selenium.[14] Analysis of NHANES 1999–2002 data revealed a dose-dependent decrease in total T4 among US adults with exposure to dioxin-like

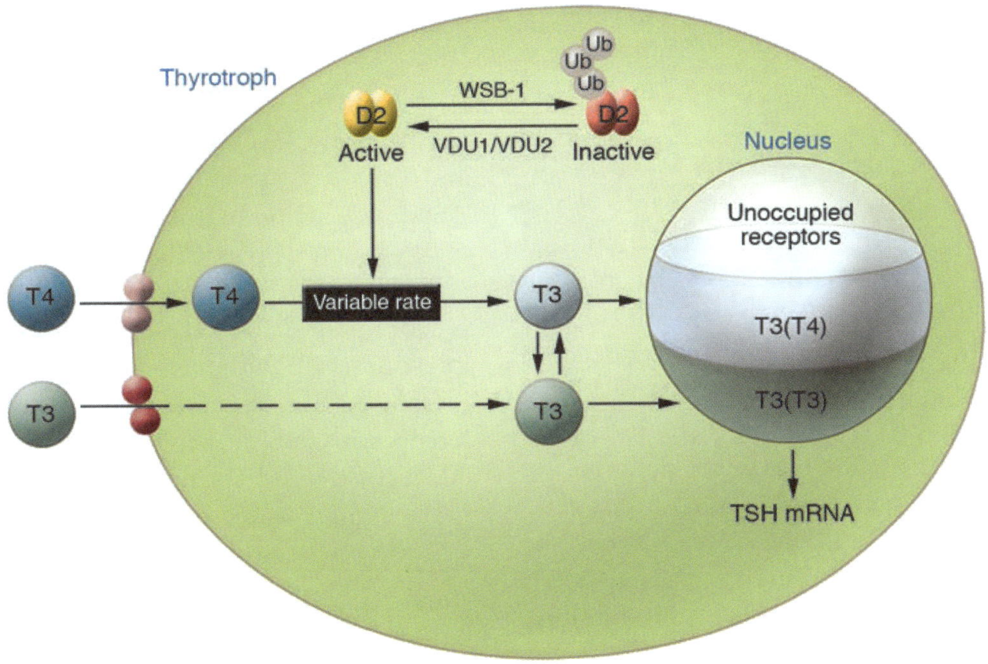

Figure 8.2 Role of D2 in TSH feedback. From: Bianco AC, Kim BW. Deiodinases: implications of the local control of thyroid hormone action. *J Clin Invest.* 2006 Oct;116(10):2571-9. Reproduced with permission from the American Society for Clinical Investigation.

toxic equivalents (TEQs) at levels similar to those found in the general U.S. population. The association was greater among women and the elderly.[15] Also, animal data suggest that thyroid hormone disrupting chemicals may work by different mechanisms and, when combined, may have synergistic effects.[16,17,18,19] Figure 8.3 shows the impact of many environmental toxins, such as PCBs, pesticides and bisphenol A, on thyroid hormone physiology.

Iodine

Inadequate availability of iodine has re-emerged as a significant factor in hypothyroidism, leading to a decrease in T4 production. While iodine deficiency is widely recognized as a cause of hypothyroidism in undeveloped countries, the iodization of salt in 1924 was thought to virtually eliminate iodine

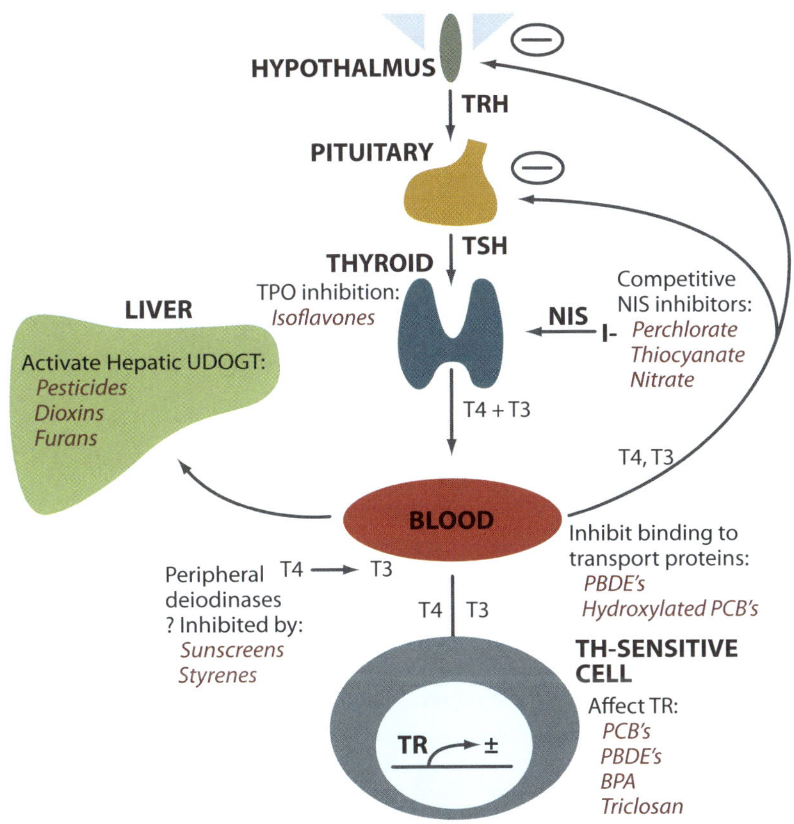

Figure 8.3 Mechanisms of various thyroid disruptors. From: Pearce EN, Braverman LE. Environmental pollutants and the thyroid. *Best Pract Res Clin Endocrinol Metab.* 2009 Dec;23(6):801-13. Review. Reproduced with permission from Elsevier.

deficiency in the United States.[20] However, a recent analysis of NHANES data suggests it is still surprisingly common. A median urinary iodine of 320 mcg/l was reported in the 1970s, but a dramatic drop to 145 mcg/l was found in the 1990s among women of reproductive age.[21] These same data indicated that 14.9% of women in their reproductive years, including 6.9% of pregnant women, have urinary iodine levels <50 mcg/l.[21] Currently, the American Thyroid Association recommends supplemental iodine intake of 150 ug during pregnancy and lactation in both Canada and the U.S., although approximately one-half of prenatal vitamins still do not contain iodine.[20,22] It has been suggested that deficiency has become more common because only 20% of food salt is iodized; with iodization of salt being voluntary in the United States, the majority of salt intake therefore is noniodized.[20]

It has also been hypothesized, but not well established, that a reduced dietary intake of iodine may be an etiological factor in cardiovascular disease, possibly because of its anti-inflammatory, antiproliferative, and antimicrobial properties.[23] In addition to a reduced iodine supply, a number of environmental toxins interfere with its uptake. Perchlorate, thiocyanate, and nitrate are competitive inhibitors of the sodium/iodine symporter (NIS). When present in sufficiently high concentrations, these substances will decrease the active transport of iodine into the thyroid and thereby decrease thyroid hormone synthesis.[24]

Goitrogens

Although rare, excessive consumption of certain foods (goitrogens) may also reduce T4 synthesis. Among these are Brassica foods (broccoli, cauliflower, turnips, cabbage, rutabagas, mustard greens, radishes, and horseradish), cassava root, soybeans, peanuts, pine nuts, and millet. For example consumption of over 30 g soybeans/day inhibits T4 production, due to the inhibition of thyroid peroxidase by genistein and daidzein.[25] This effect of soy is somewhat controversial in someone not taking thyroid medication, because the main effect of soy is to reduce absorption of exogenous thyroid medication.[26] Also, most goitrogens are rendered inert with cooking.[27]

As mentioned above, poor conversion of T4 to T3 also reduces the cellular effect of thyroid hormone, and this may partly be due to the variability in deiodinase action in different tissues. For example methylmercury, particularly when combined with an iodine or selenium deficiency, inhibits D1, the predominant deiodinase in the liver, kidney, and intestines.[28,29,30] Although D2 is the major source for plasma T3 in euthyroid patients,[31] the differences in activity may lead to reduced cellular effects of thyroid hormone in those tissues where D1 is more prevalent.

Interestingly, bile acids have been shown to stimulate D2 activity, and may be a signal for food availability, i.e., when they are secreted in response to food, it is a signal to increase metabolism. This link between nutrition and metabolism may be interrupted in those with poor digestion, particularly insufficient bile acid production.[32,33]

A decreased cellular response to T3 has been attributed to deficiencies of iron and zinc, physical inactivity, and high levels of cytokines produced by fat cells, as occurs in obesity.[34,35] Animal studies have documented arsenic's ability to disrupt thyroid hormone receptor-mediated gene regulation, at very low concentrations, and the plastic monomer bisphenol-A (BPA) has been shown to bind to the thyroid hormone receptor and antagonize its activation.[24,36]

Adrenal

Adrenal hypofunction

Etiology and epidemiology

The adrenal glands are comprised of two different portions—the medulla, which is responsible for producing catecholamines, and the larger cortex, which produces a variety of steroids, including glucocorticoids, mineralocorticoids, and sex hormones. Ultimately, the hypothalamus regulates all aspects of adrenal function. Catecholamine production is primarily regulated by sympathetic outflow from the hypothalamus, while steroidogenesis is directly controlled by ACTH secretion from the pituitary gland, which is in turn controlled by corticotrophin-releasing hormone (CRH) (and arginine vasopressin, or AVP) secretion from the hypothalamus (Figure 8.4). Endogenous cortisol binds to glucocorticoid receptors in the HPA axis, and acts as a potent negative regulator of HPA activity. These regulatory mechanisms are important in determining basal levels and circadian fluctuations in cortisol levels. While a catecholamine deficiency state is quite rare, steroid deficiency states ranging from frank adrenal failure to suboptimal steroid production are found much more frequently.[37]

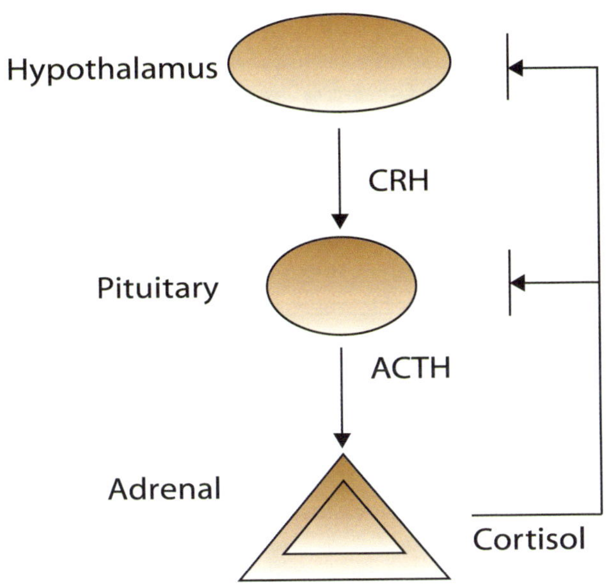

Figure 8.4 Production of ACTH (from the pituitary) and cortisol (from the adrenals), mediated by CRH from the hypothalamus. From: Arlt W, Allolio B. Adrenal insufficiency. *Lancet*. 2003 May 31;361(9372):1881-93. Reproduced with permission from Elsevier.

Addison's disease is a clear example of frank adrenal failure, characterized by insufficient production of all cortex hormones; the disease was life threatening before the introduction of glucocorticoid and mineralocorticoid replacement therapy. With a prevalence of approximately 100 cases per 1 million people in a community setting, it is fairly uncommon.[38] Although other etiologies for primary adrenal failure exist, Addison's disease represents 80–90% of all cases. Over 90% of patients with Addison's disease have adrenal autoantibodies, most commonly antibodies to the adrenal cortex (ACA) and to the enzyme 21-hydroxylase.[39] Only recently have researchers learned that there is a long preclinical period of declining function before a diagnosis of Addison's disease is made; this decline is marked by reduced adrenal function and the presence of autoantibodies. In the early stages of Addison's disease, there is demonstrable lymphocytic infiltration of the cortex, followed by atrophy in the later stages, when it becomes clinically overt. This highlights the importance of early detection, monitoring, and treatment of the underlying autoimmune process. Addison's disease may occur in isolation, but it is often part of an autoimmune process targeting several organs. For example, it carries an increased risk of celiac disease, type 1 diabetes mellitus, hypothyroidism, hypoparathyroidism, atrophic gastritis, and candidiasis. These polyendocrine syndromes are believed to result from a failure of self-tolerance to a variety of molecules in different organs and tissues.[40]

The adrenal hypofunction seen in Addison's disease can be seen along a spectrum of dysfunction, with reduced steroid output present in lesser degrees of adrenal insufficiency. In addition to autoimmune disease, the effects of environmental toxins on the adrenal gland are becoming recognized as very important.[41] Specifically, the chemical inhibition of key steroidogenic enzymes may inhibit production of adrenal hormones, and a recent review suggests that the adrenal gland is the most frequent toxicological target of all the endocrine organs, particularly the adrenal cortex.[42] In addition to environmental toxicity, other lifestyle factors such as poor nutrition, chronic or repeated stress, inadequate sleep, and insufficient exercise all contribute to impaired adrenal function.

Adrenal hyperfunction

Etiology and epidemiology

Much as Addison's disease is an example of adrenal failure, Cushing syndrome is an example of adrenal hyperfunction, specifically of elevated glucocorticoid production, resulting from excess ACTH secretion. Although Cushing's syndrome is considered quite rare, having an annual incidence ranging from 0.7 to 2.4 per million (and most commonly due to synthetic glucocorticoids), a lesser degree of hypercortisolism may be much more common, especially among some patient populations.[43] As an example, the prevalence among patients referred for evaluation of osteoporosis was almost 5%, and nearly 11% among those with fracture.[44]

Although the cause of excess endogenous cortisol production associated with Cushing's syndrome is usually a pituitary tumor (i.e., Cushing's disease, 80% of ACTH-dependent cases), adrenal tumor, carcinoid syndrome or a carcinoma, and chronic stress are often responsible for subclinical hypercortisolism.[45,46] As an adaptation to stress, increased levels of cortisol are produced with a shift away from DHEA and the sex steroid hormones, and toward glucocorticoid and mineralocorticoid production (Figure 8.5). It may be this imbalance that is responsible for many of the negative clinical consequences of stress.

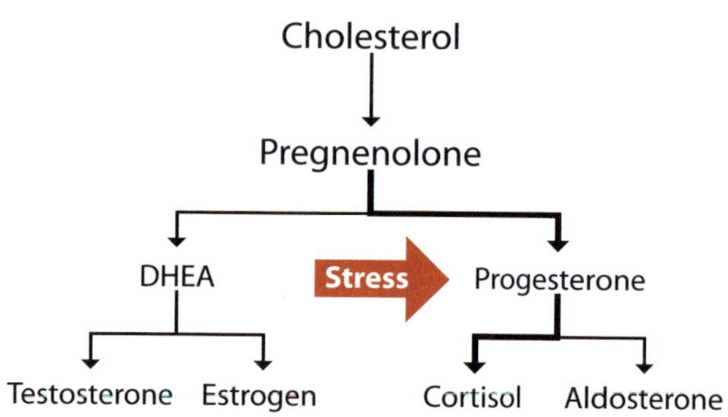

Figure 8.5 Effect of stress on steroid hormones..

Elevated cortisol-to-DHEA ratio

One consequence of adrenal hyperfunction is an imbalance in the ratio of cortisol to DHEA. Profound disturbances in this ratio occur in those experiencing chronic stress, depression, and intense exercise, particularly when the stress occurs repetitively or in an uncontrollable and unpredictable manner.[47,48] Prolonged elevations in cortisol increase epinephrine production in the adrenal gland and brain by enhancing phenylethanolamine-N-methyltransferase activity.[49]

An imbalance in this ratio may be directly responsible for neurotoxicity in the central nervous system, in part by reducing brain-derived neurotrophic factor (BDNF) levels in the brain. Cognitive decline associated with aging is partly due to the more neurotoxic milieu created by imbalanced cortisol/DHEA ratio.[50] Hypercortisolemia may also be central to the pathogenesis of depressive symptoms and cognitive deficits, and plays a role in major depression, panic disorder, and posttraumatic stress disorder.[51] Hypercortisolism is also associated with cognitive dysfunction early after ischemic stroke, as well as increased mortality after stroke.[52]

An imbalance in this ratio also has detrimental effects on immune function, including reduced NK cell activity, lymphocyte populations and proliferation, antibody production, and reactivation of latent viral infections.[53] Detrimental effects on bone health due to elevated cortisol have also been shown to increase the rates of osteoporosis and fracture. If the DHEA/cortisol ratio is balanced, this effect is minimized.[54]

Low DHEA

DHEA is the most abundant steroid hormone and is the precursor to adrenal and sex hormones. A decline in DHEA concentration is linked to a number of disorders, including obesity, insulin resistance, type 2 diabetes, and atherosclerosis.[55,56] Recently, it has also been proposed as an index of the HPA axis, at least in some populations, because low DHEA levels may reflect chronic stress or adrenal insufficiency.[57,58,59]

Because DHEA protects the immune system from stress, low DHEA levels have been associated with decreased immunity in the elderly, as well as an increased risk for atopy and chronic urticaria.[60,61,62] In elderly populations, a high cortisol/DHEA ratio is predictive of infection and impaired neutrophil function in those with bone fractures.[63] DHEA also increases fat metabolism, by increasing adiponectin gene expression, thereby inhibiting adipogenesis (through a mechanism involving peroxisome proliferator-activated receptors).[64,65,66]

DHEA levels have an inverse correlation with cardiovascular disease. DHEA-S was found to be independently associated with endothelial function in postmenopausal women, exerting a protective effect.[67] This relationship was not found in men, although low testosterone was associated with endothelial dysfunction.[68] Low levels may also predict chronic neck, shoulder, or back pain, and have been associated with more advanced nonalcoholic fatty liver disease (NAFLD).[69,70]

DHEA levels are thought to decline in response to either impaired production or increased utilization (due to chronic illness). Aging certainly affects production, with a 20% decrease per decade after age 20. People at 80 years old have 10% of a 20 year old's DHEA level. The age-related increase in the cortisol/DHEA ratio appears to be a major determinant of immunological changes observed during aging.[71] Stress also decreases DHEA and increases cortisol, with age and stress providing a double hit to the immune system over time.[71,72] Other factors known to impair DHEA production include PCBs, magnesium deficiency, hypothyroidism, and physical inactivity. In men aged 60–79, for example, DHEA-S is an independent correlate of muscle strength and calf muscle area.[73,74,75,76]

Reproductive Endocrinology

Androgen hormone regulation

The male sex hormones are collectively called androgens, and include testosterone, dihydrotestosterone, and androstenedione. These hormones are produced primarily in the Leydig cells in the testes for males, while lesser amounts are produced in the ovaries in females; they are produced in the adrenal cortex in both sexes. The hypothalamus-pituitary-gonadal axis is the major hormonal signaling cascade that controls testosterone output. Testosterone production is also regulated by a negative feedback loop, with the hypothalamus secreting gonadotropin-releasing hormone (GnRH), inducing FSH and LH production, which in turn influence spermatogenesis in the Sertoli cells and testosterone production in the testes, respectively. Testosterone, as well as aromatized estradiol, appears to have negative feedback at the level of the hypothalamus, where it reduces GnRH pulse frequency, as well as at the pituitary, where it reduces the responsiveness to GnRH; the aromatization of testosterone may be required for effect at the pituitary level. For FSH, there is additional regulation by nonsteroidal factors, essentially a negative endocrine feedback loop mediated by inhibin B secretion from Sertoli cells (Figure 8.6).[77,78,79]

Hypogonadism

Epidemiology

More than 20% of healthy men over 60 years of age present with serum total testosterone levels below the reference range for young men. Certain subpopulations of men have a higher prevalence; men with erectile dysfunction range from 23–47%,[80] and as many as 15–30% of men with type 2 diabetes mellitus have low testosterone levels.[81] Yet, it is hard to define the true prevalence of this problem, because there is no single common standard. Using data from the Boston Area Community Health (BACH) survey, 24% of subjects had total testosterone <300 ng/dl, and 11% of subjects had free testosterone <5 ng/dl. This same study tried to estimate the prevalence of testosterone deficiency symptoms, and analyze to what degree they overlapped with the laboratory findings. When combining symptoms with laboratory values, they found an overall prevalence for symptomatic androgen deficiency of 5.6% among these men, with the prevalence increasing over age.[82] Surprisingly they also found that the majority of men with symptoms of androgen deficiency had normal testosterone levels and, conversely, a considerable portion of men with low testosterone were asymptomatic. Perhaps this is more a result of poor tissue or receptor responsiveness than the

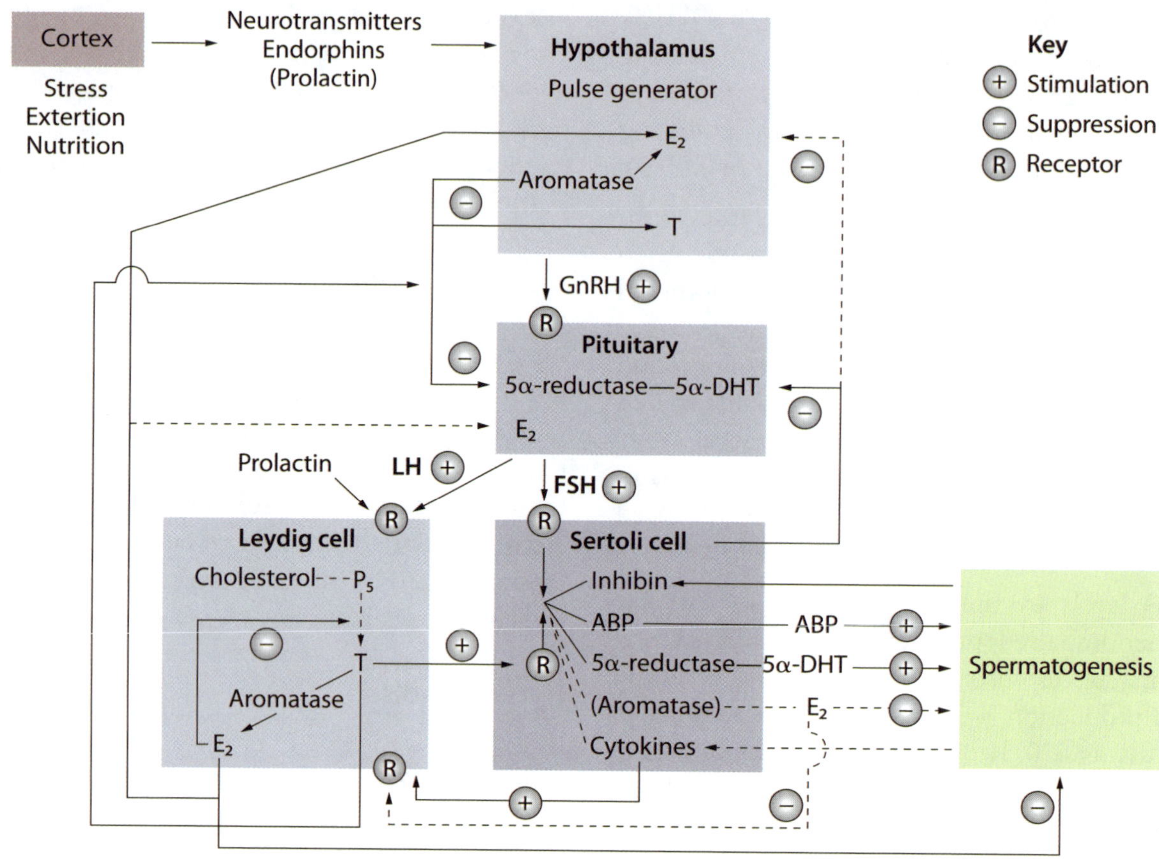

Figure 8.2 Role of D2 in TSH feedback. From: Bianco AC, Kim BW. Deiodinases: implications of the local control of thyroid hormone action. *J Clin Invest*. 2006 Oct;116(10):2571-9. Reproduced with permission from the American Society for Clinical Investigation.

low amount of available testosterone. A more recent analysis of the same data found that 87.8% with symptomatic androgen deficiency were not receiving treatment, despite access to care.[83] Common causes of androgen deficiency include age, systemic or autoimmune disease, cryptorchidism, elevated cortisol, tobacco use, nutrient deficiencies, and environmental toxicity.[84]

Androgen effects

Androgens have broad effects, ranging from increasing fertility and libido to improved mental health.[85] Low levels of testosterone are associated with greater rates of depression in men,[86] and a higher free testosterone was associated with better cognitive function in older men (though total testosterone was not similarly associated).[87] Androgens also increase muscle mass and reduce adipogenesis by encouraging pluripotent stem cells to become muscle cells through androgen receptor activity.[88] Bioavailable testosterone has been more closely associated with muscle mass than total testosterone. Androgens also affect bone tissue. Men with a low vs. high level of free testosterone have 1.5–2 times the risk of fracture, as well as a greater risk for osteopenia and osteoporosis.[89]

Testosterone is also important for cardiovascular health. Low levels are an independent risk factor for endothelial dysfunction in men,[90] and those with low free testosterone have 3–5 times the risk of coronary artery disease as those with high levels.[91] This affects mortality as well. In a prospective study of nearly 800 men, low total and bioavailable testosterone was associated with a hazard ratio of 1.40 for all-cause mortality, after adjusting for age, lifestyle, adiposity, blood pressure, and other risk factors. Specifically, cardiovascular and respiratory disease mortality increased.[92]

Finally, androgens play a role in blood sugar regulation. A robust, dose-response relationship between sex hormone levels and risk of the metabolic syndrome in men is consistent across racial/ethnic groups,[93] and testosterone has been shown to improve glucose homeostasis and visceral obesity.[94]

Causes of androgen insufficiency

Decreased androgen synthesis or a reduced cellular response to androgens both lead to insufficient androgen effects. For example, production declines significantly with age. A 20-year-old man has 700 million Leydig cells, while an 80-year-old man has only 200 million. Serum levels of sex hormone-binding globulin (SHBG) increase with age; thus, the decrease in serum free testosterone (FT) and non-SHBG-bound testosterone (often referred to as bioavailable testosterone) is even greater.[95]

Many environmental toxins also disrupt androgen function. Insecticides (chlorpyrifos, carbaryl, and naphthalene)[96] and pesticides (dieldrin) have been shown to inhibit testosterone synthesis via damage to Leydig cell activity,[97] with pesticide sprayers found to have significantly reduced age-adjusted seminal volume, percentage of motility, percentage of sperm with normal morphology, serum luteinizing hormone, serum testosterone levels, and seminal zinc concentration.[98]

Phthalates are androgen receptor antagonists, and also inhibit testosterone synthesis.[99,100,101] As a consequence, data from the NHANES national cross-section study of men found urinary concentrations of several prevalent phthalate metabolites to be significantly correlated with abdominal obesity and insulin resistance, both associated with low testosterone levels.[102] Monobutyl phthalate in urine was found to have a dose-response relationship with low sperm concentration and motility.[103] In women, prenatal urine levels of phthalates were associated with a shorter anogenital distance in their male infants, a sign of incomplete virilization and disrupted male reproductive development.[104]

Heavy metals such as lead impair sperm health, while arsenic has been shown to inhibit several enzymes involved in testosterone synthesis.[105] Arsenic exposure through well water was found to be a significant risk factor for erectile dysfunction, even after adjusting for free testosterone.[106] In animal studies, vitamin C was shown to prevent some of the oxidative damage of arsenic.[107] Cigarette smoking and alcohol use also impair testosterone synthesis in men, though alcohol may increase it in women.[108,109,110]

Other toxins interfere with the androgen receptors. Xenoestrogens, bisphenol A (BPA, heavily used in the plastics industry and in dental sealants), nitrophenols from diesel exhaust,[111,112] and other widely used surfactants have been shown to act through this mechanism, and some also act as estrogen receptor agonists. As shown Figure 8.7, increasing concentrations of these compounds reduce the effect of an androgen receptor agonist in a roughly dose-dependent manner.[113] It should also be noted that the effects of toxin mixtures are not well predicted from effects of single toxin exposure; yet, multiple simultaneous exposures are frequently found outside the laboratory.[114]

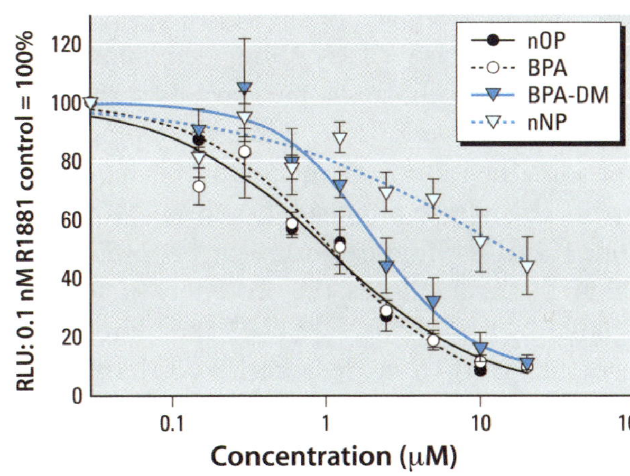

Figure 8.7 Several toxins block the action of an androgen receptor agonist in a dose-dependent manner. Legend: BPA = Bisphenol A; BPA-DM = Bisphenol A Dimethacrylate; nNP = 4-n-Nonylphenol; and nOP = 4-n-Octylphenol. From: Bonefeld-Jørgensen EC, Long M, Hofmeister MV, et al. Endocrine-disrupting potential of bisphenol A, bisphenol A dimethacrylate, 4-n-nonylphenol, and 4-n-octylphenol *in vitro*: new data and a brief review. *Environ Health Perspect*. 2007 Dec;115 Suppl 1:69-76. Reproduced from Open Access article, published online 2007 June 8. doi: 10.1289/ehp.9368.

Stress also interferes with testosterone synthesis via cortisol inhibition, as do autoimmune diseases.

For example, 38% of men with hypogonadotropic hypogonadism were found to have anti-pituitary antibodies, specifically targeting gonadotropin secreting cells.[115]

Many nutritional deficiencies have been shown to impair testosterone synthesis, including zinc, folic acid, copper, selenium, and antioxidants.[116,117] A zinc-deficient diet will decrease testosterone 75% after 20 weeks,[118] while supplementation increased testosterone 100% in older men with marginal zinc deficiency, and raised the rate of successful pregnancies in previously infertile couples.[119] Excessive fat consumption, specifically total and saturated fat, is also linked to reduced testosterone.[120] Long-term, high-dose vitamin E, PC-SPES, and mint tea have all been linked to reduced synthesis of testosterone.[121,122,123]

Estrogen and progesterone regulation

While women also produce testosterone, the production of the hormones estrogen and progesterone are much more important in influencing female reproductive health and quality of life. The balance and regulation of female hormones is very delicate and complex, with significant changes over a lifetime, as well as cycling over a menstrual cycle. The hypothalamus-pituitary-ovary (HPO) axis is the key regulator of female reproductive function. The most basic model for this regulation depicts the release of gonadotropin-releasing hormone (GnRH) in pulses from the hypothalamus, which in turn induces the secretion of follicle-stimulating hormone (FSH), and luteinizing hormone (LH) from the anterior pituitary. FSH controls follicular development and the number of follicles that mature to the preovulatory stage; it also regulates the aromatization of androgenic precursors to estradiol in the granulosa cells.

LH is required for the process of ovulation and formation of a *corpus luteum*, which produces progesterone. LH is also required for synthesis of androgens from cholesterol within the theca cells of the developing follicle. Similar to the action of ACTH on cells in the adrenal cortex, LH and FSH increase cholesterol concentration and transport to the inner mitochondrial membrane of ovarian cells by the StAR protein. There, it is converted to pregnenolone, the rate-limiting step in steroid synthesis.[124,125]

Along with the steroids, the ovaries produce nonsteroidal substances such as inhibins, which suppress basal FSH secretion from the pituitary through a negative feedback mechanism. Although inhibins are produced in other tissue, the ovaries are the main source of circulating levels. Diverse tissues produce activins (which belong to the TGF-b family) and follistatin, which appear to stimulate and inhibit FSH production, respectively.[126,127]

Each level of this 3-tiered neuroendocrine system is regulated in a complex and highly coordinated process, functioning both independently and interdependently, and influenced not only by hormone production levels but also by hormone receptor sensitivity. Thus, a dysfunction in any level of the HPO axis has consequences for all other levels.[128] Women also experience much more abrupt and profound hormonal changes with age than men, and the negative and positive feedback mechanisms involved in the balance of female reproductive hormones are not consistent throughout all of life's stages.[129] Environmental toxins, nutritional deficiencies, impaired metabolic pathways, and lifestyle patterns may affect any aspect of this tightly controlled regulation.[130]

Hormone imbalance

Epidemiology and etiology

A number of clinical conditions result in or are a consequence of either elevated or suboptimal levels of female steroid hormones, and the differential diagnosis can be quite long and challenging to refine. The problem may lie at the level of the hypothalamus, the pituitary, or the ovaries, and may be hormonal or structural. Female hypogonadism refers to deficient or abnormal function of the hypothalamus-pituitary-ovary axis, resulting in estrogen deficiency and menstrual cycle disturbances. In postpubertal females, hypogonadism typically manifests as dysfunctional uterine bleeding or amenorrhea, with an approximate prevalence between 10–30% among women of reproductive age.[131] The causes are quite diverse, and include various gynecological, endocrinological, psychiatric, genetic, chromosomal, and autoimmune conditions, as well as the menopausal loss of ovarian activity. Premature ovarian failure is an example of hypergonadotropic hypogonadism, biochemically characterized by low levels of gonadal hormones (estrogens and inhibins) and high levels of LH and FSH; it manifests with many of the symptoms typical of physiologic menopause, including infertility, heat intolerance, flushes, anxiety, depression, and fatigue. Causes include chromosomal and genetic abnormalities (including estrogen receptor and inhibin genes), autoimmune dysfunction (ovarian antibodies have been detected in 50–60% of patients with unexplained infertility), and metabolic, iatrogenic, and idiopathic triggers.[132] It has been suggested that impaired insulin sensitivity may be an early manifestation.[133]

Polycystic ovary syndrome (PCOS) is an example of normogonadotropic anovulation, characterized by gonadotropins and steroid hormone levels within the normal range. Relatively high ratios of LH to FSH and estrogen unopposed by sufficient progesterone have both been documented.[134] It is apparently not a question of an absolute progesterone deficiency, but rather a reduced sensitivity of the GnRH pulse generator to the negative feedback of progesterone. This lack of negative feedback allows the LH levels to remain relatively high compared to FSH. Although the lack of ovulation leads to lower progesterone levels, this is not sufficient to explain the anomalies seen. A relative progesterone deficiency due to reduced sensitivity of the GnRH pulse generator is a better working hypothesis, and one that may explain why additional progesterone (to overcome the reduced sensitivity) may be useful. The lack of hypothalamic sensitivity encourages androgen production, which in turn reduces hypothalamic sensitivity, a vicious cycle.[134]

Hyperprolactinemia is the most common endocrine disorder of the hypothalamus-pituitary axis; it causes hypogonadism because supraphysiological concentrations of prolactin exert an inhibitory effect on the HPO axis, inhibiting GnRH activity. Causes may be divided roughly into physiological, pathological, or pharmacological etiologies, and include hypothalamic lesions, pituitary tumors, chronic renal failure, and hypothyroidism.

In each of the imbalances of the female reproductive hormones, environmental toxins, nutritional excesses and deficiencies, stress, and lifestyle choices, such as diet and physical activity, make significant contributions. Botanical support (see *Interventions*, p. 8.19) offers symptomatic relief and helps to restore balance and endocrine function.

Estrogen insufficiency

Symptoms of low estrogen include menstrual irregularities or amenorrhea, breast atrophy, low libido, osteoporosis, vaginal dryness, vasomotor symptoms, irregular uterine bleeding, and migraine headaches. Estrogen insufficiency also is associated with a greater risk for Alzheimer's and Parkinson's disease, possibly because of lower plasma BDNF levels.[135,136,137]

Menopause

Older women of reproductive age often have a high FSH, which would in most cases indicate an estrogen insufficiency, but instead appears to be due to a natural hypothalamic-pituitary insensitivity to estrogen.[138] For example, even in the presence of adequate estrogen stimulation, perimenopausal women are known to have cycles without an LH surge.[138] Thus even though some perimenopausal women may have adequate estrogen levels, the estrogen receptor is less sensitive to estradiol, creating a relative estrogen insufficiency and its associated symptoms.

Other causes of estrogen insufficiency

Other non-menopausal causes of estrogen insufficiency inhibit estrogen production by reducing FSH levels, suggesting hypothalamic or pituitary involvement. For example, some pesticides mimic the action of estrogen at hypothalamic receptors, reducing GnRH secretion. A low FSH has been found in women exposed to pentachlorophenol (pesticide and wood preservative, such as may be used on utility poles), while heptachlor, lindane, atrazine, and simazine reduced estradiol in animals studies.[139] Other pesticides inhibit the aromatase enzyme, including fenarimol, prochloraz, and other imidazole fungicides. As a consequence, women exposed to pesticides have a 3 times greater risk for infertility (a 9 times greater risk if they have ever worked in agriculture).[140] In a study of over 500 menstrual cycles, DDT was found to lower estrogen and progesterone production at times critical for ovulation and pregnancy maintenance.[141] Another common toxin, cigarette smoke, decreases inhibin B levels and may increase FSH levels (because of impaired ovarian activity).[142,143] Aluminum (used in many antiperspirants) has been found to interfere with estrogen binding to receptors.[144,145]

Stress also contributes to estrogen insufficiency because activation of the HPA axis inhibits the HPO axis.[146] Glucocorticoids suppress gonadal axis function at the hypothalamic, pituitary, and uterine levels,[147] and inhibit estradiol-stimulated uterine growth. Indeed, cortisol levels are associated with the severity of menopausal symptoms.[148] Depression is associated with lower estrogen but higher FSH levels.[149,150]

Several nutritional factors also influence estrogen production. Zinc deficiency impairs synthesis of both FSH and LH, and lower zinc levels have been found in menopausal women with osteoporosis and osteopenia.[151] Vitamin D affects estrogen levels, partly by maintaining calcium homeostasis, but also by direct regulation of the aromatase gene and by increasing progesterone synthesis.[152,153] In healthy women, very low and very high levels of body fat have both been associated with lower estrogen levels.[154]

Estrogen excess

While insufficient levels of estrogen are associated with a number clinical disorders, excess levels may also result in pathology. PMS, endometriosis, cervical dysplasia, breast cancer, and uterine fibroids all may be influenced by increased estrogenic effects. For example, fibroid tissue is hyper-responsive to estrogen and exhibits elevated levels of estrogen receptors. Symptoms of estrogen excess include water and fat retention, headaches, anxiety, sadness, weight gain, and breast tenderness.

A number of causes exist for excessive estrogen, with poor detoxification playing an important role. CYP19, CYP17, CYP1B1, CYP1A1, and SULT1A1 polymorphisms have all been shown to affect estrogen levels, influence the production of estrogen metabolites, and modify estrogen-related cancer risk (Figure 8.8).[155,156] Phase II detoxification (including sulfation, glucuronidation, methylation, and glutathione conjugation) also influences estrogen metabolism. For example, a COMT (Val158Met) polymorphism is associated with a more than 4-fold risk for fibroid formation.[157,158]

Lifestyle behaviors also influence estrogen levels. A diet high in protein and fat and low in fiber,[159,160] inadequate exercise,[161] and poor sleep all contribute to hormone imbalance. For example, reduced parasympathetic activity during sleep was associated with an increase in PMS symptoms; as might be expected, therefore, an increase in sympathetic/parasympathetic activity is documented among women with PMS.[162,163]

Reduced levels of vitamin D and calcium,[164,165] and exposure to environmental toxins such as PCBs and cadmium, may also have estrogen effects. Elevated PCB exposure is associated with an increased risk of endometriosis, although PBBs were not.[166] PBBs have been associated with shorter menstrual cycles, particularly among women with recent weight loss.[167] Cadmium activates the estrogen receptor, and *in vitro* it induced the growth of a breast cancer cell line 5.6 fold.[168] In a prospective study of over 30,000 postmenopausal women, cadmium intake was statistically significantly associated with increased risk of endometrial cancer. A nearly 3-fold risk was found among women with a long-term cadmium intake consistently above the median.[169] In another study, cadmium intake was also associated with an increased risk of endometriosis.[170]

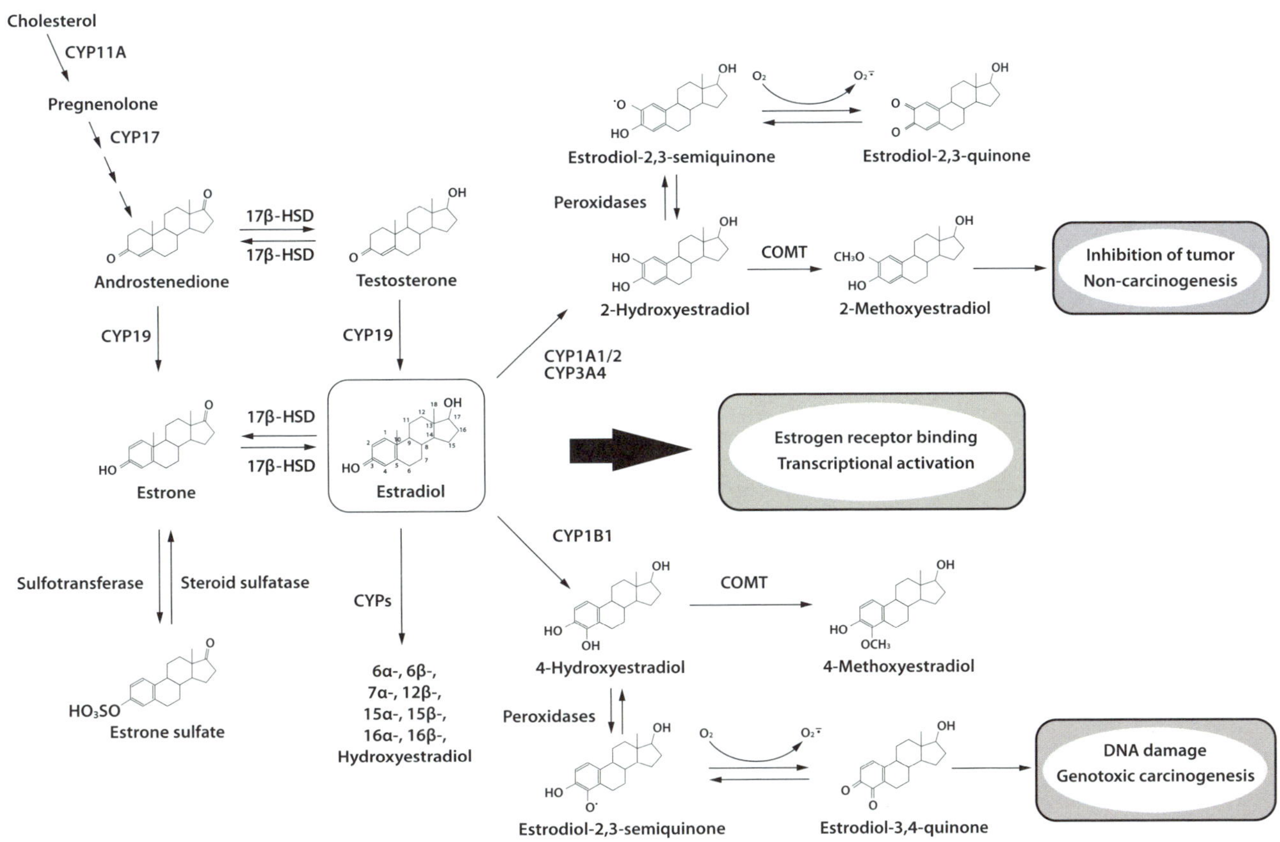

Figure 8.8 Cytochrome P450-mediated metabolic pathways of estradiol. From: Tsuchiya Y, Nakajima M, Yokoi T. Cytochrome P450-mediated metabolism of estrogens and its regulation in human. *Cancer Lett.* 2005 Sep 28;227(2):115-24. Reproduced with permission from Elsevier.

Progesterone imbalance

Although progesterone deficiency is more often seen clinically, progesterone excess has been associated with restless leg syndrome; it is unclear, however, whether the actual etiology is iron deficiency and not progesterone.[171] A progesterone metabolite, allopregnanolone, has been shown to impair memory by reducing the recruitment of those brain regions (amygdala) that support memory formation and retrieval.[172] Progesterone excess may carry a possible increased risk for breast cancer, although this risk may be limited to synthetic progestins.[173]

Progesterone deficiency has been linked to PMS, ovarian cysts, fluid retention, infertility, and recurrent pregnancy loss. For instance, in women with PCOS, there is reduced sensitivity of the GnRH pulse generator to the negative feedback of progesterone, creating a relative (not absolute) progesterone deficiency. A luteal phase defect is seen in 20% of infertility cases and up to 35% of women with recurrent pregnancy loss.[174,175]

Some of the causes of low progesterone are excess prolactin (see below), excessive weight loss or exercise, stress, alcohol, excess fat and sugar, antidepressants, exogenous toxins, and nutritional deficiencies (vitamins A, B6, and C, and zinc).[176,177,178] Vitamin C deficiency has been shown to limit the ability of the ovaries to respond to gonadotropins, while ascorbic acid stimulates production of progesterone in luteinizing granulosa cells.[179] Among the environmental causes of progesterone deficiency are bisphenol A, toluene and benzene, DDE, cadmium, and pesticides.[180] Cadmium, for example, although it stimulates ovarian progesterone production, inhibits placental production.[181] The pesticides hexachlorobenzene, methoxychlor, trichlorfon, and fenvalerate inhibit

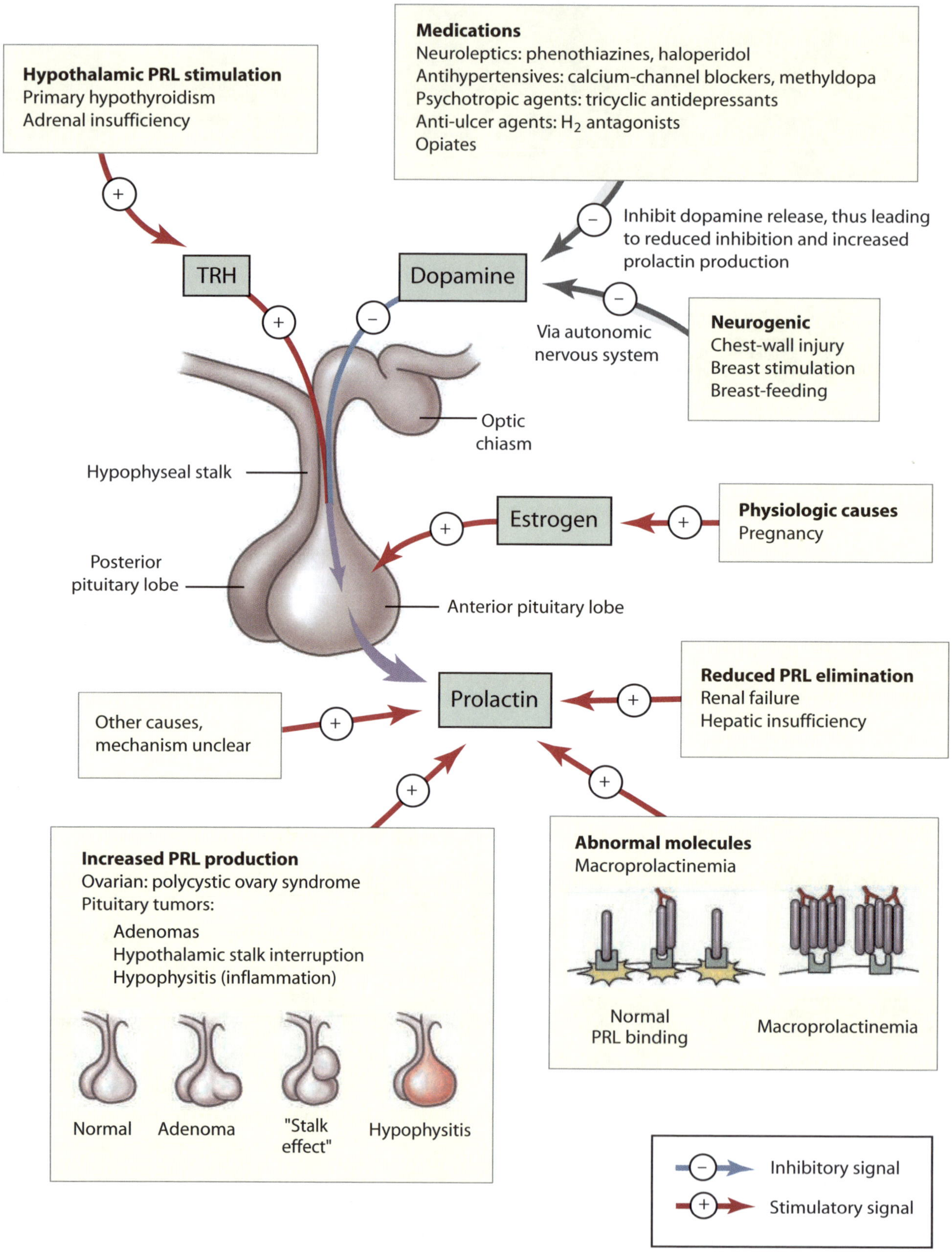

Figure 8.9 Causes of hyperprolactinemia. From: Serri O, Chik CL, Ur E, et al. Diagnosis and management of hyperprolactinemia. *CMAJ*. 2003 Sep 16;169(6):575-81.

enzymes involved in progesterone synthesis, specifically cholesterol side chain cleavage enzyme (P450scc)[182,183,184]

Prolactin excess

Symptoms of prolactin excess include galactorrhea (43% of women with this condition have hyperprolactinemia),[273] menstrual irregularities/amenorrhea (15% with anovulation), and infertility. Among individuals with elevated serum prolactin, 30% have prolactin-secreting tumors.[185] In addition to prolactinomas, a number of drugs can cause excess prolactin, including dopamine-receptor antagonists (e.g., phenothiazines, butyrophenones, thioxanthenes, risperidone, metoclopramide, sulpiride, and pimozide), dopamine-depleting agents (e.g., methyldopa, reserpine), and others (isoniazid, danazol, tricyclic antidepressants, monoamine antihypertensives, verapamil, estrogens, antiandrogens, cyproheptadine, opiates, H_2-blockers [cimetidine], and cocaine).[273] Physiological causes of prolactin excess include stress, pregnancy, and lactation, while pathological causes also include Cushing's syndrome, hypothyroidism, and renal disease.[273] See Figure 8.9 for a summary of the causes of hyperprolactinemia.

Assessment

Hypothyroidism

Laboratory

The diagnosis of hypothyroidism is often based on laboratory measures, specifically an elevated TSH accompanied by a low free T4. TSH is conventionally regarded as the single most sensitive indicator of thyroid function, although the upper limit of normal is a subject of controversy. While a TSH >10 mIU/l is universally accepted as an indicator of low thyroid function, some research suggests that an upper limit for TSH between 2.5–4.5 mIU/l may be more appropriate, with a TSH in this range referred to as subclinical hypothyroidism. Given that the T4 level in the serum provides negative feedback to the pituitary, yet does not necessarily reflect intracellular T3 levels, reliance on TSH alone has limitations for at least a subset of patients. Along with TSH, free T4, and free T3, thyroid antibodies may indicate which cases are more likely to progress to overt hypothyroidism, and may help guide the level of intervention.[186]

Functional assessment

Given the limitations of laboratory diagnosis, a more functional approach is used by some practitioners. Perhaps the most well-known is that documented by Broda Barnes, MD, who advocated measuring axillary temperature and using 97.2 °F as the lower limit of normal. While he found this to be a sensitive measure of thyroid activity, it has been criticized for lacking specificity, i.e., it may also indicate anemia (especially iron deficiency), inadequate physical activity, or nutritional deficiencies that limit metabolic processes.[187,188] Expanding upon Dr. Barnes's work, the concept of "sub-laboratory hypothyroidism" has been suggested more recently by Alan Gaby, MD, who recommends a trial of thyroid hormone in patients with signs and symptoms, but not necessarily laboratory evidence, of hypothyroidism.[189]

Adrenal hypofunction

Laboratory

Cortisol levels are often used as an index of adrenal function, often combined with DHEA. Because the hypothalamic-pituitary-adrenal (HPA) axis is activated in response to stress, adrenal gland dysfunction is often related to maladaptation to stress. Stress shifts the HPA axis away from sex hormone release and toward glucocorticoid secretion, thus the ratio of cortisol to DHEA may be used as a guide to assessing adrenal hormone balance, particularly in response to stress.

Traditionally a low morning serum cortisol and an elevated morning plasma ACTH are used to diagnose primary adrenal insufficiency. DHEA-S is often low in adrenal insufficiency.[190,191] Further evaluation may include a short corticotrophin test, during which cortisol is monitored after the administration of synthetic ACTH, with little to no change observed in those with adrenal insufficiency.[37] A recent study suggests that, in addition to measuring cortisol following an ACTH challenge, aldosterone, DHEA, and 11-deoxycortisol improve the discrimination between sufficiency and insufficiency and provide more diagnostic information as to the cause of adrenal insufficiency.[192] Salivary levels of DHEA and cortisol may offer advantages over serum, providing a clinical marker for free hormone levels using a stress-free collection method,[193] and easier monitoring of cortisol level fluctuation throughout the day.[194,195]

Functional assessment

Many symptoms of adrenal insufficiency, but not all, resolve with treatment. In some cases, evaluating the success of the treatment may be based primarily on tracking the patient's symptoms rather than on laboratory findings. Common symptoms include fatigue, reduced strength, loss of libido, insomnia, salt craving, headache, anorexia, and weight loss.[37]

Adrenal hyperfunction

Laboratory

A distinction between Cushing's syndrome and other causes of hypercortisolism should be made, with first-line screening tests to include a 24-hour urinary free cortisol and an overnight low-dose dexamethasone suppression test. Additionally, a late night salivary cortisol also has significant value for assessing hypercortisolism, with a recent study finding a sensitivity and specificity of 100% and 97.5 %, respectively, for diagnosing Cushing's syndrome.[196] Second-line tests include plasma cortisol, circadian rhythm/midnight plasma cortisol, and imaging if a tumor is suspected (pituitary, adrenal, lung).[197] For many cases of hypercortisolism, the ratio of cortisol to DHEA is equally important.

A large cohort study recently found an association between major depressive disorder (MDD) and a high morning cortisol. Interestingly, this occurred not only in those with current MDD, but also those with a past history but no current depression, indicating a potential susceptibility.[198] A second study examined morning cortisol levels among individuals without a current or past (or parental) history of depression and anxiety, and found that among numerous psychological traits, only hopelessness reactivity was associated with high morning cortisol levels (See Figure 8.10). It is known to be a risk factor for both depression and suicidality.[199]

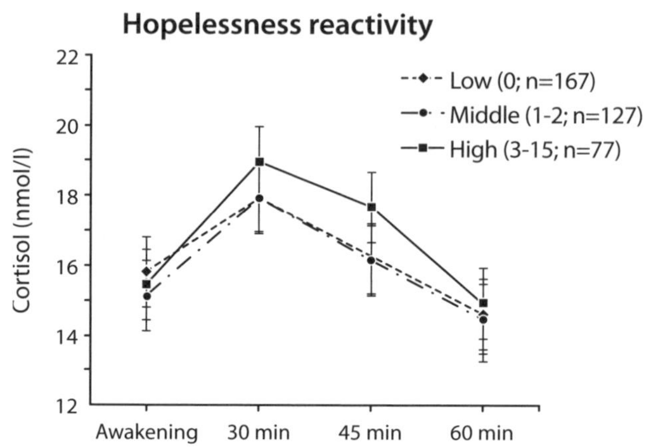

Figure 8.10 Mean salivary cortisol levels for patients with low, middle, and high scores for hopeless reactivity. From: van Santen A, Vreeburg SA, Van der Does AJ, et al. Psychological traits and the cortisol awakening response: Results from the Netherlands Study of Depression and Anxiety. *Psychoneuroendocrinology.* 2010 Aug 17 (Epub ahead of print). Reproduced with permission from Elsevier.

Androgen insufficiency

Laboratory

As mentioned above, there is no consensus for which marker of testosterone is the most useful, nor for what the cut-off for normal is. "Normal" may vary from person to person to some degree, given variations in androgen receptor sensitivity. Conventionally, total testosterone is often used, including the free (unbound) portion (2%), and the bound portion (98%, bound to either SHBG or albumin). Also relevant is "bioavailable" testosterone, which is made up of the 2% that is free, combined with the roughly 60% of the bound portion that is only loosely bound to albumin (i.e., it excludes the portion bound to SHBG). Given that SHBG levels rise with age, a greater drop in free and bioavailable testosterone than in total testosterone is usually seen. Saliva testing estimates free testosterone only. Cut-offs often employed are total testosterone <300 ng/dl (10.4 nmol/liter), <5 ng/dl for free testosterone, and <60–95 ng/dl for bioavailable testosterone.[200]

Functional/Symptomatic assessment

The Endocrine Society has published a list of symptoms indicative of androgen deficiency, comprising those that are "suggestive" signs (e.g., reduced libido, erectile dysfunction, infertility, reduced bulk and muscle strength, and osteoporosis/osteoporotic fracture) as well as those that are less specific (e.g., lethargy, sleep disturbance, depressed mood, mild anemia, and low physical performance).[201] A number of questionnaires have been developed, including the Androgen Deficiency in Aging Male (ADAM), and the Aging Male Survey (AMS); although both have fairly high sensitivity for predicting low bioavailable testosterone (97% and 83%, respectively), both have poor specificity (30% and 39%, respectively).[202]

Estrogen/progesterone/prolactin imbalance

Laboratory

The evaluation of many female endocrine abnormalities may be quite complex, often requiring laboratory and clinical procedures that are beyond the scope of this chapter. For example, evaluation of premature ovarian failure includes laboratory tests of ovarian reserve, such as early follicular FSH, basal estradiol, inhibin A and B levels, and dynamic testing with clomiphene citrate or gonadotropin analogs (with measurement of ovarian response). Serum levels of FSH and LH, along with serum, salivary, or urinary levels of estrogen and progesterone, are often useful, particularly to follow through a menstrual cycle.[203,204] If the patient is not having regular menses, but has sufficient estrogen, a 5–7 day course of progesterone may induce withdrawal bleeding (with optimal hormone testing done in the early follicular phase). Serum prolactin, pregnancy, testosterone, insulin sensitivity, and thyroid evaluations are often recommended, as well as a 24-hour urinary free cortisol to rule out hypercortisolism. Pituitary imaging is indicated if biochemical evidence of pituitary dysfunction is found, and pelvic ultrasound may be indicated to support a diagnosis of PCOS, when combined with other criteria. In some cases, genetic analysis is indicated, such as ruling out Turner's and Kallmann's syndromes as causes of hypogonadism. Screening for autoimmune disease, including autoimmune polyendocrine syndromes, may be warranted.[205]

Hypothyroid highlights

Although treatment of hypothyroidism is often accomplished with hormone replacement, a number of lifestyle and nutritional interventions can help to support healthy thyroid function. For example, for low T4 production, reducing the intake of goitrogens, decreasing stress levels, and ensuring an adequate intake of iodine, copper, zinc, and B12 may help to restore normal synthesis. As discussed above, a number of environmental toxins can impact both T4 production and its conversion to T3, as well as the cellular response to T3. Thus, testing for exposure may help guide treatment. For more information, see Clinical Focus 3—Advanced Detoxification Support.

Adrenal highlights

Interventions to increase cortisol

Lifestyle interventions shown to increase cortisol levels include stress reduction, because chronic stress may exhaust adrenal reserves over time, and improved sleep, because individuals experiencing sleep deprivation have low cortisol compared to controls.[206] Nutrients such as L-theanine, 5-HTP, and melatonin, has been shown not only to improve sleep, but to increase calmness and increase alpha brain wave activity. Both the relaxation benefit and the improved sleep contribute to healthy adrenal function. For more information, see

Clinical Focus 6—Stress, Anxiety, Depression, and Insomnia. Also, the herb *Glycyrrhiza glabra* may also be used to increase cortisol; it inhibits the enzyme 11 beta-hydroxysteroid dehydrogenase, thus prolonging the half-life of cortisol.[207] Caution should be used to avoid hypertension and hypokalemia with prolonged use.

Interventions to reduce cortisol

The most effective interventions for reducing cortisol levels are stabilizing blood sugar levels, reducing stress, and providing adrenal gland support. For example, mindfulness-based stress reduction (MBSR) has been shown to lower cortisol and to help normalize the HPA axis.[208] An 8-week program combining relaxation techniques, meditation, yoga, and daily home practice reduced cortisol levels significantly; continued reductions were noted at 6-month and 12-month follow-ups.[209]

Supporting the adrenal glands during stress is an essential part of normalizing cortisol. Herbs such as ashwagandha *(Withania somnifera),* Siberian ginseng *(Eleutherococcus senticosus),* lavender *(Lavandula angustifolia),* and rhodiola *(Rhodiola rosea)* have been shown to reduce cortisol elevation in response to stress.[210,211,212,213] Ashwagandha is also a GABA receptor agonist, further reducing the overall stress response. Siberian ginseng root contains eleutherosides known to have anti-fatigue, anti-stress, and immunomodulatory effects; clinically, it has been shown to have therapeutic efficacy for chronic fatigue, stress, and to improve athletic performance. Lavender oil is thought to act on both the central and sympathetic nervous systems; clinically, it has been shown to have a calming and relaxing effect, promoting an improved sense of well-being. *Rhodiola rosea* has been shown clinically to improve attention, cognitive function, and mental performance; decrease the cortisol response to stress; and exert an anti-fatigue affect.

For further information and additional recommendations on measures to deal with stress, see Clinical Focus 6—Stress, Anxiety, Depression, and Insomnia.

Fish oil and phosphatidyl serine blunt the effects of stress on adrenal activation, and should be used to help reduce cortisol levels.[214,215,216] Although curcumin has not been shown to affect cortisol levels, it does mitigate the damages of stress. Curcumin upregulates BDNF production, reversing damage and protecting neurons from chronic stress in animal-based studies.[217,218,219] A multivitamin containing sufficient pantothenic acid and vitamins B6, C, and E should also be a part of treatment, as these nutrients are involved in adrenal steroid production pathways.[220,221]

Interventions to increase DHEA

Lifestyle interventions, specifically meditation and exercise, both have therapeutic effects on DHEA production. Meditation increases levels by 10–20%, and improves the cortisol/DHEA ratio.[222,223] Exercise has similar benefits, showing a 30% increase in the DHEA/cortisol ratio.[224]

Melatonin was shown to increase DHEA and improve sleep during a 6-month clinical trial, with a favorable change in the ratio of DHEA to cortisol.[225]

Herbs shown to have benefits include *Tribulus terrestris* and *Panax ginseng.*[226] Protodioscin (an extract from tribulus) increased DHEA-S 29% in an animal study,[227] while *Panax ginseng* decreased the cortisol/DHEA ratio in symptomatic menopausal women by reducing cortisol and increasing DHEA.[228]

Until fairly recently, although patients with Addison's disease were treated with mineralocorticoid and glucocorticoid replacement therapy, low sex steroid hormone production was not addressed. The addition of DHEA for these patients may alleviate the symptoms often attributed to androgen deficiency, including dry skin, hair loss, reduced libido, and an overall sense of well-being. It may be that the traditional replacement of cortisol and aldosterone overlooks the physiological roles of other adrenal hormones. The goal of current treatment for patients with adrenal insufficiency is to mimic as closely as possible normal hormone production, which includes both restoring the types of hormones that are deficient, and matching the timing of their natural production.[229]

Reproductive hormone highlights

Interventions to increase testosterone

Lifestyle interventions shown to affect testosterone levels include physical activity and transcendental meditation. In a 4-month clinical trial evaluating mediation, a slight increase in testosterone levels was seen; controls, who had received only a stress education program, showed a decrease in testosterone.[230] In a one-year trial evaluating exercise, an increase was found in dihydrotestosterone, but not testosterone, in men.[231] Women actually had a decline in testosterone levels after activity, an effect related to weight loss.[232] Greater BMI and waist circumference were associated with lower free testosterone levels among men, likely related to lower LH levels, or higher levels of circulating leptin with excess BMI.[233,234]

Panax ginseng may also have benefits for androgen insufficiency. In a clinical trial involving 66 patients, FSH and LH increased in those with a low sperm count, while no change was seen in healthy controls. This may explain the benefit for Korean ginseng in treating erectile dysfunction, shown in a second clinical trial.[235,236]

A number of nutrients, including zinc and folic acid, are essential for testosterone production, while others have been shown to protect Leydig cells from environmental toxins, which impair testosterone synthesis (discussed above). Thus, in addition to reducing exposure and body burden, the use of nutrients such as vitamins C and E has a protective role against the effects of PCBs and arsenic on Leydig cells.[237]

Although supplemental DHEA does not increase testosterone significantly in men, it does so in women, particularly if they are hypoadrenal. This is likely due to a decrease in SHBG, thereby increasing free testosterone.[238] Supplemental amino acids have been found to help maintain healthy bioavailable testosterone levels, which may decrease during higher levels of resistance exercise.[239]

Interventions that facilitate estrogen function

Many botanicals with purported estrogenic effects have been used for women, although few have been proven. Some of the best research has been done on *Cimicifuga racemosa* and *Angelica sinensis*. *Cimicifuga racemosa* (black cohosh) has been shown to ameliorate a wide variety of menopausal symptoms in most studies,[240,241,242,243] though not all studies have shown benefit.[244,245] Its benefit is not due to any estrogenic effect, which has been confirmed in both breast and uterine tissue, allowing for safe administration in those at risk for estrogen-related cancer.[246,247,248] *Angelica sinensis* (dong quai) does have estrogenic effects;[249] when used with *Matricaria chamomilla*, it was shown to decrease the number and intensity of hot flushes compared to controls (90–96% vs. 15–25%).[250]

Cordyceps sinensis upregulates estrogen production and the StAR protein (the rate-limiting step of estradiol synthesis),[251] but no clinical trials have been done for estrogen-related conditions. Other therapies include gamma oryzanol, which has been shown to reduce menopausal symptoms more than 50% in the majority of patients, and zinc picolinate, known to be essential to estrogen production.[151,252]

As mentioned above, ensuring adequate vitamin D and maintaining a healthy weight both improve estrogen function.

Interventions that reduce estrogenic effects

Dietary interventions to reduce estrogenic effects should be targeted at increasing phytoestrogen content—specifically, a plant-based diet high in soy, flax, and fiber is recommended. Phytoestrogens act as competitive inhibitors at estrogen receptors, with significantly lower activity.[253,254,255]

Estradiol may be hydroxylated at either C-2 or C-16, with the latter having genotoxic effects, increasing the risk for breast cell changes and breast cancer. While pesticides, oral contraceptives,[256] and COMT and CYP1B1 polymorphisms[257] have been shown to increase this risk, nutritional interventions help to reduce the risk. Specifically, quercetin reduces the activity of CYP1B1 relative to CYP1A1, leading to C2 hydroxylation.[258] Cruciferous vegetables contain sulforaphane, which downregulates estrogen receptor transcription,[259] and indole-3-carbinol, which reduces estrogen receptor activity through the binding of its metabolite, diindolylmethane (DIM), to the nuclear aryl hydrocarbon receptor (AhR).[260] Thus, healthy detoxification, including support for phase I and II, is also an essential component of reducing estrogenic effects by increasing the efficiency of its metabolism. In addition to improving estrogen metabolism, minimizing the estrogenic effects of environmental toxins may also be indicated in some patients. For example, in animal-based studies, melatonin was able to prevent some of the estrogenic effects of cadmium.[261]

Interventions to facilitate progesterone function

As mentioned above, a number of environmental toxins interfere with progesterone function and should be avoided, including bisphenol A, pesticides, DDT, and cadmium.

Herbs used clinically to facilitate progesterone function include *Vitex agnus-castus* (chaste tree) and *Glycyrrhiza glabra*. In a trial involving 52 women with luteal phase defects due to hyperprolactinemia, *Vitex agnus-castus* was shown to decrease prolactin secretion while significantly increasing progesterone secretion.[262] Although this benefit might not apply to women without prolactin excess, two clinical trials have been done in women with PMS, with *Vitex agnus-castus* improving women's self-assessment of irritability, mood alteration, anger, headache, breast fullness, and other menstrual symptoms, including bloating.[263] The second open-label trial had 93% of patients (n=1634) reporting a decrease in the number of symptoms or even cessation of PMS complaints.[264] Adequate amounts of zinc, vitamin A, and vitamin C should be ensured.[265]

Many women with PCOS have reduced progesterone levels. N-acetylcysteine (NAC) was found to improve ovulation rates and increase progesterone levels in PCOS, when given at 1200 mg/day for 5 days, starting on the third day of the cycle.[266] Because insulin resistance is now recognized to be a significant feature of PCOS in many women, interventions to improve glucose control should be a part of therapy for these women. For more information, see Clinical Focus 4—The Spectrum of Insulin Resistance.

Interventions to decrease prolactin secretion

In addition to conventional therapies, stress management can be an important part of therapy for excess prolactin. Emotional stress may play a role in either prolactin-secreting pituitary tumors or idiopathic hyperprolactinemia.[267] Specifically, prolactin may be secreted in response to stress, particularly with "passive coping," and interventions which help to improve this coping strategy should be part of comprehensive therapy.[268]

The herb with the most evidence for reducing prolactin levels is *Vitex agnus-castus*. In clinical trials, it has demonstrated advantages in terms of better patient compliance and lower cost than bromocriptine[269]; it has an effect via dopaminergic compounds.[270,271,272] It does have the potential to mask underlying adenoma, so caution should be used.[273] Other therapies include zinc and vitamin B6, although the research is not as certain. For example, not all research confirms the benefit of B6, which may be limited to animal studies;[274] it did not decrease levels in lactating women.[275] Caution should also be used with supplemental melatonin, as elevated melatonin levels have been associated with hyperprolactinemia.[276] Finally, as part of comprehensive treatment, interventions that address long-term loss of bone mineral density should be considered, as this is a consequence of hyperprolactinemia.

References

1. Aoki Y, Belin RM, Clickner R, et al. Serum TSH and total T4 in the United States population and their association with participant characteristics: National Health and Nutrition Examination Survey (NHANES 1999-2002). *Thyroid.* 2007 Dec;17(12):1211-23.
2. Razvi S, Weaver JU, Pearce SHS. Subclinical thyroid disorders: significance and clinical impact. *J Clin Pathol.* 2010 May;63(5):379-86.
3. Nussey SS, Whitehead SA. *Endocrinology: An Integrated Approach.* Oxford: Bios Scientific Publishers; 2001.
4. Falaschi P, Martocchia A, Proietti A, et al. The hypothalamic-pituitary-thyroid axis in subjects with subclinical thyroid diseases: the impact of the negative feedback mechanism. *Neuro Endocrinol Lett.* 2004 Aug;25(4):292-6.
5. Gereben B, Zavacki AM, Ribich S, et al. Cellular and Molecular Basis of Deiodinase-Regulated Thyroid Hormone Signaling. *Endocr Rev.* 2008 Sep 24. Epub ahead of print.
6. Fliers E, Alkemade A, Wiersinga WM, et al. Hypothalamic thyroid hormone feedback in health and disease. *Prog Brain Res.* 2006;153:189-207.
7. Fliers E, Unmehopa UA, Alkemade A. Functional neuroanatomy of thyroid hormone feedback in the human hypothalamus and pituitary gland. *Mol Cell Endocrinol.* 2006 Jun 7;251(1-2):1-8.
8. Wiersinga WM. Thyroid hormone replacement therapy. *Horm Res.* 2001;56 Suppl 1:74-81.
9. Bianco AC, Kim BW. Deiodinases: implications of the local control of thyroid hormone action. *J Clin Invest.* 2006 Oct;116(10):2571-9.
10. Bános C, Takó J, Salamon F, et al. Effect of ACTH-stimulated glucocorticoid hypersecretion on the serum concentrations of thyroxine-binding globulin, thyroxine, triiodothyronine, reverse triiodothyronine and on the TSH-response to TRH. *Acta Med Acad Sci Hung.* 1979; 36(4):381-94.
11. Benker G, Raida M, Olbricht T, et al. TSH secretion in Cushing's syndrome: relation to glucocorticoid excess, diabetes, goitre, and the 'sick euthyroid syndrome'. *Clin Endocrinol* (Oxf). 1990 Dec;33(6):777-86.
12. Klein JR. The immune system as a regulator of thyroid hormone activity. *Exp Biol Med.* (Maywood). 2006 Mar;231(3):229-36.
13. Iijima K, Otake T, Yoshinaga J, et al. Cadmium, lead, and selenium in cord blood and thyroid hormone status of newborns. *Biol Trace Elem Res.* 2007 Oct;119(1):10-8.
14. Hammouda F, Messaoudi I, El Hani J, et al. Reversal of Cadmium-Induced Thyroid Dysfunction by Selenium, Zinc, or Their Combination in Rat. *Biol Trace Elem Res.* 2008 Aug 8. Epub ahead of print.
15. Turyk ME, Anderson HA, Persky VW. Relationships of thyroid hormones with polychlorinated biphenyls, dioxins, furans, and DDE in adults. *Environ Health Perspect.* 2007 Aug;115(8):1197-203.
16. Crofton KM, Craft ES, Hedge JM, et al. Thyroid-hormone-disrupting chemicals: evidence for dose-dependent additivity or synergism. *Environ Health Perspect.* 2005 Nov;113(11):1549-54.
17. Mastorakos G, Karoutsou EI, Mizamtsidi M, et al. The menace of endocrine disruptors on thyroid hormone physiology and their impact on intrauterine development. *Endocrine.* 2007 Jun;31(3):219-37.
18. Sanderson JT. The steroid hormone biosynthesis pathway as a target for endocrine-disrupting chemicals. *Toxicol Sci.* 2006 Nov;94(1):3-21.
19. Langer P, Kocan A, Tajtakova M, et al. Human thyroid in the population exposed to high environmental pollution by organochlorinated pollutants for several decades. *Endocr Regul.* 2005 Jan;39(1):13-20.
20. Washam C. Eye on iodine. *Environ Health Perspect.* 2008 May;116(5):A200.
21. Hollowell JG, Haddow JE. The prevalence of iodine deficiency in women of reproductive age in the United States of America. *Public Health Nutr.* 2007 Dec;10(12A): 1532-9;
22. Public Health Committee of the American Thyroid Association, et al. Iodine supplementation for pregnancy and lactation-United States and Canada: recommendations of the American Thyroid Association. *Thyroid.* 2006 Oct;16(10):949-51.
23. Hoption Cann SA. Hypothesis: dietary iodine intake in the etiology of cardiovascular disease. *J Am Coll Nutr.* 2006 Feb;25(1):1-11.
24. Pearce EN, Braverman LE. Environmental pollutants and the thyroid. *Best Pract Res Clin Endocrinol Metab.* 2009 Dec;23(6):801-13. Review.
25. Divi RL, Chang HC, Doerge DR. Anti-thyroid isoflavones from soybean: isolation, characterization, and mechanisms of action. *Biochem Pharmacol.* 1997 Nov 15;54(10):1087-96.
26. Messina M, Redmond G. Effects of soy protein and soybean isoflavones on thyroid function in healthy adults and hypothyroid patients: a review of the relevant literature. *Thyroid.* 2006 Mar;16(3):249-58.
27. Hathcock JN, Hattan DG, Jenkins MY, et al. Food Additives, Contaminants and Natural Toxins. In: Shils M, et al: *Modern Nutrition in Health and Disease,* 9th ed. Williams and Wilkins, Baltimore, MD 1999.
28. Ellingsen DG, Efskind J, Haug E, et al. Effects of low mercury vapour exposure on the thyroid function in chloralkali workers. *J Appl Toxicol.* 2000 Nov-Dec; 20(6):483-9.
29. Soldin OP, O'Mara DM, Aschner M. Thyroid Hormones and Methylmercury Toxicity. *Biol Trace Elem Res.* 2008 Aug 22. Epub ahead of print.

30. Takser L, Mergler D, Baldwin M, et al. Thyroid hormones in pregnancy in relation to environmental exposure to organochlorine compounds and mercury. *Environ Health Perspect.* 2005 Aug;113(8):1039-45.

31. Maia AL, Kim BW, Huang SA, et al. Type 2 iodothyronine deiodinase is the major source of plasma T3 in euthyroid humans. *J Clin Invest.* 2005 Sep;115(9):2524-33.

32. Watanabe M, Houten SM, Mataki C, et al. Bile acids induce energy expenditure by promoting intracellular thyroid hormone activation. *Nature.* 2006 Jan 26;439(7075):484-9.

33. Thomas C, Auwerx J, Schoonjans K. Bile acids and the membrane bile acid receptor TGR5—connecting nutrition and metabolism. *Thyroid.* 2008 Feb;18(2):167-74.

34. Beard JL, Borel MJ, Derr J. Impaired thermoregulation and thyroid function in iron-deficiency anemia. *Am J Clin Nutr.* 1990 Nov;52(5):813-9.

35. Toni R, Malaguti A, Castorina S, et al. New paradigms in neuroendocrinology: relationships between obesity, systemic inflammation and the neuroendocrine system. *J Endocrinol Invest.* 2004 Feb;27(2):182-6.

36. Davey JC, Nomikos AP, Wungjiranirun M, et al. Arsenic as an endocrine disruptor: arsenic disrupts retinoic acid receptor-and thyroid hormone receptor-mediated gene regulation and thyroid hormone-mediated amphibian tail metamorphosis. *Environ Health Perspect.* 2008 Feb;116(2):165-72.

37. Arlt W, Allolio B. Adrenal insufficiency. *Lancet.* 2003 May 31;361(9372):1881-93.

38. Martín Martorell P, Roep BO, Smit JW. Autoimmunity in Addison's disease. *Neth J Med.* 2002 Aug;60(7):269-75.

39. Coco G, Dal Pra C, Presotto F, et al. Estimated risk for developing autoimmune Addison's disease in patients with adrenal cortex autoantibodies. *J Clin Endocrinol Metab.* 2006 May;91(5):1637-45.

40. Eisenbarth GS, Gottlieb PA. Autoimmune polyendocrine syndromes. *N Engl J Med.* 2004 May 13;350(20):2068-79.

41. Ullerås E, Ohlsson A, Oskarsson A. Secretion of cortisol and aldosterone as a vulnerable target for adrenal endocrine disruption - screening of 30 selected chemicals in the human H295R cell model. *J Appl Toxicol.* 2008 Nov;28(8):1045-53.

42. Harvey PW, Everett DJ, Springall CJ. Adrenal toxicology: a strategy for assessment of functional toxicity to the adrenal cortex and steroidogenesis. *J Appl Toxicol.* 2007 Mar-Apr;27(2):103-15.

43. Chiodini I, Torlontano M, Carnevale V, et al. Skeletal involvement in adult patients with endogenous hypercortisolism. *J Endocrinol Invest.* 2008 Mar;31(3):267-76.

44. Chiodini I, Mascia ML, Muscarella S, et al. Subclinical hypercortisolism among outpatients referred for osteoporosis. *Ann Intern Med.* 2007 Oct 16;147(8):541-8.

45. Pivonello R, De Martino MC, De Leo M, et al. Cushing's Syndrome. *Endocrinol Metab Clin North Am.* 2008 Mar;37(1):135-49, ix.

46. Nieman LK, Ilias I. Evaluation and treatment of Cushing's syndrome. *Am J Med.* 2005 Dec;118(12):1340-6.

47. Joëls M, Karst H, Krugers HJ, et al. Chronic stress: implications for neuronal morphology, function and neurogenesis. *Front Neuroendocrinol.* 2007 Aug-Sep;28(2-3):72-96.

48. McEwen BS. Central effects of stress hormones in health and disease: Understanding the protective and damaging effects of stress and stress mediators. *Eur J Pharmacol.* 2008 Apr 7;583(2-3):174-85.

49. Wurtman RJ. Stress and the adrenocortical control of epinephrine synthesis. *Metabolism.* 2002 Jun;51(6 Suppl 1):11-4.

50. Ferrari E, Magri F. Role of neuroendocrine pathways in cognitive decline during aging. *Ageing Res Rev.* 2008 Jul;7(3):225-33.

51. Young AH. Antiglucocoticoid treatments for depression. *Aust N Z J Psychiatry.* 2006 May;40(5):402-5.

52. Marklund N, Peltonen M, Nilsson TK. Low and high circulating cortisol levels predict mortality and cognitive dysfunction early after stroke. *J Intern Med.* 2004 Jul; 256(1):15-21.

53. Webster Marketon JI, Glaser R. Stress hormones and immune function. *Cell Immunol.* 2008 Mar-Apr;252(1-2): 16-26.

54. Tauchmanovà L, Pivonello R, De Martino MC, et al. Effects of sex steroids on bone in women with subclinical or overt endogenous hypercortisolism. *Eur J Endocrinol.* 2007 Sep;157(3):359-66.

55. Herrington DM, Gordon GB, Achuff SC, et al. Plasma dehydroepiandrosterone and dehydroepiandrosterone sulfate in patients undergoing diagnostic coronary angiography, *J Am Coll Cardiol.* 16 (1990), pp. 862–870.

56. Yamaguchi Y, Tanaka S, Yamakawa T, et al. Reduced serum dehydroepiandrosterone levels in diabetic patients with hyperinsulinaemia, *Clin Endocrinol* (Oxf) 49 (1998), pp. 377–383.

57. Dorsey MJ, Cohen LE, Phipatanakul W, et al. Assessment of adrenal suppression in children with asthma treated with inhaled corticosteroids: use of dehydroepiandrosterone sulfate as a screening test. *Ann Allergy Asthma Immunol.* 2006 Aug;97(2):182-6.

58. Fischli S, Jenni S, Allemann S. Dehydroepiandrosterone sulfate in the assessment of the hypothalamic-pituitary-adrenal axis. *J Clin Endocrinol Metab.* 2008 Feb;93(2): 539-42.

59. Nasrallah MP, Arafah BM. The value of dehydroepiandrosterone sulfate measurements in the assessment of adrenal function. *J Clin Endocrinol Metab.* 2003 Nov;88(11):5293-8.

60. Martínez-Taboada V, Bartolomé MJ, Amado JA, et al. Changes in peripheral blood lymphocyte subsets in elderly subjects are associated with an impaired function of the hypothalamic-pituitary-adrenal axis. *Mech Ageing Dev.* 2002 Sep;123(11):1477-86.

61. Kasperska-Zajac A, Brzoza Z, Rogala B. Dehydroepiandrosterone and dehydroepiandrosterone sulphate in atopic allergy and chronic urticaria. *Inflammation.* 2008 Jun;31(3):141-5.

62. Kasperska-Zajac A, Brzoza Z, Rogala B. Sex hormones and urticaria. *J Dermatol Sci.* 2008 Nov;52(2):79-86.

63. Butcher SK, Killampalli V, Lascelles D, et al. Raised cortisol:DHEAS ratios in the elderly after injury: potential impact upon neutrophil function and immunity. *Aging Cell.* 2005 Dec;4(6):319-24.

64. Karbowska J, Kochan Z. Effect of DHEA on endocrine functions of adipose tissue, the involvement of PPAR gamma. *Biochem Pharmacol.* 2005 Jul 15;70(2):249-57.

65. Kochan Z, Karbowska J. Dehydroepiandrosterone upregulates resistin gene expression in white adipose tissue. *Mol Cell Endocrinol.* 2004 Apr 15;218(1-2):57-64.

66. Kajita K, Ishizuka T, Mune T, et al. Dehydroepiandrosterone down-regulates the expression of peroxisome proliferator-activated receptor gamma in adipocytes. *Endocrinology.* 2003 Jan;144(1):253-9.

67. Akishita M, Hashimoto M, Ohike Y, et al. Association of plasma dehydroepiandrosterone-sulfate levels with endothelial function in postmenopausal women with coronary risk factors. *Hypertens Res.* 2008 Jan;31(1):69-74.

68. Akishita M, Hashimoto M, Ohike Y, et al. Low testosterone level is an independent determinant of endothelial dysfunction in men. *Hypertens Res.* 2007 Nov;30(11):1029-34.

69. Charlton M, Angulo P, Chalasani N, et al. Low circulating levels of dehydroepiandrosterone in histologically advanced nonalcoholic fatty liver disease. *Hepatology.* 2008 Feb;47(2):484-92.

70. Schell E, Theorell T, Hasson D, et al. Stress biomarkers' associations to pain in the neck, shoulder and back in healthy media workers: 12-month prospective follow-up. *Eur Spine J.* 2008 Mar;17(3):393-405.

71. Bauer ME. Stress, glucocorticoids and ageing of the immune system. *Stress.* 2005 Mar;8(1):69-83.

72. Butcher SK, Lord JM. Stress responses and innate immunity: aging as a contributory factor. *Aging Cell.* 2004 Aug;3(4):151-60.

73. Valenti G, Denti L, Maggio M, et al. Effect of DHEAS on skeletal muscle over the life span: the InCHIANTI study. *J Gerontol A Biol Sci Med Sci.* 2004 May;59(5):466-72.

74. Liu Y, Apak TI, Lehmler HJ, et al. Hydroxylated polychlorinated biphenyls are substrates and inhibitors of human hydroxysteroid sulfotransferase SULT2A1. *Chem Res Toxicol.* 2006 Nov;19(11):1420-5.

75. Bonnefoy M, Kostka T, Patricot MC, et al. Physical activity and dehydroepiandrosterone sulphate, insulin-like growth factor I and testosterone in healthy active elderly people. *Age Ageing.* 1998 Nov;27(6):745-51.

76. Tagawa N, Tamanaka J, Fujinami A, et al. Serum dehydroepiandrosterone, dehydroepiandrosterone sulfate, and pregnenolone sulfate concentrations in patients with hyperthyroidism and hypothyroidism. *Clin Chem.* 2000 Apr;46(4):523-8.

77. Mahmoud A, Comhaire FH. Mechanisms of disease: late-onset hypogonadism. *Nat Clin Pract Urol.* 2006 Aug;3(8):430-8.

78. Pitteloud N, Dwyer AA, DeCruz S, et al. Inhibition of luteinizing hormone secretion by testosterone in men requires aromatization for its pituitary but not its hypothalamic effects: evidence from the tandem study of normal and gonadotropin-releasing hormone-deficient men. *J Clin Endocrinol Metab.* 2008 Mar;93(3):784-91.

79. Hayes FJ, DeCruz S, Seminara SB, et al. Differential regulation of gonadotropin secretion by testosterone in the human male: absence of a negative feedback effect of testosterone on follicle-stimulating hormone secretion. *J Clin Endocrinol Metab.* 2001 Jan;86(1):53-8.

80. Köhler TS, Kim J, Feia K, et al. Prevalence of androgen deficiency in men with erectile dysfunction. *Urology.* 2008 Apr;71(4):693-7.

81. Farrell JB, Deshmukh A, Baghaie AA. Low testosterone and the association with type 2 diabetes. *Diabetes Educ.* 2008 Sep-Oct;34(5):799-806.

82. Araujo AB, Esche GR, Kupelian V, et al. Prevalence of symptomatic androgen deficiency in men. *J Clin Endocrinol Metab.* 2007 Nov;92(11):4241-7.

83. Hall SA, Araujo AB, Esche GR, et al. Treatment of symptomatic androgen deficiency: results from the Boston Area Community Health Survey. *Arch Intern Med.* 2008 May 26;168(10):1070-6.

84. Clark BJ, Cochrum RK. The steroidogenic acute regulatory protein as a target of endocrine disruption in male reproduction. *Drug Metab Rev.* 2007;39(2-3):353-70.

85. Morley JE. Endocrine factors in geriatric sexuality. *Clin Geriatr Med.* 1991 Feb;7(1):85-93.

86. Almeida OP, Yeap BB, Hankey GJ, et al. Low free testosterone concentration as a potentially treatable cause of depressive symptoms in older men. *Arch Gen Psychiatry.* 2008 Mar;65(3):283-9.

87. Yeap BB, Almeida OP, Hyde Z, et al. Higher serum free testosterone is associated with better cognitive function in older men, while total testosterone is not. The Health In Men Study. *Clin Endocrinol* (Oxf). 2008 Mar;68(3):404-12.

88. Herbst KL, Bhasin S. Testosterone action on skeletal muscle. *Curr Opin Clin Nutr Metab Care.* 2004 May;7(3):271-7.

89. Dupree K, Dobs A. Osteopenia and male hypogonadism. 1: *Rev Urol.* 2004;6 Suppl 6:S30-4.

90. Akishita M, Hashimoto M, Ohike Y, et al. Low testosterone level is an independent determinant of endothelial dysfunction in men. *Hypertens Res.* 2007 Nov;30(11):1029-34.

91. Turhan S, Tulunay C, Güleç S, et al. The association between androgen levels and premature coronary artery disease in men. *Coron Artery Dis.* 2007 May;18(3):159-62.

92. Laughlin GA, Barrett-Connor E, Bergstrom J. Low serum testosterone and mortality in older men. *J Clin Endocrinol Metab.* 2008 Jan;93(1):68-75.

93. Kupelian V, Hayes FJ, Link CL, et al. Inverse association of testosterone and the metabolic syndrome in men is consistent across race and ethnic groups. *J Clin Endocrinol Metab.* 2008 Sep;93(9):3403-10.

94. Lunenfeld B. Testosterone deficiency and the metabolic syndrome. *Aging Male.* 2007 Jun;10(2):53-6.

95. Chu LW, Tam S, Kung AW, et al. Serum total and bioavailable testosterone levels, central obesity, and muscle strength changes with aging in healthy Chinese men. *J Am Geriatr Soc.* 2008 Jul;56(7):1286-91.

96. Meeker JD, Ryan L, Barr DB, et al. Exposure to nonpersistent insecticides and male reproductive hormones. *Epidemiology.* 2006 Jan;17(1):61-8.

97. Fowler PA, Abramovich DR, Haites NE, et al. Human fetal testis Leydig cell disruption by exposure to the pesticide dieldrin at low concentrations. *Hum Reprod.* 2007 Nov;22(11):2919-27.

98. Yucra S, Rubio J, Gasco M, et al. Semen quality and reproductive sex hormone levels in Peruvian pesticide sprayers. *Int J Occup Environ Health.* 2006 Oct-Dec;12(4):355-61.

99. Laguë E, Tremblay JJ. Antagonistic effects of testosterone and the endocrine disruptor mono-(2-ethylhexyl) phthalate on INSL3 transcription in Leydig cells. *Endocrinology.* 2008 Sep;149(9):4688-94.

100. Lee BM, Koo HJ. Hershberger assay for antiandrogenic effects of phthalates. *J Toxicol Environ Health A.* 2007 Aug;70(15-16):1365-70.

101. Ge RS, Chen GR, Tanrikut C, et al. Phthalate ester toxicity in Leydig cells: developmental timing and dosage considerations. *Reprod Toxicol.* 2007 Apr-May;23(3):366-73.

102. Stahlhut RW, van Wijngaarden E, Dye TD, et al. Concentrations of urinary phthalate metabolites are associated with increased waist circumference and insulin resistance in adult U.S. males. *Environ Health Perspect.* 2007 Jun;115(6):876-82.

103. Hauser R, Meeker JD, Duty S, et al. Altered semen quality in relation to urinary concentrations of phthalate monoester and oxidative metabolites. *Epidemiology.* 2006 Nov;17(6):682-91.

104. Swan SH, Main KM, Liu F, et al. Decrease in anogenital distance among male infants with prenatal phthalate exposure. *Environ Health Perspect.* 2005 Aug;113(8):1056-61.

105. Chiou TJ, Chu ST, Tzeng WF, et al. Arsenic trioxide impairs spermatogenesis via reducing gene expression levels in testosterone synthesis pathway. *Chem Res Toxicol.* 2008 Aug;21(8):1562-9.

106. Hsieh FI, Hwang TS, Hsieh YC. Risk of Erectile Dysfunction Induced by Arsenic Exposure through Well Water Consumption in Taiwan. *Environ Health Perspect.* 2008 Apr;116(4):532-6.

107. Chang SI, Jin B, Youn P, et al. Arsenic-induced toxicity and the protective role of ascorbic acid in mouse testis. *Toxicol Appl Pharmacol.* 2007 Jan 15;218(2):196-203.

108. Frias J, Rodriguez R, Torres JM, et al. Effects of acute alcohol intoxication on pituitary-gonadal axis hormones, pituitary-adrenal axis hormones, beta-endorphin and prolactin in human adolescents of both sexes. *Life Sci.* 2000;67(9):1081-6.

109. Kavitharaj NK, Vijayammal PL. Nicotine administration induced changes in the gonadal functions in male rats. *Pharmacology.* 1999 Jan;58(1):2-7.

110. Rinaldi S, Peeters PH, Bezemer ID, et al. Relationship of alcohol intake and sex steroid concentrations in blood in pre- and post-menopausal women: the European Prospective Investigation into Cancer and Nutrition. *Cancer Causes Control.* 2006 Oct;17(8):1033-43.

111. Li C, Taneda S, Suzuki AK, et al. Estrogenic and anti-androgenic activities of 4-nitrophenol in diesel exhaust particles. *Toxicol Appl Pharmacol.* 2006 Nov 15;217(1):1-6.

112. Furuta C, Noda S, Li C, et al. Nitrophenols isolated from diesel exhaust particles regulate steroidogenic gene expression and steroid synthesis in the human H295R adrenocortical cell line. *Toxicol Appl Pharmacol.* 2008 May 15;229(1):109-20.

113. Bonefeld-Jørgensen EC, Long M, Hofmeister MV, et al. Endocrine-disrupting potential of bisphenol A, bisphenol A dimethacrylate, 4-n-nonylphenol, and 4-n-octylphenol *in vitro*: new data and a brief review. *Environ Health Perspect.* 2007 Dec;115 Suppl 1:69-76.

114. Krüger T, Long M, Bonefeld-Jørgensen EC. Plastic components affect the activation of the aryl hydrocarbon and the androgen receptor. *Toxicology.* 2008 Apr 18;246(2-3):112-23.

115. De Bellis A, Sinisi AA, Conte M, et al. Antipituitary antibodies against gonadotropin-secreting cells in adult male patients with apparently idiopathic hypogonadotropic hypogonadism. *J Clin Endocrinol Metab.* 2007 Feb;92(2):604-7.

116. Ebisch IM, Thomas CM, Peters WH, et al. The importance of folate, zinc and antioxidants in the pathogenesis and prevention of subfertility. *Hum Reprod Update.* 2007 Mar-Apr;13(2):163-74.

117. Van Niekerk FE, Van Niekerk CH. The influence of experimentally induced copper deficiency on the fertility of rams. I. Semen parameters and peripheral plasma androgen concentration. *J S Afr Vet Assoc.* 1989 Mar;60(1):28-31.

118. Prasad AS, Mantzoros CS, Beck FW, et al. Zinc status and serum testosterone levels of healthy adults. *Nutrition.* 1996 May;12(5):344-8.

119. Netter A, Hartoma R, Nahoul K. Effect of zinc administration on plasma testosterone, dihydrotestosterone, and sperm count. *Arch Androl.* 1981 Aug;7(1):69-73.

120. Gromadzka-Ostrowska J. Effects of dietary fat on androgen secretion and metabolism. *Reprod Biol.* 2006; 6 Suppl 2:13-20.

121. Hartman TJ, Dorgan JF, Woodson K, et al. Effects of long-term alpha-tocopherol supplementation on serum hormones in older men. *Prostate.* 2001 Jan 1;46(1):33-8.

122. DiPaola RS, Zhang H, Lambert GH, et al. Clinical and biologic activity of an estrogenic herbal combination (PC-SPES) in prostate cancer. *N Engl J Med.* 1998 Sep 17;339(12):785-91.

123. Akdoğan M, Tamer MN, Cüre E, et al. Effect of spearmint (*Mentha spicata Labiatae*) teas on androgen levels in women with hirsutism. *Phytother Res.* 2007 May;21(5):444-7.

124. Petraglia F, Musacchio C, Luisi S, et al. Hormone-dependent gynaecological disorders: a pathophysiological perspective for appropriate treatment. *Best Pract Res Clin Obstet Gynaecol.* 2008 Apr;22(2):235-49.

125. Rothman MS, Wierman ME. Female hypogonadism: evaluation of the hypothalamic-pituitary-ovarian axis. *Pituitary.* 2008;11(2):163-9.

126. de Kretser DM, Hedger MP, Loveland KL, et al. Inhibins, activins and follistatin in reproduction. *Hum Reprod Update.* 2002 Nov-Dec;8(6):529-41.

127. Vadakkadath Meethal S, Atwood CS. The role of hypothalamic-pituitary-gonadal hormones in the normal structure and functioning of the brain. *Cell Mol Life Sci.* 2005 Feb;62(3):257-70.

128. Messinis IE. Ovarian feedback, mechanism of action and possible clinical implications. *Hum Reprod Update.* 2006 Sep-Oct;12(5):557-71.

129. Hall JE. Neuroendocrine changes with reproductive aging in women. *Semin Reprod Med.* 2007 Sep;25(5): 344-51.

130. Dickerson SM, Gore AC. Estrogenic environmental endocrine-disrupting chemical effects on reproductive neuroendocrine function and dysfunction across the life cycle. *Rev Endocr Metab Disord.* 2007 Jun;8(2):143-59.

131. Liu Z, Doan QV, Blumenthal P, et al. A systematic review evaluating health-related quality of life, work impairment, and health-care costs and utilization in abnormal uterine bleeding. *Value Health.* 2007 May-Jun;10(3):183-94.

132. Woad KJ, Pearson SM, Harris SE. Investigating the association between inhibin alpha gene promoter polymorphisms and premature ovarian failure. *Fertil Steril.* 2008 Feb 2. Epub ahead of print.

133. Knauff EA, Westerveld HE, Goverde AJ, et al. Lipid profile of women with premature ovarian failure. *Menopause.* 2008 Sep-Oct;15(5):919-23.

134. Blank SK, McCartney CR, Marshall JC. The origins and sequelae of abnormal neuroendocrine function in polycystic ovary syndrome. *Hum Reprod Update.* 2006 Jul-Aug;12(4):351-61.

135. Begliuomini S, Casarosa E, Pluchino N, et al. Influence of endogenous and exogenous sex hormones on plasma brain-derived neurotrophic factor. *Hum Reprod.* 2007 Apr;22(4):995-1002.

136. González C, Díaz F, Alonso A. Neuroprotective effects of estrogens: cross-talk between estrogen and intracellular insulin signaling. *Infect Disord Drug Targets.* 2008 Mar;8(1):65-7.

137. Allais G, Castagnoli Gabellari I, De Lorenzo C, et al. Menstrual migraine: clinical and therapeutical aspects. *Expert Rev Neurother.* 2007 Sep;7(9):1105-20.

138. Weiss G, Skurnick JH, Goldsmith LT. Menopause and hypothalamic-pituitary sensitivity to estrogen. *JAMA.* 2004 Dec 22;292(24):2991-6.

139. Cooper RL, Stoker TE, Tyrey L. Atrazine disrupts the hypothalamic control of pituitary-ovarian function. *Toxicol Sci.* 2000 Feb;53(2):297-307.

140. Bretveld RW, Thomas CM, Scheepers PT, et al. Pesticide exposure: the hormonal function of the female reproductive system disrupted? *Reprod Biol Endocrinol.* 2006 May 31;4:30.

141. Perry MJ, Ouyang F, Korrick SA, et al. A prospective study of serum DDT and progesterone and estrogen levels across the menstrual cycle in nulliparous women of reproductive age. *Am J Epidemiol.* 2006 Dec 1;164(11):1056-64.

142. Kinney A, Kline J, Kelly A. Smoking, alcohol and caffeine in relation to ovarian age during the reproductive years. *Hum Reprod.* 2007 Apr;22(4):1175-85.

143. Lambert-Messerlian GM, Harlow BL. The influence of depression, body mass index, and smoking on serum inhibin B levels in late reproductive-aged women. *J Clin Endocrinol Metab.* 2006 Apr;91(4):1496-500.

144. Exley C, Charles LM, Barr L, et al. Aluminium in human breast tissue. *J Inorg Biochem.* 2007 Sep;101(9):1344-6.

145. Darbre PD. Aluminium, antiperspirants and breast cancer. *J Inorg Biochem.* 2005 Sep;99(9):1912-9.

146. Chrousos GP, Torpy DJ, Gold PW. Interactions between the hypothalamic-pituitary-adrenal axis and the female reproductive system: clinical implications. *Ann Intern Med.* 1998 Aug 1;129(3):229-40.

147. Berga SL, Loucks TL. The diagnosis and treatment of stress-induced anovulation. *Minerva Ginecol.* 2005 Feb;57(1):45-54.

148. Woods NF, Carr MC, Tao EY, et al. Increased urinary cortisol levels during the menopausal transition. *Menopause.* 2006 Mar-Apr;13(2):212-21.

149. The influence of depression, body mass index, and smoking on serum inhibin B levels in late reproductive-aged women. *J Clin Endocrinol Metab.* 2006 Apr;91(4):1496-500.

150. Young EA, Midgley AR, Carlson NE. Alteration in the hypothalamic-pituitary-ovarian axis in depressed women. *Arch Gen Psychiatry.* 2000 Dec;57(12):1157-62.

151. Bedwal RS, Bahuguna A. Zinc, copper and selenium in reproduction. *Experientia.* 1994;50:626-40.

152. Kinuta K, Tanaka H, Moriwake T. Vitamin D is an important factor in estrogen biosynthesis of both female and male gonads. *Endocrinology.* 2000 Apr;141(4):1317-24.

153. Barrera D, Avila E, Hernández G, et al. Estradiol and progesterone synthesis in human placenta is stimulated by calcitriol. *J Steroid Biochem Mol Biol.* 2007 Mar;103(3-5):529-32.

154. Ziomkiewicz A, Ellison PT, Lipson SF, et al. Body fat, energy balance and estradiol levels: a study based on hormonal profiles from complete menstrual cycles. *Hum Reprod.* 2008 Nov;23(11):2555-63.

155. Tworoger SS, Chubak J, Aiello EJ, et al. Association of CYP17, CYP19, CYP1B1, and COMT polymorphisms with serum and urinary sex hormone concentrations in postmenopausal women. *Cancer Epidemiol Biomarkers Prev.* 2004 Jan;13(1):94-101.

156. Hirata H, Hinoda Y, Okayama N, et al. CYP1A1, SULT1A1, and SULT1E1 polymorphisms are risk factors for endometrial cancer susceptibility. *Cancer.* 2008 May 1;112(9):1964-73.

157. de Oliveira E, de Aquino Castro R, Gomes MT, et al. The catechol-O-methyltransferase (COMT) gene polymorphism and prevalence of uterine fibroids. *Maturitas.* 2008 Jul-Aug;60(3-4):235-8.

158. Tsuchiya Y, Nakajima M, Yokoi T. Cytochrome P450-mediated metabolism of estrogens and its regulation in human. *Cancer Lett.* 2005 Sep 28;227(2):115-24.

159. Adlercreutz H. Western diet and Western diseases: some hormonal and biochemical mechanisms and associations. *Scand J Clin Lab Invest Suppl.* 1990;201:3-23.

160. Woods MN, Gorbach SL, Longcope C, et al. Low-fat, high-fiber diet and serum estrone sulfate in premenopausal women. *Am J Clin Nutr.* 1989 Jun;49(6):1179-83.

161. Bernstein L, Henderson BE, Hanisch R, et al. Physical exercise and reduced risk of breast cancer in young women. *J Natl Cancer Inst.* 1994 Sep 21;86(18):1403-8.

162. Baker FC, Colrain IM, Trinder J. Reduced parasympathetic activity during sleep in the symptomatic phase of severe premenstrual syndrome. *J Psychosom Res.* 2008 Jul;65(1):13-22.

163. Matsumoto T, Ushiroyama T, Morimura M, et al. Autonomic nervous system activity in the late luteal phase of eumenorrheic women with premenstrual symptomatology. *J Psychosom Obstet Gynaecol.* 2006 Sep;27(3):131-9.

164. Thys-Jacobs S, McMahon D, Bilezikian JP. Cyclical changes in calcium metabolism across the menstrual cycle in women with premenstrual dysphoric disorder. *J Clin Endocrinol Metab.* 2007 Aug;92(8):2952-9.

165. Bertone-Johnson ER, Hankinson SE, Bendich A, et al. Calcium and vitamin D intake and risk of incident premenstrual syndrome. *Arch Intern Med.* 2005 Jun 13; 165(11):1246-52.

166. Hoffman CS, Small CM, Blanck HM, et al. Endometriosis among women exposed to polybrominated biphenyls. *Ann Epidemiol.* 2007 Jul;17(7):503-10.

167. Davis SI, Blanck HM, Hertzberg VS, et al. Menstrual function among women exposed to polybrominated biphenyls: a follow-up prevalence study. *Environ Health.* 2005 Aug 9;4:15.

168. Garcia-Morales P, Saceda M, Kenney N, et al. Effect of cadmium on estrogen receptor levels and estrogen-induced responses in human breast cancer cells. *J Biol Chem.* 1994 Jun 17;269(24):16896-901.

169. Akesson A, Julin B, Wolk A. Long-term dietary cadmium intake and postmenopausal endometrial cancer incidence: a population-based prospective cohort study. *Cancer Res.* 2008 Aug 1;68(15):6435-41.

170. Jackson LW, Zullo MD, Goldberg JM. The association between heavy metals, endometriosis and uterine myomas among premenopausal women: National Health and Nutrition Examination Survey 1999-2002. *Hum Reprod.* 2008 Mar;23(3):679-87.

171. Tunç T, Karadaq YS, Doğulu F, et al. Predisposing factors of restless legs syndrome in pregnancy. *Mov Disord.* 2007;22:627-31.

172. van Wingen G, van Broekhoven F, Verkes RJ, et al. How progesterone impairs memory for biologically salient stimuli in healthy young women. *J Neurosci.* 2007 Oct 17;27(42):11416-23.

173. Seeger H, Mueck AO. Are the progestins responsible for breast cancer risk during hormone therapy in the postmenopause? Experimental vs. clinical data. *J Steroid Biochem Mol Biol.* 2008 Mar;109(1-2):11-5.

174. Zawar MP, Deshpande NM, Gadgil PA, et al. Histopathological study of endometrium in infertility. *Indian J Pathol Microbiol.* 2003 Oct;46(4):630-3.

175. Arredondo F, Noble LS. Endocrinology of recurrent pregnancy loss. *Semin Reprod Med.* 2006 Feb;24(1):33-9.

176. Manore MM. Dietary recommendations and athletic menstrual dysfunction. *Sports Med.* 2002;32(14):887-901.

177. Morris FL, Payne WR, Wark JD. Prospective decrease in progesterone concentrations in female lightweight rowers during the competition season compared with the off season: a controlled study examining weight loss and intensive exercise. *Br J Sports Med.* 1999 Dec; 33(6):417-22.

178. Favier AE. The role of zinc in reproduction. Hormonal mechanisms. *Biol Trace Elem Res.* 1992 Jan-Mar;32: 363-82.

179. Murray AA, Molinek MD, Baker SJ, et al. Role of ascorbic acid in promoting follicle integrity and survival in intact mouse ovarian follicles *in vitro*. *Reproduction.* 2001 Jan;121(1):89-96.

180. Windham GC, Lee D, Mitchell P, et al. Exposure to organochlorine compounds and effects on ovarian function. *Epidemiology.* 2005 Mar;16(2):182-90.

181. Henson MC, Chedrese PJ. Endocrine disruption by cadmium, a common environmental toxicant with paradoxical effects on reproduction. *Exp Biol Med* (Maywood). 2004 May;229(5):383-92.

182. Akgul Y, Derk RC, Meighan T, et al. The methoxychlor metabolite, HPTE, directly inhibits the catalytic activity of cholesterol side-chain cleavage (P450scc) in cultured rat ovarian cells. *Reprod Toxicol.* 2008 Jan;25(1):67-75.

183. Qu JH, Hong X, Chen JF, et al. Fenvalerate inhibits progesterone production through cAMP-dependent signal pathway. *Toxicol Lett.* 2008 Jan 4;176(1):31-9.

184. Hong X, Qu J, Wang Y, et al. Study on the mechanism of trichlorfon-induced inhibition of progesterone synthesis in mouse leydig tumor cells (MLTC-1). *Toxicology.* 2007 May 5;234(1-2):51-8.

185. Sam S, Frohman LA. Normal physiology of hypothalamic pituitary regulation. *Endocrinol Metab Clin North Am.* 2008 Mar;37(1):1-22, vii.

186. Biondi B, Cooper DS. The clinical significance of subclinical thyroid dysfunction. *Endocr Rev.* 2008 Feb;29(1):76-131.

187. Beard JL, Borel MJ, Derr J. Impaired thermoregulation and thyroid function in iron-deficiency anemia. *Am J Clin Nutr.* 1990 Nov;52(5):813-9.

188. Starling RD. Energy expenditure and aging: effects of physical activity. *Int J Sport Nutr Exerc Metab.* 2001 Dec;11 Suppl:S208-17.

189. Gaby AR. Sub-laboratory hypothyroidism and the empirical use of Armour thyroid. *Altern Med Rev.* 2004 Jun;9(2):157-79.

190. Gurnell EM, Hunt PJ, Curran SE, et al. Long-term DHEA replacement in primary adrenal insufficiency: a randomized, controlled trial. *J Clin Endocrinol Metab.* 2008 Feb;93(2):400-9.

191. Arlt W, Callies F, van Vlijmen JC, et al. Dehydroepiandrosterone replacement in women with adrenal insufficiency. *N Engl J Med.* 1999 Sep 30;341(14):1013-20.

192. Holst JP, Soldin SJ, Tractenberg RE, et al. Use of steroid profiles in determining the cause of adrenal insufficiency. *Steroids.* 2007 Jan;72(1):71-84.

193. Løvås K, Thorsen TE, Husebye ES. Saliva cortisol measurement: simple and reliable assessment of the glucocorticoid replacement therapy in Addison's disease. *J Endocrinol Invest.* 2006 Sep;29(8):727-31.

194. Gallagher P, Leitch MM, Massey AE, et al. Assessing cortisol and dehydroepiandrosterone (DHEA) in saliva: effects of collection method. *J Psychopharmacol.* 2006 Sep;20(5):643-9.

195. Lewis JG. Steroid Analysis in Saliva: An overview. *Clin Biochem Rev.* 2006 Aug;27(3):139-46.

196. Cardoso EM, Arregger AL, Tumilasci OR, et al. Diagnostic value of salivary cortisol in Cushing's syndrome. *Clin Endocrinol* (Oxf). 2008 Aug 15. Epub ahead of print.

197. Nieman LK, Biller BM, Findling JW, et al. The diagnosis of Cushing's syndrome: an Endocrine Society Clinical Practice Guideline. *J Clin Endocrinol Metab.* 2008 May; 93(5):1526-40.

198. Vreeburg SA, Hoogendijk WJ, Van Pelt J, et al. Major depressive disorder and hypothalamic-pituitary-adrenal axis activity: results from a large cohort study. *Arch Gen Psychiatry.* 2009 Jun;66(6):617-26.

199. van Santen A, Vreeburg SA, Van der Does AJ, et al. Psychological traits and the cortisol awakening response: Results from the Netherlands Study of Depression and Anxiety. *Psychoneuroendocrinology.* 2010 Aug 17. Epub ahead of print.

200. Tostain JL, Blanc F. Testosterone deficiency: a common, unrecognized syndrome. *Nat Clin Pract Urol.* 2008 Jul;5(7):388-96.

201. Bhasin S, Cunningham GR, Hayes FJ, et al. Testosterone therapy in adult men with androgen deficiency syndromes: an endocrine society clinical practice guideline. *J Clin Endocrinol Metab.* 2006 Jun;91(6):1995-2010.

202. Morley JE, Perry HM 3rd, Kevorkian RT, et al. Comparison of screening questionnaires for the diagnosis of hypogonadism. *Maturitas.* 2006 Mar 20;53(4):424-9.

203. Gandara BK, Leresche L, Mancl L. Patterns of salivary estradiol and progesterone across the menstrual cycle. *Ann N Y Acad Sci.* 2007 Mar;1098:446-50.

204. Ishikawa M, Sengoku K, Tamate K. The clinical usefulness of salivary progesterone measurement for the evaluation of the *corpus luteum* function. *Gynecol Obstet Invest.* 2002;53(1):32-7.

205. Tuohy VK, Altuntas CZ. Autoimmunity and premature ovarian failure. *Curr Opin Obstet Gynecol.* 2007 Aug;19(4):366-9.

206. Wu H, Zhao Z, Stone WS, et al. Effects of sleep restriction periods on serum cortisol levels in healthy men. *Brain Res Bull.* 2008 Aug 28. Epub ahead of print.

207. van Uum SH, Lenders JW, Hermus AR. Cortisol, 11beta-hydroxysteroid dehydrogenases, and hypertension. *Semin Vasc Med.* 2004 May;4(2):121-8.

208. Witek-Janusek L, Albuquerque K, Chroniak KR, et al. Effect of mindfulness based stress reduction on immune function, quality of life and coping in women newly diagnosed with early stage breast cancer. *Brain Behav Immun.* 2008 Aug;22(6):969-81.

209. Carlson LE, Speca M, Faris P, et al. One year pre-post intervention follow-up of psychological, immune, endocrine and blood pressure outcomes of mindfulness-based stress reduction (MBSR) in breast and prostate cancer outpatients. *Brain Behav Immun.* 2007 Nov;21(8):1038-49.

210. Kulkarni SK, Dhir A. *Withania somnifera*: an Indian ginseng. *Prog Neuropsychopharmacol Biol Psychiatry.* 2008 Jul 1;32(5):1093-105.

211. Singh D, Aggarwal A, Maurya R, et al. *Withania somnifera* inhibits NF-kappaB and AP-1 transcription factors in human peripheral blood and synovial fluid mononuclear cells. *Phytother Res.* 2007 Oct;21(10):905-13.

212. Kimura Y, Sumiyoshi M. Effects of various *Eleutherococcus senticosus* cortex on swimming time, natural killer activity and corticosterone level in forced swimming stressed mice. *J Ethnopharmacol.* 2004 Dec;95(2-3):447-53.

213. Darbinyan V, Kteyan A, Panossian A, et al. *Rhodiola rosea* in stress induced fatigue—a double blind cross-over study of a standardized extract SHR-5 with a repeated low-dose regimen on the mental performance of healthy physicians during night duty. *Phytomedicine.* 2000 Oct; 7(5):365-71.

214. Delarue J, Matzinger O, Binnert C, et al. Fish oil prevents the adrenal activation elicited by mental stress in healthy men. *Diabetes Metab.* 2003 Jun;29(3):289-95.

215. Hellhammer J, Fries E, Buss C, et al. Effects of soy lecithin phosphatidic acid and phosphatidylserine complex (PAS) on the endocrine and psychological responses to mental stress. *Stress.* 2004 Jun;7(2):119-26.

216. Monteleone P, Maj M, Beinat L, et al. Blunting by chronic phosphatidylserine administration of the stress-induced activation of the hypothalamo-pituitary-adrenal axis in healthy men. *Eur J Clin Pharmacol.* 1992;42(4):385-8.

217. Xu Y, Ku B, Cui L, et al. Curcumin reverses impaired hippocampal neurogenesis and increases serotonin receptor 1A mRNA and brain-derived neurotrophic factor expression in chronically stressed rats. *Brain Res.* 2007 Aug 8;1162:9-18.

218. Xu Y, Ku B, Tie L, et al. Curcumin reverses the effects of chronic stress on behavior, the HPA axis, BDNF expression and phosphorylation of CREB. *Brain Res.* 2006 Nov 29;1122(1):56-64.

219. Wang R, Li YB, Li YH, et al. Curcumin protects against glutamate excitotoxicity in rat cerebral cortical neurons by increasing brain-derived neurotrophic factor level and activating TrkB. *Brain Res.* 2008 May 19;1210:84-91.

220. Jaroenporn S, Yamamoto T, Itabashi A, et al. Effects of pantothenic acid supplementation on adrenal steroid secretion from male rats. *Biol Pharm Bull.* 2008 Jun;31(6):1205-8.

221. Datsis SA. Effect of pyridoxine deficiency on the adrenal cortex. *Exp Pathol.* 1991;43(3-4):247-50.

222. Carlson LE, Speca M, Patel KD, et al. Mindfulness-based stress reduction in relation to quality of life, mood, symptoms of stress and levels of cortisol, dehydroepiandrosterone sulfate (DHEAS) and melatonin in breast and prostate cancer outpatients. *Psychoneuroendocrinology.* 2004 May;29(4):448-74.

223. Glaser JL, Brind JL, Vogelman JH, et al. Elevated serum dehydroepiandrosterone sulfate levels in practitioners of the Transcendental Meditation (TM) and TM-Sidhi programs. *J Behav Med.* 1992 Aug;15(4):327-41.

224. Filaire E, Duché P, Lac G. Effects of amount of training on the saliva concentrations of cortisol, dehydroepiandrosterone and on the dehydroepiandrosterone: cortisol concentration ratio in women over 16 weeks of training. *Eur J Appl Physiol Occup Physiol.* 1998 Oct;78(5):466-71.

225. Pawlikowski M, Kolomecka M, Wojtczak A, et al. Effects of six months melatonin treatment on sleep quality and serum concentrations of estradiol, cortisol, dehydroepiandrosterone sulfate, and somatomedin C in elderly women. *Neuro Endocrinol Lett.* 2002 Apr;23 Suppl 1:17-9.

226. Adimoelja A. Phytochemicals and the breakthrough of traditional herbs in the management of sexual dysfunctions. *Int J Androl.* 2000;23 Suppl 2:82-4.

227. Gauthaman K, Ganesan AP. The hormonal effects of *Tribulus terrestris* and its role in the management of male erectile dysfunction—an evaluation using primates, rabbit and rat. *Phytomedicine.* 2008 Jan;15(1-2):44-54.

228. Tode T, Kikuchi Y, Hirata J, et al. Effect of Korean red ginseng on psychological functions in patients with severe climacteric syndromes. *Int J Gynaecol Obstet.* 1999 Dec;67(3):169-74.

229. Løvås K, Husebye ES. Replacement therapy for Addison's disease: recent developments. *Expert Opin Investig Drugs.* 2008 Apr;17(4):497-509.

230. MacLean CR, Walton KG, Wenneberg SR, et al. Effects of the Transcendental Meditation program on adaptive mechanisms: changes in hormone levels and responses to stress after 4 months of practice. *Psychoneuroendocrinology.* 1997 May;22(4):277-95.

231. Hawkins VN, Foster-Schubert K, Chubak J, et al. Effect of exercise on serum sex hormones in men: a 12-month randomized clinical trial. *Med Sci Sports Exerc.* 2008 Feb;40(2):223-33.

232. McTiernan A, Tworoger SS, Rajan KB, et al. Effect of exercise on serum androgens in postmenopausal women: a 12-month randomized clinical trial. *Cancer Epidemiol Biomarkers Prev.* 2004 Jul;13(7):1099-105.

233. Lima N, Cavaliere H, Knobel M, et al. Decreased androgen levels in massively obese men may be associated with impaired function of the gonadostat. *Int J Obes Relat Metab Disord.* 2000 Nov;24(11):1433-7.

234. Allen NE, Appleby PN, Davey GK, et al. Lifestyle and nutritional determinants of bioavailable androgens and related hormones in British men. *Cancer Causes Control.* 2002 May;13(4):353-63.

235. Salvati G, Genovesi G, Marcellini L, et al. Effects of *Panax Ginseng* C.A. *Meyer saponins* on male fertility. *Panminerva Med.* 1996 Dec;38(4):249-54.

236. de Andrade E, de Mesquita AA, Claro Jde A, et al. Study of the efficacy of Korean Red Ginseng in the treatment of erectile dysfunction. *Asian J Androl.* 2007 Mar;9(2):241-4.

237. Murugesan P, Muthusamy T, Balasubramanian K, et al. Studies on the protective role of vitamin C and E against polychlorinated biphenyl (Aroclor 1254)—induced oxidative damage in Leydig cells. *Free Radic Res.* 2005 Nov; 39(11):1259-72.

238. Libè R, Barbetta L, Dall'Asta C, et al. Effects of dehydroepiandrosterone (DHEA) supplementation on hormonal, metabolic and behavioral status in patients with hypoadrenalism. *J Endocrinol Invest.* 2004 Sep;27(8):736-41.

239. Kraemer WJ, Ratamess NA, Volek JS, et al. The effects of amino acid supplementation on hormonal responses to resistance training overreaching. *Metabolism.* 2006 Mar;55(3):282-91.

240. Oktem M, Eroglu D, Karahan HB, et al. Black cohosh and fluoxetine in the treatment of postmenopausal symptoms: a prospective, randomized trial. *Adv Ther.* 2007 Mar-Apr;24(2):448-61.

241. Bai W, Henneicke-von Zepelin HH, Wang S, et al. Efficacy and tolerability of a medicinal product containing an isopropanolic black cohosh extract in Chinese women with menopausal symptoms: a randomized, double blind, parallel-controlled study versus tibolone. *Maturitas.* 2007 Sep 20;58(1):31-41.

242. Geller SE, Studee L. Botanical and dietary supplements for menopausal symptoms: what works, what does not. *J Womens Health* (Larchmt). 2005 Sep;14(7):634-49.

243. Shams T. Efficacy of black cohosh-containing preparations on menopausal symptoms: a meta-analysis. *Altern Ther Health Med.* 2010 Jan-Feb;16(1):36-44.

244. Newton KM, Reed SD, LaCroix AZ, et al. Treatment of vasomotor symptoms of menopause with black cohosh, multibotanicals, soy, hormone therapy, or placebo: a randomized trial. *Ann Intern Med.* 2006 Dec 19;145(12):869-79.

245. Geller SE, Shulman LP, van Breemen RB, et al. Safety and efficacy of black cohosh and red clover for the management of vasomotor symptoms: a randomized controlled trial. *Menopause.* 2009 Nov-Dec;16(6):1156-66.

246. Ruhlen RL, Haubner J, Tracy JK, et al. Black cohosh does not exert an estrogenic effect on the breast. *Nutr Cancer.* 2007;59(2):269-77.

247. Hirschberg AL, Edlund M, Svane G. An isopropanolic extract of black cohosh does not increase mammographic breast density or breast cell proliferation in postmenopausal women. *Menopause.* 2007 Jan-Feb;14(1):89-96.

248. Raus K, Brucker C, Gorkow C, et al. First-time proof of endometrial safety of the special black cohosh extract (*Actaea* or *Cimicifuga racemosa* extract) CR BNO 1055. *Menopause.* 2006 Jul-Aug;13(4):678-91.

249. Circosta C, Pasquale RD, Palumbo DR, et al. Estrogenic activity of standardized extract of *Angelica sinensis.* *Phytother Res.* 2006 Aug;20(8):665-9.

250. Kupfersztain C, Rotem C, Fagot R, et al. The immediate effect of natural plant extract, *Angelica sinensis* and *Matricaria chamomilla* (Climex) for the treatment of hot flushes during menopause. A preliminary report. *Clin Exp Obstet Gynecol.* 2003;30(4):203-6.

251. Huang BM, Hsiao KY, Chuang PC, et al. Upregulation of steroidogenic enzymes and ovarian 17beta-estradiol in human granulosa-lutein cells by *Cordyceps sinensis mycelium. Biol Reprod.* 2004 May;70(5):1358-64.

252. Murase Y, Iishima H. Clinical studies of oral administration of gamma-oryzanol on climacteric complaints and its syndrome. *Obstet Gynecol Prac.* 1963;12:147-149.

253. Brooks JD, Ward WE, Lewis JE, et al. Supplementation with flaxseed alters estrogen metabolism in postmenopausal women to a greater extent than does supplementation with an equal amount of soy. *Am J Clin Nutr.* 2004 Feb;79(2):318-25.

254. Bryant M, Cassidy A, Hill C, et al. Effect of consumption of soy isoflavones on behavioural, somatic and affective symptoms in women with premenstrual syndrome. *Br J Nutr.* 2005 May;93(5):731-9.

255. Xu X, Duncan AM, Wangen KE, et al. Soy consumption alters endogenous estrogen metabolism in postmenopausal women. *Cancer Epidemiol Biomarkers Prev.* 2000 Aug;9(8):781-6.

256. Jernström H, Klug TL, Sepkovic DW, et al. Predictors of the plasma ratio of 2-hydroxyestrone to 16alpha-hydroxyestrone among pre-menopausal, nulliparous women from four ethnic groups. *Carcinogenesis.* 2003 May;24(5): 991-1005.

257. McCann SE, Wactawski-Wende J, Kufel K, et al. Changes in 2-hydroxyestrone and 16alpha-hydroxyestrone metabolism with flaxseed consumption: modification by COMT and CYP1B1 genotype. *Cancer Epidemiol Biomarkers Prev.* 2007 Feb;16(2):256-62.

258. Mense SM, Chhabra J, Bhat HK. Preferential induction of cytochrome P450 1A1 over cytochrome P450 1B1 in human breast epithelial cells following exposure to quercetin. *J Steroid Biochem Mol Biol.* 2008 May;110(1-2):157-62.

259. Ramirez MC, Singletary K. Regulation of estrogen receptor alpha expression in human breast cancer cells by sulforaphane. *J Nutr Biochem.* 2008 Jul 3. Epub ahead of print.

260. Wang TT, Milner MJ, Milner JA, et al. Estrogen receptor alpha as a target for indole-3-carbinol. *J Nutr Biochem.* 2006 Oct;17(10):659-64.

261. Alonso-González C, González A, Mazarrasa O, et al. Melatonin prevents the estrogenic effects of sub-chronic administration of cadmium on mice mammary glands and uterus. *J Pineal Res.* 2007 Apr;42(4):403-10.

262. Milewicz A, Gejdel E, Sworen H, et al. *Vitex agnus castus* extract in the treatment of luteal phase defects due to latent hyperprolactinemia. Results of a randomized placebo-controlled double-blind study. *Arzneimittelforschung.* 1993 Jul;43(7):752-6.

263. Schellenberg R. Treatment for the premenstrual syndrome with agnus castus fruit extract: prospective, randomised, placebo controlled study. *BMJ.* 2001 Jan 20;322(7279):134-7.

264. Loch EG, Selle H, Boblitz N. Treatment of premenstrual syndrome with a phytopharmaceutical formulation containing *Vitex agnus castus. J Womens Health Gend Based Med.* 2000 Apr;9(3):315-20.

265. Panth M, Raman L, Ravinder P. Effect of vitamin A supplementation of plasma progesterone and estradiol levels during pregnancy. *Int J Vitam Nutr Res.* 1991;61(1):17-9.

266. Badawy A, State O, Abdelgawad S. N-acetylcysteine and clomiphene citrate for induction of ovulation in polycystic ovary syndrome: a cross-over trial. *Acta Obstet Gynecol Scand.* 2007;86(2):218-22.

267. Sonino N, Navarrini C, Ruini C. Life events in the pathogenesis of hyperprolactinemia. *Eur J Endocrinol.* 2004 Jul;151(1):61-5.

268. Sobrinho LG. Prolactin, psychological stress and environment in humans: adaptation and maladaptation. *Pituitary.* 2003;6(1):35-9.

269. Tamagno G, Burlacu MC, Daly AF, et al. *Vitex agnus castus* might enrich the pharmacological armamentarium for medical treatment of prolactinoma. *Eur J Obstet Gynecol Reprod Biol.* 2007 Nov;135(1):139-40.

270. Wuttke W, Jarry H, Christoffel V. Chaste tree (*Vitex agnus-castus*)—pharmacology and clinical indications. *Phytomedicine.* 2003 May;10(4):348-57.

271. Hu Y, Xin HL, Zhang QY, et al. Anti-nociceptive and anti-hyperprolactinemia activities of *Fructus viticis* and its effective fractions and chemical constituents. *Phytomedicine.* 2007 Oct;14(10):668-74.

272. Carmichael AR. Can *Vitex agnus castus* be Used for the treatment of mastalgia? What is the current evidence? *Evid Based Complement Alternat Med.* 2008 Sep;5(3):247-50.

273. Holt RI. Medical causes and consequences of hyperprolactinaemia. A context for psychiatrists. *J Psychopharmacol.* 2008 Mar;22(2 Suppl):28-37.

274. Ren SG, Melmed S. Pyridoxal phosphate inhibits pituitary cell proliferation and hormone secretion. *Endocrinology.* 2006 Aug;147(8):3936-42.

275. Andon MB, Howard MP, Moser PB, et al. Nutritionally relevant supplementation of vitamin B6 in lactating women: effect on plasma prolactin. *Pediatrics.* 1985 Nov; 76(5):769-73.

276. Karasek M, Stawerska R, Hilczer M, et al. Melatonin circadian rhythm in women with idiopathic hyperprolactinemia. *Neuro Endocrinol Lett.* 2004 Dec;25(6):411-4.

Cardiovascular Disease

Overview

Cardiovascular disease (CVD) is estimated to be responsible for 38% of all deaths in North America. It is the number one cause of death in the United States, where it is responsible for one of every 2.8 deaths.[1,2] In 2006, >630,000 deaths were attributed to heart disease and nearly 140,000 deaths to stroke in the U.S.[3] CVD includes all diseases that affect the heart and blood vessels, such as coronary heart disease (CHD), coronary artery disease (CAD), congestive heart failure (CHF), dyslipidemia, stroke, peripheral arterial disease (PAD), and hypertension.

We know that CVD usually stems from vascular dysfunction—for example, as a result of atherosclerosis, thrombosis, or high blood pressure, which then compromises organ function.[4] Atherosclerosis specifically is thought to underlie the vast majority of CVD; although clinical manifestations often do not occur until adulthood, it is a progressive process that begins in childhood.[14] Low-level inflammation and poor glycemic control have a significant impact on cardiovascular dysfunction.

Both CVD and atherosclerosis have been closely linked with preventable factors such as smoking, dietary habits, physical activity, and exposure to environmental toxins. For example, in a prospective cohort study of >7000 women followed for an average of >30 years, researchers found that nonsmokers without diabetes and with a healthy cholesterol, blood pressure, and weight had a multivariate-adjusted CVD mortality hazard of 0.19 compared to women with two or more risk factors.[5] Similarly, a prospective trial enrolling over 20,000 men and women found that four healthy behaviors combined (non-smoking, not physically inactive, moderate alcohol intake, and a plasma vitamin C indicative of at least five servings of fruit per day) had a 4-fold effect on total mortality (See Figure 9.1).[6] Fortunately, there are many effective natural interventions to both prevent and treat CVD and reduce risks associated with its development.

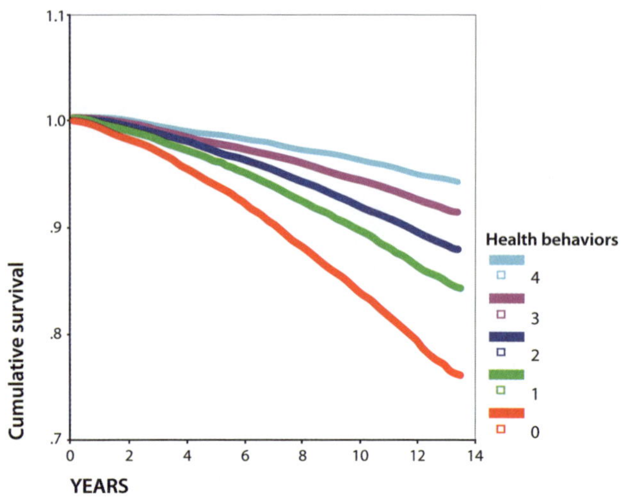

Figure 9.1 Survival function according to number of health behaviors in men and women aged 45–79 years. From: Khaw KT, Wareham N, Bingham S, et al. Combined impact of health behaviours and mortality in men and women: the EPIC-Norfolk prospective population study. *PLoS Med.* 2008 Jan 8;5(1):e12. Reproduced from Open Access article distributed under the terms of the Creative Commons Attribution License, doi:10.1371/journal.pmed.0050012.g001.

Epidemiology

Prevalence

Cardiovascular disease is very common among adults, with nearly 81 million individuals in the U.S. estimated to have one or more forms.[2] Among this number, ~73 million have hypertension (nearly 30% of adults), ~16 million have coronary heart disease, ~5 million have heart failure, and ~5 million have peripheral arterial disease.[7,8,9] Nearly 50% of U.S. adults have at least one lipid abnormality (Figure 9.2), and >83% of those with CVD or related comorbidities (e.g., the metabolic syndrome) do not meet the recommendations of the National Cholesterol Education Program guidelines for all lipids.[10]

Comorbidities are quite common in CVD. Analysis of NHANES data found that, among the elderly, the combined incidence of hypercholesterolemia and hypertension is greater than 50%.[11] This combination of risk factors has a powerful impact on cardiovascular morbidity and mortality. For example, data from >4000 participants in the Cardiovascular Health Study revealed an approximate 2-fold increase in CHD and CVD events from the lowest to highest combined blood pressure/LDL-C levels, and a 4-fold increase in event rates from the lowest blood pressure/highest HDL-C to the highest BP/lowest HDL-C categories (Figure 9.3).[12] As will be discussed in more depth below, poor glycemic control is a significant contributor to CVD. Indeed, researchers found that among U.S. adults over age 30 with diabetes, more than 85% had hypertension, obesity, or hyperlipidemia, while 21% had all 3 cormorbidities.[13]

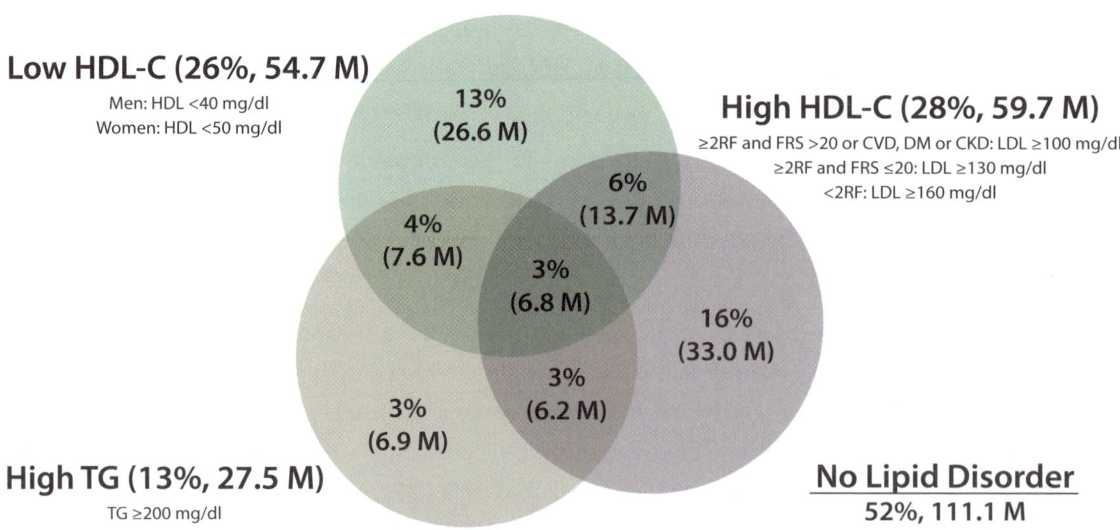

Figure 9.2 Proportion and projected number of U.S. adults in 2007 with lipid abnormalities. From: Ghandehari H, Kamal-Bahl S, Wong ND. Prevalence and extent of dyslipidemia and recommended lipid levels in US adults with and without cardiovascular comorbidities: the National Health and Nutrition Examination Survey 2003-2004. *Am Heart J.* 2008 Jul;156(1):112-9. Reproduced with permission from Elsevier.

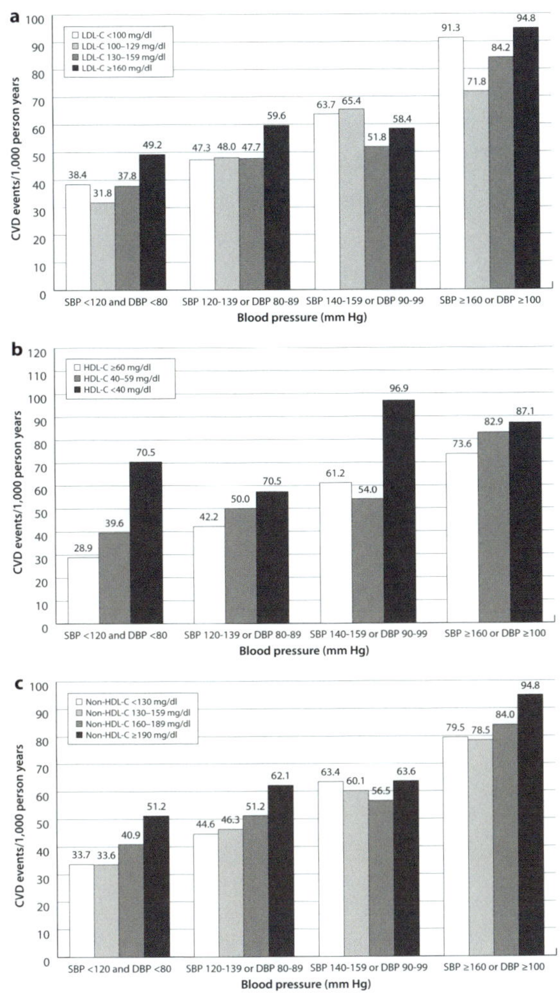

Figure 9.3 Age- and sex-adjusted CVD event rates (per 1000 person years) by (a) blood pressure and LDL-C, (b) blood pressure and HDL-C, and (c) blood pressure and non-HDL-C. From: Wong ND, Lopez VA, Roberts CS, et al. Combined association of lipids and blood pressure in relation to incident cardiovascular disease in the elderly: the cardiovascular health study. *Am J Hypertens*. 2010 Feb;23(2):161-7. Reproduced with permission from Macmillan Publishers Ltd.

Pathophysiology of CVD

Atherosclerosis

Atherosclerotic lesions (atheromata) underlie the majority of cardiovascular pathology. These lesions are asymmetric focal thickenings of the innermost layer of the artery (the intima); they are characterized by lipid accumulation, an inflammatory response, cell death, and fibrosis in the arterial wall (Figure 9.4).

It should also be noted that the initiation of atherosclerosis begins quite early in life, with fatty streaks found in young children.[14] As determined by the Fate of Early Lesions in Children (FELIC) study, maternal hypercholesterolemia determines the long-term susceptibility of children to fatty-streak formation and subsequent atherosclerosis. Those fatty steaks that do not fully regress predetermine the rate of progression of atherosclerosis throughout childhood.[14]

The major cause of morbidity and mortality due to atherosclerosis is a vascular event, such as myocardial infarction (MI) or stroke. However, the risk of vascular events is not primarily a function of the size of the atherosclerotic plaque, i.e., gradual blockage of an arterial lumen. Instead, the risk is more strongly associated with the tendency for a plaque to rupture. For example, 70–85% of all myocardial infarctions occur with >30% stenosis. Rupture is a more frequent cause

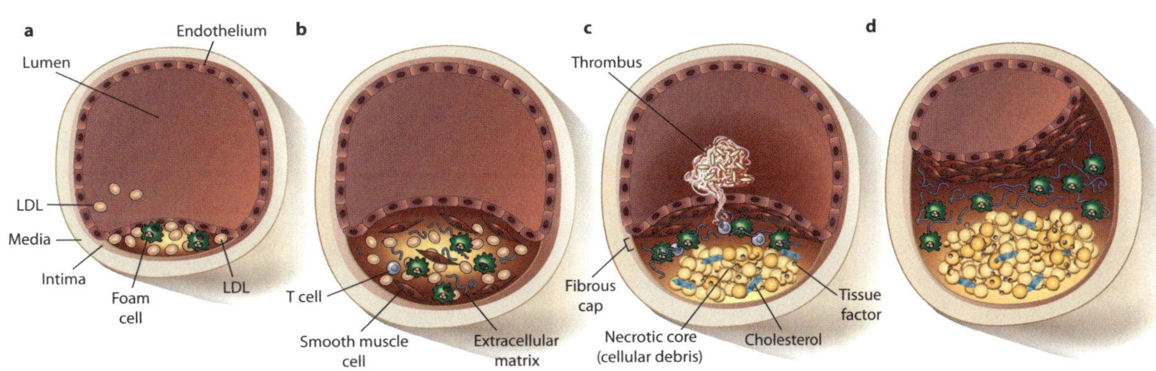

Figure 9.4 Initiation and progression of atherosclerosis. From: Rader DJ, Daugherty A. Translating molecular discoveries into new therapies for atherosclerosis. *Nature*. 2008 Feb 21;451(7181):904-13. Reproduced with permission from Macmillan Publishers Ltd.

of coronary thrombosis in men than women.[15,16] Thus, *targeting plaque stabilization appears to be more clinically important than simply enlarging the lumen.*

To develop a strategic approach to plaque stabilization, it is important to understand the factors that lead to plaque instability. These factors include increased local and systemic inflammation, increased reactive oxygen species, the activation of mast cells, and the infiltration and activation of macrophages.[17] Addressing the endothelial dysfunction which contributes to atherosclerosis should be part of a comprehensive approach.

Endothelial dysfunction

The endothelium plays a pivotal role in the regulation of vascular tone and structure as well as vascular inflammation and thrombosis.[18] We now know that atherosclerotic lesions first begin to develop under an intact but leaky, activated, and dysfunctional endothelium.[16]

Endothelial damage may occur via a number of mechanisms, including insulin resistance, reactive oxygen and nitrogen species, impaired repair processes, heavy metal toxicity, hyperhomocysteinemia, and inhibition of either nitric oxide production or availability.[19] One of the ways that hyperlipidemia and hypertension contribute to atherosclerosis is by impairing endothelial repair. Endothelial progenitor cells (EPCs) are reduced by both of these conditions, inhibiting normal repair mechanisms.[18] Similarly, heavy metals are known to contribute to endothelial damage. Arsenic, lead, and cadmium have all been shown to cause direct toxicity to vascular tissue.[20] As a result, arsenic exposure is associated with increased rates of hypertension, carotid atherosclerosis, ischemic heart disease, and vascular mortality.[21] Similarly, urinary cadmium has been associated with myocardial infarction in women (but not men), with an odds ratio of 1.[80,22] as well as an increased risk for peripheral vascular disease.[23] One suggested mechanism is the inhibition of nitric oxide synthase, thus limiting the availability of NO.[24]

Endogenous toxins are also known to cause endothelial dysfunction. Homocysteine, for example, reduces nitric oxide availability and increases the levels of reactive oxygen species, leading to endothelial dysfunction and platelet activation and aggregation.[25] Homocysteine has also been shown to induce NF-kB and CD40 ligand expression; inhibit apoA-I synthesis (leading to an overall reduction in HDL-C); impair mitochondrial function by activating NMDA-R (N-methyl-D-aspartate (NMDA) receptor); and induce mitochondrial permeability transition (MPT), leading to a decrease in myocyte contractility.[26,27,28,29,30,31,32]

Nitric oxide availability

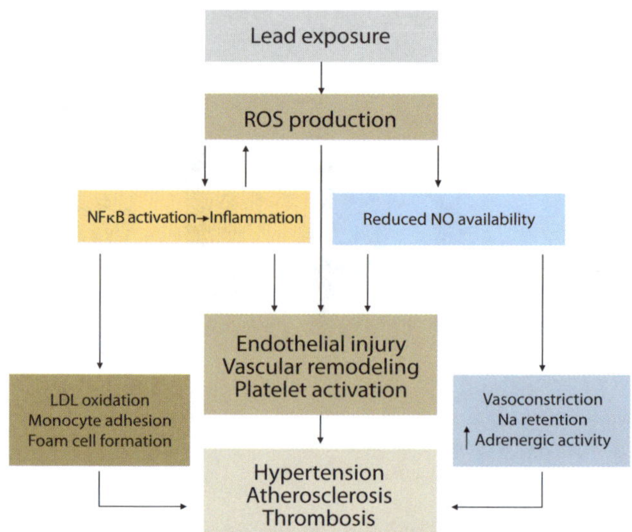

Figure 9.5 Lead exposure increases oxidative stress and inflammation, reduces availability of NO, and increases endothelial dysfunction, thus contributing to increased risk of hypertension. From: Vaziri ND. Mechanisms of lead-induced hypertension and cardiovascular disease. *Am J Physiol Heart Circ Physiol.* 2008 Aug;295(2):H454 65. Reproduced with permission from the American Physiological Society.

The inhibition of nitric oxide production is a common mechanism of endothelial dysfunction, often due to an excess of reactive oxygen species. As noted earlier, many heavy metals cause endothelial damage. Lead, by increasing reactive oxygen species production, increases inflammation and inhibits NO availability (Figure 9.5). As a consequence, lead has been definitively linked as causal for hypertension[33] and is associated with an increased risk for all-cause and cardiovascular mortality at surprisingly low levels. Analysis of the 3rd NHANES data found increased risk for myocardial infarction and stroke with blood lead levels greater than 2 mcg/dl.[34,35] Cumulative exposure, reflected more accurately in bone lead levels, increases the risk for hypertension.[36]

Another common environmental toxin is cigarette smoke, considered the most important cause of myocardial infarction globally.[37] Figure 9.6 traces the pathways by which cigarette smoke induces cardiovascular dysfunction. Cigarette smoke inhibits the L-arginine nitric oxide synthase pathway, leading to elevated levels of asymmetrical dimethylarginine (ADMA), as do cadmium and arsenic, two components of cigarette smoke.[38,39,40] Much of this effect is thought to be due to an increase in reactive oxygen species.[41]

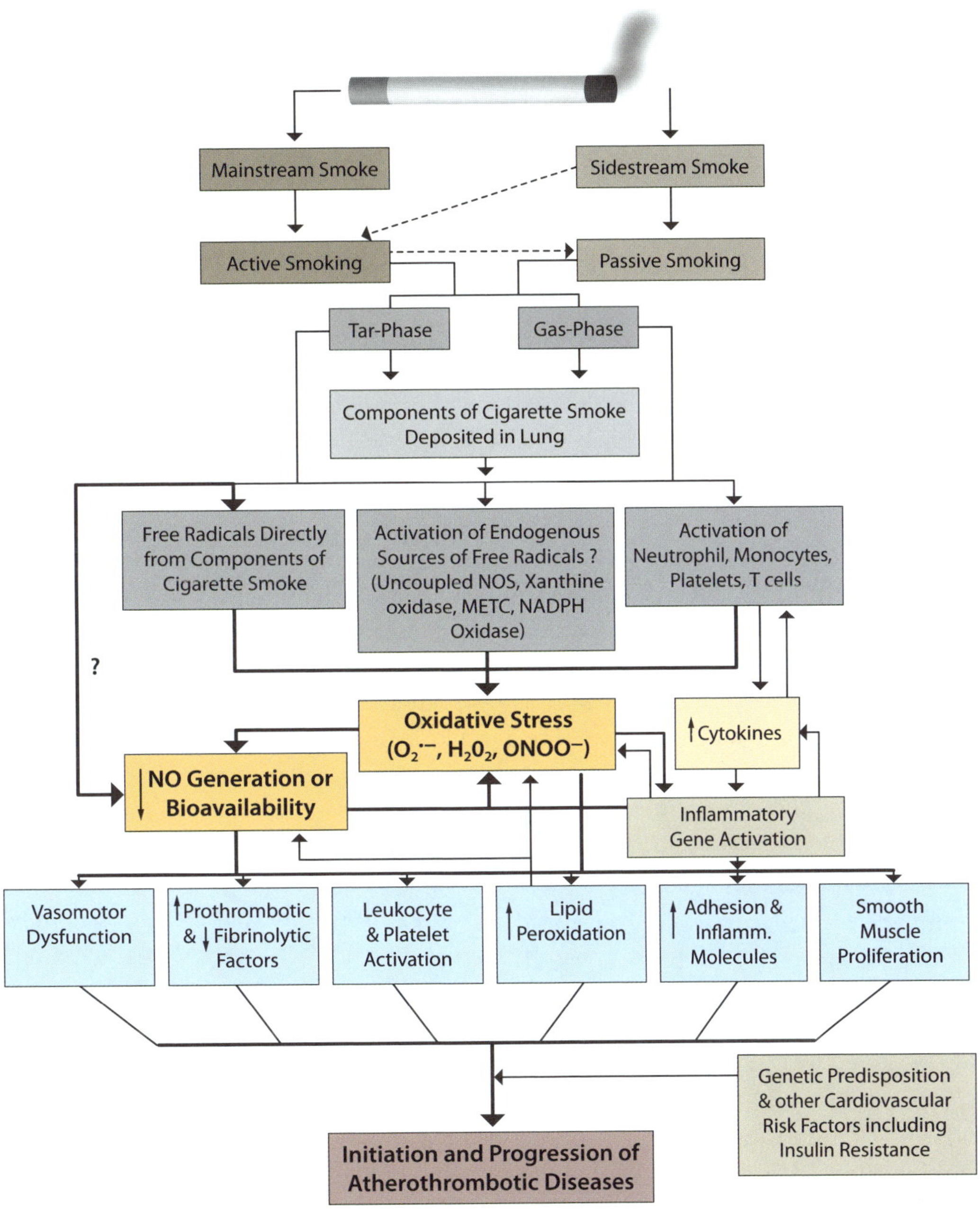

Figure 9.6 Potential pathways and mechanisms for cigarette smoking-mediated cardiovascular dysfunction. From: Ambrose JA, Barua RS. The pathophysiology of cigarette smoking and cardiovascular disease: an update. *J Am Coll Cardiol.* 2004 May 19;43(10):1731-7. Reproduced with permission from Elsevier.

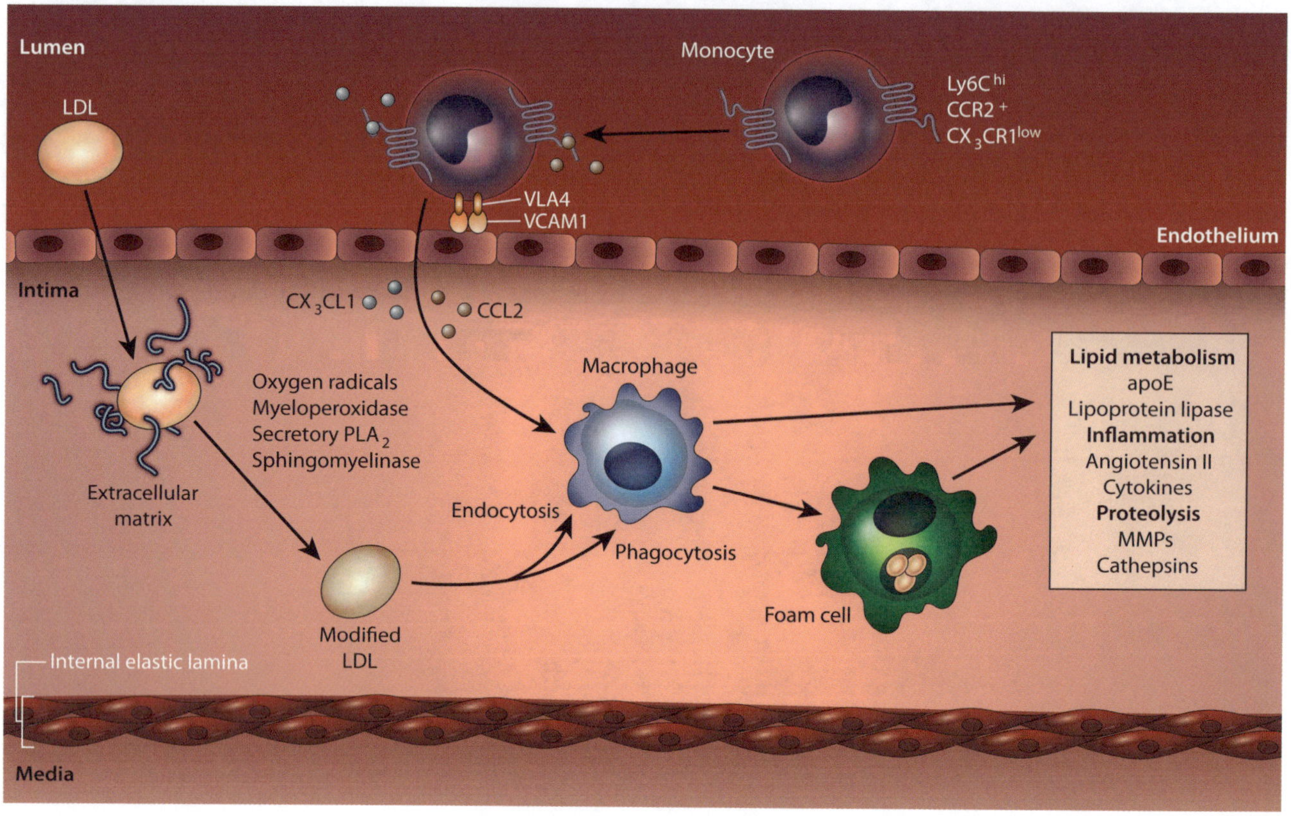

Figure 9.7 Recruitment of monocytes and formation of foam cells. From: Rader DJ, Daugherty A. Translating molecular discoveries into new therapies for atherosclerosis. *Nature*. 2008 Feb 21;451(7181):904-13. Reproduced with permission from Macmillan Publishers Ltd.

Dyslipidemia

Lesion initiation and progression in atherosclerosis both appear to be associated with markedly increased levels of plasma LDL.[42] Human studies and animal studies have shown that lipoproteins containing apolipoprotein B (such as LDL) are required for atherosclerosis development. LDLs are modified upon reaching the intima, and are taken up by macrophages which then become foam cells (Figure 9.7).

In an environment of elevated triglycerides and low HDL-C, LDL-C tends to become small and dense, a pattern more closely associated with cardiovascular risk.[43,44] HDL-C carries excess cholesterol from peripheral cells to the liver for removal (the process termed reverse cholesterol transport), reduces oxidative modification of LDL-C, and inhibits cytokine-induced expression of cellular adhesion molecules on endothelial cells.[45] Plasma levels of HDL-C are strongly and inversely correlated with atherosclerotic CVD.[46]

Inflammation

Chronic inflammation is now known to play an important role in the promotion of atherosclerosis and its thrombotic complications.[47,48] Substantial evidence supports a pivotal role for inflammation in all phases of atherosclerosis, from initiation of the fatty streak to final culmination in acute coronary syndromes.[49] Indeed, although once thought to be completely different processes, it has recently been reported that "the boundaries between inflammation and coagulation can now hardly be distinguished."[50] Figure 9.8 shows the triggers of arterial and venous thrombosis.

C-reactive protein (CRP) has emerged as a robust marker and independent risk factor in the prediction of primary and secondary adverse cardiovascular events. Although preliminary data suggest that elevated CRP plays a causal role in atherogenesis and atherothrombosis, this remains uncertain.[51] Elevated CRP has been associated with a relative risk (RR) of 1.45 for

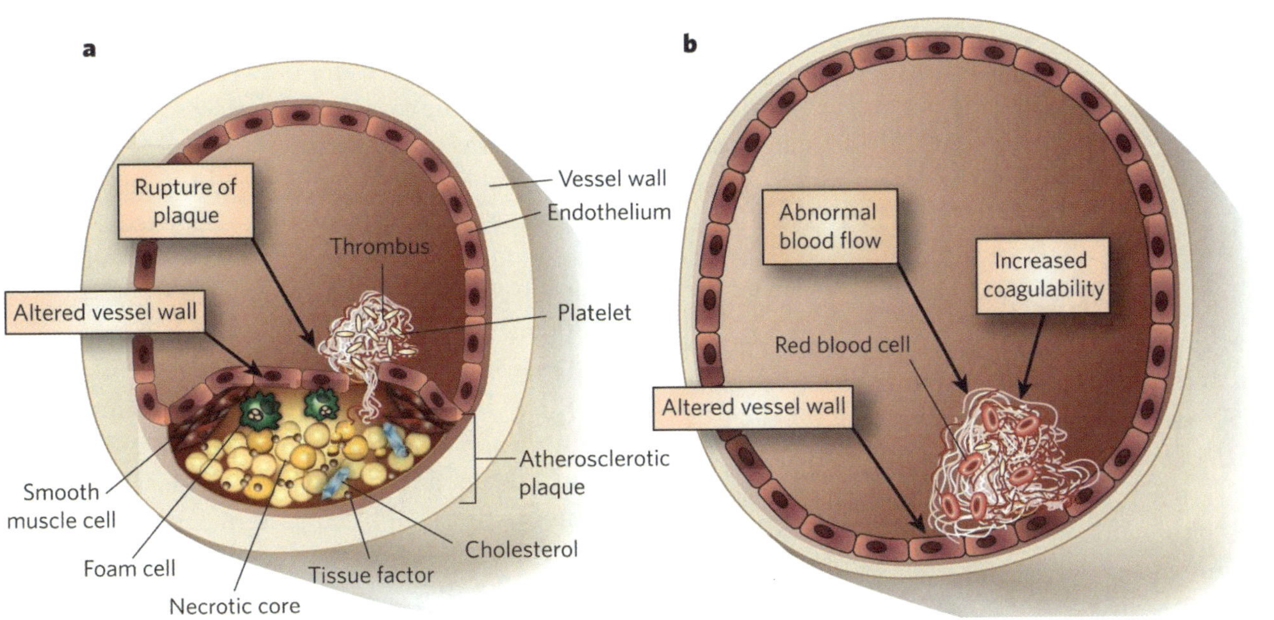

Figure 9.8 Triggers of arterial and venous thrombosis. From: Mackman N. Triggers, targets and treatments for thrombosis. *Nature*. 2008 Feb 21;451(7181):914-8. Reprinted with permission from Macmillan Publishers Ltd.

coronary heart disease for men and women in the Framingham study, after adjusting for age, ethnicity, sex, and traditional risk factors.[52] Similarly, a recent analysis of >10,000 individuals of Danish descent found that elevated CRP levels increased the risk of ischemic heart and cerebrovascular disease, and that polymorphisms in the CRP gene increased CRP levels. Surprisingly, the polymorphisms themselves were not associated with increased ischemic vascular disease.[53]

Another marker of inflammation associated with atherosclerosis is fibrinogen. In the Coronary Artery Risk Development in Young Adults (CARDIA) study, nearly 1400 participants were followed, and researchers found that an elevated fibrinogen level between the ages of 25–37 was independently associated with subclinical atherosclerosis a decade later.[54] Fibrinogen is a coagulation factor, a marker of the acute phase response (inflammation), a platelet activator, a major determinant of plasma viscosity, and a component of atherosclerotic plaque. Systemic levels may be a potential marker of peripheral arterial disease progression, and possibly a target for therapy.[55]

Insulin resistance and obesity

Insulin resistance and poor glucose control have both been shown to have a dramatic impact on CVD incidence and progression. Insulin resistance has been associated with CVD in the general population and in patients with diabetes, independently of other risk factors.[56,57] Among patients with diabetes, carotid artery intima-media thickness (IMT) has been found to be 0.13 mm larger than in control groups, corresponding to approximately 10 years in age, and patients with impaired glucose tolerance have an increase in IMT about one-third of that observed in diabetic patients.[58] The risk of CVD among diabetics has been found to be at least 2- to 3-fold higher than for those without CVD, as determined using data from the ongoing Framingham study.[59,60] For those with the metabolic syndrome, a meta-analysis of longitudinal studies with >90,000 participants found a relative risk of cardiovascular events and death of 1.78, with a higher risk in women.[61] HOMA-IR has also been found to be associated with peripheral arterial disease, with a nearly 2-fold increase in risk for those in the highest quartile.[62] A recent prospective trial with >48,000 participants highlighted the importance of good glycemic control for preventing CVD. Following a study population for an average of 8 years, researchers found that consumption of foods with a high glycemic load increased the risk of coronary heart disease (CHD) in women by 68%; women in the highest glycemic load quartile had a relative risk of 2.2 for CHD compared to those in the lowest quartile.[63]

Obesity and overweight, which often accompany poor glycemic control, are also significant risk factors for CVD and contribute to atherosclerotic development and progression. An overview of 33 cohort studies involving >300,000 participants found that body mass index was directly associated with ischemic and hemorrhagic stroke, and ischemic heart disease; for each 2 kg/m^2 lower the BMI measurement, the risk was reduced 12%, 8%, and 11%, respectively.[64]

While a variety of indexes may be used to assess weight, a recent analysis of >16,000 men in the Physicians' Health Study and >32,000 women from the Nurses' Health Study found the *waist-to-height ratio* to have the strongest association with incident CVD.

Obesity during childhood is also a risk for CVD, perhaps by increasing insulin resistance. In a trial comparing obese pre-pubertal children to controls, the obese children were found to have a greater degree of insulin resistance, and increased carotid intima-media thickness (IMT).[65] Fortunately, a hypocaloric low glycemic index diet has been shown to improve carotid artery IMT and stiffness, reduce weight, and increase insulin sensitivity among obese children.[66]

Other risk/contributing factors

Diet and physical activity

The dietary pattern most consistently associated with a reduction in CVD is predominantly plant based, emphasizing fruits, vegetables, whole grains, nuts, fiber, and a source of omega-3 fatty acids. A "Western diet," high in meats, refined grains, saturated fat, omega-6 oils, French fries, and sugars, is associated with a greater risk of CVD.[67,68]

INTERHEART is a standardized case-control study involving participants from 52 countries that analyzed the associations between food groups and myocardial infarction. An inverse and graded association was found between MI and the intake of raw vegetables, green leafy vegetables, other cooked vegetables, and fruits, while a positive association was found between salty and fried foods and, to a lesser degree, meat intake.[69] Similarly, a study of >5000 men and women in the Multi-Ethnic Study of Atherosclerosis (MESA) defined a "Simplified Healthy Dietary Pattern," emphasizing whole grains, fruit, and nuts, while minimizing intake of added fats and oils, processed meat, and fried potatoes. This simplified pattern compared well to the more complex pattern associated with reduced markers of CVD.[70]

Analysis of >28,000 U.S. women health professionals (Women's Health Study) found that hypertension was directly associated with increasing red meat intake, while poultry was unassociated.[71] Data from the Nurses' Health Study, a prospective cohort of >72,000 women, found that greater adherence to a Western diet was associated with increased cardiovascular, cancer, and overall mortality risk.[72]

Greater physical activity is consistently associated with lower cardiovascular risk among apparently healthy individuals and also among those with CVD. Mild benefits seen at low levels of activity do increase with higher physical activity patterns in a dose-response fashion.[73,74]

Vitamin D deficiency

Data from >8000 individuals enrolled in the NHANES 2001–2004 study indicated that individuals with vitamin D (25-OH) levels <30 ng/ml were more likely to be at high risk for CVD (OR 1.32), for coronary heart disease (OR 1.48), and for both coronary heart disease and heart failure (OR 3.52), after controlling for other variables and as compared to those at low risk for CVD.[75] Similar analysis from the 3rd NHANES study showed an increased risk for hypertension, diabetes, obesity, and elevated triglycerides.[76] A prospective cohort study of >3000 men and women found that those in the lowest quartile of 25-hydroxy vitamin D had a hazard ratio of 2.22 for cardiovascular mortality and 2.08 for all-cause mortality.[77] Lastly, data from the Framingham offspring study found significant increase in risk for cardiovascular events in those with a 25-OH vitamin D <15 ng/ml, particularly those with hypertension.[78]

Vitamin D status is also important in younger populations. In a study following >3500 U.S. adolescents, low levels were found to increase the risk of hypertension (OR 2.36), hyperglycemia (OR 2.54), low HDL cholesterol (1.54), and metabolic syndrome (OR 3.88), independently of adiposity.[79] And as shown below in Figure 9.9, vitamin D status is also predictive of cardiovascular mortality (as well as overall mortality) in older populations (data from the InCHIANTI study, over 1000 adults age 65+).[80]

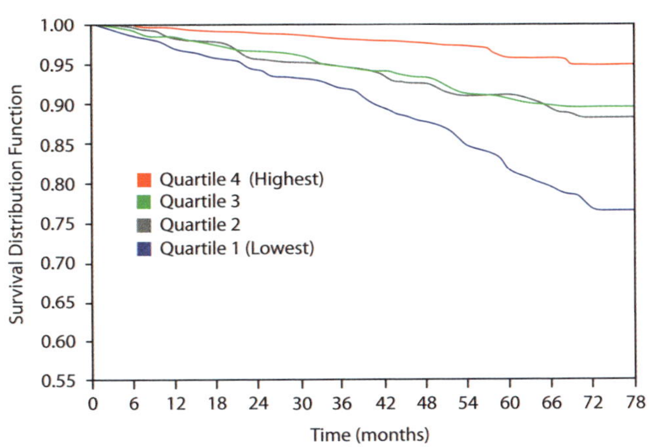

Figure 9.9 Kaplan-Meier plots of cardiovascular disease mortality by quartiles of serum 25-hydroxyvitamin D. From: Semba RD, Houston DK et al. Relationship of 25-hydroxyvitamin D with all-cause and cardiovascular disease mortality in older community-dwelling adults. *Eur J Clin Nutr.* 2010 Feb;64(2):203-9. Reproduced with permission from Macmillan Publishers Ltd.

Hypo/hyperthyroid

Overt hypo- and hyperthyroidism are well established causes of CVD. Hyperthyroidism is known to induce a hyperdynamic cardiovascular state that is associated with a faster heart rate, enhanced left ventricular systolic and diastolic function, and increased prevalence of atrial fibrillation, whereas overt hypothyroidism is characterized by the opposite changes.[81] Less certain is the effect of subclinical hyper- and hypothyroidism, although carotid artery intima thickness has been inversely associated with serum free thyroxine in euthyroid subjects.[82,83] Not all studies have found an association with subclinical thyroid disease and CVD.[84]

Toxin exposure

Other toxin exposures with known adverse cardiovascular risks include mercury, persistent organic pollutants, bisphenol A, and polychlorinated biphenyls (PCBs).[85,86,87,88]

Assessment

Traditional risk factors

Traditional risk factor assessment for CVD includes a comprehensive lipid panel containing total cholesterol (TC), LDL-C, HDL-C, and triglycerides. LDL is recommended as the primary target of therapy by the 3rd Report of the National Cholesterol Education Program (NCEP), with optimal levels below 100 mg/dl.[89] Non-lipid risk factors should also be assessed, including blood pressure (including pulse pressure),[90] weight, smoking, diabetes, physical activity, age, and family history.

Inflammation and glycemic control

In addition to traditional risk factors, there are other factors that help to assess cardiovascular risk. For example, given the impact that hyperglycemia has on CVD initiation and progression, both fasting glucose and either an oral glucose tolerance test or (preferably) a 24-hour continuous blood glucose monitoring can help to identify pathology and guide treatment. For more information, see Clinical Focus 4—The Spectrum of Insulin Resistance. Similarly, hsCRP and fibrinogen are both valuable tools to assess cardiovascular risk, particularly given the importance of inflammation in the development CVD. For more information, see Clinical Focus 5—A Comprehensive Approach to Inflammation.

Framingham Risk Score and ankle-brachial index

Another helpful tool is the Framingham Risk Score, a calculated score based on gender-specific points for age, smoking, diabetes, blood pressure, LDL cholesterol, and HDL cholesterol. The score is used to predict risk of CHD over the subsequent 10 years. It correlates well with other markers of subclinical atherosclerosis, such as carotid plaques and common carotid artery intima-media thickness, and may help to guide the aggressiveness of treatment.[91,92] The national cholesterol education program provides a free online resource to calculate risk: http://hp2010.nhlbihin.net/atpiii/calculator.asp?usertype=prof.

Ankle-brachial index has also proven to be an important marker of risk. Analysis of nearly 25,000 men and 24,000 women from 16 population cohort studies found that a low ABI (<0.9) was associated with a 10-year cardiovascular mortality hazard ratio of 4.2 in men and 3.5 in women. Use of this index improves the predictive value of the Framingham Risk Score.[93] It was also associated with an increased risk of stroke when data from the NHANES 2001–2004 data were analyzed.[94]

Omega-3 index

The omega-3 index is defined as the sum of EPA and DHA expressed as a percentage of the total fatty acid content of red blood cell membranes. Because the omega-3 index half-life is 4–6 times longer than serum or plasma EPA and DHA, it is analogous to the measurement of HbA1c in red blood cells in patients with diabetes mellitus, i.e., it better reflects long-term exposure to these fatty acids than do serum and plasma. It also has the advantage of not being influenced by the fasting or fed state.[95]

An analysis of related laboratory and clinical data found that the omega-3 index was inversely associated with risk for CHD mortality (Figure 9.10). An omega-3 index of ≥8% was associated with the greatest cardioprotection, whereas an index of ≤4% was associated with the least.[96] While less precise, whole blood omega-3 content was also significantly associated with risk for sudden death. In a prospective trial using data from the Physicians' Health Study, men whose blood levels of omega-3 fatty acids were in the 3rd and 4th quartiles had relative risks of sudden death of 0.28 and 0.19, respectively, compared to those in the lowest quartile.[97]

Interestingly, the omega-3 index was associated with improved cardiovascular risk factors independently of body fatness in younger overweight and obese individuals, suggesting that achieving an optimal omega-3 index may negate some of the risk associated with excess weight.[98]

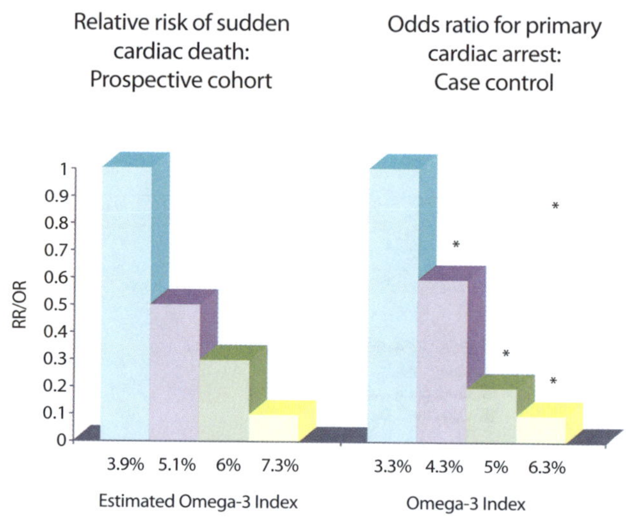

Figure 9.10 Relationship of the omega-3 index to risk of cardiac death and cardiac arrest. From: Harris WS. The omega-3 index as a risk factor for coronary heart disease. *Am J Clin Nutr.* 2008 Jun;87(6):1997S-2002S. Reproduced with permission from the American Society for Nutrition.

Cholesterol subfractions/assays

A number of cholesterol subfractions have emerged with potentially more clinically useful information than traditional lipid risk factors alone. For example, in a systematic review of LDL subfractions, a small particle number was consistently associated with increased risk for CVD, independent of other lipid measurements (although this same review did not find benefit for other LDL subfractions).[99] Oxidized LDL is a persistent pro-inflammatory trigger for the progression of atherosclerosis and plaque rupture, and recently has been shown to play a role in ventricular remodeling. This impact on cardiac structure and function was found to be independent of other classic risk factors.[100]

The size and density of cholesterol subfractions also appears to be prognostic, because the structure of these subfractions influences their physiological effects. For example, it has been established that plasma levels of small dense LDL-C (indicating greater content of apolipoprotein CIII (apo-CIII) and apoB particles) are associated with plasma triglyceride (TG) concentrations, are more atherogenic than larger and less dense LDL-C, and are markers for CVD risk.[101,102] Indeed, the ratio of apoB to apoA-1 (found in HDL-C) may be a better risk indicator than the ratio of LDL to HDL.[103] But the reason that small dense LDLs are more atherogenic appears to relate to their glycation. In a small trial of nondiabetic subjects, researchers determined that these smaller particles (LDL3) were *more heavily and preferentially glycated* over the larger more buoyant LDL, strongly suggesting an explanation for why these particles are more likely to participate in atherogenesis.[104] The study authors emphasized that maintaining optimal glucose control and reducing glycation of these more atherogenic particles is a good clinical strategy.

Subfractions for VLDL and HDL also have clinical importance. For example, high levels of apo-CIII have been associated with increased risk of arteriosclerosis and cardiovascular events, and have also been found in subjects with hypertriglyceridemia as part of the metabolic syndrome, most likely because apo-CIII inhibits the lipolysis of TG-rich

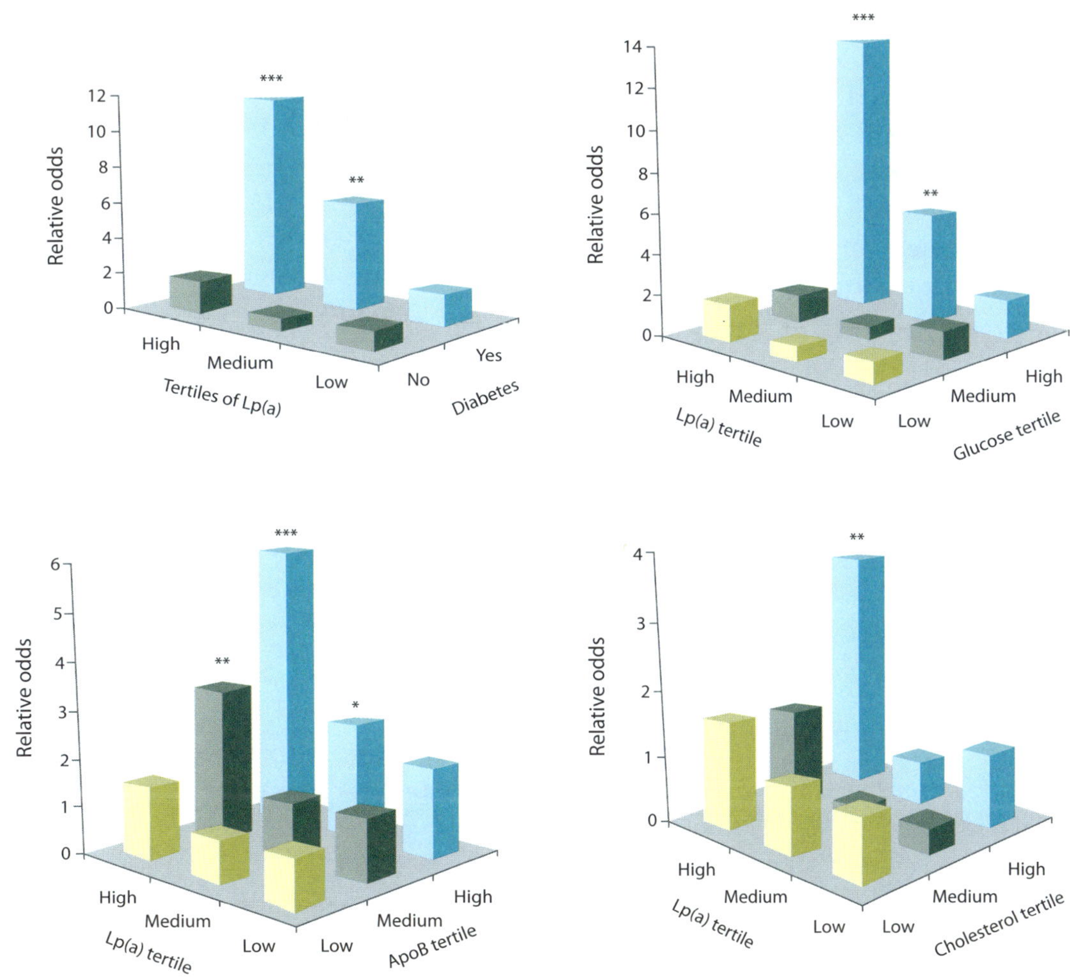

Figure 9.11 Relative odds for CAD associated with tertiles of Lp(s) and the presence or absence of diabetes and tertiles of glucose, apoB, and cholesterol. From: Rasouli M, Nesarhosseini V, Kiasari AM, et al. *Clin Chem Lab Med.* 2008;46(5):667-73. Reproduced with permission from Walter De Gruyter and Company.

lipoproteins (TRLs) and interferes with their clearance from the circulation.[105] Finally, higher levels of Lp(a) have been associated with an increased risk for coronary artery disease, and individuals with elevated Lp(a) accompanied by diabetes or high levels of serum glucose, apoB, and cholesterol have an amplified risk for CAD (Figure 9.11).[106]

Homocysteine

A recent meta-analysis found that for each increase of 5 micromol/l in homocysteine, the risk of CHD events increased by approximately 20%, independently of traditional CHD risk factors.[107] Elevated homocysteine has been associated with smaller brain size and silent infarcts in a sample of nearly 2000 healthy adults.[108]

Coronary artery calcification

Coronary artery calcification has been found to predict coronary artery disease accurately and independently of standard risk factors in at least four different ethnic groups.[109,110] Data from the Multi-Ethnic Study of Atherosclerosis also found it to be a better predictor of CVD incidence than carotid intima-media thickness.[111]

Vitamin D

As noted above, low levels of vitamin D are associated with increased risk, thus assessment of 25-hydroxyvitamin D should be part of routine evaluation.

Interventions

General lifestyle recommendations

Given the many ways that CVD may manifest, and the complexity of care, it is often practical to start with general goals that have the broadest benefit. For example, achieving normal body weight and improving insulin sensitivity may have tremendous impact and can largely be achieved by lifestyle modifications and nutritional supplementation. Reducing systemic inflammation, oxidative stress, and the environmental toxin load may be accomplished by implementing many of the same interventions. Beginning with lifestyle changes, evaluating for specific risk factors, and introducing individualized treatments should be done as part of a comprehensive treatment plan. Below are general recommendations for treating and preventing CVD, followed by specific recommendations to address abnormal findings.

General recommendations for CVD

Diet

In general, the adoption of a more plant-based, high fiber, whole grain, vegetable and fruit-rich diet, with emphasis on monounsaturated fats such as olive oil, and omega-3 rich oils is the most appropriate for treatment and prevention of CVD. One of the most frequently studied diets is the Mediterranean diet, for which numerous studies have documented benefit, including a reduction in the risk of diet-related cardiovascular risk factors (lipids, diabetes, hypertension, dyslipidemia, and obesity),[112,113] a reduction in markers of inflammation,[114] and a reduction in cardiovascular and overall mortality.[115]

The benefits of the Mediterranean diet appear to be at least partly due to reduced oxidative stress. A study of >130 pairs of twins found a robust association between the diet and plasma oxidative stress, not confounded by genetic or shared environmental factors.[116] A Mediterranean diet supplemented with either nuts or olive oil has been shown to reduce markers of inflammation, even in individuals with polymorphisms of COX-2 that put them at higher risk for CVD.[117]

In addition to the Mediterranean diet, the Portfolio diet (comprised of plant-based cholesterol-lowering foods, such as soy, plant sterols, almonds, and viscous fibers) has also emerged as a powerful therapeutic intervention for CVD. It has been shown to cause significant reductions in LDL-C and blood pressure,[118] with lipid-lowering effects similar to statins in terms of both LDL-C and LDL size.[119]

Finally, a low glycemic index/load diet is an essential part of any dietary intervention. A recent study published in *JAMA* found a direct association between sugar intake and dyslipidemia, particularly with a low HDL-C.[120] Also, a study following youth ages 10–23 found that both poor glycemic control (per HbA1c) and duration of diabetes both affect the thickness of the carotid artery IMT.[121] Given the impact of insulin resistance and obesity on CVD progression, maintaining optimal glycemic control and a healthy weight should be part of CVD treatment and prevention.

In addition to a low glycemic load diet, fiber supplementation which specifically targets postprandial hyperglycemia is of particular importance. Indeed, the DECODE (Diabetes Epidemiology: Collaborative Analysis of Diagnostic Criteria) study in Europe found that postprandial hyperglycemia is a greater risk factor for CVD than is fasting hyperglycemia.[122] Postprandial hyperglycemia has also been shown to be a risk factor for arterial stiffness.[123] These studies emphasize the importance of achieving stable glucose levels before and after a meal, as well as the need to diagnose insulin resistance and non-fasting hyperglycemia. Adding to this evidence is a strong correlation between fiber intake and both coronary heart disease and all-cause mortality.[124]

Physical activity

Physical activity has been associated with subclinical atherosclerosis. In a prospective study with 18 years' average follow-up, exercise training was found to reduce all-cause and cardiovascular mortality in men and women with CHD.[125,126] Recently published recommendations by the American Heart Association and the American College of Sports Medicine for the promotion and maintenance of health include aerobic activity of moderate intensity (brisk walk) for at least 30 minutes per day, 5 days each week or vigorous activity (jogging) for 20 or more minutes, 3 days per week; combinations of the two may be performed to meet the goals.[127] The benefits of physical activity appear to be dose-related, particularly in regard to weight control.[73] For those with elevated amounts of smaller denser LDL-C, endurance exercise may have additional benefit. In a study following 100 sedentary older adults, adoption of an aerobic exercise program not only increased HDL-C, but it reduced the denser subfractions of LDL independently of body fat phenotypes.[128]

Certainly one of the most powerful and well-documented lifestyle interventions is the Ornish program, which combines a low-fat, primarily plant-based diet, physical activity, stress reduction, and smoking cessation. The Ornish intervention has been shown to regress atherosclerosis, improve cardiovascular risk profiles, and decrease angina pectoris and cardiac events in a number of studies.[129] Other studies have also demonstrated the importance of comprehensive lifestyle change involving physical activity, diet, smoking reduction, and weight control.[130] In one prospective study of >20,000 men and women, four factors (current nonsmoking, not physically inactive, moderate alcohol intake (1–14 units a week) and plasma vitamin C >50 mmol/l indicating fruit and vegetable intake of at least five servings a day) predicted >4-fold difference in mortality, equivalent to 14 years of life.[131] Lifestyle modification programs have also been shown to improve cholesterol subfractions, including reducing LDL particles, small dense LDL particles, and increasing LDL particle size.[132]

Omega-3 fatty acids

Consumption of DHA and EPA, usually from fish oil, has been associated with reductions in subclinical atherosclerosis[133] and subclinical brain abnormalities[134] and a significant improvement in a number of cardiovascular risk factors, including lipid measures, myocardial contractility, blood pressure, platelet function, arterial cholesterol delivery, vascular function, and inflammatory responses.[135,136] A review of previous trials found that consumption of omega-3s from fish or fish-oil supplements, but not of alpha-linolenic acid, reduced the rates of all-cause mortality, cardiac and sudden death, and possibly stroke.[137]

Numerous epidemiologic studies continue to substantiate the correlation between consumption of fish rich in EPA and DHA and a lower incidence of fatal or nonfatal cardiovascular events.[138] Particular benefit has been documented for preventing sudden cardiac death (risk reductions of 45–81%).[139] In hypercholesterolemic patients, EPA reduced the incidence of CAD, and was particularly effective in patients with the potent risk factor combination of low HDL-C and elevated triglycerides, reducing the risk of CAD in this group by 53%.[140] Daily dosage of EPA/DHA (combined) sufficient to offer protection against CV-related death is 1000 mg. Dosage to lower triglyceride levels is 3000 mg.

Vitamin D

Widespread vitamin D deficiency and its numerous cardiovascular benefits call for regular monitoring of 25-hydroxy vitamin D levels. Optimal serum levels are considered to be 75–80 nmol/l,[141] and dosage varies from 1000–4000 IU per day to achieve sufficient intake.

Specific recommendations for CVD

In addition to interventions with broad-based benefit, such as making dietary changes, increasing physical activity, supplementing with omega-3 fatty acids and vitamin D, and maintaining healthy glucose levels, a number of specific interventions may be needed to address underlying dysfunctions.

Dyslipidemia

Elevated LDL-C is considered the primary target for treatment, although we now know that subfractions of LDL-C, specifically a small particle number, high apo-CIII and apoB particles, smaller denser LDL-C, and increased ox-LDL are all independently associated with elevated risk. Dietary interventions shown to lower LDL-C include increasing monounsaturated fat (e.g., olive oil) and nut intake (including tree nuts, macadamia nuts, almonds and pistachios).[142,143,144,145]

As discussed earlier, postprandial hyperglycemia is a significant risk factor for CVD. Postprandial hyperlipidemia (the postprandial increase in triglycerides following a high-fat meal) has been associated with smaller, denser LDL.[146] Eating a low glycemic load diet and fiber supplementation is critical in reducing postprandial hyperglycemia. For more information see Clinical Focus 4—The Spectrum of Insulin Resistance.

For those patients with small particle LDL-C, niacin has been shown to increase the large particle LDL-C by 82%, while reducing small particle LDL-C by 12%. In addition to its benefit for LDL-C, niacin is also considered the most effective pharmacological agent currently available for raising HDL-C, elevating levels by 15–35% at clinical doses (1.5–3 g/day) while also reducing triglycerides in subjects with coronary artery disease.[147,148] In a trial of intermediate-release niacin in patients with the metabolic syndrome, improvement in endothelial function and a reduction in carotid intimal medial thickness were reported.[149] In recent animal-based studies, niacin has been shown to reduce vascular inflammation and improve endothelial function independently of its effect on lipids.[150]

Berry consumption was shown to have favorable effects on HDL, blood pressure, and platelet function in a randomized single-blinded trial.[153] Pomegranate juice specifically has been shown to reduce common carotid intima-media thickness, blood pressure, and LDL-C oxidation when consumed for up to 3 years.[151] It may reverse the inhibition of nitric oxide synthase caused by ox-LDL-C.[152,153] Cranberry juice supplementation has been shown to reduce the oxidation of LDL-C.[154]

For patients taking statin medications, coenzyme Q10 is indicated at a dosage of 100–200 mg/day. It has been shown to reduce the myopathy associated with statin use, and has several cardiovascular benefits.[155] For example, CoQ10 improves endothelium-dependent vasodilation through bioenergetic effects and by counteracting nitric oxide oxidation.[156] It is an independent predictor of mortality in patients with chronic heart failure.[157]

Hypertriglyceridemia

A large body of accumulating evidence indicates that hypertriglyceridemia (HTG) is an independent risk factor for CVD. An 88 mg/dl (1.0 mmol/l) increase in plasma triglyceride levels significantly increases the relative risk of CVD by approximately 30% in men and 75% in women.[158] This increased risk is mediated through the metabolic interrelationships between serum triglyceride (TG) levels and other risk factors, such as the atherogenic lipid profile (low HDL-C levels and elevated small dense LDL levels), insulin resistance, a prothrombotic propensity, and low-grade systemic inflammation. An effective TG-lowering strategy in patients with HTG is an important clinical goal to reduce the risk of atherosclerosis, the metabolic syndrome, and diabetes.

One of the most effective means for reducing triglyceride levels is to maintain normoglycemia and prevent postprandial hyperglycemia, most effectively achieved through a low glycemic load diet and fiber supplementation. Fish oil supplements are also particularly effective for reducing triglyceride levels at dosages providing 3000 mg of EPA/DHA daily. These long-chain omega-3 fatty acids act by accelerating chylomicron triglyceride clearance,[159] are effective when combined with statins, and are indicated after myocardial infarction.[160] When additional support is required, niacin has been shown to significantly reduce triglycerides by inhibiting their synthesis and their secretion from VLDL-C.[161] L-arginine has also been shown to prevent the endothelial dysfunction brought on by postprandial hypertriglyceridemia,[162] and to improve endothelium-dependent, flow-mediated dilatation in hypertensive patients.[163]

Hyperhomocysteinemia

Although it is unclear whether lowering of homocysteine levels with B vitamins reduces cardiovascular risk, the mechanisms by which homocysteine promotes atherosclerosis are compelling, as is the reduction in stroke risk seen with folic acid supplementation.[164,165] Homocysteine also induces NF-κB expression,[166] an effect which may be blunted by folic acid even if homocysteine levels are not reduced.[167] A combination of vitamins B6, B12, and folic acid as well as choline and betaine is the most effective way to lower homocysteine levels.[168]

Hypertension

Lifestyle interventions—particularly those that help to achieve weight loss, are high in fiber, and restrict sodium content—are particularly effective for maintaining a healthy blood pressure. For example, a recent meta-analysis concluded that, in hypertensive patients, increased fiber intake was associated with a significant reduction in both systolic and diastolic blood pressure, although it may take up to 8 weeks to begin to see the maximum effects.[169] Similarly, even small amounts of weight loss can help to improve metabolic abnormalities that contribute to blood pressure elevation. For example, in a recent study comparing arterial stiffness in both weight loss and control groups, the weight loss group experienced reduced blood pressure and reduced arterial stiffness in proportion to both total and abdominal weight lost.[170] The DASH diet, discussed below, was also recently found to produce greater blood pressure reductions, greater improvements in vascular and autonomic function, and reduced left ventricular mass when combined with weight loss than when used alone.[171]

The Dietary Approaches to Stop Hypertension (DASH) diet (high in fruits, vegetables, and low-fat dairy products and reduced in fat) can reduce blood pressure significantly, especially if combined with sodium restriction and, as mentioned above, with weight loss.[172] The DASH research group found that coupling the original DASH diet with sodium restriction is more effective than dietary manipulation alone. In the first trial, the DASH diet produced a net blood pressure reduction of 11.4 and 5.5 mmHg systolic and diastolic, respectively, in patients with hypertension. In the second trial, sodium intake was quantified at a "higher" intake of 3300 mg/day; an "intermediate" intake of 2400 mg/day; and a "lower" intake of 1500 mg/day. Compared to the control diet, the DASH diet was associated with a significantly lower systolic blood pressure at each sodium level. The DASH diet with the lower sodium level led to a mean systolic blood pressure that was 7.1 mmHg lower in participants without hypertension, and 11.5 mmHg lower in participants with hypertension.

A recent review reported that a sodium intake exceeding 1150–2300 mg/day is necessary but not sufficient for the development of primary hypertension. Isolated populations eating natural foods (and having an insignificant incidence of hypertension) have an individual potassium intake that exceeds 5850 mg/day and a sodium intake of only 460–920 mg/day; the ratio of dietary potassium to sodium is >3 and usually closer to 10. By contrast, people in industrialized nations eat many processed foods and thereby ingest 1170–2730 mg of potassium per day and as much as 2300–9200 mg of sodium per day (the usual dietary potassium to sodium ratio is <0.4).[173]

CoQ10 can be a useful nutrient for treating hypertension. A recent meta-analysis of 12 clinical trials found that CoQ10 has the potential in hypertensive patients to lower systolic blood pressure by up to 17 mmHg, and diastolic blood pressure by up to 10 mmHg, without significant side effects.[174]

Antioxidants have particular efficacy for treating hypertension. Trials with vitamins C and E have shown reductions in markers of oxidative stress and blood pressure,[175] and the antioxidant Pycnogenol has been shown to increase NO availability, and is particularly effective for the microangiopathy that is due to diabetes and vascular insufficiency.[176,177] It has been used to reduce hypertension, to prevent vascular damage, and also to control the edema often seen as a consequence of hypertensive medications such as calcium antagonists.[178]

Garlic also has efficacy for lowering blood pressure. A recent analysis of 10 clinical trials found that garlic reduced systolic blood pressure (SBP) by 16.3 mmHg and diastolic blood pressure by 9.3 mmHg compared with placebo, but only in those patients with elevated SBP.[179] A meta-analysis of 11 studies also found garlic to be superior to placebo in helping to normalize blood pressure.[180]

N-acetylcysteine and L-arginine also address underlying causes of hypertension, as they have been shown to improve oxidative stress and NO availability in a double-blind study of diabetic hypertensive patients. This outcome was accompanied by a reduction of both systolic and diastolic pressure, total cholesterol, LDL-C, oxidized LDL-C, hsCRP, intracellular adhesion molecule, vascular cell adhesion molecule, nitrotyrosine, fibrinogen, and plasminogen activator inhibitor-1, and an increase in HDL-C.[181]

Screening for vitamin D status, as part of routine examination, is also important for blood pressure control. Plasma 25(OH)D levels have been found to be inversely and independently associated with the risk of developing hypertension, likely because vitamin D is a potent negative endocrine regulator of renin gene expression.[182,183]

Additional factors

An increased intake of omega-3 fatty acids for those with a genetic polymorphism of the 5-lipoxygenase gene is especially warranted. The variant 5-lipoxygenase (5-LO) genotype was identified in a randomly sampled cohort of 470 men and women; it was associated with increased atherosclerosis, an effect promoted by dietary omega-6 fatty acids, and *inhibited by omega-3 fatty acids*.[184] A larger study of >1800 case-control pairs confirmed the higher expression of 5-LO associated with the variant genotype, and the greater risks in the context of a high arachidonic acid diet.[185]

Omega-3 fatty acid supplementation is indicated for those with elevated levels of lipoprotein-associated phospholipase A(2) (Lp-PLA[2]), an emerging cardiovascular risk factor. Omega-3 fatty acids appear to reduce Lp-PLA(2), mitigating its effects.[186] Similarly, a polymorphism in the PPAR-alpha (PPARA) gene interacts with polyunsaturated fat intake, with high omega-3 consumption triggering a low triglyceride level in those with the variant. Alternatively, low consumption resulted in high triglycerides and apoC-III levels in those with the variant.[187]

For patients with peripheral arterial disease, the use of omega-3 fatty acids, possibly in combination with folic acid, B6, and vitamin E, is indicated. This combination was shown to increase pain-free walking distance and reduce total cholesterol, apoB concentrations, and homocysteine (if initially elevated) compared to controls.[188] Omega-3 fatty acids alone were shown to improve endothelial function in these patients.[189] A low glycemic load diet is highly recommended in those with peripheral arterial disease, given recent findings that insulin resistance is strongly and independently associated with PAD incidence and modifies the association of inflammation and PAD.[190]

References

1. Hansson GK. Inflammation, atherosclerosis, and coronary artery disease. *N Engl J Med.* 2005 Apr 21;352(16):1685-95.
2. http://www.americanheart.org/presenter.jhtml?identifier =4478, accessed 1-15-2009.
3. Centers for Disease Control and Prevention: Leading Causes of Death. Available at: http://www.cdc.gov/nchs/FASTATS/lcod.htm. Accessed 4-13-2010.
4. Basson M. Cardiovascular disease. *Nature.* 2008 Feb 21; 451(7181):903.
5. Daviglus ML, Stamler J, Pirzada A, et al. Favorable cardiovascular risk profile in young women and long-term risk of cardiovascular and all-cause mortality. *JAMA.* 2004 Oct 6; 292(13):1588-92.
6. Khaw KT, Wareham N, Bingham S, et al. Combined impact of health behaviours and mortality in men and women: the EPIC-Norfolk prospective population study. *PLoS Med.* 2008 Jan 8;5(1):e12.
7. Cutler JA, Sorlie PD, Wolz M. Trends in hypertension prevalence, awareness, treatment, and control rates in United States adults between 1988-1994 and 1999-2004. *Hypertension.* 2008 Nov;52(5):818-27.
8. Kannel WB, Benjamin EJ. Current perceptions of the epidemiology of atrial fibrillation. *Cardiol Clin.* 2009 Feb;27(1):13-24, vii.
9. Selvin E, Erlinger TP. Prevalence of and risk factors for peripheral arterial disease in the United States: results from the National Health and Nutrition Examination Survey, 1999-2000. *Circulation.* 2004 Aug 10;110(6):738-43.
10. Ghandehari H, Kamal-Bahl S, Wong ND. Prevalence and extent of dyslipidemia and recommended lipid levels in U.S. adults with and without cardiovascular comorbidities: the National Health and Nutrition Examination Survey 2003-2004. *Am Heart J.* 2008 Jul;156(1):112-9.
11. Wong ND. Prevalence, treatment, and control of combined hypertension and hypercholesterolemia in the United States. *Am J Cardiol.* 2006 Jul 15;98(2):204-8.
12. Wong ND, Lopez VA, Roberts CS, et al. Combined association of lipids and blood pressure in relation to incident cardiovascular disease in the elderly: the cardiovascular health study. *Am J Hypertens.* 2010 Feb;23(2):161-7.
13. Suh DC, Choi IS, Plauschinat C. Impact of comorbid conditions and race/ethnicity on glycemic control among the U.S. population with type 2 diabetes, 1988-1994 to 1999-2004. *J Diabetes Complications.* 2009 Aug 26. Epub ahead of print.
14. Napoli C, Glass CK, Witztum JL, et al. Influence of maternal hypercholesterolaemia during pregnancy on progression of early atherosclerotic lesions in childhood: Fate of Early Lesions in Children (FELIC) study. *Lancet.* 1999 Oct 9;354(9186):1234-41.
15. Mallika V, Goswami B, Rajappa M. Atherosclerosis pathophysiology and the role of novel risk factors: a clinicobiochemical perspective. *Angiology.* 2007 Oct-Nov; 58(5):513-22.
16. Falk E. Pathogenesis of atherosclerosis. *J Am Coll Cardiol.* 2006 Apr 18;47(8 Suppl):C7-12.
17. Halvorsen B, Otterdal K, Dahl TB. Atherosclerotic plaque stability—what determines the fate of a plaque? *Prog Cardiovasc Dis.* 2008 Nov-Dec;51(3):183-94.
18. Mannarino E, Pirro M. Endothelial injury and repair: a novel theory for atherosclerosis. *Angiology.* 2008 Apr-May;59(2 Suppl):69S-72S.
19. Boueiz A, Hassoun PM. Regulation of endothelial barrier function by reactive oxygen and nitrogen species. *Microvasc Res.* 2008 Nov 7. Epub ahead of print.
20. Prozialeck WC, Edwards JR, Nebert DW, et al. The vascular system as a target of metal toxicity. *Toxicol Sci.* 2008 Apr;102(2):207-18.
21. States JC, Srivastava S, Chen Y, et al. Arsenic and cardiovascular disease. *Toxicol Sci.* 2009 Feb;107(2):312-23.
22. Everett CJ, Frithsen IL. Association of urinary cadmium and myocardial infarction. *Environ Res.* 2008 Feb;106(2):284-6.
23. Navas-Acien A, Silbergeld EK, Sharrett R, et al. Metals in urine and peripheral arterial disease. *Environ Health Perspect.* 2005 Feb;113(2):164-9.
24. Kolluru GK, Tamilarasan KP, Geetha Priya S, et al. Cadmium induced endothelial dysfunction: consequence of defective migratory pattern of endothelial cells in association with poor nitric oxide availability under cadmium challenge. *Cell Biol Int.* 2006 May;30(5):427-38.
25. Weiss N. Mechanisms of increased vascular oxidant stress in hyperhomocysteinemia and its impact on endothelial function. *Curr Drug Metab.* 2005 Feb;6(1):27-36.
26. Cheung GT, Siow YL, O K. Homocysteine stimulates monocyte chemoattractant protein-1 expression in mesangial cells via NF-kappaB activation. *Can J Physiol Pharmacol.* 2008 Mar;86(3):88-96.
27. Au-Yeung KK, Yip JC, Siow YL. Folic acid inhibits homocysteine-induced superoxide anion production and nuclear factor kappa B activation in macrophages. *Can J Physiol Pharmacol.* 2006 Jan;84(1):141-7.
28. Prontera C, Martelli N, Evangelista V, et al. Homocysteine modulates the CD40/CD40L system. *J Am Coll Cardiol.* 2007 Jun 5;49(22):2182-90.
29. Vishnevetsky D, Kiyanista VA, Gandhi PJ. CD40 ligand: a novel target in the fight against cardiovascular disease. *Ann Pharmacother.* 2004 Sep;38(9):1500-8.
30. Mikael LG, Genest J Jr, Rozen R. Elevated homocysteine reduces apolipoprotein A-I expression in hyperhomocysteinemic mice and in males with coronary artery disease. *Circ Res.* 2006 Mar 3;98(4):564-71.
31. Moshal KS, Metreveli N, Frank I, et al. Mitochondrial MMP activation, dysfunction and arrhythmogenesis in hyperhomocysteinemia. *Curr Vasc Pharmacol.* 2008 Apr;6(2):84-92.

32. Moshal KS, Tipparaju SM, Vacek TP, et al. Mitochondrial matrix metalloproteinase activation decreases myocyte contractility in hyperhomocysteinemia. *Am J Physiol Heart Circ Physiol.* 2008 Aug;295(2):H890-7.
33. Navas-Acien A, Guallar E, Silbergeld EK, et al. Lead exposure and cardiovascular disease—a systematic review. *Environ Health Perspect.* 2007 Mar;115(3):472-82.
34. Menke A, Muntner P, Batuman V, et al. Blood lead below 0.48 micromol/L (10 microg/dL) and mortality among U.S. adults. *Circulation.* 2006 Sep 26;114(13):1388-94.
35. Schober SE, Mirel LB, Graubard BI, et al. Blood lead levels and death from all causes, cardiovascular disease, and cancer: results from the NHANES III mortality study. *Environ Health Perspect.* 2006 Oct;114(10):1538-41.
36. Cheng Y, Schwartz J, Sparrow D, et al. Bone lead and blood lead levels in relation to baseline blood pressure and the prospective development of hypertension: the Normative Aging Study. *Am J Epidemiol.* 2001 Jan 15;153(2):164-71.
37. Teo KK, Ounpuu S, Hawken S, et al. Tobacco use and risk of myocardial infarction in 52 countries in the INTERHEART study: a case-control study. *Lancet.* 2006 Aug 19;368(9536):647-58.
38. Zhang WZ, Venardos K, Chin-Dusting J, et al. Adverse effects of cigarette smoke on NO bioavailability: role of arginine metabolism and oxidative stress. *Hypertension.* 2006 Aug;48(2):278-85.
39. Bhatnagar A. Environmental cardiology: studying mechanistic links between pollution and heart disease. *Circ Res.* 2006 Sep 29;99(7):692-705.
40. Kolluru GK, Tamilarasan KP, Geetha Priya S, et al. Cadmium induced endothelial dysfunction: consequence of defective migratory pattern of endothelial cells in association with poor nitric oxide availability under cadmium challenge. *Cell Biol Int.* 2006 May;30(5):427-38.
41. Ambrose JA, Barua RS. The pathophysiology of cigarette smoking and cardiovascular disease: an update. *J Am Coll Cardiol.* 2004 May 19;43(10):1731-7.
42. Expert Panel on Detection, Evaluation, and Treatment of High Blood Cholesterol in Adults. Executive Summary of The Third Report of The National Cholesterol Education Program (NCEP) Expert Panel on Detection, Evaluation, And Treatment of High Blood Cholesterol In Adults (Adult Treatment Panel III). *JAMA.* 2001 May 16;285(19):2486-97.
43. Shoji T, Hatsuda S, Tsuchikura S, et al. Small dense low-density lipoprotein cholesterol concentration and carotid atherosclerosis. *Atherosclerosis.* 2008 May 1. Epub ahead of print.
44. Bradley RD, Oberg EB. Are Additional Lipid Measures Useful? *Integrative Medicine*, Vol. 7, No. 6, 2009.
45. Brewer HB Jr, Santamarina-Fojo S. Clinical significance of high-density lipoproteins and the development of atherosclerosis: focus on the role of the adenosine triphosphate-binding cassette protein A1 transporter. *Am J Cardiol.* 2003 Aug 21;92(4B):10K-16K.
46. Tabet F, Rye KA. High-density lipoproteins, inflammation and oxidative stress. *Clin Sci* (Lond). 2009 Jan;116(2):87-98.
47. Ridker PM, Silvertown JD. Inflammation, C-reactive protein, and atherothrombosis. *J Periodontol.* 2008 Aug; 79(8 Suppl):1544-51.
48. Wilson PW. Evidence of systemic inflammation and estimation of coronary artery disease risk: a population perspective. *Am J Med.* 2008 Oct;121(10 Suppl 1): S15-20.
49. Devaraj S, Singh U, Jialal I. The Evolving Role of C-Reactive Protein in Atherothrombosis. *Clin Chem.* 2008 Dec 18. Epub ahead of print.
50. Viles-Gonzalez JF, Fuster V, Badimon JJ. Links between inflammation and thrombogenicity in atherosclerosis. *Curr Mol Med.* 2006 Aug;6(5):489-99.
51. Wilson AM, Ryan MC, Boyle AJ. The novel role of C-reactive protein in cardiovascular disease: risk marker or pathogen. *Int J Cardiol.* 2006 Jan 26;106(3):291-7.
52. Cushman M, Arnold AM, Psaty BM, et al. C-reactive protein and the 10-year incidence of coronary heart disease in older men and women: the cardiovascular health study. *Circulation.* 2005 Jul 5;112(1):25-31.
53. Zacho J, Tybjaerg-Hansen A, Jensen JS, et al. Genetically elevated C-reactive protein and ischemic vascular disease. *N Engl J Med.* 2008 Oct 30;359(18):1897-908.
54. Green D, Foiles N, Chan C, et al. Elevated fibrinogen levels and subsequent subclinical atherosclerosis: The CARDIA Study. *Atherosclerosis.* 2008 Jul 2. Epub ahead of print.
55. Paraskevas KI, Baker DM, Vrentzos GE, et al. The role of fibrinogen and fibrinolysis in peripheral arterial disease. *Thromb Res.* 2008;122(1):1-12.
56. Bonora E, Kiechl S, Willeit J, et al. Insulin resistance as estimated by homeostasis model assessment predicts incident symptomatic cardiovascular disease in caucasian subjects from the general population: the Bruneck study. *Diabetes Care.* 2007 Feb;30(2):318-24.
57. Bonora E, Formentini G, Calcaterra F, et al. HOMA-estimated insulin resistance is an independent predictor of cardiovascular disease in type 2 diabetic subjects: prospective data from the Verona Diabetes Complications Study. *Diabetes Care.* 2002 Jul;25(7):1135-41.
58. Brohall G, Odén A, Fagerberg B. Carotid artery intima-media thickness in patients with type 2 diabetes mellitus and impaired glucose tolerance: a systematic review. *Diabet Med.* 2006 Jun;23(6):609-16.
59. Fox CS, Coady S, Sorlie PD, et al. Trends in cardiovascular complications of diabetes. *JAMA.* 2004 Nov 24;292(20):2495-9.
60. Fox CS, Coady S, Sorlie PD, et al. Increasing cardiovascular disease burden due to diabetes mellitus: the Framingham Heart Study. *Circulation.* 2007 Mar 27; 115(12):1544-50.

61. Gami AS, Witt BJ, Howard DE, et al. Metabolic syndrome and risk of incident cardiovascular events and death: a systematic review and meta-analysis of longitudinal studies. *J Am Coll Cardiol.* 2007 Jan 30;49(4):403-14. 17258085.

62. Pande RL, Perlstein TS, Beckman JA, et al. Association of insulin resistance and inflammation with peripheral arterial disease: the National Health and Nutrition Examination Survey, 1999 to 2004. *Circulation.* 2008 Jul 1;118(1):33-41.

63. Sieri S, Krogh V, Berrino F, et al. Dietary glycemic load and index and risk of coronary heart disease in a large italian cohort: the EPICOR study. *Arch Intern Med.* 2010 Apr 12;170(7):640-7.

64. Ni Mhurchu C, Rodgers A, Pan WH, et al. Body mass index and cardiovascular disease in the Asia-Pacific Region: an overview of 33 cohorts involving 310 000 participants. *Int J Epidemiol.* 2004 Aug;33(4):751-8. Epub 2004 Apr 22.

65. Giannini C, de Giorgis T, Scarinci A, et al. Obese related effects of inflammatory markers and insulin resistance on increased carotid intima-media thickness in pre-pubertal children. *Atherosclerosis.* 2008 Mar;197(1):448-56. Epub 2007 Aug 6.

66. Iannuzzi A, Licenziati MR, Vacca M. Comparison of two diets of varying glycemic index on carotid subclinical atherosclerosis in obese children. *Heart Vessels.* 2009 Nov;24(6):419-24. Epub 2009 Nov 22.

67. Van Horn L, McCoin M, Kris-Etherton PM, et al. The evidence for dietary prevention and treatment of cardiovascular disease. *J Am Diet Assoc.* 2008 Feb;108(2):287-331.

68. Heidemann C, Schulze MB, Franco OH, et al. Dietary patterns and risk of mortality from cardiovascular disease, cancer, and all causes in a prospective cohort of women. *Circulation.* 2008 Jul 15;118(3):230-7.

69. Iqbal R, Anand S, Ounpuu S, et al. Dietary patterns and the risk of acute myocardial infarction in 52 countries: results of the INTERHEART study. *Circulation.* 2008 Nov 4;118(19):1929-37.

70. Nettleton JA, Schulze MB, Jiang R, et al. A priori-defined dietary patterns and markers of cardiovascular disease risk in the Multi-Ethnic Study of Atherosclerosis (MESA). *Am J Clin Nutr.* 2008 Jul;88(1):185-94.

71. Wang L, Manson JE, Buring JE, et al. Meat intake and the risk of hypertension in middle-aged and older women. *J Hypertens.* 2008 Feb;26(2):215-22.

72. Heidemann C, Schulze MB, Franco OH, et al. Dietary patterns and risk of mortality from cardiovascular disease, cancer, and all causes in a prospective cohort of women. *Circulation.* 2008 Jul 15;118(3):230-7.

73. Kokkinos P. Physical activity and cardiovascular disease prevention: current recommendations. *Angiology.* 2008 Apr-May;59(2 Suppl):26S-9S.

74. Moholdt T, Wisløff U, Nilsen TI. Physical activity and mortality in men and women with coronary heart disease: a prospective population-based cohort study in Norway (the HUNT study). *Eur J Cardiovasc Prev Rehabil.* 2008 Dec;15(6):639-45.

75. Kim DH, Sabour S, Sagar UN, et al. Prevalence of hypovitaminosis D in cardiovascular diseases (from the National Health and Nutrition Examination Survey 2001 to 2004). *Am J Cardiol.* 2008 Dec 1;102(11):1540-4.

76. Martins D, Wolf M, Pan D, et al. Prevalence of cardiovascular risk factors and the serum levels of 25-hydroxyvitamin D in the United States: data from the Third National Health and Nutrition Examination Survey. *Arch Intern Med.* 2007 Jun 11;167(11):1159-65.

77. Dobnig H, Pilz S, Scharnagl H, et al. Independent association of low serum 25-hydroxyvitamin d and 1,25-dihydroxyvitamin d levels with all-cause and cardiovascular mortality. *Arch Intern Med.* 2008 Jun 23;168(12): 1340-9.

78. Wang TJ, Pencina MJ, Booth SL. Vitamin D deficiency and risk of cardiovascular disease. *Circulation.* 2008 Jan 29;117(4):503-11.

79. Reis JP, von Mühlen D, Miller ER, et al. Vitamin D Status and Cardiometabolic Risk Factors in the United States Adolescent Population. *Pediatrics.* 2009 Aug 3. Epub ahead of print.

80. Semba RD, Houston DK, Bandinelli S, et al. Relationship of 25-hydroxyvitamin D with all-cause and cardiovascular disease mortality in older community-dwelling adults. *Eur J Clin Nutr.* 2010 Feb;64(2):203-9.

81. Fazio S, Palmieri EA, Lombardi G, et al. Effects of thyroid hormone on the cardiovascular system. *Recent Prog Horm Res.* 2004;59:31-50.

82. Dullaart RP, de Vries R, Roozendaal C, et al. Carotid artery intima media thickness is inversely related to serum free thyroxine in euthyroid subjects. *Clin Endocrinol* (Oxf). 2007 Nov;67(5):668-73.

83. Takamura N, Akilzhanova A, Hayashida N, et al. Thyroid function is associated with carotid intima-media thickness in euthyroid subjects. *Atherosclerosis.* 2008 Sep 27. Epub ahead of print.

84. Cappola AR, Fried LP, Arnold AM, et al. Thyroid status, cardiovascular risk, and mortality in older adults. *JAMA.* 2006 Mar 1;295(9):1033-41.

85. Virtanen JK, Rissanen TH, Voutilainen S, et al. Mercury as a risk factor for cardiovascular diseases. *J Nutr Biochem.* 2007 Feb;18(2):75-85.

86. Ha MH, Lee DH, Jacobs DR. Association between serum concentrations of persistent organic pollutants and self-reported cardiovascular disease prevalence: results from the National Health and Nutrition Examination Survey, 1999-2002. *Environ Health Perspect.* 2007 Aug;115(8):1204-9.

87. Lang IA, Galloway TS, Scarlett A, et al. Association of urinary bisphenol A concentration with medical disorders

and laboratory abnormalities in adults. *JAMA*. 2008 Sep 17;300(11):1303-10.

88. Everett CJ, Mainous AG 3rd, Frithsen IL, et al. Association of polychlorinated biphenyls with hypertension in the 1999-2002 National Health and Nutrition Examination Survey. *Environ Res*. 2008 Sep;108(1):94-7.
89. National Cholesterol Education Program (NCEP) Expert Panel on Detection, Evaluation, and Treatment of High Blood Cholesterol in Adults (Adult Treatment Panel III). Third Report of the National Cholesterol Education Program (NCEP) Expert Panel on Detection, Evaluation, and Treatment of High Blood Cholesterol in Adults (Adult Treatment Panel III) final report. *Circulation*. 2002 Dec 17; 106(25):3143-421.
90. Panagiotakos DB, Kromhout D, Menotti A, et al. The relation between pulse pressure and cardiovascular mortality in 12,763 middle-aged men from various parts of the world: a 25-year follow-up of the seven countries study. *Arch Intern Med*. 2005 Oct 10;165(18):2142-7.
91. Wilson PW, D'Agostino RB, Levy D, et al. Prediction of coronary heart disease using risk factor categories. *Circulation*. 1998 May 12;97(18):1837-47.
92. Karim R, Hodis HN, Detrano R, et al. Relation of Framingham risk score to subclinical atherosclerosis evaluated across three arterial sites. *Am J Cardiol*. 2008 Oct 1;102(7):825-30.
93. Fowkes FG, Murray GD, Butcher I, et al. Ankle Brachial Index Collaboration. Ankle brachial index combined with Framingham Risk Score to predict cardiovascular events and mortality: a meta-analysis. *JAMA*. 2008 Jul 9;300(2): 197-208.
94. Ovbiagele B. Association of ankle-brachial index level with stroke. *J Neurol Sci*. 2009 Jan 15;276(1-2):14-7.
95. Abu EO, Oluwatowoju I. Omega-3 index determined by gas chromatography with electron impact mass spectrometry. *Prostaglandins Leukot Essent Fatty Acids*. 2009 Apr; 80(4):189-94.
96. Harris WS. The omega-3 index as a risk factor for coronary heart disease. *Am J Clin Nutr*. 2008 Jun;87(6):1997S-2002S.
97. Albert CM, Campos H, Stampfer MJ, et al. Blood levels of long-chain n-3 fatty acids and the risk of sudden death. *N Engl J Med*. 2002 Apr 11;346(15):1113-8.
98. Ramel A, Pumberger C, et al. Cardiovascular risk factors in young, overweight, and obese European adults and associations with physical activity and omega-3 index. *Nutr Res*. 2009 May;29(5):305-12.
99. Ip S, Lichtenstein AH, Chung M. Systematic review: association of low-density lipoprotein subfractions with cardiovascular outcomes. *Ann Intern Med*. 2009 Apr 7; 150(7):474-84.
100. Rietzschel ER, Langlois M, De Buyzere ML, et al. Oxidized low-density lipoprotein cholesterol is associated with decreases in cardiac function independent of vascular alterations. *Hypertension*. 2008 Sep;52(3):535-41.
101. Davidson MH. Apolipoprotein measurements: is more widespread use clinically indicated? *Clin Cardiol*. 2009 Sep;32(9):482-6.
102. Shin MJ, Krauss RM. Apolipoprotein CIII bound to apoB-containing lipoproteins is associated with small, dense LDL independent of plasma triglyceride levels in healthy men. *Atherosclerosis*. 2010 Feb 24. Epub ahead of print.
103. Walldius G, Jungner I. The apoB/apoA-I ratio: a strong, new risk factor for cardiovascular disease and a target for lipid-lowering therapy—a review of the evidence. *J Intern Med*. 2006 May;259(5):493-519.
104. Davidson MH. Apolipoprotein measurements: is more widespread use clinically indicated? *Clin Cardiol*. 2009 Sep;32(9):482-6.
105. Tian L, Wu J, Fu M, et al. Relationship between apolipoprotein C-III concentrations and high-density lipoprotein subclass distribution. *Metabolism*. 2009 May;58(5):668-74.
106. Rasouli M, Kiasari AM. Interactions of lipoprotein(a) with diabetes mellitus, apolipoprotein B and cholesterol enhance the prognostic values for coronary artery disease. *Clin Chem Lab Med*. 2008;46(5):667-73.
107. Humphrey LL, Fu R, Rogers K, et al. Homocysteine level and coronary heart disease incidence: a systematic review and meta-analysis. *Mayo Clin Proc*. 2008 Nov;83(11):1203-12.
108. Seshadri S, Wolf PA, Beiser AS, et al. Association of plasma total homocysteine levels with subclinical brain injury: cerebral volumes, white matter hyperintensity, and silent brain infarcts at volumetric magnetic resonance imaging in the Framingham Offspring Study. *Arch Neurol*. 2008 May;65(5):642-9.
109. Arad Y, Goodman KJ, Roth M, et al. Coronary calcification, coronary disease risk factors, C-reactive protein, and atherosclerotic cardiovascular disease events: the St. Francis Heart Study. *J Am Coll Cardiol*. 2005 Jul 5;46(1):158-65.
110. Detrano R, Guerci AD, Carr JJ, et al. Coronary calcium as a predictor of coronary events in four racial or ethnic groups. *N Engl J Med*. 2008 Mar 27;358(13):1336-45.
111. Folsom AR, Kronmal RA, Detrano RC, et al. Coronary artery calcification compared with carotid intima-media thickness in the prediction of cardiovascular disease incidence: the Multi-Ethnic Study of Atherosclerosis (MESA). *Arch Intern Med*. 2008 Jun 23;168(12):1333-9.
112. Sánchez-Taínta A, Estruch R, Bulló M, et al. Adherence to a Mediterranean-type diet and reduced prevalence of clustered cardiovascular risk factors in a cohort of 3,204 high-risk patients. *Eur J Cardiovasc Prev Rehabil*. 2008 Oct;15(5):589-93.
113. Estruch R, Martínez-González MA, Corella D, et al. Effects of a Mediterranean-style diet on cardiovascular risk factors: a randomized trial. *Ann Intern Med*. 2006 Jul 4;145(1):1-11.

114. Salas-Salvadó J, Garcia-Arellano A, Estruch R, et al. Components of the Mediterranean-type food pattern and serum inflammatory markers among patients at high risk for cardiovascular disease. *Eur J Clin Nutr.* 2008 May;62(5):651-9.

115. Sofi F, Cesari F, Abbate R, et al. Adherence to Mediterranean diet and health status: meta-analysis. *BMJ.* 2008 Sep 11;337:a1344.

116. Dai J, Jones DP, Goldberg J, et al. Association between adherence to the Mediterranean diet and oxidative stress. *Am J Clin Nutr.* 2008 Nov;88(5):1364-70.

117. Corella D, González JI, Bulló M, et al. Polymorphisms cyclooxygenase-2 -765G>C and interleukin-6 -174G>C are associated with serum inflammation markers in a high cardiovascular risk population and do not modify the response to a Mediterranean diet supplemented with virgin olive oil or nuts. *J Nutr.* 2009 Jan;139(1):128-34.

118. Jenkins DJ, Kendall CW, Faulkner DA, et al. Long-term effects of a plant-based dietary portfolio of cholesterol-lowering foods on blood pressure. *Eur J Clin Nutr.* 2008 Jun;62(6):781-8.

119. Gigleux I, Jenkins DJ, Kendall CW, et al. Comparison of a dietary portfolio diet of cholesterol-lowering foods and a statin on LDL particle size phenotype in hypercholesterolaemic participants. *Br J Nutr.* 2007 Dec;98(6):1229-36.

120. Welsh JA, Sharma A, Abramson JL, et al. Caloric Sweetener Consumption and Dyslipidemia Among U.S. Adults. *JAMA* 2010;303(15):1490-1497.

121. Shah AS, Dolan LM, Kimball TR, et al. Influence of duration of diabetes, glycemic control, and traditional cardiovascular risk factors on early atherosclerotic vascular changes in adolescents and young adults with type 2 diabetes mellitus. *J Clin Endocrinol Metab.* 2009 Oct; 94(10):3740-5. Epub 2009 Sep 1.

122. Gao W, Qiao Q, Tuomilehto J. Post-challenge hyperglycaemia rather than fasting hyperglycaemia is an independent risk factor of cardiovascular disease events. *Clin Lab.* 2004;50(9-10):609-15.

123. Ohshita K, Yamane K, Ishida K, et al. Post-challenge hyperglycaemia is an independent risk factor for arterial stiffness in Japanese men. *Diabet Med.* 2004 Jun;21(6):636-9.

124. Streppel MT, Ocké MC, Boshuizen HC, et al. Dietary fiber intake in relation to coronary heart disease and all-cause mortality over 40 y: the Zutphen Study. *Am J Clin Nutr.* 2008 Oct;88(4):1119-25.

125. Bertoni AG, Whitt-Glover MC, Chung H, et al. The association between physical activity and subclinical atherosclerosis: the Multi-Ethnic Study of Atherosclerosis. *Am J Epidemiol.* 2009 Feb 15;169(4):444-54.

126. Moholdt T, Wisløff U, Nilsen TI, Slørdahl SA. Physical activity and mortality in men and women with coronary heart disease: a prospective population-based cohort study in Norway (the HUNT study). *Eur J Cardiovasc Prev Rehabil.* 2008 Dec;15(6):639-45.

127. Haskell WL, Lee IM, Pate RR, et al. Physical activity and public health: updated recommendation for adults from the American College of Sports Medicine and the American Heart Association. *Med Sci Sports Exerc.* 2007 Aug;39(8):1423-34.

128. Halverstadt A, Phares DA, Wilund KR, et al. Endurance exercise training raises high-density lipoprotein cholesterol and lowers small low-density lipoprotein and very low-density lipoprotein independent of body fat phenotypes in older men and women. *Metabolism.* 2007 Apr;56(4):444-50.

129. Dod HS, Bhardwaj R, Sajja V, et al. Effect of intensive lifestyle changes on endothelial function and on inflammatory markers of atherosclerosis. *Am J Cardiol.* 2010 Feb 1;105(3):362-7.

130. van Dam RM, Li T, Spiegelman D, et al. Combined impact of lifestyle factors on mortality: prospective cohort study in U.S. women. *BMJ.* 2008 Sep 16;337:a1440. doi: 10.1136/bmj.a1440.

131. Khaw KT, Wareham N, Bingham S, et al. Combined impact of health behaviours and mortality in men and women: the EPIC-Norfolk prospective population study. *PLoS Med.* 2008 Jan 8;5(1):e12.

132. Decewicz DJ, Neatrour DM, Burke A, et al. Effects of cardiovascular lifestyle change on lipoprotein subclass profiles defined by nuclear magnetic resonance spectroscopy. *Lipids Health Dis.* 2009 Jun 29;8:26.

133. He K, Liu K, Daviglus ML, et al. Intakes of long-chain n-3 polyunsaturated fatty acids and fish in relation to measurements of subclinical atherosclerosis. *Am J Clin Nutr.* 2008 Oct;88(4):1111-8.

134. Virtanen JK, Siscovick DS, Longstreth WT Jr, et al. Fish consumption and risk of subclinical brain abnormalities on MRI in older adults. *Neurology.* 2008 Aug 5;71(6):439-46.

135. Jung UJ, Torrejon C, Tighe AP, et al. n-3 Fatty acids and cardiovascular disease: mechanisms underlying beneficial effects. *Am J Clin Nutr.* 2008 Jun;87(6):2003S-9S.

136. Bhatnagar D, Durrington PN. Omega-3 fatty acids: their role in the prevention and treatment of atherosclerosis related risk factors and complications. *Int J Clin Pract.* 2003 May;57(4):305-14.

137. Wang C, Harris WS, Chung M, et al. n-3 Fatty acids from fish or fish-oil supplements, but not alpha-linolenic acid, benefit cardiovascular disease outcomes in primary- and secondary-prevention studies: a systematic review. *Am J Clin Nutr.* 2006 Jul;84(1):5-17.

138. von Schacky C. Omega-3 fatty acids and cardiovascular disease. *Curr Opin Clin Nutr Metab Care.* 2007 Mar;10(2):129-35.

139. Khavandi A, Khavandi K, Greenstein A, et al. n-3 polyunsaturated fatty acids are still underappreciated and underused post myocardial infarction. *Heart.* 2009 Jan 8. Epub ahead of print.

140. Saito Y, Yokoyama M, Origasa H, et al. Effects of EPA on coronary artery disease in hypercholesterolemic patients with multiple risk factors: sub-analysis of primary prevention cases from the Japan EPA Lipid Intervention Study (JELIS). *Atherosclerosis.* 2008 Sep;200(1):135-40.

141. Zittermann A, Schleithoff SS, Koerfer R. Putting cardiovascular disease and vitamin D insufficiency into perspective. *Br J Nutr.* 2005 Oct;94(4):483-92.

142. Gebauer SK, West SG, Kay CD, et al. Effects of pistachios on cardiovascular disease risk factors and potential mechanisms of action: a dose-response study. *Am J Clin Nutr.* 2008 Sep;88(3):651-9.

143. Kris-Etherton PM, Yu-Poth S, Sabaté J, et al. Nuts and their bioactive constituents: effects on serum lipids and other factors that affect disease risk. *Am J Clin Nutr.* 1999 Sep;70(3 Suppl):504S-511S.

144. Nash SD, Nash DT. Nuts as part of a healthy cardiovascular diet. *Curr Atheroscler Rep.* 2008 Dec;10(6):529-35.

145. Griel AE, Cao Y, Bagshaw DD, et al. A macadamia nut-rich diet reduces total and LDL-cholesterol in mildly hypercholesterolemic men and women. *J Nutr.* 2008 Apr;138(4):761-7.

146. Blackburn P, Côté M, Lamarche B, et al. Impact of postprandial variation in triglyceridemia on low-density lipoprotein particle size. *Metabolism.* 2003 Nov; 52(11):1379-86.

147. Hausenloy DJ, Yellon DM. Targeting residual cardiovascular risk: raising high-density lipoprotein cholesterol levels. *Heart.* 2008 Jun;94(6):706-14.

148. Kuvin JT, Dave DM, Sliney KA, et al. Effects of extended-release niacin on lipoprotein particle size, distribution, and inflammatory markers in patients with coronary artery disease. *Am J Cardiol.* 2006 Sep 15;98(6):743-5.

149. Thoenes M, Oguchi A, Nagamia S, et al. The effects of extended-release niacin on carotid intimal media thickness, endothelial function and inflammatory markers in patients with the metabolic syndrome. *Int J Clin Pract.* 2007 Nov;61(11):1942-8.

150. Wu BJ, Yan L, Charlton F, et al. Evidence that niacin inhibits acute vascular inflammation and improves endothelial dysfunction independent of changes in plasma lipids. *Arterioscler Thromb Vasc Biol.* 2010 May;30(5):968-75. Epub 2010 Feb 18.

151. Aviram M, Rosenblat M, Gaitini D, et al. Pomegranate juice consumption for 3 years by patients with carotid artery stenosis reduces common carotid intima-media thickness, blood pressure and LDL oxidation. *Clin Nutr.* 2004 Jun;23(3):423-33.

152. de Nigris F, Williams-Ignarro S, Botti C, et al. Pomegranate juice reduces oxidized low-density lipoprotein downregulation of endothelial nitric oxide synthase in human coronary endothelial cells. *Nitric Oxide.* 2006 Nov;15(3):259-63.

153. Erlund I, Koli R, Alfthan G, et al. Favorable effects of berry consumption on platelet function, blood pressure, and HDL cholesterol. *Am J Clin Nutr.* 2008 Feb;87(2):323-31.

154. Ruel G, Pomerleau S, Couture P, et al. Low-calorie cranberry juice supplementation reduces plasma oxidized LDL and cell adhesion molecule concentrations in men. *Br J Nutr.* 2008 Feb;99(2):352-9.

155. Caso G, Kelly P, McNurlan MA, et al. Effect of coenzyme Q10 on myopathic symptoms in patients treated with statins. *Am J Cardiol.* 2007 May 15;99(10):1409-12. Epub 2007 Apr 3.

156. Tiano L, Belardinelli R, Carnevali P, et al. Effect of coenzyme Q10 administration on endothelial function and extracellular superoxide dismutase in patients with ischaemic heart disease: a double-blind, randomized controlled study. *Eur Heart J.* 2007 Sep;28(18):2249-55. Epub 2007 Jul 19.

157. Molyneux SL, Florkowski CM, George PM, Coenzyme Q10: an independent predictor of mortality in chronic heart failure. *J Am Coll Cardiol.* 2008 Oct 28;52(18):1435-41.

158. Hokanson JE, Austin MA. Plasma triglyceride level is a risk factor for cardiovascular disease independent of high-density lipoprotein cholesterol level: a meta-analysis of population-based prospective studies. *J Cardiovasc Risk.* 1996 Apr;3(2):213-9.

159. Park Y, Harris WS. Omega-3 fatty acid supplementation accelerates chylomicron triglyceride clearance. *J Lipid Res.* 2003 Mar;44(3):455-63. Epub 2002 Dec 1.

160. Nambi V, Ballantyne CM. Combination therapy with statins and omega-3 fatty acids. *Am J Cardiol.* 2006 Aug 21;98(4A):34i-38i. Epub 2006 May 30.

161. Meyers CD, Kamanna VS, Kashyap ML. Niacin therapy in atherosclerosis. *Curr Opin Lipidol.* 2004 Dec;15(6):659-65.

162. Lin CC, Tsai WC, Chen JY, et al. Supplements of L-arginine attenuate the effects of high-fat meal on endothelial function and oxidative stress. *Int J Cardiol.* 2008 Jul 21;127(3):337-41.

163. Lekakis JP, Papathanassiou S, Papaioannou TG, et al. Oral L-arginine improves endothelial dysfunction in patients with essential hypertension. *Int J Cardiol.* 2002 Dec;86(2-3):317-23.

164. Albert CM, Cook NR, Gaziano JM, et al. Effect of folic acid and B vitamins on risk of cardiovascular events and total mortality among women at high risk for cardiovascular disease: a randomized trial. *JAMA.* 2008 May 7;299(17):2027-36.

165. Wang X, Qin X, Demirtas H, et al. Efficacy of folic acid supplementation in stroke prevention: a meta-analysis. *Lancet.* 2007 Jun 2;369(9576):1876-82.

166. Cheung GT, Siow YL, O K. Homocysteine stimulates monocyte chemoattractant protein-1 expression in mesangial cells via NF-kappaB activation. *Can J Physiol Pharmacol.* 2008 Mar;86(3):88-96.

167. Au-Yeung KK, Yip JC, Siow YL. Folic acid inhibits homocysteine-induced superoxide anion production and nuclear factor kappa B activation in macrophages. *Can J Physiol Pharmacol.* 2006 Jan;84(1):141-7.

168. Chiuve SE, Giovannucci EL, Hankinson SE, et al. The association between betaine and choline intakes and the plasma concentrations of homocysteine in women. *Am J Clin Nutr.* 2007 Oct;86(4):1073-81.

169. Whelton SP, Hyre AD, Pedersen B, et al. Effect of dietary fiber intake on blood pressure: a meta-analysis of randomized, controlled clinical trials. *J Hypertens.* 2005 Mar;23(3):475-81.

170. Dengo AL, Dennis EA, Orr JS, et al. Arterial destiffening with weight loss in overweight and obese middle-aged and older adults. *Hypertension.* 2010 Apr;55(4):855-61. Epub 2010 Mar 8.

171. Blumenthal JA, Babyak MA, Hinderliter A, et al. Effects of the DASH diet alone and in combination with exercise and weight loss on blood pressure and cardiovascular biomarkers in men and women with high blood pressure: the ENCORE study. *Arch Intern Med.* 2010 Jan 25;170(2):126-35.

172. Craddick SR, Elmer PJ, Obarzanek E, et al. The DASH diet and blood pressure. *Curr Atheroscler Rep.* 2003 Nov;5(6):484-91.

173. Adrogué HJ, Madias NE. Sodium and potassium in the pathogenesis of hypertension. *N Engl J Med.* 2007 May 10;356(19):1966-78.

174. Rosenfeldt FL, Haas SJ, Krum H, et al. Coenzyme Q10 in the treatment of hypertension: a meta-analysis of the clinical trials. *J Hum Hypertens.* 2007 Apr;21(4):297-306.

175. Rodrigo R, Prat H, Passalacqua W, et al. Decrease in oxidative stress through supplementation of vitamins C and E is associated with a reduction in blood pressure in patients with essential hypertension. *Clin Sci* (Lond). 2008 May;114(10):625-34.

176. Cesarone MR, Belcaro G, Rohdewald P, et al. Comparison of Pycnogenol and Daflon in treating chronic venous insufficiency: a prospective, controlled study. *Clin Appl Thromb Hemost.* 2006 Apr;12(2):205-12.

177. Cesarone MR, Belcaro G, Rohdewald P, et al. Improvement of diabetic microangiopathy with pycnogenol: A prospective, controlled study. *Angiology.* 2006 Aug-Sep;57(4):431-6.

178. Belcaro G, Cesarone MR, Ricci A, et al. Control of edema in hypertensive subjects treated with calcium antagonist (nifedipine) or angiotensin-converting enzyme inhibitors with Pycnogenol. *Clin Appl Thromb Hemost.* 2006 Oct;12(4):440-4.

179. Reinhart KM, Coleman CI, Teevan C, et al. Effects of garlic on blood pressure in patients with and without systolic hypertension: a meta-analysis. *Ann Pharmacother.* 2008 Dec;42(12):1766-71.

180. Ried K, Frank OR, Stocks NP, et al. Effect of garlic on blood pressure: a systematic review and meta-analysis. *BMC Cardiovasc Disord.* 2008 Jun 16;8:13.

181. Martina V, Masha A, Gigliardi VR, et al. Long-term N-acetylcysteine and L-arginine administration reduces endothelial activation and systolic blood pressure in hypertensive patients with type 2 diabetes. *Diabetes Care.* 2008 May;31(5):940-4.

182. Li YC. Vitamin D regulation of the renin-angiotensin system. *J Cell Biochem.* 2003 Feb 1;88(2):327-31.

183. Forman JP, Curhan GC, Taylor EN. Plasma 25-hydroxyvitamin D levels and risk of incident hypertension among young women. *Hypertension.* 2008 Nov;52(5):828-32. Epub 2008 Oct 6.

184. Dwyer JH, Allayee H, Dwyer KM, et al. Arachidonate 5-lipoxygenase promoter genotype, dietary arachidonic acid, and atherosclerosis. *N Engl J Med.* 2004 Jan 1;350(1):29-37.

185. Allayee H, Baylin A, Hartiala J, et al. Nutrigenetic association of the 5-lipoxygenase gene with myocardial infarction. *Am J Clin Nutr.* 2008 Oct;88(4):934-40.

186. Schmidt EB, Koenig W, Khuseyinova N, et al. Lipoprotein-associated phospholipase A2 concentrations in plasma are associated with the extent of coronary artery disease and correlate to adipose tissue levels of marine n-3 fatty acids. *Atherosclerosis.* 2008 Jan;196(1):420-4. Epub 2006 Dec 8.

187. Tai ES, Corella D, Demissie S, et al. Polyunsaturated fatty acids interact with the PPARA-L162V polymorphism to affect plasma triglyceride and apolipoprotein C-III concentrations in the Framingham Heart Study. *J Nutr.* 2005 Mar;135(3):397-403.

188. Carrero JJ, López-Huertas E, Salmerón LM, et al. Daily supplementation with (n-3) PUFAs, oleic acid, folic acid, and vitamins B-6 and E increases pain-free walking distance and improves risk factors in men with peripheral vascular disease. *J Nutr.* 2005 Jun;135(6):1393-9.

189. Schiano V, Laurenzano E, Brevetti G, et al. Omega-3 polyunsaturated fatty acid in peripheral arterial disease: effect on lipid pattern, disease severity, inflammation profile, and endothelial function. *Clin Nutr.* 2008 Apr;27(2):241-7. Epub 2008 Jan 31.

190. Pande RL, Perlstein TS, Beckman JA, et al. Association of insulin resistance and inflammation with peripheral arterial disease: the National Health and Nutrition Examination Survey, 1999 to 2004. *Circulation.* 2008 Jul 1;118(1):33-41. Epub 2008 Jun 16.

Regeneration/Healthy Aging

Overview

Aging is a complex process in which organisms undergo general or specific degeneration, as well as the death of cell populations within vital organs. Aging has been characterized as a "collision between destructive processes that act on cells and organs over the lifetime and the responses that promote homeostasis, vitality, and longevity."[1] While the precise causes of aging have not been definitely established, current research points to a combination of excessive damage and impaired regenerative processes. The accumulation of damage over time, particularly DNA damage, causes a decline in cellular function that is associated with aging. Thus, regenerative and healthy aging treatments are aimed at reducing the causes of excess damage, such as reactive oxygen and nitrogen species, inflammation, environmental toxins, and metabolic byproducts (e.g., advanced glycation end-products and homocysteine), while improving cellular function and regenerative processes through lifestyle changes and targeted supplemental therapies.

Causes of Excessive Degeneration

Reactive oxygen species (ROS)

Many factors may contribute to accelerated degeneration. While not universally accepted, the free-radical theory of aging has had the most support since it was first articulated in the 1950s. According to this theory, when oxidative stress overwhelms antioxidant defenses, the resulting damage causes degeneration over time. While certainly environmental toxins and other exogenous sources create reactive oxygen species (ROS), intracellular production by mitochondrial respiration is now thought to be the most significant generator of ROS.[60]

Indeed, while the metabolic rate of an organism might be expected to predict ROS production and thus lifespan, it has been shown that mitochondrial ROS production is a much better marker for overall longevity than metabolic rate.[2] For example, birds have a much longer lifespan than would be predicted by their high metabolic rate, but their mitochondria produce much fewer

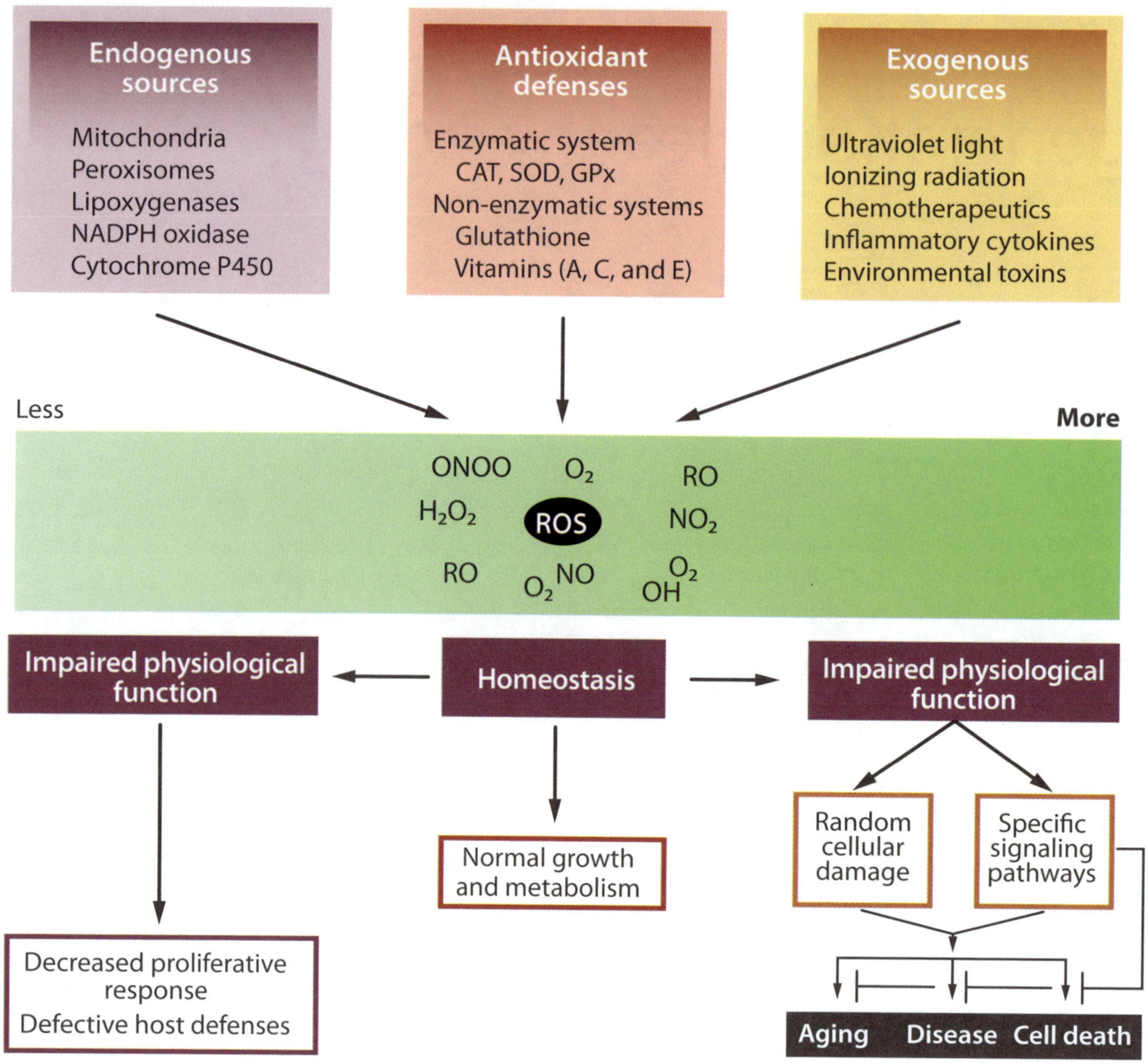

Figure 10.1 Sources of, and cellular responses to, reactive oxygen species (ROS). From: Finkel T, Holbrook NJ. Oxidants, oxidative stress and the biology of aging. *Nature*. 2000 Nov 9;408(6809):239-47. Reproduced with permission from Macmillan Publishers Ltd.

ROS than other species.[2] Although not all studies have found this correlation between lifespan and mitochondrial ROS production, oxidative stress may still play a crucial role in other mechanisms of aging, such as accumulation of mutations in genes, telomere shortening, damage in mitochondrial DNA, inflammation, and the neuroendocrine theory of aging.[3] (The neuroendocrine theory of aging posits that changes in the hormonal and neurological functions which coordinate physiological adaptations to stress are behind the aging process.)[4] Figure 10.1 shows common sources of ROS, and the resultant cellular responses.

AGEs (advanced glycation end-products)

In addition to ROS, compounds known as advanced glycation end-products (AGEs) are also thought to contribute to the aging process.[7] AGEs are formed by a non-enzymatic reaction between a ketone group of glucose (or aldehydes) and the amino groups of proteins, lipids, or nucleic acids. If the rate of AGE formation is fairly low, AGEs may only form with long-lived molecules, such as collagen or crystallins (proteins found in the lens of the eye).

The hyperglycemia resulting from poor glucose control, seen in both metabolic syndrome and

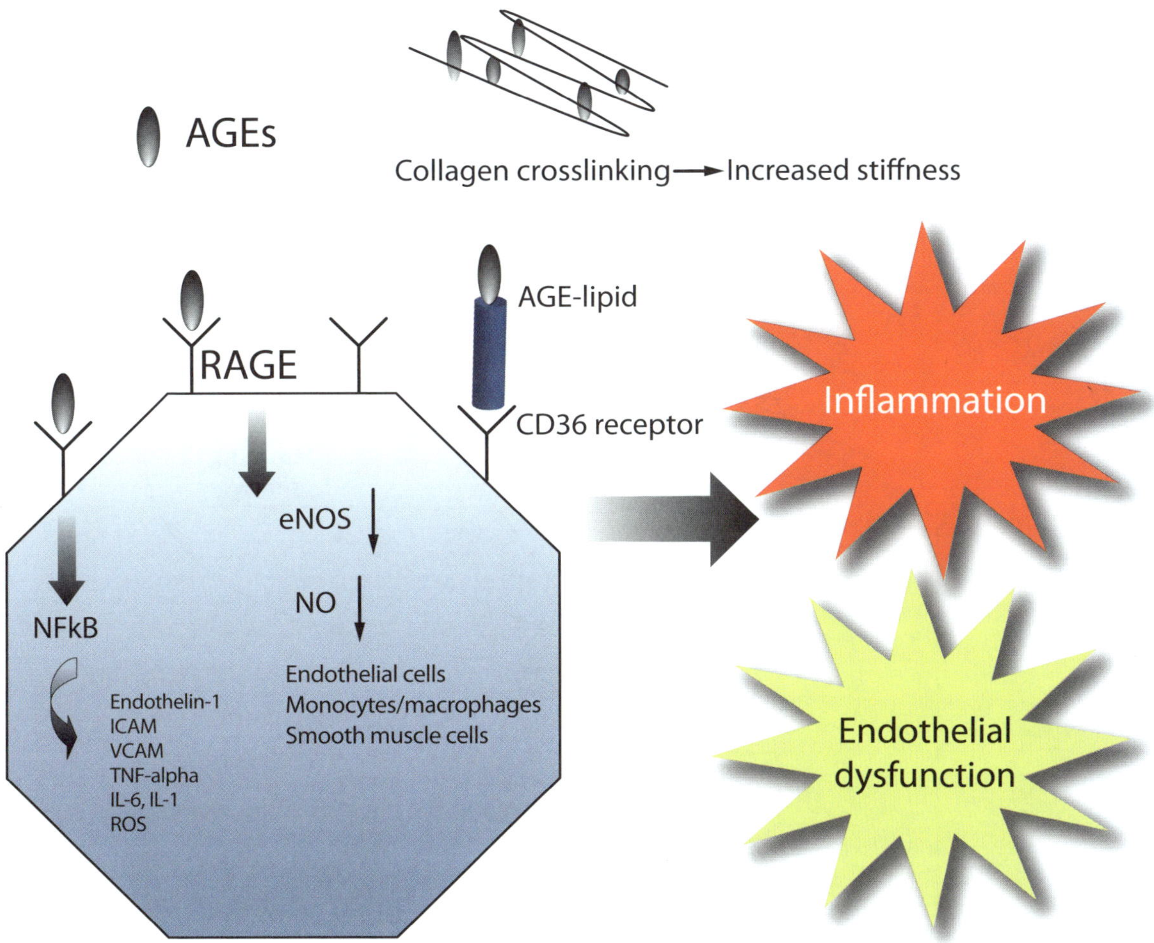

Figure 10.2 AGE-induced mechanisms for increased vascular stiffness. From: Meerwaldt R, Links T, Zeebregts C, et al. Clinical relevance of advanced glycation end-products for vascular surgery. *Eur J Vasc Endovasc Surg*. 2008;36(2):125-31. Reproduced with permission from Elsevier.

diabetes, creates an abundance of glucose and thus an accelerated rate of formation and accumulation of AGEs. This leads to greater modification of long-lived molecules, and also to modification of shorter-lived molecules, such as apolipoproteins and LDL, linking AGE formation to cardiovascular disease as well as accelerated degeneration.[5]

The damage of AGEs

AGEs are known to cause damage through several mechanisms. They accumulate on a number of proteins (collagen, fibronectin, tubulin, hemoglobin, albumin and apolipoproteins), causing changes in their structural integrity and cellular function, accelerating cardiovascular disease.[6] AGE cross-linking to collagens decreases vascular elasticity and reduces vascular compliance, resulting in increased vascular stiffness (see Figure 10.2). AGEs are also able to quench nitric oxide (NO) and generate ROS by stimulating NADPH oxidase activity.[6]

Along with direct effects, AGEs also cause damage by binding to AGE-specific receptors, or RAGE (receptor of AGEs). These receptors have been shown to mediate much of the damage associated with AGE accumulation by impairing endothelial function and inducing inflammatory (NF-KappaB) and profibrotic pathways.[7] Activation of these pathways may also be responsible for a more chronic inflammation, as NF-KappaB may trigger AGE-specific receptors, creating a positive feedback loop (see Figure 10.3).

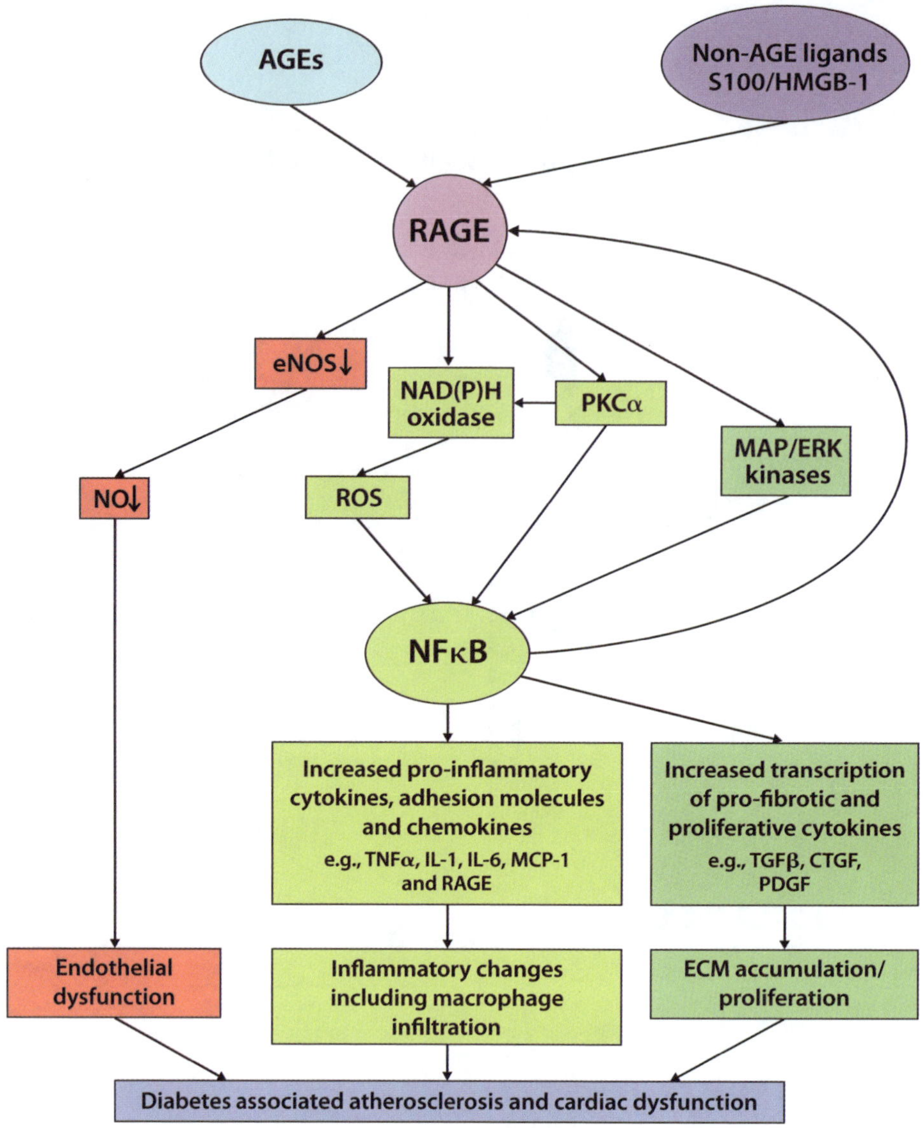

Figure 10.3 Interaction of AGEs with RAGE. From: Jandeleit-Dahm K, Cooper ME. The role of AGEs in cardiovascular disease. *Curr Pharm Des*. 2008;14(10):979-86. Reproduced with permission from Bentham Science Publishers Ltd.

Sources of AGEs

The largest contributor to AGE formation is hyperglycemia, with diabetes being the greatest risk factor. Indeed, glycosylated hemoglobin is a product of the non-enzymatic reaction between hemoglobin and glucose, and is used as a diagnostic marker for diabetes as well as a measure of average glucose concentrations.[8] AGEs are thought to be very significant contributors to the complications of diabetes, such as retinopathy and neuropathy, and are also thought to exacerbate the etiology. AGEs have been shown to inhibit the conversion of proinsulin to insulin, measured as the P/I ratio, and to inhibit the production of insulin by pancreatic beta cells, in part by blocking the formation of ATP.[9,10]

In addition to the damage caused by hyperglycemia, other lifestyle behaviors such as smoking and food choices can increase AGE formation.[11] The contribution of diet to the body's AGE pool can be quite significant, with a direct association shown between the AGE content of the diet and systemic markers of inflammation, such as CRP, among healthy individuals.[12] The foods highest in AGEs appear to be those with the highest fat and protein content; for example, fat and meat foods contain 30- and 12-fold higher AGE content, respectively, than do carbohydrate foods.[13] In addition to the types of foods, the cooking method also significantly influences AGE content. The temperature and method used are much better predictors than the duration of time that heat is applied. For example, as shown in Table 1, broiling a food (tuna) for only 10 minutes at 225 °C produces nearly 10 times the AGE content as does roasting it for 40 minutes at 177 °C. The higher temperatures used when boiling, grilling, deep-frying, and roasting meats produce a very high AGE content compared to less intense methods of cooking such as steaming.

Dietary AGE content is thought to contribute to a number of disorders, including insulin resistance, atherosclerosis, and neurodegenerative disease. AGEs in food are absorbed in the intestine and AGE content is directly correlated with blood levels. For example, human studies have shown a significant increase in plasma AGE levels within 2 hours following the oral administration of a single AGE-rich meal.[14] Those with diabetes or renal disease have greater difficulty with urinary elimination of AGEs, resulting in higher and longer-lasting levels as a result of an AGE-rich diet.[14]

Reversing the damage of AGEs

It has been shown that a 50% reduction in AGEs ingested with foods decreases AGE plasma levels by 30% within a month.[15] Diabetic patients consuming a diet low in AGEs for 6 weeks decreased their C-reactive protein levels by 20%, whereas a diet rich in AGEs increased C-reactive protein by 35%.[15] In addition to consuming foods low in AGEs, both cooking at lower temperatures and consuming foods with a low glycemic index will help to reduce the overall AGE burden. Foods containing the flavonoid rutin, such as tomatoes and other fruits and vegetables, have been shown to inhibit AGE formation.[16,17,18]

Since hyperglycemia is the greatest contributor to AGE formation, interventions that normalize blood sugar are essential to reducing the impact of AGEs. A combination of diet and exercise has been shown to be a powerful tool for improving glycemic control.[19,20,21] In addition to lifestyle changes, a number of nutritional supplements have been shown to improve insulin resistance and reduce hyperglycemia. See Clinical Focus 4—The Spectrum of Insulin Resistance for more complete information.

Table 10.1 AGE content of selected foods

Food Item	AGE* (kU/g or /ml of food)
Fats	
Almonds, roasted	66.5 kU/g
Oil, olive	120 kU/ml
Butter	265 kU/g
Mayonnaise	94 kU/g
Proteins	
Chicken breast, broiled x 15 min	58 kU/g
Chicken breast, fried x 15 min	61 kU/g
Beef, boiled x 1 h	22 kU/g
Beef, broiled x 15 min	60 kU/g
Tuna, roasted x 40 min	6 kU/g
Tuna, broiled x 10 min	51 kU/g
Cheese, American	87 kU/g
Cheese, Brie	56 kU/g
Egg, fried	27 kU/g
Egg yolk, boiled	12 kU/g
Tofu, raw	8 kU/g
Tofu, broiled	41 kU/g
Carbohydrates	
Bread, whole-wheat center	0.54 kU/g
Pancake, homemade	10 kU/g
Milk, cow, whole	0.05 kU/ml
Milk, human, whole	0.05 kU/ml
Enfamil (infant formula)	4.86 kU/ml
Apple	0.13 kU/g
Banana	0.01 kU/g
Carrots	0.1 kU/g
Green beans	0.18 kU/g

*AGE denotes N-carboxymethyl-lysine (CML)-like immunoreactivity, assessed by enzyme-linked immunosorbent assay based on monoclonal antibody (4G9)

Advanced glycation end-products in commonly consumed foods. From: Goldberg T, Cai W, et al. *J Am Diet Assoc.* 2004 Aug;104(8):1287-91. Reproduced with permission from Elsevier.

In addition to a diet low in AGE content, a number of pharmaceutical agents have been shown to reduce the total load of AGEs in the body, or modify them into inactive forms. These include ACE inhibitors, angiotensin receptor antagonists, metformin, metal chelators, and peroxisome proliferator receptor agonists.[22] Some compounds, such as aminoguanidine, have been shown to be potent inhibitors of AGE formation, and also have the benefit of normalizing protein kinase C activity and improving mitochondrial respiration. Its clinical usefulness has been limited by adverse effects, however.[23]

Several natural "AGE-breakers" have also been shown to prevent AGE formation. Thiamine, for example, was found to be as effective as, or more effective than, aminoguanidine in inhibiting the formation of AGEs.[24] Even more effective may be thiamine derivatives, such as benfotiamine, a garlic-derived, lipid-soluble form of thiamine that results in up to a 120-fold increase in intracellular thiamine compared to an equivalent amount of thiamine itself.[25] Benfotiamine has been shown to prevent both micro- and macrovascular complications of a meal rich in AGEs when given to patients with type 2 diabetes.[26] A second thiamine analog (a thiazolium derivative), alagebrium (ALT-711), has been shown to break established AGE crosslinks, and attenuate diabetic renal disease, cardiac dysfunction, and atherosclerosis in animal models.[27] In human trials, it reduced pulse pressure and improved vascular compliance in patients with systolic hypertension, though safety and efficacy trials are in process.[27] One of the active forms of vitamin B6, pyridoxamine, was found to prevent arterial stiffening in an animal model of diabetes, at least partly by inhibiting the formation of AGEs and their accumulation on aortic collagen.[28] Other compounds shown to be of benefit in animal models include lipoic acid, L-carnitine, and astragalosides.[29,30,31] Additionally, some glycation repair enzymes have been shown to require magnesium as a cofactor.[32]

Telomeres

Aging is also associated with a change in telomere length (Figure 10.4). Telomeres are specialized DNA sequences that cap the ends of linear chromosomes; they are comprised of repeated sequences of TTAGGG, reiterated in tandem for up to 15 kilobases at birth, and are bound to specialized proteins.[33,34] They stabilize chromosomal ends by preventing them from being processed as double-stranded breaks by repair enzymes.[35] However, cell division results in a shortening of telomere length, with the loss leading to breaks in DNA and cellular senescence. When telomere shortening reaches a critical point, a cell can no longer divide and becomes apoptotic or senescent.

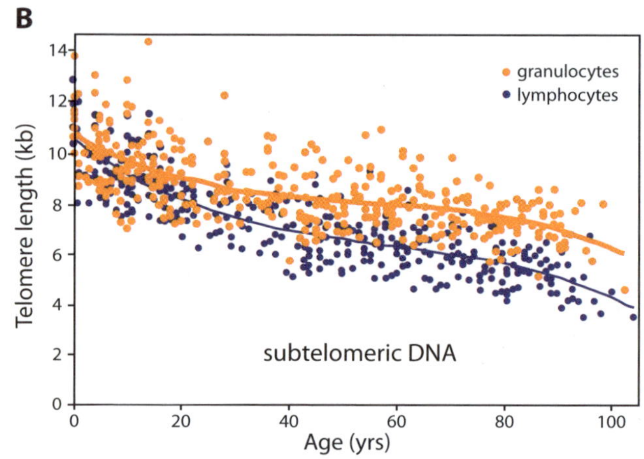

Figure 10.4 Telomere length in lymphocytes and granulocytes during human lifespan. From: Aubert G, Lansdorp PM. Telomeres and aging. *Physiol Rev.* 2008 Apr;88(2):557-79. Reproduced with permission from the American Physiological Society.

Thus, the number of times a cell may divide has long been assumed to be finite. Interestingly, a growing body of evidence suggests that, in contrast to earlier theories, the shortening in telomere length may not be automatic in healthy cells, and a number of interventions may prevent telomeres from shortening in healthy cells.[36] Telomere shortening appears to be due to decreased expression of telomerase, the enzyme responsible for maintaining telomere length, in response to cellular damage, such as oxidative stress. This establishes a mechanism for identifying and removing cells that may be dysfunctional—when cells reach a critical telomere length due to increased cellular stress and damage, they can be identified as ready for apoptosis or senescence. Shorter telomeres are therefore not only associated with a shorter lifespan but are also a marker for an increased risk of disease. From an evolutionary standpoint, this mechanism would have a protective effect on a younger organism, because directing a cell to become senescent or apoptotic prevents it from becoming neoplastic. Notably, 80–90% of all cancer cells either express telomerase or have found alternate ways to maintain their telomere length, considerably extending their lifespan.[37] Figure 10.5 depicts some of the outcomes of telomere dysfunction.

There is research supporting the theory that the health of the cell influences telomerase activity; interventions that increase or maintain telomere length appear to work by upregulating genes known as sirtuins (SIR2 in yeast, SIRT1-7 in mammals, with SIRT1 the most extensively studied).[42] SIRT1 plays a major role in energy homeostasis in key metabolic tissues, apparently linking metabolic status to transcriptional output. In other words, sirtuins may act as metabolic sensors, affecting telomere length and cellular lifespan accordingly. For example, calorie restriction is one of the most well-documented methods of extending lifespan in essentially all species studied.[42] It is thought that the increase in lifespan is mediated at least partly through a pathway involving SIRT1 (see Figure 10.6). The polyphenol resveratrol is thought to have an effect on sirtuin expression and has been shown to mimic numerous aspects of calorie restriction in all eukaryotic cells studied, including the increase in lifespan; in yeast cells, however, calorie restriction did not further augment the increase in lifespan caused by resveratrol.[38]

Among other interventions shown to increase telomerase activity, comprehensive lifestyle changes

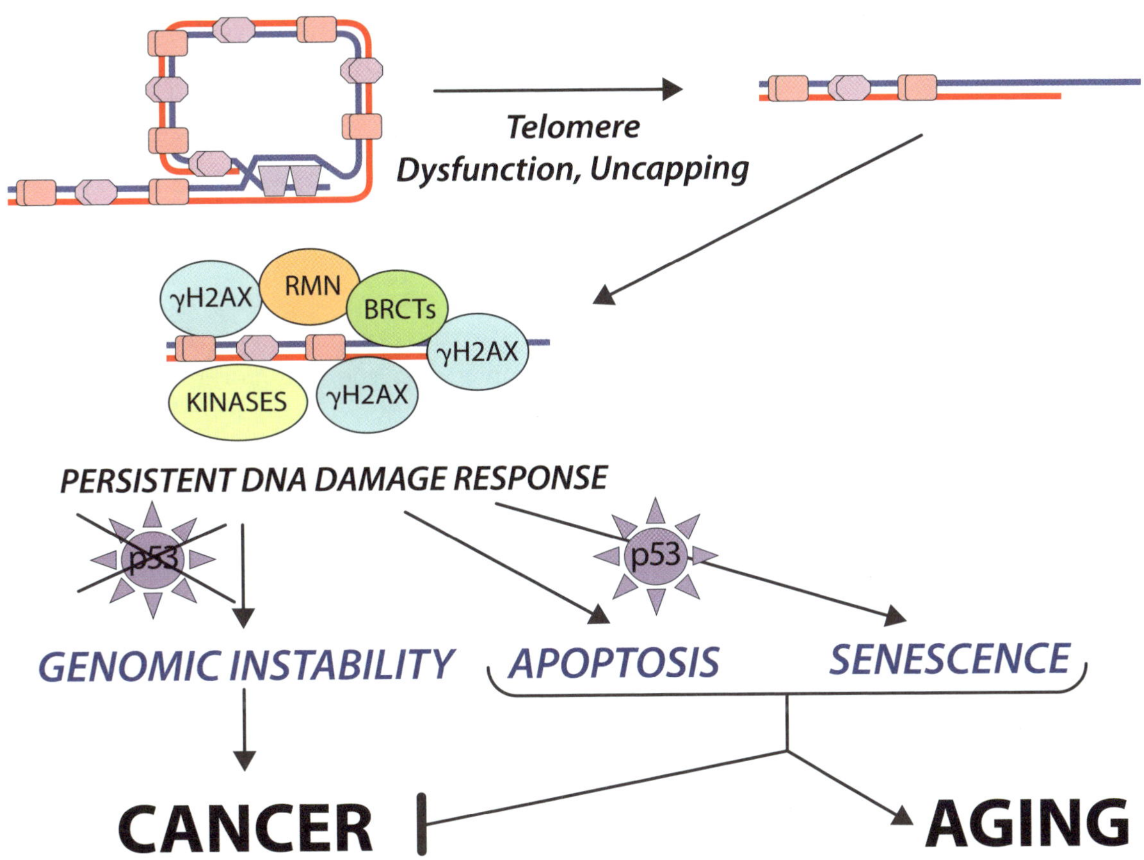

Figure 10.5 Outcomes of telomere dysfunction. From: Rodier F, Kim SH, Nijjar T, et al. Cancer and aging: the importance of telomeres in genome maintenance. *Int J Biochem Cell Biol.* 2005 May;37(5):977-90. Reproduced with permission from Elsevier Science & Technology Journals.

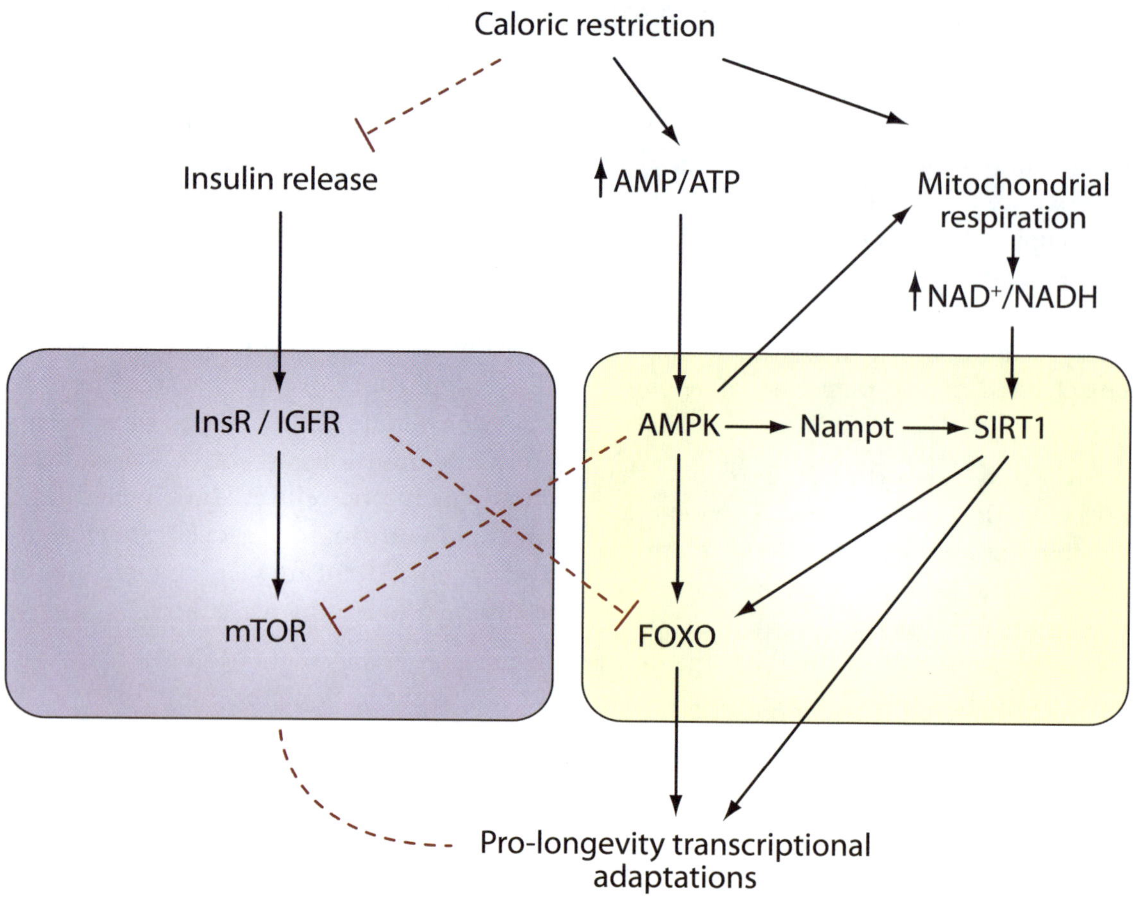

Figure 10.6 Signaling pathways involved in regulating the effects of calorie restriction. From: Cantó C, Auwerx J. Caloric restriction, SIRT1 and longevity. *Trends Endocrinol Metab.* 2009 Sep;20(7):325-31. Reproduced with permission from Elsevier Science & Technology Journals.

(e.g., the Ornish program) were recently shown to increase activity and thus telomere maintenance capacity in immune cells in a 3-month trial of 30 men with prostate cancer.[39] Physical exercise has been shown to be associated with preserving telomere length,[40] and some forms of meditation may have salutary effects on telomere length by reducing cognitive stress and stress arousal.[41] Vitamin D was recently found to be directly associated with telomere length in a study of over 2000 women, even after adjusting for age, menopausal status, use of hormone replacement therapy, and physical activity. Telomere length was even greater in those with low CRP levels across all levels of serum vitamin D (see Figure 10.7).[42]

Telomeres also appear to be more susceptible to oxidative damage than to other types of DNA damage, possibly explaining the associations between markers of oxidation and longevity.[43] For example, the most important defense system against oxidative stress is the glutathione system; an age-related decline in intracellular glutathione concentration—and therefore a decrease of cellular antioxidative capacity—has been demonstrated.[44] A direct relationship between mtDNA damage and mitochondrial glutathione oxidation has also been documented, indicating its importance in the aging process.[45] Furthermore, in a sample of community-dwelling elderly, higher glutathione levels were associated with higher levels of physical health, fewer illnesses, and higher levels of self-rated health.[46]

Recent studies have also reported that both diabetes and prediabetes are associated with shorter telomeres.[47] This association may be mediated by the damaging effects of hyperglycemia; a recent report linked the increase in oxidative stress, particularly mitochondrial ROS production, to shorter telomeres among diabetics.[48] Other endogenous and exogenous sources of toxicity, such as elevated homocysteine levels and exposure to traffic pollution, have also been shown to be associated with shorter telomeres.[49,50]

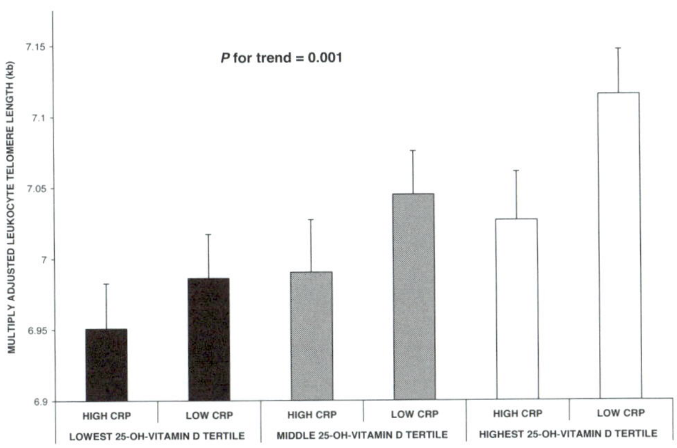

Figure 10.7 Associations between 25-OH-vitamin D levels and leukocyte telomere length, stratified by CRP. From: Richards JB, Valdes AM, Gardner JP, et al. Higher serum vitamin D concentrations are associated with longer leukocyte telomere length in women. *Am J Clin Nutr.* 2007 Nov;86(5):1420-5. Reproduced with permission from the American Society for Nutrition.

Extracts from *Astragalus membranaceous* may have benefit in counteracting telomere shortening. In an *in vitro* study, these extracts were found to slow down the rate of telomere shortening, to reduce DNA damage, and to improve DNA repair ability.[51]

Mitochondrial DNA

DNA is the only biological molecule that relies solely on repair of existing molecules, rather than remanufacture; hence, the accumulation of damage to DNA increases with age, contributing to sub-optimal cellular function and to the aging process. Combining spontaneous damage with exogenous (UV) and endogenous (reactive oxygen, nitrogen, and carbonyl species) sources, it is estimated that close to 105 lesions per cell per day may occur.[52]

Perhaps more important than the damage to nuclear DNA is the damage to mitochondrial DNA (mtDNA). In one study, researchers measured the levels of the oxidative marker 8-oxo-7,8-dihydro-2'-deoxyguanosine (8-oxodG) in heart and brain tissue of 8 different mammalian species of varying lifespans. They found that 8-oxodG in mtDNA was inversely correlated with the maximum life span (MLSP), i.e., slow-aging mammals showed lower 8-oxodG levels in mtDNA than fast-aging ones (Figure 10.8). However, this inverse relationship was restricted to mtDNA, since 8-oxodG levels in nuclear DNA were not significantly correlated with MLSP.[53]

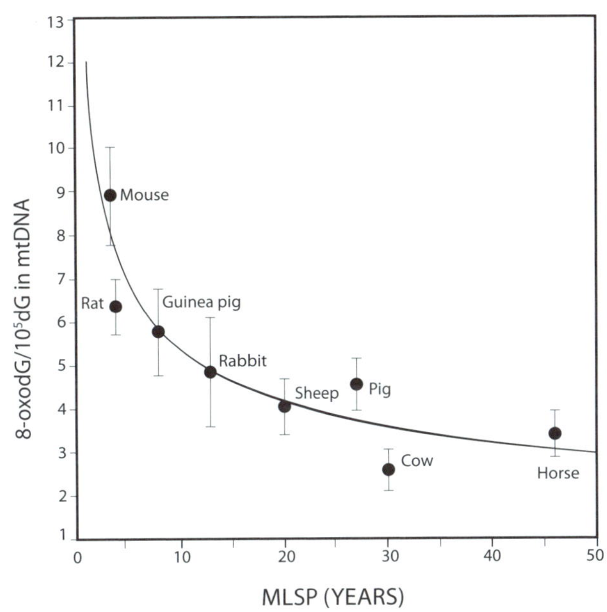

Figure 10.8 Inverse correlation between heart 8-oxodG in mtDNA and maximum life span. From: Barja G, Herrero A. Oxidative damage to mitochondrial DNA is inversely related to maximum life span in the heart and brain of mammals. *FASEB J.* 2000 Feb;14(2):312-8. Reproduced with permission from the Federation of American Societies for Experimental Biology (FASEB).

A recent study of 146 healthy men and women reported that the abundance of mtDNA, as well as mitochondrial function in skeletal muscle, decreased with age, an effect associated with aerobic capacity and glucose tolerance.[54] However, it has also been shown that mitochondrial biogenesis can be induced with physical activity, preventing some of the age-associated decline.[55]

As discussed earlier, the mitochondrial production of ROS is one of the better predictors of maximal lifespans. Dysfunctional mitochondria and mtDNA damage appear to generate a feed-forward cycle. As more damage is done to mtDNA, mitochondria become less efficient at producing ATP and create more ROS as a consequence (Figure 10.9). The additional ROS burden may accelerate the rate of mtDNA damage, though this has not been well-confirmed. Treatments aimed at improving mitochondrial respiration and reducing mtDNA damage may halt this vicious cycle.[56]

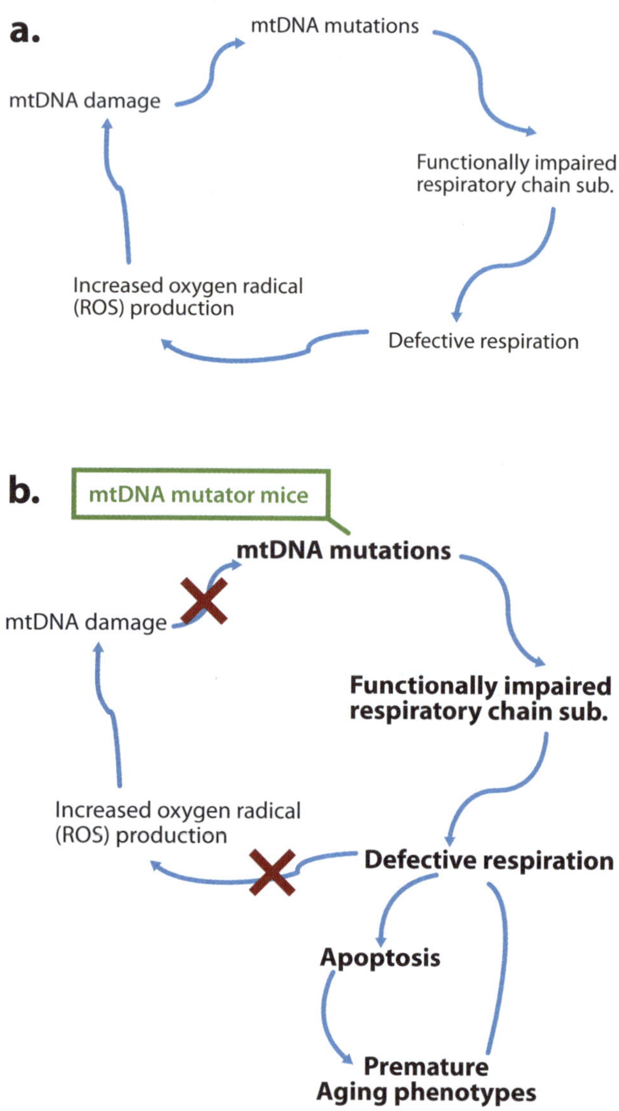

Figure 10.9 Accumulations of mtDNA increase ROS. From: Trifunovic A. Mitochondrial DNA and ageing. *Biochim Biophys Acta.* 2006 May-Jun;1757(5-6):611-7. Reproduced with permission from Elsevier Science & Technology Journals.

Many nutrients improve mitochondrial function through diverse mechanisms. Transport of fatty acids across the inner mitochondrial membrane can be enhanced by L-carnitine or by providing cofactors for the enzymes of respiration, such as riboflavin. By avoiding mitochondrial toxins, and providing nutrients necessary for energy production and useful for reducing oxidative stress, the ROS generated by oxidative phosphorylation should be reduced, with a consequent reduction in mtDNA damage. Steps to improve mitochondrial function are outlined in detail in Clinical Focus 1—A Cellular Approach to Health.

Neurological Degeneration

Neurodegenerative disease increases in prevalence with age, and may be accompanied by symptoms such as memory loss, cognitive impairment, loss of taste and smell, as well as more devastating pathologies such as Alzheimer's and Parkinson's diseases and senile dementia. Neurological degeneration is characterized by declines in the number and function of neurons, and by damaged interconnections between them. In a very recent study, more than 140 healthy elderly participants were followed with MRI; researchers found significant reductions in many parts of the brain in healthy individuals within just 1 years' time. Atrophy accelerated with age and occurred in parts of the brain not associated with Alzheimer's disease, suggesting that a different degenerative process occurs in healthy adults.[57]

There are many known risk factors for neurodegeneration, including stress/glucocorticoid use, the *APOE* e4 allele, insomnia, vitamin D insufficiency, poor glucose control, toxin exposure, hyperhomocysteinemia. Although much remains to be learned about neurodegenerative disease, some common etiologies include mitochondrial dysfunction, inflammation, dysfunctional or misfolded proteins, and excessive reactive oxygen species.[58]

Causes of neurological degeneration are thought to include abnormal protein folding. Common to many neurodegenerative diseases are misfolded proteins that aggregate, resulting in synapse degeneration, apoptosis, and excitotoxicity, all of which contribute to neuronal dysfunction. For example, Alzheimer's disease is characterized by the presence of neurofibrillary tangles (composed of a hyperphosphorylated form of the microtubular protein tau) and the peptide β-amyloid (Aβ), which is known to cause cell death by directly triggering apoptogenic signaling and ROS production and by indirectly activating astrocytes and microglia to produce excess amounts of inflammatory cytokines, including NF-KappaB.[59] Elevated levels of Aβ have been directly correlated with dementia and the rate of cognitive decline.[60]

Although the precise causes for the abnormal protein folding found in many neurodegenerative disorders are not completely understood, cellular stress from a variety of sources certainly plays a role. For example, oxidative stress has clearly been shown to damage biological molecules, initiating a cascade of events that includes dysfunction of mitochondrial respiration, excitotoxicity, and a fatal rise in cytosolic calcium; these events lead to cellular dysfunction, and nitric oxide (NO) and reactive nitrogen species (RNC) production. Oxidative stress is considered a major factor in the cytopathology of many neurodegenerative disorders, and it may be a fundamental molecular mechanism in the early-stage protein aggregation which underlies their pathogenesis.[62] The generation of excessive nitric oxide and ROS can mediate protein misfolding in the absence of genetic predisposition (through excessive activation of the NMDA receptor).[61]

Other sources of neuronal stress include glucocorticoids, which have been shown to reduce the volume of the amygdala and hippocampus compared to healthy controls, in proportion to duration of use (Figure 10.10).[62] This is thought to be due to their effect on glutamate release.[63]

Hyperhomocysteinemia has also been shown to be toxic to nerve cells. Elevated homocysteine levels have been found among patients with Parkinson's disease (particularly those taking L-dopa), an effect accentuated in those with low folic acid

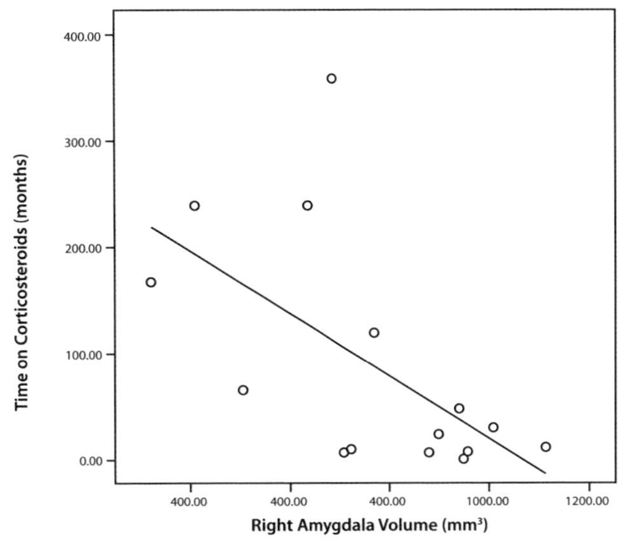

Figure 10.10 Relationship of time on corticosteroids to amygdala volume. From: Brown ES, Woolston DJ, Frol AB. Amygdala volume in patients receiving chronic corticosteroid therapy. *Biol Psychiatry.* 2008;63:705-9. Reproduced with permission from Elsevier.

levels.[64,65] Elevated homocysteine and low B12 and folate levels are also directly linked to risk of Alzheimer's disease, dementia, and multiple sclerosis (Figure 10.11).[66,67,68] Elevated homocysteine levels have been shown to reduce nitric oxide availability and increase the level of reactive oxygen species, perhaps contributing to protein misfolding.[69] Additionally, homocysteine induces NF-KappaB expression,[70] an effect which may be blunted by folic acid even if homocysteine levels are not reduced.[71] Optimal treatment for elevated homocysteine levels includes supplementation with folic acid, B6, and B12.[72,73] There may also be benefit from a greater intake of choline and betaine, as these two nutrients are involved in the remethylation of homocysteine and their intakes have been associated with a reduction in inflammatory markers such as CRP.[74,75]

Lack of sleep is another risk factor with a significant association to neurodegeneration. With age, the percentage of deep, slow wave sleep has been shown to decrease, and sleep fragmentation increases, effects associated with higher evening cortisol concentrations independent of age.[76] Sleep disturbances are also found early in many neurodegenerative disease processes, even in the presence of mild cognitive impairment.[77] A number

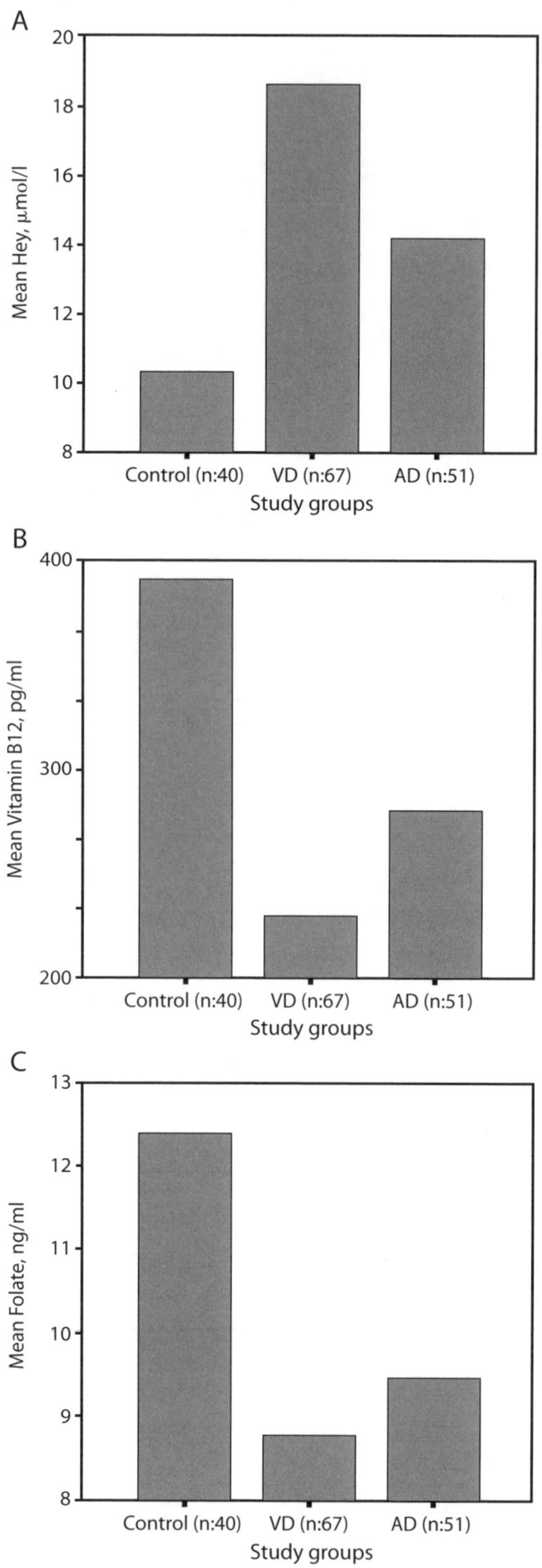

Figure 10.11 Comparison of patients with Alzheimer's disease, vascular dementia, and controls with respect to their mean Hcy, vitamin B12 and folate levels. From: Köseoglu E, Karaman Y. Relations between homocysteine, folate and vitamin B12 in vascular dementia and in Alzheimer disease. *Clin Biochem* 2007;40:859-63. Reproduced with permission from Elsevier Science & Technology Journals.

of lifestyle interventions, such as taking short daytime naps, maintaining a routine and using bright light therapy, as well as supplemental interventions have been found to increase deep wave sleep, improve sleep onset latency, and prolong overall sleep time, as well as to reduce the stress that often accompanies sleep disturbances.[78,79,80] Supplementation with melatonin,[81] vitamin B12,[82] 5-HTP,[83] and L-theanine[84] have all shown significant clinical benefit. For more information, see Clinical Focus 6—Stress, Anxiety, Depression, and Insomnia.

Hyperglycemia is also a significant risk factor for neurodegenerative disease. In a prospective study of over 6000 participants, diabetes was found to almost double the risk of dementia, and those being treated with insulin had more than quadruple the risk (Figure 10.12). The authors concluded that diabetes may account for nearly 10% of the population with dementia.[85] In a recent study of more than 2500 participants, diabetes was also found to increase the risk of Alzheimer's disease, particularly in those with the *APOE* 4 (e4) allele (discussed further below). Compared to those individuals without diabetes and with no copies of the e4 allele, those with both had a nearly 5-fold risk for developing Alzheimer's.[86]

Vitamin D plays an important role in preventing neurodegeneration. It is thought to have a beneficial effect by increasing neurotrophic factors, providing antioxidant protection, and regulating neuronal calcium metabolism. Polymorphisms in the vitamin D receptor (VDR) gene have been shown to increase the risk for Alzheimer's disease by more than 2-fold.[87] Lower vitamin D levels have been shown to increase the risk of multiple sclerosis (MS), at least among the Caucasian population.[88] And while polymorphisms in the VDR gene were not found to be associated with risk for MS in all studies, the season of birth was found to affect risk, suggesting that higher vitamin D levels in the third trimester of pregnancy may reduce risk.[89] Some studies have found an association between VDR genotype and risk, particularly when linked to past sun exposure.[90]

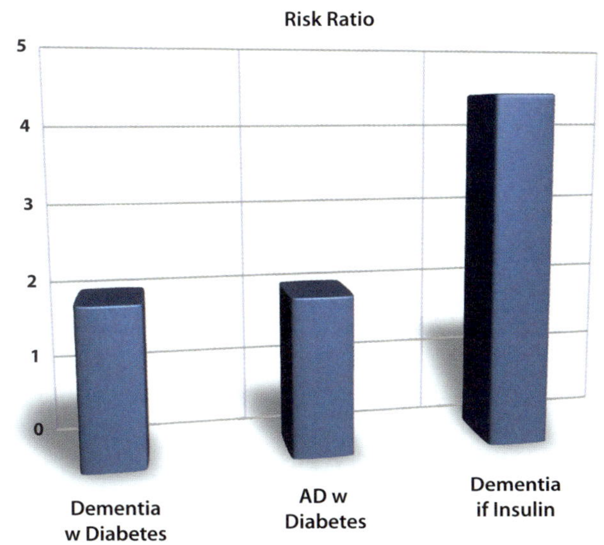

Figure 10.12 Risk of Alzheimer's disease (AD) and dementia for those with diabetes. Created using data from: Ott A, Stolk RP, van Harskamp F, et al. Diabetes mellitus and the risk of dementia: The Rotterdam Study. *Neurology*. 1999 Dec 10;53(9):1937-42.

Finally, the *APOE* gene deserves special mention, because it increases the risk of neurodegenerative disease and cognitive decline, and modulates the risk from other factors, such as diabetes. The E4 allele has been found to substantially increase the risk of cognitive decline in combination with atherosclerosis, peripheral vascular disease, or diabetes mellitus. Individuals with one or more E4 alleles of the *APOE* gene have been shown to have a reduced amygdala volume, as well as an increased risk for dementia, Alzheimer's disease, and even mild cognitive impairment.[91,92] Early studies found that heterozygotes have been shown to have an onset of Alzheimer's 5–10 years earlier, and homozygotes 10–20 years earlier, than those with no copies.[93] More recent research using advanced ultra-high-density SNP genotyping found that a SNP located 14 kilobase pairs distal to the *APOE* epsilon variant distinguished between cases and controls with an OR of 4.01, and was far more strongly associated with Alzheimer's disease than any of the over 500,000 SNPs tested.[94] While it has been known for some time that apoE modulates extracellular lipid transport, only very recently has it been shown that apoE4 also binds to mitochondrial complex III and complex IV, inhibiting their activity.[95]

Assessment

While no single laboratory or clinical marker absolutely identifies risk for neurodegeneration or accelerated aging, a number of assessments may identify individuals at greater risk. For example, given the close association between hyperglycemia and AGE formation, as well as diabetes and neurodegeneration, screening for prediabetes and insulin resistance is certainly indicated. Homocysteine levels should certainly be evaluated with any indication of a neurodegenerative disorder. A more extensive list of tests for assessing the risk of accelerated aging is provided in Table 10.2.

Table 10.2 Key tests for assessing the risk of accelerated aging

Test
BMI
Waist circumference
Oral glucose tolerance or HOMA-IR
Serum lipids
HbA1c
Homocysteine
Serum folic acid
Methylmalonic acid (B12)
25-OH Vitamin D
Urinary levels of 8-oxo-7,8-dihydro-2'-deoxyguanosine (8-oxodG)
GGT (gamma glutamyltransferase)
APOE gene testing
C-reactive protein
Mitochondrial assessment (see Clinical Focus 1)

Several nutrient assessments may be part of a full evaluation. For example, folic acid and B12 levels (methylmalonic acid) should be measured. Similarly, 25-OH vitamin D levels should be obtained to assure sufficient vitamin D to prevent neurodegeneration and accelerated telomere loss; a genetic screen of VDR polymorphisms might be useful.

Evaluating mitochondrial function and cellular senescence may be indicated; a range of minimally intrusive to more invasive testing is available, from urinary organic acid analysis to muscle biopsy (see Clinical Focus 1). Assessment of oxidative status is also of value, given the many aspects of aging affected by ROS generation.

Screening for *APOE* alleles may also identify those with a greater risk of cognitive impairment and neurodegeneration, allowing for earlier treatment. Monitoring markers of systemic inflammation, such as CRP, allows for more targeted anti-inflammatory interventions.

Oxidative stress markers: 8-oxodG and GGT

Urinary analysis of 8-oxo-7,8-dihydro-2'-deoxyguanosine (8-oxodG), an oxidized nucleoside of DNA, is indicative of damaged nuclear or mitochondrial DNA; it is a good marker for assessing oxidative damage, as well as risk of atherosclerosis, cancer, and other disease complications.[96] 8-oxodG is used to estimate exposure to cancer-causing agents, such as tobacco smoke, asbestos fibers, heavy metals, and polycyclic aromatic hydrocarbons; its presence, therefore, is largely determined by environmental toxin exposure.[97] For example, smokers have up to 300% more 8-oxodG than nonsmokers, and those living in polluted cities have almost twice the levels of those living in rural settings.[98,99] Mercury exposure has been directly correlated to urinary 8-oxodG levels. Among the most useful interventions to reduce 8-oxodG is a diet rich in colorful fruits and vegetables, particularly purple sweet-potato leaves and almonds.[100] Indeed, one study found that increasing fruits and vegetables to 12 servings a day decreased urinary 8-oxodG by a remarkable 57% after only 2 weeks, with those eating the poorest diets beforehand improving the most.[101] Supplemental CoQ10, curcumin, lycopene, and green tea have all been shown to significantly reduce levels of this oxidative biomarker.[102,103,104,105]

A second marker of oxidative stress is the serum level of the enzyme gamma-glutamyltransferase (GGT). Epidemiologic studies have found GGT to be a significant marker of disease risk and a predictor of mortality from all causes, including liver disease, cancer, and diabetes.[106] Within its normal range, GGT has a clear dose-response association with a variety of chemicals, including lead, cadmium, mercury, organochlorine pesticides, and dioxin.[107] It is also a marker for oxidative stress, perhaps because it is closely linked to metabolism of glutathione (GSH), metabolizing extracellular GSH and allowing precursor amino acids to be reutilized for intracellular GSH re-synthesis, a pathway known as the gamma-glutamyl cycle. Paradoxically, however, there is a strong inverse association between extracellular GSH levels and serum GGT. High-normal or elevated levels of GGT are an indication for interventions that increase glutathione levels, such as N-acetylcysteine.[108,109]

Therapies and Prevention

Regeneration

In addition to therapies that reduce oxidant burden and inflammation and improve cellular function, interventions that increase regeneration also promote healthy aging. Some of the factors inhibiting regeneration include poor diet, lack of physical activity, inadequate sleep, excessive stress, nutrient deficiencies, poor circulation, and genetic predispositions.

Diet and physical activity

The Mediterranean diet—known to be useful in reducing the risk of cardiovascular disease, diabetes, inflammation, and insulin resistance—would logically also be useful for healthy aging. Research has shown that those following most closely this dietary pattern have a longer lifespan and a reduced risk of neurodegenerative disease, including Alzheimer's.[110] As mentioned earlier, the Ornish program increased telomerase activity in men, suggesting that it would also be an effective dietary approach to increasing lifespan. A calorie-restricted diet has also been shown to improve markers of longevity, such as fasting insulin levels, in a 6-month program.[111] Among the many benefits of regular physical activity, a recent trial found that adoption of an exercise endurance training program prevented age-related cognitive decline among healthy adults. Indeed, they were nearly 3 times as likely to have a stable cognitive status after 1 year as were controls.[112] Also, when resistance training was combined with supplemental DHEA in a placebo-controlled trial, an enhanced effect was seen on muscle strength and mass (Figure 10.13).[113]

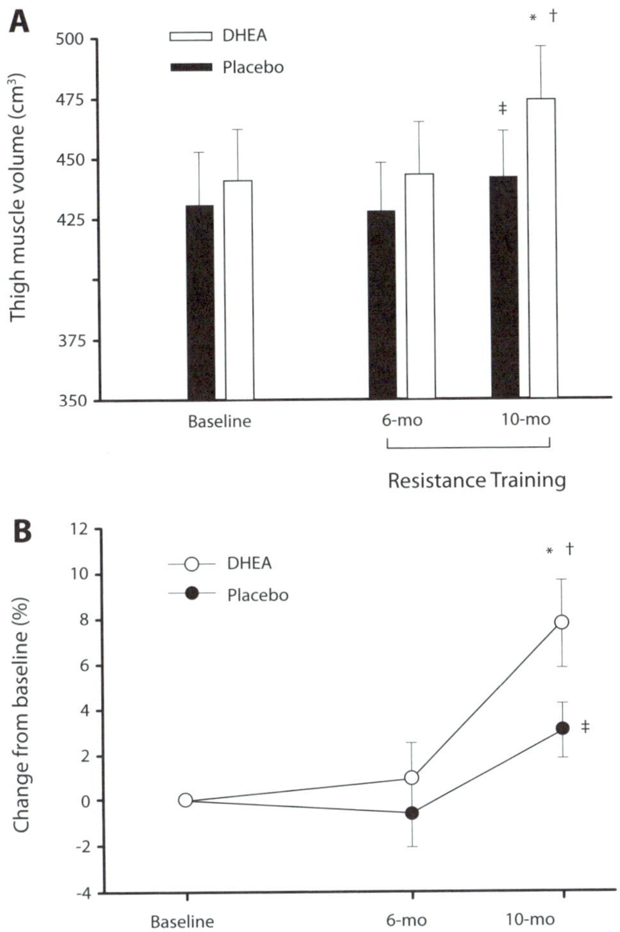

Figure 10.13 Improvements in muscle strength and mass with use of DHEA and resistance training. From: Villareal DT, Holloszy JO. DHEA enhances effects of weight training on muscle mass and strength in elderly women and men. *Am J Physiol Endocrinol Metab.* 2006 Nov;291(5):E1003-8. Reproduced with permission from the American Physiological Society.

Adequate sleep

Inadequate sleep increases the risk of neurodegeneration, as well as the risk of inflammation. Indeed, loss of as little as one night of sleep triggers a stress response, increasing both pro- and anti-inflammatory proteins.[114] Longer periods of sleep restriction (5 days) were found to increase a number of inflammatory markers, including CRP and heart rate, which remained elevated after two nights of recovery sleep.[115] Interventions to improve a delayed sleep onset include melatonin and phototherapy, while individuals who wake early benefit from a cooler temperature, magnesium, GABA, 5-HTP, taurine, and melatonin.[85,116,117,118,119]

Melatonin may have other benefits in addition to promoting healthy sleep rhythms. It is a ROS scavenger in the brain, and can counteract glucocorticoid damage; unfortunately, it decreases with age.[120,121] Some very interesting research has linked melatonin to sirtuin production, a relationship which may in part explain its cancer-preventive properties, and its potential to promote healthy aging.

Interventions to reduce AGEs

The powerful effects of diabetes and hyperglycemia on AGE formation compel the clinician to help patients normalize blood glucose levels, a step that is essential for controlling AGE accumulation and associated cellular damage. This should include choosing foods low in AGE content, particularly for those with preexisting diabetes.

Additionally, Alagebrium (ALT-711) may help to repair tissues by removing existing crosslinks. Animal studies have reported benefit for its use in diabetic renal disease, cardiac dysfunction, and atherosclerosis.[122] In human trials, it reduced pulse pressure and improved vascular compliance in patients with systolic hypertension.[27] Other compounds with potential therapeutic benefit include aged garlic extract, lipoic acid, L-carnitine, and extracts from astragalus.[123]

Interventions to improve mitochondrial function

Mitochondrial function and mtDNA are closely tied to aging, and interventions that support these organelles help to increase efficient energy production and reduce ROS generation. Several nutrients have shown significant benefit for optimizing mitochondrial function, including lipoic acid, carnitine, CoQ10, and magnesium.[124,125,126,127] See Clinical Focus 1—A Cellular Approach to Health for more information.

Neurological degeneration treatment

As discussed earlier, a number of treatments may help to reduce the risk of neurodegenerative disease and its progression. Therapies should aim to improve blood sugar regulation, reduce stress and inflammation, and provide targeted nutritional supplementation to reduce pathology.

Glutathione boost

Foremost in fighting neurological aging is boosting neural glutathione levels. As mentioned earlier, glutathione levels decrease with age, and have been associated with the overall health of older adults. Given the strong association between telomere length and oxidative stress, interventions that increase glutathione levels are likely to protect both telomeres and mtDNA from damage; both are strongly associated with longevity and aging. Supplementation with NAC has been shown to increase plasma levels of glutathione and decrease some of the toxicity of beta-amyloid in an *in vitro* trial.[112,113,128,129] Other interventions known to increase glutathione levels include inhaled or IV glutathione, milk thistle, pomegranate juice, lipoic acid, and SAMe.[130,131,132,133,134,135] IV glutathione has also been shown to reduce symptoms of Parkinson's disease, with benefits lasting 2–4 months after an infusion.[136]

Coenzyme Q10

CoQ10 has also shown benefit for neurodegenerative disease, particularly Parkinson's and Huntington's diseases. In a placebo-controlled trial lasting 16 months, CoQ10 was found to slow the progressive deterioration of Parkinson's disease in a dose-dependent manner, with increased platelet mitochondrial function of complexes I, II, and III, compared with placebo.[137,138,139] Data from subsequent trials suggests that doses of at least 2000 mg per day may be required for benefit.[140,141] Animal studies suggest that a combination of CoQ10 and carnitine may have additive neuroprotective benefit in Huntington's and Parkinson's diseases.[142]

Melatonin

Melatonin has broad neuroprotective functions, and appears to have benefit for stroke, Alzheimer's disease, Parkinson's disease, Huntington's disease, and ALS.[143] Animal studies have shown that it may even have the potential to facilitate removal of beta-amyloid from the brain.[144]

L-theanine

L-theanine, one of the major peptides from green tea, is also neuroprotective, at least partly as a function of reducing the toxicity of beta-amyloid. It has also been shown to reduce memory impairment in animal studies, prevent neuronal death, have antioxidant properties, and prevent depletion of glutathione levels.[145]

Resveratrol

As discussed earlier, resveratrol has many of the same physiological benefits as calorie restriction. It appears to have free radical scavenging properties, to inhibit the formation of beta-amyloid and the induction of inflammatory pathways, and it may increase telomerase activity.[146,147]

References

1. Calderwood SK, Murshid A, Prince T. The shock of aging: molecular chaperones and the heat shock response in longevity and aging—a mini-review. *Gerontology.* 2009;55(5):550-8.
2. Finkel T, Holbrook NJ. Oxidants, oxidative stress and the biology of aging. *Nature.* 2000 Nov 9;408(6809):239-47.
3. Bassi P, Sacco E. Cancer and aging: the molecular pathways. *Urol Oncol.* 2009 Nov-Dec;27(6):620-7.
4. Tosato M, Zamboni V, Ferrini A, et al. The aging process and potential interventions to extend life expectancy. *Clin Interv Aging.* 2007;2(3):401-12.
5. Yamagishi S, Ueda S, Matsui T, et al. Role of advanced glycation end products (AGEs) and oxidative stress in diabetic retinopathy. *Curr Pharm Des.* 2008;14(10):962-8.
6. Jandeleit-Dahm K, Cooper ME. The role of AGEs in cardiovascular disease. *Curr Pharm Des.* 2008;14(10):979-86.
7. Grillo MA, Colombatto S. Advanced glycation end-products (AGEs): involvement in aging and in neurodegenerative diseases. *Amino Acids.* 2008 Jun;35(1):29-36.
8. International Expert Committee. International Expert Committee report on the role of the A1C assay in the diagnosis of diabetes. *Diabetes Care.* 2009 Jul;32(7):1327-34.
9. Saisho Y, Maruyama T, Hirose H, et al. Relationship between proinsulin-to-insulin ratio and advanced glycation endproducts in Japanese type 2 diabetic subjects. *Diabetes Res Clin Pract.* 2007 Nov;78(2):182-8.
10. Zhao Z, Zhao C, Zhang XH, et al. Advanced glycation end products inhibit glucose-stimulated insulin secretion through nitric oxide-dependent inhibition of cytochrome c oxidase and adenosine triphosphate synthesis. *Endocrinology.* 2009 Jun;150(6):2569-76.
11. Yamagishi S, Matsui T, Nakamura K. Possible involvement of tobacco-derived advanced glycation end products (AGEs) in an increased risk for developing cancers and cardiovascular disease in former smokers. *Med Hypotheses.* 2008 Aug;71(2):259-61.
12. Uribarri J, Cai W, Sandu O, et al. Diet-derived advanced glycation end products are major contributors to the body's AGE pool and induce inflammation in healthy subjects. *Ann N Y Acad Sci.* 2005 Jun;1043:461-6.
13. Goldberg T, Cai W, Peppa M. Advanced glycoxidation end products in commonly consumed foods. *J Am Diet Assoc.* 2004 Aug;104(8):1287-9.
14. Koschinsky T, He CJ, Mitsuhashi T, et al. Orally absorbed reactive glycation products (glycotoxins): an environmental risk factor in diabetic nephropathy. *Proc Natl Acad Sci U S A.* 1997 Jun 10;94(12):6474-9.
15. Xanthis A, Hatzitolios A, Koliakos G, et al. Advanced glycosylation end products and nutrition—a possible relation with diabetic atherosclerosis and how to prevent it. *J Food Sci.* 2007 Oct;72(8):R125-9.
16. Kiho T, Usui S, Hirano K, et al. Tomato paste fraction inhibiting the formation of advanced glycation end-products. *Biosci Biotechnol Biochem.* 2004 Jan;68(1):200-5.
17. Cervantes-Laurean D, Schramm DD, Jacobson EL, et al. Inhibition of advanced glycation end product formation on collagen by rutin and its metabolites. *J Nutr Biochem.* 2006 Aug;17(8):531-40. Epub 2005 Oct 28.
18. Pashikanti S, de Alba DR, Boissonneault GA, et al. Rutin metabolites: Novel inhibitors of nonoxidative advanced glycation end products. *Free Radic Biol Med.* 2009 Dec 4. Epub ahead of print.
19. Panagiotakos DB, Tzima N, Pitsavos C, et al. The association between adherence to the Mediterranean diet and fasting indices of glucose homoeostasis: the ATTICA Study. *J Am Coll Nutr.* 2007 Feb;26(1):32-8. 17353581.
20. Panagiotakos DB, Chrysohoou C, Pitsavos C, et al. Association between the prevalence of obesity and adherence to the Mediterranean diet: the ATTICA study. *Nutrition.* 2006 May;22(5):449-56. 16457990.
21. Martínez-González MA, de la Fuente-Arrillaga C, Nunez-Cordoba JM, et al. Adherence to Mediterranean diet and risk of developing diabetes: prospective cohort study. *BMJ.* 2008 Jun 14;336(7657):1348-51. 18511765.
22. Desai K, Wu L. Methylglyoxal and advanced glycation endproducts: new therapeutic horizons? *Recent Pat Cardiovasc Drug Discov.* 2007 Jun;2(2):89-99.
23. Jandeleit-Dahm K, Cooper ME. The role of AGEs in cardiovascular disease. *Curr Pharm Des.* 2008;14(10): 979-86.
24. Thomas MC, Baynes JW, Thorpe SR, et al. The role of AGEs and AGE inhibitors in diabetic cardiovascular disease. *Curr Drug Targets.* 2005 Jun;6(4):453-74.
25. Woelk H, Lehrl S, Bitsch R, et al. Benfotiamine in treatment of alcoholic polyneuropathy: an 8-week randomized controlled study (BAP I Study). *Alcohol.* 1998 Nov-Dec;33(6):631-8.
26. Stirban A, Negrean M, Stratmann B, et al. Benfotiamine prevents macro- and microvascular endothelial dysfunction and oxidative stress following a meal rich in advanced glycation end products in individuals with type 2 diabetes. *Diabetes Care.* 2006 Sep;29(9):2064-71.
27. Coughlan MT, Forbes JM, Cooper ME. Role of the AGE crosslink breaker, alagebrium, as a renoprotective agent in diabetes. *Kidney Int Suppl.* 2007 Aug;(106): S54-60.
28. Chang KC, Liang JT, Tsai PS, et al. Prevention of arterial stiffening by pyridoxamine in diabetes is associated with inhibition of the pathogenic glycation on aortic collagen. *Br J Pharmacol.* 2009 Aug;157(8):1419-26.
29. Rajasekar P, Anuradha CV. L-Carnitine inhibits protein glycation *in vitro* and *in vivo*: evidence for a role in diabetic management. *Acta Diabetol.* 2007 Jun;44(2):83-90. Epub 2007 May 27.

30. Thirunavukkarasu V, Anitha Nandhini AT, Anuradha CV. Lipoic acid improves glucose utilisation and prevents protein glycation and AGE formation. *Pharmazie.* 2005 Oct;60(10):772-5.

31. Motomura K, Fujiwara Y, Kiyota N, et al. Astragalosides isolated from the root of astragalus radix inhibit the formation of advanced glycation end products. *J Agric Food Chem.* 2009 Sep 9;57(17):7666-72.

32. Fortpied J, Maliekal P, Vertommen D, et al. Magnesium-dependent phosphatase-1 is a protein-fructosamine-6-phosphatase potentially involved in glycation repair. *J Biol Chem.* 2006 Jul 7;281(27):18378-85.

33. Oeseburg H, de Boer RA, van Gilst WH, et al. Telomere biology in healthy aging and disease. *Pflugers Arch.* 2009 Sep 10. Epub ahead of print.

34. Ahmed A, Tollefsbol T. Telomeres and telomerase: basic science implications for aging. *J Am Geriatr Soc.* 2001 Aug;49(8):1105-9.

35. de Lange T. 1992. Human telomeres are attached to the nuclear matrix. *EMBO J.* 11:717-24.

36. Rodier F, Kim SH, Nijjar T, et al. Cancer and aging: the importance of telomeres in genome maintenance. *Int J Biochem Cell Biol.* 2005 May;37(5):977-90.

37. Shay JW, Bacchetti S. A survey of telomerase activity in human cancer. *Eur J Cancer.* 1997 Apr;33(5):787-91.

38. Cantó C, Auwerx J. Caloric restriction, SIRT1 and longevity. *Trends Endocrinol Metab.* 2009 Sep;20(7):325-31.

39. Ornish D, Lin J, Daubenmier J, et al. Increased telomerase activity and comprehensive lifestyle changes: a pilot study. *Lancet Oncol.* 2008 Nov;9(11):1048-57.

40. Cherkas LF, Hunkin JL, Kato BS, et al. The association between physical activity in leisure time and leukocyte telomere length. *Arch Intern Med.* 2008 Jan 28;168(2):154-8.

41. Epel E, Daubenmier J, Moskowitz JT. Can meditation slow rate of cellular aging? Cognitive stress, mindfulness, and telomeres. *Ann N Y Acad Sci.* 2009 Aug;1172:34-53.

42. Richards JB, Valdes AM, Gardner JP, et al. Higher serum vitamin D concentrations are associated with longer leukocyte telomere length in women. *Am J Clin Nutr.* 2007 Nov;86(5):1420-5.

43. Rubio MA, Davalos AR, Campisi J. Telomere length mediates the effects of telomerase on the cellular response to genotoxic stress. *Exp Cell Res.* 2004 Aug 1;298(1):17-27.

44. Voss P, Siems W. Clinical oxidation parameters of aging. *Free Radic Res.* 2006 Dec;40(12):1339-49.

45. de la Asuncion JG, Millan A, Pla R, et al. Mitochondrial glutathione oxidation correlates with age-associated oxidative damage to mitochondrial DNA. *FASEB J.* 1996 Feb;10(2):333-8.

46. Julius M, Lang CA, Gleiberman L, et al. Glutathione and morbidity in a community-based sample of elderly. *J Clin Epidemiol.* 1994 Sep;47(9):1021-6.

47. Adaikalakoteswari A, Balasubramanyam M, Ravikumar R, et al. Association of telomere shortening with impaired glucose tolerance and diabetic macroangiopathy. *Atherosclerosis.* 2007 Nov;195(1):83-9.

48. Salpea KD, Talmud PJ, Cooper JA, et al. Association of telomere length with type 2 diabetes, oxidative stress and UCP2 gene variation. *Atherosclerosis.* 2009 Oct 6. Epub ahead of print.

49. Richards JB, Valdes AM, Gardner JP, et al. Homocysteine levels and leukocyte telomere length. *Atherosclerosis.* 2008 Oct;200(2):271-7.

50. Hoxha M, Dioni L, Bonzini M, Pesatori AC, et al. Association between leukocyte telomere shortening and exposure to traffic pollution: a cross-sectional study on traffic officers and indoor office workers. *Environ Health.* 2009 Sep 21;8:41.

51. Wang P, Zhang Z, Sun Y, et al. The two isomers of HDTIC compounds from Astragali Radix slow down telomere shortening rate via attenuating oxidative stress and increasing DNA repair ability in human fetal lung diploid fibroblast cells. *DNA Cell Biol.* 2010 Jan;29(1):33-9.

52. Hoeijmakers JH. DNA damage, aging, and cancer. *N Engl J Med.* 2009 Oct 8;361(15):1475-85.

53. Barja G, Herrero A. Oxidative damage to mitochondrial DNA is inversely related to maximum life span in the heart and brain of mammals. *FASEB J.* 2000 Feb;14(2):312-8.

54. Short KR, Bigelow ML, Kahl J. Decline in skeletal muscle mitochondrial function with aging in humans. *Proc Natl Acad Sci U S A.* 2005 Apr 12;102(15):5618-23.

55. Ljubicic V, Joseph AM, Saleem A, et al. Transcriptional and post-transcriptional regulation of mitochondrial biogenesis in skeletal muscle: Effects of exercise and aging. *Biochim Biophys Acta.* 2009 Aug 12. Epub ahead of print.

56. Trifunovic A. Mitochondrial DNA and aging. *Biochim Biophys Acta.* 2006 May-Jun;1757(5-6):611-7.

57. Fjell AM, Walhovd KB, Fennema-Notestine C, et al. One-year brain atrophy evident in healthy aging. *J Neurosci.* 2009 Dec 2;29(48):15223-31.

58. Jellinger KA. Recent advances in our understanding of neurodegeneration. *J Neural Transm.* 2009 Sep;116(9):1111-62. Epub 2009 Jun 5.

59. Chiarini A, Dal Pra I, Whitfield JF, Armato U. The killing of neurons by beta-amyloid peptides, prions, and pro-inflammatory cytokines. *Ital J Anat Embryol.* 2006 Oct-Dec;111(4):221-46.

60. Näslund J, Haroutunian V, Mohs R, et al. Correlation between elevated levels of amyloid beta-peptide in the brain and cognitive decline. *JAMA.* 2000 Mar 22-29;283(12):1571-7.

61. Nakamura T, Lipton SA. Cell death: protein misfolding and neurodegenerative diseases. *Apoptosis.* 2009 Apr;14(4):455-68.

62. Brown ES, Woolston DJ, Frol AB, et al. Amygdala volume in patients receiving chronic corticosteroid therapy. *Biol Psychiatry*. 2008;63:705-9.
63. Desai S, Khanani S, Shad MU, et al. Attenuation of amygdala atrophy with lamotrigine in patients receiving corticosteroid therapy. *J Clin Psychopharmacol*. 2009 Jun;29(3):284-7.
64. Zesiewicz TA, Wecker L, Sullivan KL, et al. The controversy concerning plasma homocysteine in Parkinson disease patients treated with levodopa alone or with entacapone: effects of vitamin status. *Clin Neuropharmacol*. 2006 May-Jun;29(3):106-11.
65. dos Santos EF, Busanello EN, Miglioranza A, et al. Evidence that folic acid deficiency is a major determinant of hyperhomocysteinemia in Parkinson's disease. *Metab Brain Dis*. 2009 Jun;24(2):257-69. Epub 2009 Mar 18.
66. Seshadri S. Alzheimer's disease. *NEJM* 2002; 346:476-83
67. Köseoglu E, Karaman Y. Relations between homocysteine, folate and vitamin B12 in vascular dementia and in Alzheimer disease. *Clin Biochem* 2007;40:859-63.
68. Obeid R, McCaddon A, Herrmann W. The role of hyperhomocysteinemia and B-vitamin deficiency in neurological and psychiatric diseases. *Clin Chem Lab Med*. 2007;45(12):1590-606.
69. Weiss N. Mechanisms of increased vascular oxidant stress in hyperhomocysteinemia and its impact on endothelial function. *Curr Drug Metab*. 2005 Feb;6(1):27-36.
70. Cheung GT, Siow YL, O K. Homocysteine stimulates monocyte chemoattractant protein-1 expression in mesangial cells via NF-kappaB activation. *Can J Physiol Pharmacol*. 2008 Mar;86(3):88-96.
71. Au-Yeung KK, Yip JC, Siow YL. Folic acid inhibits homocysteine-induced superoxide anion production and nuclear factor kappa B activation in macrophages. *Can J Physiol Pharmacol*. 2006 Jan;84(1):141-7.
72. Albert CM, Cook NR, Gaziano JM, et al. Effect of folic acid and B vitamins on risk of cardiovascular events and total mortality among women at high risk for cardiovascular disease: a randomized trial. *JAMA*. 2008 May 7;299(17):2027-36.
73. Wang X, Qin X, Demirtas H, et al. Efficacy of folic acid supplementation in stroke prevention: a meta-analysis. *Lancet*. 2007 Jun 2;369(9576):1876-82.
74. Chiuve SE, Giovannucci EL, Hankinson SE, et al. The association between betaine and choline intakes and the plasma concentrations of homocysteine in women. *Am J Clin Nutr*. 2007 Oct;86(4):1073-81.
75. Detopoulou P, Panagiotakos DB, Antonopoulou S, et al. Dietary choline and betaine intakes in relation to concentrations of inflammatory markers in healthy adults: the ATTICA study. *Am J Clin Nutr*. 2008 Feb;87(2):424-30.
76. Van Couter E, Leproult R, Plat L. Age-related changes in slow wave sleep and REM sleep and relationship with growth hormone and cortisol levels in healthy men. *JAMA* 2000;284: 861-8.
77. Chokroverty S. Sleep and neurodegenerative diseases. *Semin Neurol*. 2009 Sep;29(4):446-67.
78. Dhand R, Sohal H. Good sleep, bad sleep! The role of daytime naps in healthy adults. *Curr Opin Pulm Med*. 2006 Nov;12(6):379-82.
79. Tanaka H, Shirakawa S. Sleep health, lifestyle and mental health in the Japanese elderly: ensuring sleep to promote a healthy brain and mind. *J Psychosom Res*. 2004 May;56(5):465-77.
80. Zisberg A, Gur-Yaish N, Shochat T, et al. Contribution of routine to sleep quality in community elderly. *Sleep*. 2010 Apr 1;33(4):509-14.
81. Lemoine P, Nir T, Laudon M, et al. Prolonged-release melatonin improves sleep quality and morning alertness in insomnia patients aged 55 years and older and has no withdrawal effects. *J Sleep Res*. 2007 Dec;16(4):372-80.
82. Ohta T, Ando K, Iwata T. Treatment of persistent sleep-wake schedule disorders in adolescents with methylcobalamin (vitamin B12). *Sleep*. 1991 Oct;14(5):414-8.
83. Bruni O, Ferri R, Miano S, et al. L -5-Hydroxytryptophan treatment of sleep terrors in children. *Eur J Pediatr*. 2004 Jul;163(7):402-7. Epub 2004 May 14.
84. Shell W, Bullias D, Charuvastra E, May LA, Silver DS. A Randomized, Placebo-Controlled Trial of an Amino Acid Preparation on Timing and Quality of Sleep. *Am J Ther*. 2009 May 15. Epub ahead of print.
85. Ott A, Stolk RP, van Harskamp F, et al. Diabetes mellitus and the risk of dementia: The Rotterdam Study. *Neurology*. 1999 Dec 10;53(9):1937-42.
86. Irie F, Fitzpatrick AL, Lopez OL, et al. Enhanced risk for Alzheimer disease in persons with type 2 diabetes and APOE epsilon4: the Cardiovascular Health Study Cognition Study. *Arch Neurol*. 2008 Jan;65(1):89-93.
87. Gezen-Ak D, Dursun E, Ertan T, et al. Association between vitamin D receptor gene polymorphism and Alzheimer's disease. *Tohoku J Exp Med*. 2007;212:275-82
88. Munger KL, Levin LI, Hollis BW, et al. Serum 25-hydroxyvitamin D levels and risk of multiple sclerosis. *JAMA* 2006;296:2832-8.
89. Fernandes de Abreu DA, Babron MC, Rebeix I, et al. Season of birth and not vitamin D receptor promoter polymorphisms is a risk factor for multiple sclerosis. *Mult Scler*. 2009 Oct;15(10):1146-52. Epub 2009 Sep 21.
90. Dickinson JL, Perera DI, van der Mei AF, et al. Past environmental sun exposure and risk of multiple sclerosis: a role for the Cdx-2 Vitamin D receptor variant in this interaction. *Mult Scler*. 2009 May;15(5):563-70. Epub 2009 Apr 21.
91. Boyle PA, Buchman AS, Wilson RS, et al. The APOE epsilon4 Allele Is Associated with Incident Mild Cognitive Impairment among Community-Dwelling Older Persons. *Neuroepidemiology*. 2009 Nov 11;34(1):43-49. Epub ahead of print.

92. Fleisher A, Grundman M, Jack CR Jr, et al. Sex, apolipoprotein E epsilon 4 status, and hippocampal volume in mild cognitive impairment. *Arch Neurol* 2005;62:953-7.

93. Corder EH, Saunders AM, Strittmatter WJ, et al. Gene dose of apolipoprotein E type 4 allele and the risk of Alzheimer's disease in late onset families. *Science*. 1993 Aug 13;261(5123):921-3.

94. Coon KD, Myers AJ, Craig DW, et al. A high-density whole-genome association study reveals that APOE is the major susceptibility gene for sporadic late-onset Alzheimer's disease. *J Clin Psychiatry*. 2007 Apr;68(4):613-8.

95. Nakamura T, Watanabe A, Fujino T, et al. Apolipoprotein E4 (1-272) fragment is associated with mitochondrial proteins and affects mitochondrial function in neuronal cells. *Mol Neurodegener*. 2009 Aug 20;4:35.

96. Wu LL, Chiou CC, Chang PY, et al. Urinary 8-OHdG: a marker of oxidative stress to DNA and a risk factor for cancer, atherosclerosis and diabetics. *Clin Chim Acta*. 2004 Jan;339(1-2):1-9.

97. Valavanidis A, Vlachogianni T, Fiotakis C. 8-hydroxy-2' -deoxyguanosine (8-OHdG): A critical biomarker of oxidative stress and carcinogenesis. *J Environ Sci Health C Environ Carcinog Ecotoxicol Rev*. 2009 Apr;27(2):120-39.

98. Yano T, Shoji F, Baba H, et al. Significance of the urinary 8-OHdG level as an oxidative stress marker in lung cancer patients. *Lung Cancer*. 2009 Jan;63(1):111-4.

99. Buthbumrung N, Mahidol C, Navasumrit P, et al. Oxidative DNA damage and influence of genetic polymorphisms among urban and rural schoolchildren exposed to benzene. *Chemico-Biological Interactions* 2008; 172:185-194.

100. Chen CM, Lin YL, Chen CY, et al. Consumption of purple sweet potato leaves decreases lipid peroxidation and DNA damage in humans. *Asia Pac J Clin Nutr*. 2008; 17(3):408-14.

101. Thompson HJ, Heimendinger J, Haegele A, et al. Effect of increased vegetable and fruit consumption on markers of oxidative cellular damage. *Carcinogenesis*. 1999 Dec; 20(12):2261-6.

102. Niklowitz P, Sonnenschein A, Janetzky B, et al. Enrichment of coenzyme Q10 in plasma and blood cells: defense against oxidative damage. *Int J Biol Sci*. 2007 Apr 5;3(4):257-62.

103. Kowluru RA, Mamta Kanwar M. Effects of curcumin on retinal oxidative stress and inflammation in diabetes. *Nutr Metab* (Lond). 2007;4:8.

104. Hakim IA, Harris RB, Brown S, et al. Effect of increased tea consumption on oxidative DNA damage among smokers: A randomized controlled study. *J. Nutr.* 133:3303S-3309S, 2003.

105. Devaraj S, Mathur S, Basu A, et al. A dose-response study on the effects of purified lycopene supplementation on biomarkers of oxidative stress. *J Am Coll Nutr*. 2008 Apr; 27(2):267-73.

106. Ruhl CE, Everhart JE. Elevated Serum Alanine Aminotransferase and Gamma-Glutamyltransferase and Mortality in the United States Population. *Gastroenterology* 2009;136:477-85.

107. Lee DH, Jacobs DR Jr. Serum gamma-glutamyltransferase: new insights about an old enzyme. *J Epidemiol Community Health*. 2009 Nov;63(11):884-6.

108. Soltan-Sharifi MS, Mojtahedzadeh M, Najafi A, et al. Improvement by N-acetylcysteine of acute respiratory distress syndrome through increasing intracellular glutathione, and extracellular thiol molecules and anti-oxidant power: evidence for underlying toxicological mechanisms. *Hum Exp Toxicol*. 2007 Sep;26(9):697-703.

109. Will Y, Kaetzel RS, Brown MK, et al. *In vivo* reversal of glutathione deficiency and susceptibility to *in vivo* dexamethasone-induced apoptosis by N-acetylcysteine and L-2-oxothiazolidine-4-carboxylic acid, but not ascorbic acid, in thymocytes from gamma-glutamyltranspeptidase-deficient knockout mice. *Arch Biochem Biophys*. 2002 Jan 15; 397(2):399-406.

110. Pérez-López FR, Chedraui P, Haya J, et al. Effects of the Mediterranean diet on longevity and age-related morbid conditions. *Maturitas*. 2009 Oct 20;64(2):67-79. Epub 2009 Aug 31.

111. Heilbronn LK, de Jonge L, Frisard MI, et al. Effect of 6-month calorie restriction on biomarkers of longevity, metabolic adaptation, and oxidative stress in overweight individuals: a randomized controlled trial. *JAMA*. 2006 Apr 5;295(13):1539-48.

112. Muscari A, Giannoni C, Pierpaoli L, et al. Chronic endurance exercise training prevents aging-related cognitive decline in healthy older adults: a randomized controlled trial. *Int J Geriatr Psychiatry*. 2009 Dec 23. Epub ahead of print.

113. Villareal DT, Holloszy JO. DHEA enhances effects of weight training on muscle mass and strength in elderly women and men. *Am J Physiol Endocrinol Metab*. 2006 Nov; 291(5):E1003-8. Epub 2006 Jun 20.

114. Frey DJ, Fleshner M, Wright KP Jr. The effects of 40 hours of total sleep deprivation on inflammatory markers in healthy young adults. *Brain Behav Immun*. 2007 Nov; 21(8):1050-7. Epub 2007 May 23.

115. van Leeuwen WM, Lehto M, Karisola P, et al. Sleep restriction increases the risk of developing cardiovascular diseases by augmenting proinflammatory responses through IL-17 and CRP. *PLoS One*. 2009;4(2):e4589. Epub 2009 Feb 25.

116. Raymann RJ, Swaab DF, Van Someren EJ. Skin temperature and sleep-onset latency: changes with age and insomnia. *Physiol Behav*. 2007 Feb 28;90(2-3):257-66.

117. Soulairac A, Lambinet H. Effect of 5-hydroxytryptophan, a serotonin precursor, on sleep disorders. *Ann Med Psychol* (Paris). 1977;1(5):792-798.

118. Eschenauer G, Sweet BV. Pharmacology and therapeutic uses of theanine. *Am J Health Syst Pharm*. 2006;63(1):26-30.

119. Shirani A, St Louis EK. Illuminating rationale and uses for light therapy. *J Clin Sleep Med.* 2009 Apr 15;5(2):155-63.

120. Konakchieva R, Mitev Y, Almeida OF, et al. Chronic melatonin treatment counteracts glucocorticoid-induced dysregulation of the hypothalamic-pituitary-adrenal axis in the rat. *Neuroendocrinology.* 1998 Mar;67(3):171-80.

121. Karasek M. Does melatonin play a role in aging processes? *J Physiol Pharmacol.* 2007;58s:105-13.

122. Coughlan MT, Forbes JM, Cooper ME. Role of the AGE crosslink breaker, alagebrium, as a renoprotective agent in diabetes. *Kidney Int Suppl.* 2007 Aug;(106):S54-60.

123. Ahmad MS, Pischetsrieder M, Ahmed N. Aged garlic extract and S-allyl cysteine prevent formation of advanced glycation endproducts. *Eur J Pharmacol.* 2007 Apr 30; 561(1-3):32-8.

124. Malaguarnera M, Gargante MP, Cristaldi E, et al. Acetyl L-carnitine (ALC) treatment in elderly patients with fatigue. *Arch Gerontol Geriatr.* 2008 Mar-Apr;46(2):181-90.

125. Long J, Gao F, Tong L. Mitochondrial decay in the brains of old rats: ameliorating effect of alpha-lipoic acid and acetyl-L-carnitine. *Neurochem Res.* 2009 Apr;34(4):755-63.

126. Rosenfeldt F, Marasco S, Lyon W, et al. Coenzyme Q10 therapy before cardiac surgery improves mitochondrial function and *in vitro* contractility of myocardial tissue. *J Thorac Cardiovasc Surg.* 2005 Jan;129(1):25-32.

127. Kubota T, Shindo Y, Tokuno K, et al. Mitochondria are intracellular magnesium stores: investigation by simultaneous fluorescent imagings in PC12 cells. *Biochim Biophys Acta.* 2005 May 15;1744(1):19-28.

128. Soltan-Sharifi MS, Mojtahedzadeh M, Najafi A, et al. Improvement by N-acetylcysteine of acute respiratory distress syndrome through increasing intracellular glutathione, and extracellular thiol molecules and antioxidant power: evidence for underlying toxicological mechanisms. *Hum Exp Toxicol.* 2007;26(9):697-703.

129. Wang R, Malter JS, Wang DS. N-acetylcysteine prevents 4-hydroxynonenal- and amyloid-beta-induced modification and inactivation of neprilysin in SH-SY5Y cells. *J Alzheimers Dis.* 2010 Jan;19(1):179-89.

130. Hagen TM, Ingersoll RT, Lykkesfeldt J, et al. (R)-Lipoic acid-supplemented old rats have improved mitochondrial function, decreased oxidative damage, and increased metabolic rate. *FASEB J* 1999;13:411-8.

131. Liu J. The effects and mechanisms of mitochondrial nutrient alpha-lipoic acid on improving age-associated mitochondrial and cognitive dysfunction: overview. *Neurochem Res* 2008;33:194-203.

132. Jariwalla RJ, Lalezari J, Cenko D, et al. Restoration of blood total glutathione status and lymphocyte function following alpha-lipoic acid supplementation in patients with HIV infection. *J Altern Complement Med.* 2008;14(2):139-46.

133. Alidoost F, Gharagozloo M, Bagherpour B, et al. Effects of silymarin on the proliferation and glutathione levels of peripheral blood mononuclear cells from beta-thalassemia major patients. *Int Immunopharmacol.* 2006;6(8):1305-10.

134. Rosenblat M, Hayek T, Aviram M. Antioxidative effects of pomegranate juice (PJ) consumption by diabetic patients on serum and on macrophages. *Atherosclerosis.* 2006; 187(2):363-71.

135. Liber CS, Packer L (November 2002). "S-Adenosylmethionine: molecular, biological, and clinical aspects—an introduction". *Am J Clin Nutr.* 76 (5): 1148S-50S.

136. Sechi G, Deledda MG, Bua G, et al. Reduced intravenous glutathione in the treatment of early Parkinson's disease. *Prog Neuropsychopharmacol Biol Psychiatry.* 1996; 20(7):1159-70.

137. Shults CW, Oakes D, Kieburtz K, et al . Effects of coenzyme Q10 in early Parkinson disease: evidence of slowing of the functional decline. *Arch Neurol.* 2002;59:1541-50.

138. Spindler M, Beal MF, Henchcliffe C. Coenzyme Q10 effects in neurodegenerative disease. *Neuropsychiatr Dis Treat.* 2009;5:597-610. Epub 2009 Nov 16.

139. Huntington Study Group. A randomized, placebo-controlled trial of coenzyme Q10 and remacemide in Huntington's disease. *Neurology.* 2001 Aug 14;57(3): 397-404.

140. Spindler M, Beal MF, Henchcliffe C. Coenzyme Q10 effects in neurodegenerative disease. *Neuropsychiatr Dis Treat.* 2009;5:597-610. Epub 2009 Nov 16.

141. Huntington Study Group. A randomized, placebo-controlled trial of coenzyme Q10 and remacemide in Huntington's disease. *Neurology.* 2001 Aug 14;57(3): 397-404.

142. Yang L, Calingasan NY, Wille EJ, et al. Combination therapy with coenzyme Q10 and creatine produces additive neuroprotective effects in models of Parkinson's and Huntington's diseases. *J Neurochem.* 2009 Jun;109(5):1427-39. Epub 2009 Mar 28.

143. Wang X. The antiapoptotic activity of melatonin in neurodegenerative diseases. *CNS Neurosci Ther.* 2009 Winter; 15(4):345-57.

144. Olcese JM, Cao C, Mori T, et al. Protection against cognitive deficits and markers of neurodegeneration by long-term oral administration of melatonin in a transgenic model of Alzheimer disease. *J Pineal Res.* 2009 Aug;47(1): 82-96. Epub 2009 Jun 17.

145. Kim TI, Lee YK, Park SG, et al. L-theanine, an amino acid in green tea, attenuates beta-amyloid-induced cognitive dysfunction and neurotoxicity: reduction in oxidative damage and inactivation of ERK/p38 kinase and NF-kappaB pathways. *Free Radic Biol Med.* 2009 Dec 1;47(11):1601-10.

146. Kim J, Lee HJ, Lee KW. Naturally occurring phytochemicals for the prevention of Alzheimer's disease. *J Neurochem.* 2009 Dec 26. Epub ahead of print.

147. Pearce VP, Sherrell J, Lou Z, et al. Immortalization of epithelial progenitor cells mediated by resveratrol. *Oncogene.* 2008 Apr 10;27(17):2365-74. Epub 2007 Oct 29.

Appendix A
Disease Reference Chart

SYSTEM IMPLICATED	Cellular	Digestion	Detoxification	Insulin Resistance	Inflammation	Stress/Anxiety/ Insomnia	Immune	Endocrine	Regeneration/ Aging	Cardiovascular
DISEASE										
Acne vulgaris			●					●		
Addison's disease								●		
ADHD			●							
Adrenal insufficiency						●		●		
Allergic rhinitis							●			
Alzheimer's disease	●		●		●				●	
Andropause								●		
Asthma					●		●			
Atherosclerosis	●		●	●	●		●			●
Atopic dermatitis		●			●					
Atrial fibrillation										●
Autoimmune disease		●					●			
Cancer	●		●		●		●			
Celiac disease		●					●			
Chronic fatigue syndrome	●		●						●	
Coronary artery disease					●					●
Dementia	●				●				●	
Dermatitis herpetiformis		●					●			
Diabetes	●		●	●	●					●
Endometriosis			●					●		

SYSTEM IMPLICATED	Cellular	Digestion	Detoxification	Insulin Resistance	Inflammation	Stress/Anxiety/ Insomnia	Immune	Endocrine	Regeneration/ Aging	Cardiovascular
DISEASE										
Food allergy		•					•			
Fungal infection, persistent							•			
Hypertension										•
Hypochlorhydria		•								
Hypogonadism								•		
Hypothyroidism			•				•	•		
Inflammatory bowel disease		•			•					
Intestinal permeability, increased		•								
Irritable bowel syndrome		•								
Ischemic heart disease					•					•
Metabolic syndrome			•	•	•					•
Migraine	•	•								
Multiple chemical sensitivity			•							
Multiple sclerosis			•				•			
Nonalcoholic steatohepatitis			•		•			•		
Obesity	•	•	•	•						•
Obstructive sleep apnea						•				
Osteoarthritis			•		•					
Osteoporosis/Osteopenia	•		•					•		
Otitis media		•					•			
Pancreatic insufficiency		•								
Parkinson's disease			•						•	
Peptic ulcer		•								
Periodontal disease					•					•
Peripheral arterial disease					•					•
Polycystic ovary syndrome				•				•		
Premature ovarian failure								•		
Rheumatoid arthritis			•		•		•			
Small bowel bacterial overgrowth		•								
Systemic lupus erythematosus			•				•			
Upper respiratory tract infection, recurrent							•			
Urolithiasis	•									
Uterine fibroids								•		

Appendix B
Symptom Reference Chart

SYSTEM IMPLICATED	Cellular	Digestion	Detoxification	Insulin Resistance	Inflammation	Stress/Anxiety/ Insomnia	Immune	Endocrine	Regeneration/ Aging	Cardiovascular
SYMPTOM / SIGNS										
Abdominal bloating/gas		●								
Acid-blocking medication		●								
Acute coronary syndrome	●									●
Angina					●					●
Anxiety						●		●		
Back pain					●				●	
Caffeine sensitivity			●							
Chest, pressure/heaviness					●					●
Cognitive function, impaired			●			●			●	
Common cold, recurrent							●			
Constipation		●								
Cough, recurrent							●			
C-reactive protein, elevated					●					●
Dental amalgams, silver			●							
Depression			●			●		●		
Diarrhea		●								
Dyslipidemia				●	●					●
Earache					●		●			
Erectile dysfunction					●			●		●
Fatigue	●									●

SYSTEM IMPLICATED	Cellular	Digestion	Detoxification	Insulin Resistance	Inflammation	Stress/Anxiety/ Insomnia	Immune	Endocrine	Regeneration/ Aging	Cardiovascular
SYMPTOM / SIGNS										
Fingernails, week, peeling		•					•			
Fluid retention					•			•		•
Food hypersensitivity		•					•			
Gums receding					•				•	•
Halitosis		•								
Hayfever	•						•			
Headache	•		•		•			•		
Hearing loss									•	
Heartburn		•								
Homocysteine, elevated					•					•
Hot flashes								•		
Hyperglycemia	•			•	•					
Indigestion		•								
Infertility			•					•		
Insomnia						•				
Insulin resistance	•		•	•	•					•
Joint pain			•		•				•	
Learning difficulties			•							
Libido, low								•		
Memory loss									•	
Menopausal symptoms								•		
Menstrual cycle, abnormalities								•		
Muscle weakness	•								•	
Polyuria/polydipsia				•	•			•		•
Premature aging									•	
Shortness of breath							•			•
Stress, chronic						•				
Sulfite sensitivity			•							
Urination, frequent				•				•		
Urticaria, chronic			•				•			
Weight gain		•	•	•						
Wheeze, recurrent					•		•			

Index

Italic page numbers refer to figures and tables.

A

B

C

D

E

F

G

H

I

J

K

L

M

N

O

P

Q

R

S

T

U

V

W

X

Y

Z